NOVICK & MORROW'S
PUBLIC HEALTH
ADMINISTRATION

Principles for Population-Based Management

EDITED BY

Leiyu Shi, DrPH, MBA, MPA

Professor
The Johns Hopkins Bloomberg School of Public Health
Director
The Johns Hopkins Primary Care Policy Center
Baltimore, Maryland

James A. Johnson, PhD, MPA, MSc

Professor
School of Health Sciences
Dow College of Health Professions
Central Michigan University
Mount Pleasant, Michigan

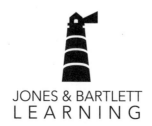

JONES & BARTLETT
LEARNING

World Headquarters
Jones & Bartlett Learning
5 Wall Street
Burlington, MA 01803
978-443-5000
info@jblearning.com
www.jblearning.com

Jones & Bartlett Learning books and products are available through most bookstores and online booksellers. To contact Jones & Bartlett Learning directly, call 800-832-0034, fax 978-443-8000, or visit our website, www.jblearning.com.

Substantial discounts on bulk quantities of Jones & Bartlett Learning publications are available to corporations, professional associations, and other qualified organizations. For details and specific discount information, contact the special sales department at Jones & Bartlett Learning via the above contact information or send an email to specialsales@jblearning.com.

Production Credits

Executive Publisher: William Brottmiller
Publisher: Michael Brown
Editorial Assistant: Kayla Dos Santos
Editorial Assistant: Chloe Falivene
Production Manager: Tracey McCrea
Senior Marketing Manager: Sophie Fleck Teague

Manufacturing and Inventory Control Supervisor: Amy Bacus
Composition: Cenveo© Publisher Services
Cover Design: Scott Moden
Cover Image: © Dinga/ShutterStock, Inc.
Printing and Binding: McNaughton & Gunn
Cover Printing: McNaughton & Gunn

To order this product, use ISBN: 978-1-4496-8833-2

Library of Congress Cataloging-in-Publication Data
Novick & Morrow's public health administration : principles for population-based management.—3rd ed. / edited by Leiyu Shi, James Johnson.
   p. ; cm.
Public health administration
Rev. ed. of: Public health administration / edited by Lloyd F. Novick, Cynthia B. Morrow, Glen P. Mays. 2nd ed. c2008.
Includes bibliographical references and index.
ISBN 978-1-4496-5741-3 (pbk.)
I. Novick, Lloyd F.   II. Shi, Leiyu.   III. Johnson, James A., 1954-   IV. Public health administration.   V. Title: Public health administration.
[DNLM: 1. Public Health Administration. WA 525]
RA425
362.1068—dc23
                                                                                          2013004172

6048
Printed in the United States of America
21 20 19 18   10 9 8 7 6

Table of Contents

Chapter 1

Overview of Public Health Administration 1

James A. Johnson and Leiyu Shi

Chapter 2

Historical Developments in Public Health in the 21st Century 11

James Allen Johnson III, James A. Johnson, and Cynthia B. Morrow

Chapter 3

Public Health and Social Determinants of Health 33
Leiyu Shi

Chapter 4

Public Health Administration and Practice Framework 53
Cynthia B. Morrow and James A. Johnson

Chapter 5

Organization of the Public Health System **79**
Glen P. Mays and Alene Kennedy-Hendricks

Chapter 8

Public Health Policy **159**
Walter J. Jones

Chapter 9

Public Health Finance. **181**
Peggy A. Honoré and Louis Gapenski

Chapter 10

Gerald M. Barron, Linda Duchak, and Margaret A. Potter

Chapter 11

Human Resource Management for Public Health 221
Janet E. Porter

Chapter 12

Chapter 13

Chapter 14

Alan L. Melnick and Brendon Haggerty

Chapter 15

Chapter 16

Chapter 17

Performance Management in Public Health 357

Leslie M. Beitsch, Laura B. Landrum, Bernard J. Turnock,
and Arden S. Handler

Chapter 20

Advancing Public Health Systems Research 431
Leiyu Shi

Chapter 21

**Social Marketing and Consumer-Based Approaches
in Public Health** **449**

Moya Alfonso and Mary P. Martinasek

Chapter 22

Prevention, Health Education, and Health Promotion **477**
Lawrence W. Green, Judith M. Ottoson, and Maria L. Roditis

Chapter 23

Chapter 24

Social Entrepreneurship and Public Health

*Kristine Marin Kawamura, Nailya O. DeLellis, and
Ormanbek T. Zhuzzhanov*

Chapter 25

Linda Young Landesman and Cynthia B. Morrow

Chapter 26

Public Health and Healthcare Quality. 599
Cheryll D. Lesneski, Peggy A. Honoré, and Carolyn Clancy

Chapter 27

Global Health Challenges and Opportunities 627
Leiyu Shi and James A. Johnson

Preface

The First Edition of *Public Health Administration: Principles for Population-Based Management* was published in 2001 by Aspen Publishers and reprinted by Jones and Bartlett Publishers in 2005. The leaders in the book's conceptualization and inaugural edition were Lloyd F. Novick and publisher Michael Brown. The First Edition of the book was coedited by Lloyd F. Novick and Glen P. Mays and included 30 chapters contributed by a wide range of public health scholars and practitioners. The Second Edition was published in 2008 with the addition of Cynthia B. Morrow as coeditor. The text has since become a cornerstone of public health education across the United States, becoming the most widely adopted book on the subject of public health administration.

At the 2010 American Public Health Association (APHA) meeting in Denver, Colorado, Michael Brown approached me about editing another edition of this text. The founding editor, Lloyd Novick, had planned to retire from the project and someone else was needed. Having previously worked with Jones & Bartlett Learning on three other books, I was comfortable accepting the challenge. The one condition was that I could select a coeditor, as was the tradition for this text. The first person to come to mind was a 20-year-long colleague and friend, Leiyu Shi, at The Johns Hopkins University. He too has a multibook record of publishing with Jones & Bartlett Learning. Mike Brown readily agreed and so did Leiyu. The two-person editing team we formed was well suited for the task ahead. Not only did we have a history of working together, we also brought somewhat different skill sets and colleague networks to the project. Leiyu's background has primarily been in health services research, healthcare delivery systems, and population health, while mine has focused on health policy, health organizations, and comparative health systems. Both of us had already published more than 10 books each, so we were quite seasoned for the task of revising this text.

Now, over a decade since the publication of the original book, the Third Edition of *Public Health Administration: Principles of Population-Based Management* has been published. We have maintained some continuity with previous editions, with many past chapter contributors still involved and two of the past editors, Drs. Morrow and Mays, also contributing. However, new elements and topics have been added. We have streamlined the book somewhat with generally shorter chapters and have added chapter objectives and discussion questions. These elemental changes were made to enhance the classroom experience for students. As for substantive changes, we have added chapters on public health policy, social determinants of health, public health systems research, social marketing, social entrepreneurship for public health, and global health. Leiyu and I feel these reflect the ever-expanding scope and scale of public health practice and scholarship.

This is an exciting time for you to be studying public health. The world is full of challenges and opportunities, many of which are emergent and will continue to unfold in unexpected ways. The growth of knowledge in the medical and social sciences is more vibrant than ever. Likewise, our understanding of public health organizations, management, and leadership is more sophisticated and better informed than in the past. Our embrace of evidence-based decision making and data-informed policy and practice is moving to become the new normal. The public health community's realization of the centrality of systems thinking and global perspectives continues to lead us to more comprehensive solutions and a deeper understanding of public health. It is my wish, and that of the entire team of editors and authors, that you find great utility, value, and perhaps inspiration in this text.

James A. Johnson

About the Editors

Dr. Leiyu Shi, DrPH, MBA, MPA, is professor of health policy and health services research in the Department of Health Policy and Management, Bloomberg School of Public Health at The Johns Hopkins University. He is also director of The Johns Hopkins Primary Care Policy Center. Prior to his academic positions, Dr. Shi worked in the public health field focusing on community-based primary care and vulnerable populations. He received his doctoral education from the University of California, Berkeley, majoring in health policy and services research. He also has a master's in business administration focusing on finance. Dr. Shi's research focuses on primary care, health disparities, and vulnerable populations. He has conducted extensive studies about the association between primary care and health outcomes, particularly on the role of primary care in mediating the adverse impact of income inequality on health outcomes. Dr. Shi is also well known for his extensive research on the nation's vulnerable populations, in particular community health centers that serve vulnerable populations, including their sustainability, provider recruitment and retention experiences, financial performance, experience under managed care, and quality of care. Dr. Shi is the author of 9 textbooks and more than 150 scientific journal articles.

    Dr. James A. Johnson, PhD, MPA, MSc, is a medical social scientist who specializes in international health and organization development in public health. He is the former chair of the Department of Health Administration and Policy at the Medical University of South Carolina and currently professor of health administration and health sciences in the Herbert H. and Grace A. Dow College of Health Professions at Central Michigan University. Additionally, he is visiting professor in the Department of Preventive Medicine and Public Health at St. George's University in Grenada, West Indies, and adjunct professor of health policy at Auburn University. Dr. Johnson has also been an active researcher and health science writer, with more than 100 journal articles and 15 books published. His book, *Comparative Health Systems: Global Perspectives* involves coresearchers from around the world and analyzes the health systems of

20 countries. He is also the author of *Introduction to Public Health Management, Organization, and Policy*; pasteditor of the *Journal of Healthcare Management*; and currently contributing editor for the *Journal of Health and Human Services Administration*. Dr. Johnson works closely with the World Health Organization (WHO) and ProWorld Service Corps and is a regular delegate to the World Health Congress and member of the Global Health Council. He has been an invited lecturer at Oxford University (England), Beijing University (China), University of Dublin (Ireland), University of Colima (Mexico), St. George's University (Grenada), and University of Pretoria (South Africa). Additionally, he has served on many boards, including the board of the Association of University Programs in Health Administration (AUPHA), advisory board of the Alliance for the Blind and Visually Impaired, board president of Lowcountry AIDS Services (Charleston, SC), scientific advisory board of the National Diabetes Trust Foundation, advisory board of the Joint Africa Working Group, board of directors of the Africa Research and Development Center, advisory board of the Center for Collaborative Health Leadership, and board of advisors for Health Systems of America. He completed a Master of Public Administration (MPA) in healthcare administration at Auburn University and his PhD at the College of Social Sciences and Public Policy, Florida State University.

Acknowledgment

We want to thank Lloyd F. Novick, MD, MPH, for his vision and intrepid dedication to the initiation and development of this book. It is upon his shoulders that the *Third Edition* is built.

Dr. Novick brought so much experience and intellect to the project from its inception over a decade ago. During his career, he has been a professor of public health and medicine at East Carolina University, SUNY Upstate Medical University, and University of Albany. He has been a health commissioner in New York, Vermont, and Arizona. Dr. Novick was the chair of the Council on Linkages Between Academia and Public Health Practice. He has been president of the Association for Prevention Teaching and Research (APTR), the Association of State and Territorial Health Officials (ASTHO), and is founder and editor of the *Journal of Public Health Management and Practice*. He has received numerous national awards, including the Special Recognition Award from the American College of Preventive Medicine; the Duncan Clark Award, Association of Teachers of Preventive Medicine; Distinguished Service Award, Yale University; Excellence Award, American Public Health Association (APHA); and the Arthur T. McCormack Award, ASTHO.

Always the visionary for this text and its core focus, Dr. Novick states: "The population-based approach, the hallmark of public health activities, will retain its importance in future efforts to improve the health of communities." All of us who work in public health—whether in teaching, research, or service—continue to embrace his vision and learn from his experience.

Contributors

Moya Alfonso, PhD, MSPH
Assistant Professor
Jiann-Ping Hsu College of Public Health
Georgia Southern University
Statesboro, Georgia

Gerald M. Barron, MPH
Deputy Director
Center for Public Health Practice
Associate Professor
Department of Health Policy and
    Management
University of Pittsburgh
Pittsburgh, Pennsylvania

Leslie M. Beitsch, MD, JD
Director
Center for Medicine and Public Health
Associate Dean for Health Affairs
College of Medicine
Florida State University
Tallahassee, Florida

Ruth Berkelman, MD
Rollins Professor and Director
Center for Public Health Preparedness
    and Research

Emory University
Atlanta, Georgia

Ruth Gaare Bernheim, JD, MPH
Associate Director
Institute for Practical Ethics
    and Public Life
Professor and Chair
Department of Public Health Sciences
University of Virginia
Charlottesville, Virginia

Ross C. Brownson, PhD
Professor
George Warren Brown School
    of Social Work
Siteman Cancer Center
School of Medicine
Washington University in St. Louis
St. Louis, Missouri

Carolyn Clancy, MD
Director
Agency for Healthcare Research and Quality
U.S. Department of Health and
    Human Services
Washington, DC

Nailya O. DeLellis, PhD, MPH
Assistant Professor
Herbert H. and Grace A. Dow College
of Health Professions
Central Michigan University
Mount Pleasant, Michigan

Linda Duchak, EdM
Associate Director
Center for Public Health Practice
University of Pittsburgh
Pittsburgh, Pennsylvania

Michael C. Fagen, PhD, MPH
Clinical Assistant Professor
Community Health Sciences Division
School of Public Health
University of Illinois at Chicago
Chicago, Illinois

Elizabeth Fenton, PhD, MPH
University of Virginia
Norfolk, Virginia

Claudia S. P. Fernandez, DrPH, MS
Director
Public Health and Healthcare Leadership
Institute
University of North Carolina
Chapel Hill, North Carolina

Louis Gapenski, PhD, MBA, MS
Professor
College of Public Health and Health
Professions
University of Florida
Gainesville, Florida

Lawrence O. Gostin, JD, LLD (Hon)
Professor
Center for Law and the Public's Health
Georgetown University
Washington, DC

Lawrence W. Green, DrPH, MPH
Professor
Department of Epidemiology
and Biostatistics
School of Medicine
University of California, San Francisco
San Francisco, California

Brendon Haggerty, MURP
Health Planner
Clark County Public Health Department
Vancouver, Washington

Arden S. Handler, DrPH
Professor
Community Health Sciences Division
School of Public Health
University of Illinois at Chicago
Chicago, Illinois

Michael T. Hatcher, DrPH, MPH
Chief
Environmental Medicine Branch
Agency for Toxic Substances and
Disease Registry
Atlanta, Georgia

Theresa Hatzell Hoke, PhD, MPH
Health Services Research Scientist
Family Health International
Research Triangle Park, North Carolina

Peggy A. Honoré, DHA, MHA
Director
Public Health System, Finance and Quality
Program
U.S. Department of Health and Human
Services
Washington, DC
Associate Professor
School of Public Health
Louisiana State University Health Sciences
Center
New Orleans, Louisiana

L. Michele Issel, PhD, RN
Clinical Professor
Community Health Sciences Division
School of Public Health
University of Illinois at Chicago
Chicago, Illinois

James Allen Johnson, III, MPH, DrPH(c)
Karl E. Peace Endowed Research Assistant
Jiann-Ping Hsu College of Public Health
Georgia Southern University
Statesboro, Georgia

Walter J. Jones, PhD, MHSA
Professor
Department of Healthcare Leadership
    and Management
Medical University of South Carolina
Charleston, South Carolina

Kristine Marin Kawamura, PhD, MBA
Professor and Director
Multi-Sector Health Management Program
St. George's University
Grenada, West Indies

Alene Kennedy-Hendricks, PhD(c)
Research Assistant
Bloomberg School of Public Health
The Johns Hopkins University
Baltimore, Maryland

Bernard J. Kerr, Jr., EdD, MPH
Professor
Health Administration Division
Herbert H. and Grace A. Dow College of
    Health Professions
Central Michigan University
Mount Pleasant, Michigan

Linda Young Landesman, DrPH, MSW
President
Landesman Consulting
Rye Brook, New York

Laura B. Landrum, MUPP
Public Health Consultant
Laura Landrum Consultancy
Chicago, Illinois

Gerald R. Ledlow, PhD, MHA
Professor
Jiann-Ping Hsu College of Public Health
Georgia Southern University
Statesboro, Georgia

Cheryll D. Lesneski, DrPh, MA
Assistant Professor
Public Health Leadership Program
Gillings School of Global Public Health
University of North Carolina at Chapel Hill
Chapel Hill, North Carolina

Mary P. Martinasek, PhD, MPH
Assistant Professor
Department of Health Science
University of Tampa
Tampa, Florida

Glen P. Mays, PhD, MPH
Professor
College of Public Health
University of Kentucky
Lexington, Kentucky

Alan L. Melnick, MD, MPH
Health Officer
Clark County Public Health Department
Vancouver, Washington
Associate Professor
Oregon Health and Sciences University
Portland, Oregon

Cynthia B. Morrow, MD, MPH
Commissioner of Health
Onondaga County, New York
Assistant Professor
Public Health and Preventive Medicine
SUNY Upstate Medical University
Syracuse, New York

Ray M. Nicola, MD, MHSA
Field Assignee
Centers for Disease Control and Prevention
Affiliate Professor
Northwest Center for Public Health Practice
University of Washington
Seattle, Washington

Judith M. Ottoson, EdD, MPH
Evaluation Consultant
San Francisco, California

Jean Popiak-Goodwin, DHA, MPH
Project Officer
Centers for Disease Control and Prevention
Atlanta, Georgia

Janet E. Porter, PhD, MBA, MHA
Chief Operating Officer
Dana-Farber Cancer Institute
Harvard Medical Center
Boston, Massachusetts

Margaret A. Potter, JD, MSc
Director
Center for Public Health Practice
Professor and Associate Dean
Graduate School of Public Health
University of Pittsburgh
Pittsburgh, Pennsylvania

Maria L. Roditis, PhD, MPH, MA
Postdoctoral Fellow
Center for Tobacco Control, Research,
    and Education
University of California, San Francisco
San Francisco, California

Benjamin Silk, PhD, MPH
Research Project Manager
Center for Public Health Preparedness
    and Research

Rollins School of Public Health
Emory University
Atlanta, Georgia

David P. Steffen, DrPH, MSN
Director, Leadership Concentration
Public Health Leadership Program
Clinical Assistant Professor
Gillings School of Global Public Health
University of North Carolina at Chapel Hill
Chapel Hill, North Carolina

James H. Stephens, DHA, MHA
Assistant Professor
Jiann-Ping Hsu College of Public Health
Georgia Southern University
Statesboro, Georgia

Barry Thatcher, PhD, MA
Founder
Border Writing
Professor
Department of English
New Mexico State University
Las Cruces, New Mexico

Bernard J. Turnock, MD, MPH
Clinical Professor
Community Health Sciences Division
School of Public Health
University of Illinois at Chicago
Chicago, Illinois

Andrew T. Westrum, DHA, MBA
Program Manager
TRICARE Management Activity
Falls Church, Virginia

Ormanbek T. Zhuzzhanov, MD, PhD
Professor
Public Health Institute
Astana Medical University
Astana, Kazakhstan

Overview of Public Health Administration

James A. Johnson and Leiyu Shi

LEARNING OBJECTIVES

- To be able to define public health and population health
- To describe public health functions and essential services
- To understand the systems perspective in public health and the utility of systems thinking
- To understand the roles and responsibilities of public health administrators
- To be familiar with core competencies for public health managers and leaders
- To identify the purpose and goals of *Healthy People 2020* and how this relates to public health administration

Chapter Overview

From the beginning of public health activities in the ancient world there has been a need for organization and management. Coordination of effort to accomplish goals necessitates certain skills and abilities. This chapter defines public health and population health to establish the context in which public health administration takes place. It also addresses important perspectives and needed competencies, along with future goals and challenges.

Public Health and Population Health Definitions

As described by Novick, Morrow, Mays[1] in the previous edition of this text, **public health** consists of organized efforts to improve the health of populations. The operative components of this definition are that public health efforts are directed to populations rather than to individuals. Public health practice does not rely on a specific body of knowledge and expertise, but rather relies on a dynamic, multidisciplinary approach that often combines the natural and social sciences. The definition of public health reflects its central goal, the reduction of disease and the improvement of health in a population. In 1920, famed American bacteriologist and public health expert Charles-Edward Amory Winslow provided the following seminal definition of public health practice:[2]

> Public health is the science and art of preventing disease, prolonging life, and promoting physical health and efficiency through organized community efforts for the sanitation of the environment, the control of community infections, the education of the individual in principles of personal hygiene, the organization of medical and nursing services for the early diagnosis and preventive treatment of disease, and the development of social machinery which will ensure to every individual in the community a standard of living adequate for the maintenance of health.
>
> Charles-Edward Amory

Since Winslow's definition, the Institute of Medicine (IOM) published its classic 1988 report, *The Future of Public Health*, which similarly defined public health as an "organized community effort to address the public interest in health by applying scientific and technical knowledge to prevent disease and promote health."[3] Thus, the mission of public health, both historically and contemporarily, is to ensure the necessary conditions that promote the health of the population.

Richard Riegelman, founding dean of the School of Public Health and Health Services at George Washington University, stated:[4]

> Public health is about what makes us sick, what keeps us healthy, and what we can do TOGETHER about it. When we think about health, what comes to mind first is individual health and wellness. In public health, what should come to mind first is the health of communities and society as a whole. Thus, in public health the focus shifts from the individual to the population, from me to us.

Population-based strategies for improving health include, but are not limited to, efforts to control epidemics, ensure safe drinking water and food, reduce vaccine-preventable diseases, improve maternal and child health, and conduct surveillance of health problems. In addition to long-standing efforts to protect populations from infectious disease and environmental health hazards, the public health mission has expanded to address contemporary health risks such as obesity, injury, violence, substance abuse, sexually transmitted infections (STIs), human immunodeficiency virus (HIV) infection, acquired immune deficiency syndrome (AIDS), natural disasters, and bioterrorism. To effectively address both historical and contemporary health concerns and sustain improved health outcomes, public health approaches involve multilevel interventions that address the individual, the community, and public policy.

The importance of public health and population-based interventions is underscored by achievements in the 20th century during which individuals living in developed countries increased life expectancy from 45 to 75 years. Now in the 21st century we have seen this increase to 78 years in the United States and 82 years in Japan.[5] The majority of this gain, 25 of the 30-plus years, can be attributed to public health measures such as better nutrition, improved air quality, sanitation, and clean drinking water. Medical care focusing on individual patients, though important, is estimated to have contributed about 5 years of the gain in life expectancy.

Both science and social factors form the basis for an effective public health intervention. For example, successfully eradicating a vaccine-preventable disease from a community requires more than the development of an effective vaccine. Acceptance and widespread use of the vaccine in the community depends on a successful public health initiative providing public information and facilitating delivery. Policies to support the initiative, such as the Vaccines for Children Program and school/daycare requirements for vaccinations, further increase the likelihood of success. Too often, scientific advances are not fully translated into improved health outcomes. For example, in the United States perinatal transmission of HIV decreased because of aggressive approaches for testing and treatment of HIV during pregnancy and delivery, whereas congenital syphilis, though decreased, has not achieved the same level of success despite the fact that the scientific means (penicillin) to eradicate it was discovered in 1928. A comprehensive public health approach, combining science with practical approaches to address cultural and socioeconomic factors affecting health, is essential for the reduction and ultimately the elimination of preventable diseases.

The focus on the health of populations as the most contemporary way of expanding the definition of public health is further underscored, by Kindig's perspective on population health as "the distribution of health outcomes within a population, the health determinants that influence distribution and the policies and interventions that impact those determinants."[6] Further along this line of thinking, Nash adds:[7]

> It spans wellness and health promotion, chronic disease management, care of the frail and elderly, and palliative and end-of-life care. In essence, broad population health approaches are designed to preserve wellness and minimize the physical and financial impact of illness.

The concept of **population health** can be described as a comprehensive way of thinking about the current and future scope of public health. It utilizes an evidence-based approach to analyze the determinants of health and disease, along with options for intervention and prevention to preserve and improve health. The interconnection of public health, public policy, and health systems is demonstrated by Riegelman[4] in **Figure 1.1**.

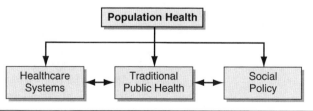

Figure 1.1   A Full Spectrum of Population Health
Source: Reproduced from Riegelman, Richard, *Public Health 101: Healthy People-Healthy Populations,* 2012: Jones & Bartlett Learning, Burlington MA. www.jblearning.com. Reprinted with permission.

Public Health Functions

The 1988 Institute of Medicine report mentioned earlier, *The Future of Public Health*, defined three core functions that public health agencies need to perform.[3] These functions remain the responsibility of governments and should not be delegated to nongovernmental organizations. While population health does engage the full spectrum of stakeholders, public health agencies at the local, state, and federal levels are responsible for accomplishing the essential health services. While much work may be contracted out to other sectors, the responsibility remains with the government public health agencies. The core functions, assessment, policy development, and assurance, are defined by the IOM as follows:

- **Assessment** involves obtaining data to define the health of populations and the nature of health problems
- **Assurance** includes the oversight responsibility for ensuring that essential components of an effective health system are in place
- **Policy development** includes developing evidence-based recommendations and analysis to guide public policy as it pertains to health

Building on the IOM recommendations the U.S. Public Health Service put forth the "Public Health in America Statement" in 1994. This was supported and promoted by the American Public Health Association and most other groups advocating for a consistent and unified approach to public health. The 10 essential services are presented in **Table 1.1**. **Figure 1.2** can help to better visualize how the core functions and essential services for public health fit together. This framework is used by local, state, and federal agencies throughout the country. It serves as a guide and framework for public health organization design and development, workforce planning and staffing, strategic management, resource allocation, information systems design, and staff training.

Table 1.1   Essential Public Health Services

1. **Monitor** health status to identify community health problems.
2. **Diagnose and investigate** health problems and health hazards in the community.
3. **Inform, educate, and empower** people about health issues.
4. **Mobilize** community partnerships to identify and solve health problems.
5. **Develop policies and plans** that support individual and community health efforts.
6. **Enforce** laws and regulations that protect health and ensure safety.
7. **Link** people to needed personal health services and assure the provision of health care when otherwise unavailable.
8. **Assure** a competent public health and personal healthcare workforce.
9. **Evaluate** effectiveness, accessibility, and quality of personal and population-based health services.
10. **Research** for new insights and innovative solutions to health problems.

Source: Reproduced from Centers for Disease Control and Prevention (CDC), Atlanta, GA. Available at: http://www.cdc.gov/nphpsp/essentialservices.html. Accessed December 16, 2012.

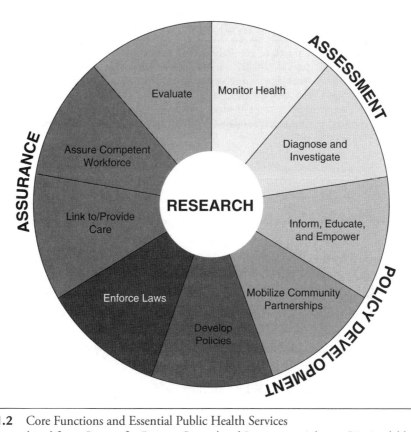

Figure 1.2   Core Functions and Essential Public Health Services
Source: Reproduced from Centers for Disease Control and Prevention, Atlanta, GA. Available at:
http://www.cdc.gov/nceh/ehs/ephli/core_ess.htm. Accessed December 1, 2012.

Systems Perspective in Public Health

Public health is best understood from a **systems perspective**. As described by Johnson:[8]

> Public health is highly interconnected and interdependent in its relationship to individuals, communities, and the larger society, including the global community. Using the language of systems theory, public health is a complex adaptive system. It is complex in that it is composed of multiple, diverse, interconnected elements, and it is adaptive in that the system is capable of changing and learning from experience and its environment.

Johnson further explains the systems approach in public health is more than the relationships that support and facilitate the organization and actions of public health, but also includes "the mindset of public health professionals." This is often referred to as systems thinking and is especially salient in public health management, practice, and research. The National Cancer Institute (NCI) sums up their understanding and embrace of systems thinking as presented in **Box 1.1**. It was one of the first public health agencies to fully embrace systems thinking and has found it a most useful paradigm in its Tobacco Control Research Branch.

Box 1.1   National Cancer Institute (NCI) Statement on Systems Thinking

Public health researchers and practitioners often work to solve complex population and health issues, such as obesity and chronic disease, which are deeply embedded within the fabric of society. As such, the solutions often require intervention and engagement with key stakeholders and organizations across many levels ranging from local entities (schools, churches, and work environments) to regional systems (health departments and hospital networks) to entire countries (national agencies). This multilevel, multiparticipant view is at the heart of systems thinking, a process of understanding how parts influence one another within a whole.

Source: Reproduced from National Cancer Institute, Washington, DC. Available at: https://researchtoreality.cancer.gov /cyber-seminars/using-systems-thinking-and-tools-solve-public-health-problems. Accessed December 1, 2012.

Other systems thinking applications and efforts in public health have been identified by Trochim, Cabrera, Milstein, Gallagher, and Leischow.[9] These include the Syndemics Prevention Network, supported by the CDC, which studies how recognition of mutually reinforcing health problems (substance abuse, violence, HIV/AIDS) expands the conceptual, methodological, and moral dimensions of public health work and ways of thinking about health as a system. Examples of other relevant efforts include the Institute of Medicine report, *Crossing the Quality Chasm: A New Health System for the 21st Century*;[10] the Community–University Partnerships Initiative sponsored by the W. K. Kellogg Foundation; community-based participatory research efforts sponsored jointly by the Agency for Healthcare Research and Quality and the W. K. Kellogg Foundation; the Community–Campus Partnerships for Health; the Healthy Cities movement; and the efforts of the World Health Organization's Commission on Social Determinants of Health.

The World Health Organizations published a report in 2009 titled *Systems Thinking for Health Systems Strengthening* in which they claim systems thinking is a "paradigm shift" for public health. As stated in the report, "Systems thinking offers a more comprehensive way of anticipating synergies and mitigating negative emergent behaviors, with direct relevance for creating more system-ready policies."[11]

Trochim, et al.[9] assert that systems thinking is consonant with ecological models familiar to public health professionals, including the ideas of human ecology, population health, and the social determinants of health. But it goes beyond these models, incorporating advances in fields such as organizational behavior,[12] system dynamics,[13] emergence theory,[14] and complexity theory.[15] The system thinking approach emphasizes how everything fits into the larger social, cultural, economic, and political system. As Johnson and Breckon[16] claim, the importance placed on interconnectedness cannot be underestimated in the world of the 21st century.

Role of the Public Health Administrator and Manager

The work of public health could not be done nor its goals accomplished without managers and administrators. These individuals often obtain a graduate degree, either master of public health (MPH) or master of public administration (MPA) during which time they study management, administration, and policy. Others learn management skills on the job or take coursework in other related fields of **management** such as business and health services administration. Burke and Friedman define management in the following ways:[17]

- It is first and foremost an interdisciplinary, rigorous, and valid endeavor that is integral to all human enterprise, including public health.
- It is both a necessary and sufficient condition to ensure the goals of public health programs are met.

Johnson and Breckon identify seven interconnected processes and responsibilities commonly associated with the administrative role:[16]

1. **Planning** is the process of specifying goals, establishing priorities, and otherwise identifying and sequencing action steps to accomplish goals.
2. **Organizing** involves establishing a structure or set of relationships so plans can be implemented and goals accomplished.
3. **Staffing** is the assignment of personnel to specific roles or functions so the organization works as designed.
4. **Directing** involves making decisions and communicating them so they can be implemented.
5. **Coordinating** is the task of assuring effective interrelationships.
6. **Reporting** is the transfer of information and assurance of accountability.
7. **Budgeting** is fiscal planning, accounting, and control.

The Council on Education for Public Health (CEPH) places considerable importance on management and administration by identifying "Management Competencies" for public health education and practice. The Association of Schools of Public Health provides a list of core competencies in the managerial and leadership domains, as shown in **Tables 1.2** and **1.3**.

Johnson defines management as "the process or working with and through others to achieve organizational or program objectives in an efficient and ethical manner."[8] One of the goals of this text is to address and elaborate upon every element of this definition and all of the competencies listed in Tables 1.2 and 1.3.

Future Outlook

Public health administrators and practitioners will face many challenges in the 21st century while also having an opportunity to shape public health practice and policy. One way of gaining insight into the kinds of issues to be faced is to look at the *Healthy People 2020* initiative. As described by Shi and Singh,[18] since 1980 the United States has undertaken 10-year plans outlining certain key national objectives to be accomplished during each subsequent decade. The process and achievements of these plans are explored further later; however, in our discussion of the role of public health administrators, it is important to realize how these objects for the coming years will help galvanize efforts and guide policy. The mission is as follows:[18]

> *Healthy People 2020* strives to: (1) Identify nationwide health improvement priorities; (2) Increase public awareness and understanding of the determinants of health, disease and disability and the opportunities for progress; (3) Provide measurable objectives and goals

Table 1.2   Management Competencies, Health Policy and Management

D. Health Policy and Management*

Health policy and management is a multidisciplinary field of inquiry and practice concerned with the delivery, quality, and costs of health care for individuals and populations. This definition assumes both a managerial and a policy concern with the structure, process, and outcomes of health services including the costs, financing, organization, outcomes, and accessibility of care.

Competencies: Upon graduation, a student with an MPH should be able to…

D.1 Identify the main components and issues of the organization, financing, and delivery of health services and public health systems in the United States.

D.2 Describe the legal and ethical bases for public health and health services.

D.3 Explain methods of ensuring community health safety and preparedness.

D.4 Discuss the policy process for improving the health status of populations.

D.5 Apply the principles of program planning, development, budgeting, management, and evaluation in organizational and community initiatives.

D.6 Apply principles of strategic planning and marketing to public health.

D.7 Apply quality and performance improvement concepts to address organizational performance issues.

D.8 Apply "systems thinking" for resolving organizational problems.

D.9 Communicate health policy and management issues using appropriate channels and technologies.

D.10 Demonstrate leadership skills for building partnerships.

*In this series, *health policy* is treated as a separate text and area of inquiry. As such, this text addresses only the health management competencies.

Source: ASPH.

Table 1.3   Management Competencies, Leadership

H. Leadership

The ability to create and communicate a shared vision for a changing future, champion solutions to organizational and community challenges, and energize commitment to goals.

Competencies: Upon graduation, it is increasingly important that a student with an MPH be able to…

H.1 Describe the attributes of leadership in public health.

H.2 Describe alternative strategies for collaboration and partnership among organizations, focused on public health goals.

H.3 Articulate an achievable mission, set of core values, and vision.

H.4 Engage in dialogue and learning from others to advance public health goals.

H.5 Demonstrate team building, negotiation, and conflict management skills.

H.6 Demonstrate transparency, integrity, and honesty in all actions.

H.7 Use collaborative methods for achieving organizational and community health goals.

H.8 Apply social justice and human rights principles when addressing community needs.

H.9 Develop strategies to motivate others for collaborative problem solving, decision making, and evaluation.

Source: ASPH.

that can be used at national, state, and local levels; (4) Engage multiple sectors to take actions that are driven by the best available evidence and knowledge; (5) Identify critical research and data collection needs.

Figure 1.3 presents an action model that may be used by public health planners, administrators, and policymakers to better achieve overarching goals.

As described by Shi and Singh,[18] *Healthy People 2020* is differentiated from previous *Healthy People* initiatives by including multiple new topic areas to its objective list, such as adolescent health; blood disorders and blood safety; dementias; genomics; global health; healthcare-associated infections; quality of life and wellbeing; lesbian, gay, bisexual, and transgender health; older adults; preparedness; sleep health; and social determinants of health. *Healthy People 2020* also establishes four foundational health measures to monitor progress toward achieving its goals. These measures include general health status, health-related quality of life and wellbeing, determinants of health, and health disparities.

This text addresses a wide range of public health administration and population health management topics including ethics, law, finance, policy, human resources, leadership, information systems, strategic planning, performance management, evaluation, social marketing, health education and prevention, social entrepreneurship, disaster preparedness, public health quality, and global health. The intent is to facilitate a comprehensive understanding of this subject matter and an appreciation for the complex role of public health administrators and managers in the promotion and assurance of the nation's health.

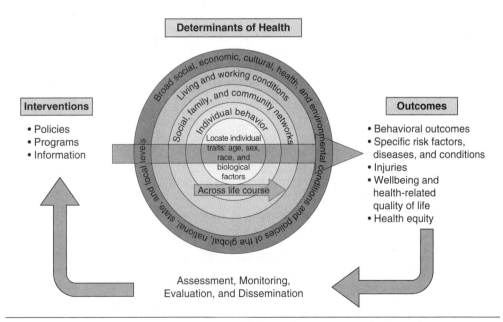

Figure 1.3   Action Model to Achieve U.S. *Healthy People 2020* Overarching Goals
Source: Reproduced from the Department of Health and Human Services.

Discussion Questions

1. Define public health and define population health. How are the two concepts related?
2. What are the core functions of public health?
3. Describe the 10 essential services of public health.
4. What is systems thinking, and why is it useful for public health?
5. What are the tasks and processes managers are commonly involved in?
6. Identify several core competencies needed by public health managers and leaders. How does your degree program address these?
7. What is *Healthy People 2020* and what does it seek to accomplish? How might it serve to guide public health administrators in their program planning?

References

1. Novick LF, Morrow CB, Mays GP. *Public Health Administration: Principles of Population-Based Management*, 2nd ed. Sudbury, MA: Jones and Bartlett Publishers; 2008.
2. Winslow CE. The untilled fields of public health. *Science*. 1920;51(1306):23–33.
3. Institute of Medicine. *The future of public health*. Available at: http://iom.edu/Reports/1988/The-Future-of-Public-Health.aspx. Accessed November 13, 2012.
4. Riegelman R. *Public Health 101: Healthy People–Healthy Populations*. Sudbury, MA: Jones & Bartlett Learning; 2010.
5. Johnson JA, Stoskopf CH. *Comparative Health Systems: Global Perspectives*. Sudbury, MA: Jones & Bartlett Learning; 2010.
6. Kindig D. Understanding population health terminology. *Milbank Q.* 2007;85(1):139–61.
7. Nash DB. Population health and health reform-Inseparable concepts. *Prescriptions for Excellence in Health Care.* 2012;1(16):1.
8. Johnson JA. *Introduction to Public Health Management, Organizations, and Policy*. Clifton Park, NY: Delmar-Cengage Learning; 2013;184.
9. Trochim WM, Cabrera DA, Milstein B, et al. Practical challenges of systems thinking and modeling in public health. *American Journal of Public Health*. 2006;96(3):538–46.
10. Institute of Medicine. *Crossing the Quality Chasm: A New Health System for the 21st Century*. Available at: http://www.iom.edu/Reports/2001/Crossing-the-Quality-Chasm-A-New-Health-System-for-the-21st-Century.aspx. Accessed December 1, 2012.
11. World Health Organization. *Systems Thinking for Health Systems Strengthening*. Geneva: WHO Press; 2009.
12. Johnson JA. *Health Organizations: Theory, Behavior, and Development*. Sudbury, MA: Jones and Bartlett Publishers; 2009.
13. Meadows DH. *Thinking in Systems*. White River, VT: Chelsea Green Publishing; 2008.
14. Johnson S. *Emergence: The Connected Lives of Ants, Brains, Cities, and Software*. New York: Scribner; 2001.
15. McDaniel RR, Jordan ME. Complexity and postmodern theory. In: Johnson JA, *Health Organizations: Theory, Behavior, and Development*. Sudbury, MA: Jones and Bartlett Publishers; 2008.
16. Johnson JA, Breckon DJ. *Managing Health Education and Promotion Programs: Leadership Skills for the 21st Century*. Sudbury, MA: Jones and Bartlett Publishers; 2007.
17. Burke RE, Friedman LH. *Essentials of Management and Leadership in Public Health*. Sudbury, MA: Jones & Bartlett Learning; 2011.
18. Shi L, Singh, DA. *Delivering Health Care in America: A Systems Approach*. Burlington, MA: Jones & Bartlett Learning; 2012.

Historical Developments in Public Health and the 21st Century

James Allen Johnson III, James A. Johnson, and Cynthia B. Morrow

---

LEARNING OBJECTIVES

- To better understand the historical context of public health
- To gain perspective on the role of public health in society
- To grasp the key milestones in the evolution of public health practice and policy
- To understand recent reform and its implications for the future of public health

---

Chapter Overview

Public health administration and practice comprises organized efforts to improve the health of populations. Public health prevention strategies target populations rather than individuals. Throughout history, public health efforts have focused on the control of communicable diseases, reducing environmental hazards, and providing safe drinking water. Because social, environmental, and biologic factors interact to determine health, public health practice must utilize a broad set of skills and interventions. During the 20th century, the historic emphasis of public health on protecting populations from infectious disease and environmental threats expanded to include the prevention and reduction of chronic disease through behavioral and lifestyle interventions. As we move forward in the 21st century new challenges will emerge and new strategies and initiatives will need to be developed. The role of public health will undoubtedly be central to the wellbeing of the nation and the world.

Early History of Public Health

Little is known about the health of the hunting and gathering people of prehistoric times. Paleopathology has shown that disease not only existed in antiquity, but that it has always occurred in humans in the same basic forms such as infection, inflammation, disturbance of development and metabolism, and tumors.[1] When humans began to aggregate into larger, more permanent settlements with the introduction of agricultural techniques and the domestication of animals, they fundamentally altered the way they lived. With the adoption of an agrarian society, humans began to live in closer contact in communities supported by the production of food. These new types of human settlements reconstructed the ecosystems over which they presided, ushering a fundamental shift in how humans interacted with each other and their environments. These new denser living arrangements afforded innumerable microorganisms a new ecological niche to exploit, paving the way for pestilence, epidemics, and disease.[2,3,4] For example, human settlements offered greater opportunity for constant contact with intestinal parasites carried through human feces, whereas constantly mobile bands of hunters and gatherers were less likely to acquire such infections.[2] Permanent and semipermanent settlements, the domestication of plants and animals, and the urbanization of human society forever altered the disease environment of the human species.[2,3,5] From the most ancient times of recorded history, all human societies have been affected by the contingencies of illness and health.[1,2,6]

Although little is known about the disease regimes of prehistoric societies, it is generally assumed that the early settlements of Mesopotamia, the Indus valley, and the Peruvian coastal region were plagued by tropical diseases such as malaria and schistosomiasis.[2,3] Ancient medical systems relied predominantly on mystical and religious explanations for disease and often stressed the importance of evading illness through ritual and practical methods of prevention grounded in spiritual and temporal purity through various codes of behavior and dietary protocols.[1,2,7] Chinese physicians under the Chou Dynasty (1122–250 BCE) advocated for the preservation of health through a mixture of dietary restrictions, temperance, and physical and spiritual exercises.[2] Similarly, in ancient Egypt the consensus was that illness and disease were a result of an imbalance between temporal and spiritual existence. The ancient Egyptians used techniques such as prayers, magic, ritual, and pharmacopoeia to restore health.[2,8] Regulations governing food preparation, hygiene, and sexual relations were largely ritualistic and widely practiced throughout ancient Egyptian society.[2,9] Furthermore, archaeological excavations in Egypt have provided evidence that several ancient cities from around the 14th century BCE were planned and had relatively sophisticated stone masonry drainage systems.[1] In ancient India, planned cities, in which bathrooms and drains in buildings were commonplace, were also constructed around 4,000 years ago in the Indus valley. These cities also routinely enjoyed broad, paved streets and covered sewers.[1] In Mesopotamia, many societies, including the Babylonians, Assyrians, and Hebrews, embraced regulatory hygiene customs in the form of established codes. The aims of these codes were to encourage spiritual purity; although, the hygiene regulations often latently prevented disease.[9] Furthermore, Hebrew rabbi-physicians formulated elaborate rules for disease prevention based on the belief that some diseases were communicable through foods, bodily discharge, clothing, water, and air.[2] The Hebrews and Babylonians also believed that plagues spread through contaminated water[2] and connected epidemics with certain animals such as rats, flies, and gnats.[10] Both of these groups isolated individuals during epidemics and fumigated and disinfected their houses and belongings. The Hebrew and Babylonian codes also demanded that no well was to be dug near a cemetery or waste dump; water was to be boiled before drinking; and food had to be clean, fresh, and thoroughly cooked.[2] The association between ritualistic cleanliness and health was not limited to the "old world"; the Incas instituted an annual health ceremony which included the cleaning of all homes.[11] These examples provide evidence of early understanding of the importance of protecting the public from disease.

Hellenistic Health

Between the 7th and 5th centuries BCE new philosophies that separated the temporal and divine causes of disease began to emerge in ancient Greece. However, these philosophies were the exception and their influence was only minuscule; much of the ancient Greek understanding of health was still dominated by mysticism until the emergence of Hippocrates and the **Hippocratic tradition**. Hippocrates was an honored and celebrated physician who probably lived sometime between 460 and 360 BCE. He was one of the authors and namesake of the Hippocratic Corpus, from which the Hippocratic Oath pledged by physicians today was derived. The Corpus is a compilation of works by many authors that presented a radical departure from the religious and mystical traditions of healing. The Corpus and more generally the Hippocratic tradition concentrated on the patient rather than the disease and emphasized prevention.[2] The Hippocratic tradition represented medicine as a professional vocation that used and adapted healing methods and regimes that were based on empirical observation.[2,12] Hippocratic physiology recognized the body as consisting of four fluids or *humours*: blood, black bile, yellow bile, and phlegm. Health was achieved when all four were in perfect balance or equilibrium. The *humours* reflected the essential elements of the physical universe: fire, earth, air, and water.

Hippocratic tradition recognized that health was affected by seasons and the quality of the environment. *On Airs, Waters, and Places*, a central Hippocratic text, analyzed the environmental determinants of health and divided diseases into ones that were **endemic**, always present, and ones that were **epidemic**, occurring occasionally.[1,2] These terms and concepts are still used today. *On Airs, Waters, and Places* was not limited to a theoretical treatise, but rather it served as a practical guide used in Hellenistic colonial expansion. The text recommended that before a place was colonized and building commenced, a physician should conduct a detailed investigation of the environment's integrity. Building settlements on or near marshes and swamps was discouraged, whereas it was recommended to erect houses on dry, elevated areas warmed by the sun.[1] Another practical application of *On Airs, Waters, and Places* was to assist physicians in setting up practices in unfamiliar towns or areas.

Greek medicine never exclusively relied on curative methods, but rather embraced a tradition of combining therapeutic treatments with prevention measures. Because disease was believed to reflect an imbalance in the *humours*, preventing the disturbance of equilibrium was thought to be essential. To preserve equilibrium, physicians proposed an ideal model of life that required that nutrition, excretion, exercise, and rest remain in perfect balance. However, very few people in ancient Greece could afford to live such a life and this recommended regimen was limited to the upper classes whose lives consisted of leisure. In ancient Greece, the upper classes were supported by a slave economy; thus, for most Greeks the recommended equilibrium was virtually unattainable.[1] The theoretical idea of equilibrium proposed by the ancient Greeks has had a profound impact on the perceptions of health and healing throughout the ages. Today it remains at the conceptual core of homeostasis, the foundation of modern allopathic medicine.

Latin Engineering and Administration

Hellenistic expansion through the conquests of Alexander the Great spread Hippocratic traditions throughout parts of Europe, the Middle East, and North Africa. However, nothing had as profound an impact on the spread of Hippocratic traditions and the abandonment of religious and mystical healing techniques as the emergence of the Roman Empire. Rome conquered the Mediterranean world and embraced the legacy of Greek culture. Although the Romans adopted the philosophies proposed by Hippocratic traditions, they added to them components that were distinctly Roman. The Roman clinician was, in most respects, an imitation of the Greek physician, embracing the Hippocratic traditions. Roman elites frequently hired Greek physicians as their personal healers. In fact, the famed Roman physician Galen (129–200 CE) was ethnically Greek. Where the Romans differed from the Greeks was in their abilities in engineering and administration, as builders of complex sewage systems and baths, and as providers of water supplies and other health facilities.[1] Through the construction of complex engineering projects and the establishment of sophisticated administration systems, the Romans forever changed how the world addressed health.

Sanitation reform in Rome was catalyzed by the growth of the bureaucratic imperial state and the development of sophisticated civil engineering to provide rapid communication across the empire.[2] By the 2nd century BCE, an elaborate system of aqueducts was bringing fresh water into the city of Rome; eventually most cities throughout the empire would have systems in place that were on par with Rome's. Many cities also had sophisticated baths, public fountains, piped water, drainage systems, underground sewage systems, and public pay lavatories located in the busier sections of town.[1,2,13] The public routinely retrieved water from communal water sources, whereas aristocrats and the ruling elite typically had their own private water supplies.[1] The administration of public health services was a responsibility of the imperial state. In Rome, government supervision and regulations extended to public baths, water supplies, street cleaning, and the sale of spoiled food.[14] The state also commissioned and oversaw innumerable building projects that contributed to health and sanitation. By the early 2nd century, physicians were given immunity from taxation by most civil authorities.[2] Furthermore, physicians were employed by many municipalities to provide medical services for the poor; however, these services were limited and inadequate for addressing the needs of the expansive poor populations.[1,2,15] Infirmaries were established in the 1st century CE throughout the empire to service sick slaves; occasionally these facilities were utilized by free citizens, although, this was rare. Also, military hospitals were established at large fortresses to services the expansive military.[16] While hospitals were provided for soldiers and slaves, the duel engines of the imperial economy, such provisions for the poor members of Roman society were virtually nonexistent.[1,2] Although the

Roman state provided a salubrious metropolitan environment for its aristocracy and ruling elite, most citizens lived in overcrowded squalid conditions in burgeoning cities.[14]

In addition to their revolutionary sanitation reforms, the Romans recognized the connection between swamps and marshes and disease, especially malaria. In the 1st century BCE, the Roman scholar and writer Marcus Terentius Varro advised against establishing farms near swamps and marshes because "there are bred certain minute creatures which cannot be seen by the eyes, which float in the air and enter the body through the mouth and nose and there cause serious disease."[1, p. 19] Despite all of the public engineering projects and sanitation regulations and reforms, Rome was burdened by the many endemic and epidemic diseases similarly experienced by other peoples of the Mediterranean basin.

The Middle Ages

In the Middle Ages (500–1500 CE), continual epidemics of infectious diseases spurred collective activities by communities to promote the public's health, presaging the later formation of boards of health and public health departments in the 1800s. The Middle Ages were marked by two major epidemics of bubonic plague, the Plague of Justinian (543 CE) and the Black Death (1348 CE), with smaller outbreaks of various diseases in the intervening period including leprosy, smallpox, tuberculosis, and measles.[17]

The decline of the Roman Empire was most pervasive in the City of Rome and the empire's western provinces. The emperor Constantine accelerated this decline when he relocated the administrative capital of Rome to Byzantium, current day Istanbul. The Western Roman Empire eventually dissolved, unofficially ushering in the Middle Ages. However, the Eastern Roman Empire, often referred to as the Byzantine Empire, thrived for several hundred more years. During the Middle Ages, the Eastern Roman Empire, Persia, and Arab city-states became economically interrelated fostering the exchange of knowledge and ideas, including health and healing methods. The disintegration of the Roman Empire in the west led to the decentralization of government and administration. The sophisticated cities built by the Romans were largely abandoned and their maintenance and upkeep went unattended. This decentralization of civic power coupled with mass emigration from the dilapidated cities dissolved the administrative health reforms established by the empire. The absence of centralized governance gave rise to the expansive power of the Christian Church. The Church became the presiding authority over Europe during this period and thus inherited the responsibilities required by such a position, including public health administration. The Church, unlike the Roman Empire, had no established bureaucracy in place to administrate complex public health measures. This led to a reliance on municipal initiatives that were endorsed by the Church. With the emergence of the Church over the Roman State, cultural preoccupations with health in this period began to focus less upon the comfort of aristocrats and ruling elites and more upon the dangerous effects disease had on the general population.[1,2] The needs and health of the poor became objects of Christian welfare provisions.

Changing patterns in agriculture production during this period led to a substantial increase in the population. Furthermore, there was increased trade with the densely urbanized societies of the Middle East. These two developments contributed to the urbanization of Europe, and people began to aggregate in and around old Roman cities and newly established settlements. These new cities relied on encircling fortifications for security and consequently suffered from overcrowding in the confined spaces.[2] As social, economic, and demographic factors began to change, there were new opportunities for pestilence and disease to exploit, and approaches to disease prevention faced new challenges.

The Black Death, a bubonic plague that peaked in 1348, had devastating consequences on medieval Europe. At the time, it was unknown that bubonic plague was transmitted to humans via the fleas of rodents; consequently, it was regarded as a communicable disease. One countermeasure employed to combat the pestilence was the isolation of individuals who were ill. In addition, victims of the disease had to be reported to authorities, an antecedent of the basic public health functions of disease reporting and surveillance. **Quarantine** measures were instituted to prevent entry of the plague from outside regions. Quarantine consists of the systematic isolation of travelers and ships for a period of 40 days, hence the name quarantine. The period of 40 days was believed to separate acute infection from chronic illness.[1] Italian administrative measures to prevent the import of disease became the model eventually adopted by the rest of Europe.[18] In 1348, Venice, a chief port of entry for commerce from Asia, was the first city to institute quarantine, requiring the inspection and segregation of ships and individuals suspected of carrying disease. These early efforts of isolation remain relevant today, as they are precedents to the contemporary public health practice of quarantine.

Industrialization and the Influence of Great Britain

Public health activities in Great Britain were greatly influenced by the growing urbanization and industrialization of the 1800s. Conditions in England and the responsive social reforms and public health policies had a profound influence on how the United States addressed similar problems. London more than tripled in size from approximately 200,000 inhabitants in 1600 to 675,000 in 1700. During the 1700s, London grew only by approximately one-third and still had less than 1 million residents, but between 1800 and 1840, London doubled in size to nearly 2 million residents.[19] Malnutrition, overcrowding, filth, and poor working conditions contributed to severe disease outbreaks.[20] Similarly, in New York City, the rise of typhus as a significant cause of death was attributed in part to the large increase in the number of immigrants in the 1840s and 1850s. In New York, the rise of tenement housing transformed typhus into an endemic slum disorder, but because it affected the poorest groups of society, it aroused little public concern.[21]

In 1842, Edwin Chadwick published the "General Report on the Sanitary Condition of the Laboring Population of Great Britain."[17] This and follow-up reports became essential public health documents, stimulating sanitary awareness and social reforms.[17,20,22,23] Chadwick described the prevalence of disease among the laborer populations, showing that the poor exhibited a preponderance of disease and disability compared to more affluent populations,[22] an observation that remains true throughout the world today. Chadwick's report concluded that unsanitary environments caused the poor health of working people. At the time, disease was often attributed to miasma and foul odors,[22] and epidemics such as typhus, typhoid, and cholera were attributed to filth, stagnant pools of water, rotting animals and vegetables, and garbage.[19]

As chief administrator of the Poor Law Commission, Chadwick was responsible for providing relief to impoverished populations in England and Wales. He championed sanitary reform, which became the basis for public health activities in Great Britain and the United States alike.

Chadwick was also the chief architect of the 1848 Public Health Act, which created a general board of health empowered to establish local boards of health and appoint an officer of health.[17,24] The latter was required to be a medically qualified practitioner and inspector of sanitary conditions. The board of health incurred opposition from those with property interests who, for economic reasons, were against proposals for the improvement of drainage and water systems. In 1854, only 5 years after its commencement, Parliament refused to renew the Public Health Act, thereby dissolving England's first national board of health.[17]

Although repealed, the 1848 Public Health Act was instrumental in improving public health and remains relevant to current population-based preventive efforts.[24] Based on available morbidity and mortality data, the Act identified major public health issues of the time and assigned responsibility to national and local boards including inspectors and officers of health.[24] The identified issues included poverty, housing, water, sewerage, the environment, safety, and food. Public health in England and Wales was thus organized with the primary purpose of improving the sanitary conditions of towns. The drafters of the Public Health Act, concerned with population health, assigned the responsibility of public health to national and local governments.[24] The sanitation reforms in Great Britain had profound influence on the development of public health administration in America as the two nations confronted similar problems throughout the 19th century.

The Emergence and Impact of Bacteriology

During the latter part of the 1800s and the early 1900s, scientific advances, particularly in microbiology, ushered in a new era for the fields of public health and medicine.[20] Sometimes referred to as the bacteriologic phase of the public health movement, this era was led by the discoveries of Louis Pasteur and Robert Koch and the subsequent germ theory of disease. Pasteur discovered aerobic and anaerobic organisms and began to consider the possibility of a causal relationship between germs and disease. Koch, a country physician, discovered the bacillus responsible for anthrax and was able to demonstrate that the disease was transmissible in mice. He later discovered other disease-causing bacteria, including those that caused tuberculosis and cholera. This new germ theory afforded new opportunities for infectious diseases control, including improved diagnosis, understanding of carrier states, and insight into the importance of vectors with respect to the transmission of disease. Furthermore, in New York City in the 1920s, the development of antitoxin and immunizations against diphtheria were harbingers of the abilities of organized public health programs to prevent a wide range of communicable diseases.[17]

The bacteriologic discoveries of Pasteur and Koch became a marker between the "old" and the "new" public health.[25] The association between bacteria and disease causation drew attention away from the sanitary problems of water supply, street cleaning, housing, and living conditions of the poor.[25,26,27] Disease-oriented approaches to public health were adopted by health officers and local health agencies.[27] Polluted water was demonstrated to be responsible for the transmission of typhoid fever, and methods were developed to measure bacteria in air, water, and milk.[25]

Although disease-oriented approaches became the standard during this period, public health professionals continued to emphasize social reform with the realization that diseases, even those caused by germs, could not be separated from living and working conditions.[10]

Public Health in the United States

> The specters cholera, yellow fever, and smallpox recoil in fear as their way through the port of New York is blocked by a barrier labeled "Quarantine" and by an angel holding a sword and a shield on which is written "Cleanliness."[28, p. 139]
>
> **—Description of "At the Gates," an etching printed by Harper and Brothers, New York, September 5, 1885**

The American Colonies and the Early United States

The early American colonists struggled with hunger and malnutrition, their respective diseases, and infectious diseases such as smallpox, cholera, measles, diphtheria, and typhoid fever.[29] Malaria was endemic in parts of the colonies and smallpox was epidemic throughout the 1600s, yellow fever in the 1700s, and the pervasive disease of the 1800s was cholera.[22] The major public health measure employed by the colonies was the control of communicable diseases through legal efforts regarding quarantine and sanitation. The early colonies consisted of a series of seaports connected by ships. In 1699, William Penn, concerned about yellow fever in the colony he had established, passed the Act to Prevent Sickly Vessels from Coming into This Government.[22] The Massachusetts Quarantine Act of July 1701 required parties bringing infectious diseases within the colony to pay all associated costs and damages and compelled confinement of individuals who were infected with pestilential illnesses. Quarantine laws were enacted in all major cities and towns along the eastern seaboard. Other laws that protected the health of the community included sanitary laws regulating such matters as privies and disposal of wastes and of animals.

In addition to the passage of these laws, another notable public health intervention of the colonial period was smallpox inoculation. Reverend Cotton Mather, known for his involvement in the Salem Witch trials, provided an account of the smallpox epidemic of 1689–1690 in New England: "In about a twelvemonth, one thousand of our neighbors have been carried to their long home."[22, p. 22] The total population of Boston at that time was only 6,000. In 1721, during a smallpox epidemic in Boston, Mather suggested the use of smallpox inoculation. As with many public health interventions, initially there was considerable controversy concerning smallpox inoculation; however, inoculation efforts eventually prevailed. Years later, when smallpox again struck Massachusetts, the death rate was 1.8% in individuals who were vaccinated, compared to 14% in those who were not.[22]

Yellow fever, an acute mosquito-borne viral infectious disease of short duration and varying severity, was the scourge of the 1700s.[30] In 1702, following importation of the disease from the Virgin Islands, New York City was particularly affected by the yellow fever epidemic, although numerous other cities, including Philadelphia, Norfolk, Charleston, New Orleans, and Boston, also fell victim to the disease. When a ship was quarantined in a harbor because it was a suspected carrier of yellow fever, it was required to fly a yellow flag upon its mast; hence, the name of the disease was derived. Yellow fever epidemics were experienced in cities throughout the century with some cities experiencing multiple epidemics.[31] An example is Philadelphia in which nearly 50,000 people were reported to have contracted yellow fever (with 4,044 reported deaths) in 1793 only to be devastated by the disease again 5 years later, when another 3,506 deaths were attributed to the disease.[26] In the northern colonies the disease was noted to occur only in summer, after ships arrived from ports affected by yellow fever, whereas when the fall frost arrived the epidemics ended. This underscored the importance of the environment in epidemic disease and improved understanding of the opportunity and necessity for public health measures.

Public Health in the 19th Century

In the 1800s, New York City was ravaged by several epidemics, including cholera, smallpox, typhus, dysentery, and diphtheria.[26] In addition to epidemics, the health of the public was threatened by the constant presence of tuberculosis (TB), the leading cause of death in the United States at that time. In 1890, nearly one out of every four dwellings in New York City experienced a TB-related death. The toll was much higher in poorer neighborhoods, leaving these communities devastated by the disease.[26]

As in Britain, public health activities in the United States were greatly influenced by the growing urbanization and industrialization of the 1800s. Early health reformers in the United States, including Lemuel Shattuck of Boston, identified environmental improvement to prevent epidemic disease as a moral mission.[32] Shattuck was the foremost American advocate for community action in the area of environmental health. In the report, Census of Boston, Shattuck reported on high mortality rates, including maternal and infant mortality rates, and the prevalence of communicable diseases.[33] He described these findings as directly related to living conditions and low income. In 1850, Shattuck published *General Plan for the Promotion of Public and Personal Health*, describing health and social conditions in Massachusetts and extolling the sanitary movements taking place in Britain and Europe.[33] Sewage, refuse, and waste disposal and drainage were identified as priority public health measures; of these, sewage disposal was considered the most important.[34]

C. E. A. Winslow characterized **sanitation**, ensuring healthful environmental conditions, as the first stage in public health. He stated:

> To a large section of the public, I fear that the health authorities are still best known as the people to whom one complains of unpleasant accumulations of rubbish in the backyard of a neighbor, accumulations which possess such offensive characteristics which somehow can only originate in a neighbor's yard and never in one's own.[35, p. 5]

Early public health interventions in the United States, like those enacted in Europe and Great Britain, often required government authority to address environmental factors thought to be compromising the health of communities. Local public health agencies in the United States developed from the local boards of health dating to the 1700s.[36] Various claims have been made asserting community formation of the first board of health in the United States with Baltimore, Charleston, New York City, and Philadelphia all contending for the honor. New York City, for example, established a board of health in 1796, which consisted of three commissioners and a health officer. The term *health officer* designated the responsibilities of a quarantine officer. From 1832, repeated cholera epidemics stimulated the creation of boards of health in the eastern United States, and port cities instituted a 40-day quarantine of ships entering harbors.[27] In his 1850 report, Shattuck emphasized the importance of government involvement in public health when he recommended the establishment of a state health department and local boards of health in each town.[33] In 1865, the Association of New York issued a report, Sanitation of the City, pressuring New York (both the city and state) to organize a Metropolitan Board of Health the following year.[26] The report documented the intimate relationship between social and economic forces contributing to ill health. A newly organized New York City Department of Public Health followed, focusing on cleaning the streets, regulating sewage and waste disposal, and mandating tenement reforms.[26] It soon became a model that many other cities emulated.

Subsequent development of local health departments was sporadic until around 1910 when severe epidemics of typhoid fever occurred in a number of cities. In response, the federal government recommended the establishment of full-time local health departments throughout the United States. In the meantime, the New York City Health Department continued to address environmental concerns during the 1900s. In a 1912 annual report, the health department described the removal of 20,000 dead horses, mules, donkeys, and cattle from the streets of New York in addition to nearly half a million smaller animals such as pigs, hogs, calves, and sheep. In total, the disposal of more than 5 million pounds of spoiled poultry, fish, pork, and beef was accomplished. The report also noted that there were records of 343,000 complaints from the public with respect to poor ventilation, waste disposal, and unlicensed manure dumps.[26]

The development and spread of state health departments were similar to that of local health departments. The first state board of health was established by the Louisiana State Legislature in 1855 in response to yellow fever, but this proved not to be a functional organization. The first successful board of health was established in Massachusetts in 1869; it followed Shattuck's earlier recommendation.[22,33] Other states quickly followed: California (1870), Minnesota (1872), Virginia (1872), Michigan (1873), Maryland (1874), and Alabama (1875). By 1900, all but eight states had boards of health. With the formation of the New Mexico board of health in 1919, all states had boards of health.[22]

Public Health in the 20th Century

In the early part of the 1900s, the public health workforce had gained skills in understanding the impact of the environment on the community's health and was beginning to understand the relationship between bacteria and infectious diseases. An example of a city-wide public health effort pertaining to the control of influenza can be seen in **Exhibit 2.1**. Over the next several decades, public health realized tremendous gains with interventions such as improved sanitation, water purity, nutrition, control of infectious disease, and immunization.[37] This translated into major gains in health. Life expectancy increased by more than 30 years, and the quality of life remarkably improved. Much of the increase was experienced in the first 25 years of the century. For example, the death rate from all causes in New York City was 31 per 1,000 in 1825; this rate had dramatically fallen to 12 per 1,000 a century later in 1925. Similarly, in 1880, the

| Exhibit 2.1 | Early Influenza Warning |

INFLUENZA

FREQUENTLY COMPLICATED WITH

PNEUMONIA

IS PREVALENT AT THIS TIME THROUGHOUT AMERICA.

THIS THEATRE IS CO-OPERATING WITH THE DEPARTMENT OF HEALTH.

YOU MUST DO THE SAME

IF YOU HAVE A COLD AND ARE COUGHING AND SNEEZING. DO NOT ENTER THIS THEATRE

GO HOME AND GO TO BED UNTIL YOU ARE WELL

Coughing, Sneezing or Spitting Will Not Be Permitted In The Theatre. In case you must cough or Sneeze, do so in your own handkerchief, and if the Coughing or Sneezing Persists Leave The Theatre At Once.

This Theatre has agreed to co-operate with the Department Of Health in disseminating the truth about Influenza. and thus serve a great educational purpose.

HELP US TO KEEP CHICAGO THE HEALTHIEST CITY IN THE WORLD

JOHN DILL ROBERTSON

COMMISSIONER OF HEALTH

Source: Reproduced from National Library of Medicine. Office of Public Health Historian.

average life expectancy in New York City and Brooklyn was 36 years; by 1920, life expectancy had increased to 53 years, an increase of 47% in a 40-year period.[38] As exclaimed by Winslow and others, public health activities were responsible for reducing environmental and infectious disease threats and that such "achievements were almost wholly based on the organized application of the sciences of sanitary engineering and bacteriology."[38, p. 1079]

Attempts to replicate the successes achieved with infectious and environmentally related diseases have been extended to the contemporary health challenges of obesity, diabetes, injury prevention, violence, substance abuse, HIV infection, tobacco-related diseases, and other noncommunicable diseases. As early as 1926, Winslow argued early for this extension in a speech delivered before the American Public Health Association in Buffalo, New York:

> We may . . . say that the health officer should concern himself only with communicable disease. Or we may say that the field of the health department includes all the health problems of the infant and the child plus the communicable diseases of the adult. This is a second clear and defensible position and one that approximates current-day practice. Or we may take a still wider view and envisage the whole field of the prevention of disease and the promotion of physical and mental health and efficiency.[38, p. 1080]

As Americans began to live longer, the impact of injuries and noncommunicable diseases and the potential for prevention of these health threats became a priority for public health professionals, with positive outcomes including a substantial decrease in cigarette smoking, declines in the rates of heart disease mortality and motor vehicle–associated fatalities, and improved quality of the workplace.[39] While King James I of England had written and published an anti-smoking treatise in 1604, titled *A Counterblaste to Tobacco*, certainly the first public health document on smoking to be promoted by a national leader, in 1966 the United States enacted legislation to require warning labels on cigarette packages. This effort to address one of the world's greatest noncommunicable public health problems was further advanced by the U.S. Surgeon General, C. Everet Koop who advocated for a smoke-free America by the year 2000 and began the practice of rotating messages on warning labels, as shown in **Exhibit 2.2**.

The 10 great public health achievements in the United States in the 1900s include advances in both communicable and chronic disease prevention, as listed in **Exhibit 2.3**.

The public may not recognize many of these gains because it has become accustomed to the accrual of long-standing benefits from communal efforts to protect against hazards to health. Quentin Young, former president of the American Public Health Association, remarked: "Turning on any kitchen faucet for a glass of drinking water without hesitation or peril is a silent homage to public health success, which would not have been possible at the start of the twentieth century."[40, p. 1]

It is ironic that the very accomplishments in population-based prevention have probably resulted in decreased visibility for public health activities in our communities. When these protective activities work well, illnesses from water, food, and environmental toxins do not occur. In the absence of clearly visible problems, the public knows little about the methods of assurance, and, historically, collective support for public health resources and programs has been nominal.

One of the biggest public health challenges that emerged toward the end of the 20th century was HIV/AIDS. Since first being reported in the Unites States in 1981, more than 600,000 men, women, and children have died as a result of HIV disease, and, globally, according to UNAIDS, the estimate of HIV-related deaths is 30 million. Many public health interventions have been used over the decades since 1981, and there has been considerable success in slowing the spread of HIV in the general population and major advances in treating the associated

---

Exhibit 2.2   Surgeon General's Warning

SURGEON GENERAL'S WARNING:
Smoking Causes Lung Cancer,
Heart Disease, Emphysema, And
May Complicate Pregnancy.

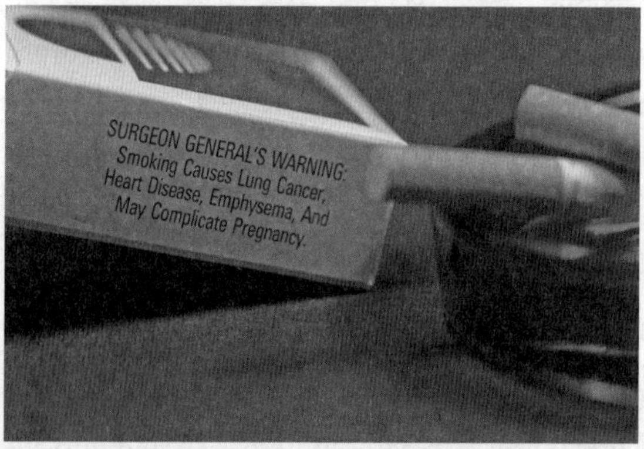

Source: CDC/Debora Cartagena.

Exhibit 2.3   Ten Great Public Health Achievements

1. Vaccines: Few treatments were effective in the prevention of infectious diseases in 1900. Now, smallpox, measles, diphtheria, pertussis, rabies, typhoid, cholera, and the plague are preventable through widespread use of vaccines.

2. Recognition of tobacco use as a health hazard: Since the 1964 surgeon general's report on risks associated with smoking, smoking among adults has decreased, saving lives.

3. Motor vehicle safety: Improved engineering of vehicles and roads plus the use of seat belts, car seats, and helmets have reduced the number of deaths, as has decreased drinking and driving.

4. Safer workplaces: A 40% decrease in fatal occupational injuries (since 1980) has resulted through efforts to control work-related disease such as pneumoconiosis (black lung) and silicosis, which are associated with coal mining, and to improve safety in manufacturing, construction, transportation, and mining.

5. Control of infectious diseases: Efforts to protect the water supply and keep it clean with improved sanitation methods have greatly improved health, particularly curbing the spread of cholera and typhoid. The discovery of antimicrobial therapy has helped to control tuberculosis and sexually transmitted diseases (STDs).

6. Fewer deaths from heart disease and stroke: Smoking cessation, blood pressure control, early detection, and better treatments have resulted in a 51% decrease in death rates for coronary heart disease since 1972.

7. Safer and healthier foods: Major nutritional deficiency diseases such as rickets, goiter, and pellagra have been virtually eliminated in the United States through greater recognition of essential nutrients, increases in nutritional content, food fortification, and decreases in microbial contamination.

8. Healthier mothers and babies: Better hygiene, nutrition, access to health care, antibiotics, and technologic advances have helped to reduce infant mortality by 90% and maternal mortality by 99%.

9. Family planning and contraceptive services: These services have altered the social and economic roles of women. Access to counseling and screening has resulted in fewer infant, child, and maternal deaths. Contraceptives have provided protection from human immunodeficiency virus and other STDs.

10. Fluoridation of drinking water: Nearly 150 million people have access to treated water, a safe and effective way to prevent tooth decay. Fluoridation has helped reduce tooth decay in children 40–70% and tooth loss in adults 40–60%.

Source: Adapted from Centers for Disease Control and Prevention. Ten great public health achievements—United States, 1900–1999. *MMWR.* 1999;48(12):1–3.

diseases. Jones and Johnson have described a range of successful education and prevention programs and initiatives.[41] (Additionally, a timeline of AIDS developments and milestones was published on the 30th anniversary of the first cases identified in the United States, which can be viewed at http://aids.gov/hiv-aids-basics/hiv-aids-101/aids-timeline/.) The White House Office of National AIDS Policy has also identified strategies designed to reduce HIV-related disparities and health inequities. The Director of the Office of HIV/AIDS Policy commented:

> There is no doubt we have made substantial progress in confronting HIV/AIDS . . . but we continue to face challenges. Identifying effective prevention packages for at-risk populations and bringing them to scale, modifying health care and other systems so they can work efficiently across organizational boundaries, and altering the social determinants that impede individuals and communities from living healthy, disease-free lives.[42, p. 5]

Public Health in the 21st Century

From the early understanding of the importance of covering sewers in ancient India to the practice of isolation and quarantine in the Middle Ages to the recognition of poverty as a significant determinant of health in the 1800s to the increasing recognition of the impact of social, behavioral, and environmental determinants and of the need for evidence-based, systematic approaches to improve the public health in the 1900s along with meeting the ever-vexing challenge of HIV/AIDS, the field of public health is rapidly evolving. Despite this increasing recognition and the commensurate increase in the public's expectations of public health, the economic crisis of the first decade of the 21st century resulted in dramatic reductions in the public health workforce at federal, state, and local levels, threatening the successes in improving the public's health. In a May 2012 research brief, "Local Health Department Job Losses and Program Cuts," the National Association of County and City Health Officials estimated that more than 40,000 employees have lost their jobs in local public health since 2008.[43] When combined with cuts at state agencies, the total loss of public health jobs reached 55,000.[44] Concurrently, at the federal level, there has been an astounding 21.5% decrease in funding for the Centers for Disease Control and Prevention since 2009, with other federal agencies in the public health system experiencing similar cuts.[44]

In addition to the assault on the public health workforce and programs, another challenge facing public health administrators is evidence that gains made in life expectancy over the past 100 years are actually being reversed in certain demographics. In a 2012 publication, Olshansky identified that white men and women with fewer than 12 years of education had a shorter life expectancy in 2008 than they did in 1990. For example, the life expectancy of women with low educational achievement decreased by more than 5 years in this timeframe. Furthermore, the author describes widening disparities in life expectancy with highly educated white males now living more than 14 years longer than black males with fewer than 12 years of education.[45] Low educational achievement is a leading determinant of poor health outcomes for numerous reasons, including, but not limited to, increased prevalence of behaviors (e.g., tobacco use, poor nutrition, low physical activity) associated with chronic diseases, decreased effectiveness and fewer resources to manage such diseases, and less access to health care and related services.

A third challenge for public health administrators is that even in the face of fewer resources for public health, there are greater expectations for the discipline. The public understandably expects that public health will not only address the widening disparities and the impact of chronic and emerging diseases but that it will also play a prominent role in understanding and mitigating the impact of natural and man-made disasters including, among others, the effects of climate change.

Despite these daunting challenges, there are many reasons to be optimistic about the future of public health in the United States in the 21st century. All of the work of generations of public health leaders has led to a much better understanding of the determinants of health and opportunities for impact (Thomas Frieden's "Health Impact Pyramid," see **Figure 2.1**),[46] a potentially important role for public health in the field of genomics, exciting new information technology advances that may dramatically change public health surveillance and evaluation, new openings

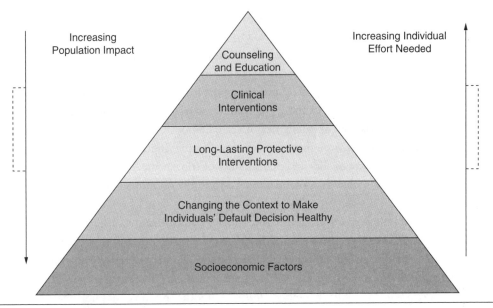

Figure 2.1   Health Impact Pyramid
Source: Reproduced from Figure 1, "State Legislative and Regulatory Action to Prevent Obesity and Improve Nutrition and Physical Activity." Published by the National Center for Chronic Disease Prevention and Health Promotion, Division of Nutrition, Physical Activity & Obesity.

with social media to effect behavioral change, a greater appreciation for the importance of evidence-based public health and public health systems research, and a new emphasis on accreditation and quality improvement. These are just some of the factors that show promise for the field.

A recent series of reports by the Institute of Medicine, "For the Public's Health," provides a roadmap for future public health efforts. The first in the series, "The Role of Measurement in Action and Accountability"[47] addresses the need to improve data collection and analysis and communication of information about health outcomes and of social, economic, and environmental determinants of health. Furthermore, it calls for a "cohesive national strategy" and a "measurement framework that provides the clear accountability needed to enable communities and policy makers to understand, monitor, and improve the contributions of various partners in the health system."[47]

The brief on the second report, "Revitalizing Law and Policy to Meet New Challenges," begins with, "Good health is not merely the result of good medical care but the result of what we do as a society to create the conditions in which people can be healthy."[3] This report proposes to create such conditions by modernizing laws and policies, improving use of legal and policy tools, and being more proactive by challenging all public health partners to "explore and implement '*health in all policies*' (HIAP)."[48] The third and final report, "Investing in a Healthier Future" addresses the problems that currently exist with funding of public health efforts in the United States, the disconnect between the level of funding and the scope of the mission for public health, and the need for significantly increased investment in public health. Collectively, this series provides guidance that has the potential to significantly improve the public's health in the 21st century.[49] One of the reports includes a recommendation to "ensure that all public health agencies have the mandate and the capacity to effectively deliver the Ten Essential Public Health Services."[48, p. 5] Furthermore, in a great show of support for the move toward standardization in public health practice across the country, the committee recommended that "states revise their laws to *require* [emphasis added] public health accreditation for state and local health departments."[48, p. 6] Accreditation, through its emphasis on "improving and protecting the health of the public by advancing the quality and performance of tribal, state, local, and territorial public health departments," truly has the potential to transform the traditional public health system in the 21st century.

To fully realize improvement in health outcomes at both the individual and population levels, however, public health and the clinical healthcare delivery system must work in concert to improve health outcomes. Successful integration of the two disciplines has not yet occurred. The 2012 publication of the Institute of Medicine's report on *Primary Care and Public Health: Exploring Integration to Improve Population Health*[50] is another resource for public health administrators and as such, has the potential to galvanize the relationship between these currently distinct systems.

While all of the described advances and reports will contribute to a healthier nation in the 21st century, President Barack Obama's signing of the **Patient Protection and Affordable Care Act (ACA)** in 2010 has arguably the greatest potential to improve the public's health. The Supreme Court's June 2012 decision about the Act and President Obama's reelection in November 2012 ensured that healthcare delivery and public health in the United States have forever changed.

It is widely accepted that the ACA will result in increased access to health insurance, however, many of the other provisions in the ACA are less well understood. The National Association of County and City Health Officials (NACCHO) has an excellent overview of the "Public Health and Prevention Provisions of the Affordable Care Act."[51] **Box 2.1** provides descriptions of selected funded provisions detailed in the report:

While the provisions listed in Box 2.1 will not result in restoration of the public health workforce that was lost in the economic downturn at the beginning of the century, the scope of the provisions and their potential to significantly impact the public's health are exciting. For example, in 2011, Community Transformation Grants were awarded to 61 state and local government agencies, tribes and territories, and nonprofit organizations in 36 states, in addition to 6 national networks of community-based organizations, potentially impacting 120 million people.[52] In 2012, another 40 grants were awarded to smaller communities, potentially impacting an additional 9 million people. Another example of how the ACA has already impacted public health is the June 2012 publication of the National Prevention Council Action Plan. This plan provides specific plans federal agencies are currently implementing "to move America from a system of sick care to one based on wellness and prevention."[53] While there is an overall vision for the plan (see **Figure 2.2**) the action plan provides specific details about what agencies will be doing. One example of a project highlight in the report is Promise Neighborhoods,

---

Box 2.1   Affordable Care Act Public Health Elements

- Investments in public health and prevention:
  - Prevention and Public Health Fund (PPHF): Provides the greatest amount of funding for public health initiatives including Community Transformation Grants; Epidemiology and Lab Capacity Grants; National Public Health Improvement Initiatives; and National Diabetes Prevention Programs
  - National Prevention, Health Promotion, and Public Health Council: Establishes a council to coordinate and lead federal government's prevention, wellness, and health-promotion efforts
  - Maternal, Infant, and Early Childhood Home Visitation Programs: Authorizes funds for evidence-based home visitation programs for this target population
- Public health workforce:
  - Fellowship Training in Public Health (partially funded by PPHF)
  - Public Health and Preventive Medicine Programs (partially funded by PPHF)
- Expansion of coverage, awareness, and access to clinical preventive services:
  - Contains numerous provisions to improve insurance coverage of family planning services and U.S. Preventive Services Task Force (USPSTF)–recommended services, in addition to many areas of expanded coverage under Medicare and Medicaid specifically
  - Authorizes funding for Personal Responsibility Education (adolescent abstinence, contraception, and prevention of sexually transmitted infections), Pregnancy Assistance Fund (support of victims of domestic violence and sexual assault), school-based health centers, and oral health activities
  - Provides recommendations with respect to the USPSTF and the Community Preventive Service Task Force (Community Guide) with funding from PPHF
- Wellness programs:
  - Authorizes grants to small businesses to provide comprehensive workplace wellness programs
  - Requires the Centers for Disease Control and Prevention (CDC) to provide employers with assistance to evaluate worksite wellness programs
- Public health research and data:
  - Directs the CDC to fund research on effectiveness of evidence-based practices that relate to public health initiatives
  - Authorizes funds for a childhood obesity demonstration project through the Centers for Medicare and Medicaid Services (CMS)
- Other:
  - Requires the U.S. Department of Health and Human Services (HHS) to develop a national quality improvement plan
  - Requires nutrition labeling at restaurants with more than 20 locations

Source: Adapted from NACCHO. Public Health and Prevention Provisions of the Affordable Care Act. Available at: http://www.naccho.org/advocacy/upload/PH-and-Prevention-Provisions-in-the-ACA-Revised.pdf. Accessed February 8, 2013.

---

a collaboration among the White House, DHHS, and the Departments of Education (ED), Housing and Urban Development, Justice, and the Treasury that:

> aims to transform high-poverty neighborhoods. Led by ED, Promise Neighborhoods aims to address significant challenges faced by students and families living in distressed communities by providing resources to plan and implement a continuum of services from early learning to college and career with the goal of improving educational and developmental outcomes for children and youth.[8, p. 23]

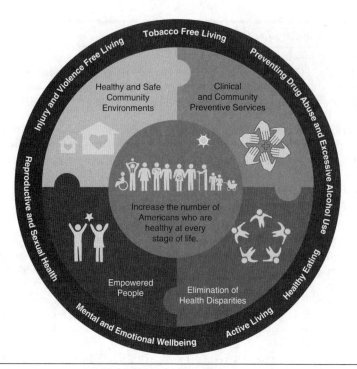

Figure 2.2   National Prevention Council Action Plan
Source: Reproduced from National Prevention Council. National Prevention Council Action Plan
2012. Available at: http://www.healthcare.gov/prevention/nphpphc/2012-npc-action-plan.pdf.
Accessed December 4, 2012.

As stated by James A. Johnson, coeditor of this text, "Public health policy in the twenty-first
century is still emerging, but many of the older themes of democracy, federalism, social justice,
human rights, and dignity continue to provide a link to the Nation's founding principles."[54]
Yet, the 21st century promises to be a uniquely challenging time for public health with fewer
resources and greater expectations in a rapidly transforming healthcare and public health system. However, a new political mandate and new standards for evidence-based public health, in
addition to an energizing emphasis on quality improvement and accreditation, set the stage for
public health to achieve tremendous gains.

Discussion Questions

1. Identify 10 milestones in the evolution of public health and discuss each one.
2. Describe the focus of the various Institute of Medicine reports discussed in this chapter.
3. How does public health align with the nation's founding principles?
4. Describe the public health elements of the Affordable Care Act.

5. As a future public health administrator, why do you feel it is important to know the history presented in this chapter? What are some emerging challenges that you might face in your public health role?

6. As a cross-disciplinary exercise, choose an event you studied in one of your history classes and revisit it from a public health perspective. What did you learn?

References

1. Rosen G. *A History of Public Health, Expanded Edition.* Baltimore, MD: The Johns Hopkins University Press; 1993.
2. Porter D. *Health, Civilization and the State: A History of Public Health from Ancient to Modern Times.* New York: Routledge; 1999.
3. Cohen MN. *Health and the Rise of Civilization.* New Haven: Yale University Press; 1989.
4. McKeown T. *The Origin of Human Disease.* Oxford: Basil Blackwell; 1988.
5. Cockburn A. Where did our infectious diseases come from? The evolution of infectious diseases, *CIBA Foundation Symposium.* 1977;49:103–112.
6. McNeill W. *Plagues and Peoples.* New York: Anchor Press/Doubleday; 1976.
7. Lloyd GER. *Magic, Reason and Experience.* Cambridge: Cambridge University Press; 1979.
8. Whitney J. *Healing and Resonance in Ancient Egypt.* London: Open Door; 1996.
9. Risse G. Imhotep and medicine: A re-evaluation. *Western Journal of Medicine.* 1986;144:622–4.
10. Preuss J. *Biblical and Talmudic Medicine.* New York: Sanhedrin Press; 1978.
11. Garrison FH. *An Introduction to the History of Medicine.* 4th ed. Philadelphia: W. B. Saunders; 1929.
12. Smith WD. *The Hippocratic Tradition.* Ithaca, NY: Cornell University Press; 1979.
13. Bruun C. *The Water Supply of Ancient Rome. A Study of Roman Imperial Administration.* Helsinki: Societas Scientiarium Fennica; 1991.
14. Robinson OF. *Ancient Rome City Planning and Administration.* London: Routledge; 1992.
15. Nutton V. Continuity or rediscovery? The city physician in classical antiquity and medieval Italy. In: Russell AW. ed., *The Town and State Physician in Europe.* Wolfenbüttel, Germany: Herzong August Bibliothek; 1981.
16. Davies RW. In: Breeze D, Maxfield VA, eds., *Service in the Roman Army.* Edinburgh: Edinburgh University Press; 1989.
17. Rosen G. *A History of Public Health.* New York: MD Publications; 1958.
18. Palmer R. *The Control of Plague in Venice and Northern Italy, 1348–1600.* PhD. thesis, University of Kent; 1978.
19. Bynum W, Porter R. *Living and Dying in London.* London: Wellcome Institute for the History of Medicine; 1991.
20. Affi A, Breslow L. A maturing paradigm of public health. *Annu Rev Public Health.* 1994;15:223–35.
21. Duffy J. *A History of Public Health in New York City, 1866–1966.* New York: Russell Sage Foundation; 1968.
22. Smillie W. *Public Health: Its Promise for the Future.* New York: The Macmillan Co; 1955.
23. Kottek S. Gems from the Talmud: public health I—water supply. *Isr J Med Sci.* 1995;31:255–6.
24. Ashton J, Sram I. Millennium report to Sir Edwin Chadwick. *BMJ.* 1998;317:592–6.
25. Fee E. Public health and the state: the United States. *Clio Medica.* 1994;26:224–75.
26. Rosner D. *Hives of Sickness.* New Brunswick, NJ: Rutgers University Press; 1995.
27. Fee E. The origins and development of public health in the United States. In: Holland WW, Detels R, Knox G, et al., eds. *Oxford Textbook of Public Health.* 2nd ed. Oxford, UK: Oxford University Press; 1991:3–21.
28. Byrne JP, ed. *Encyclopedia of Pestilence, Pandemics, and Plagues* (Vol. 1). Westport, CT: Greenwood Press; 2008.

29. Duffy J. *Epidemics in Colonial America*. Baton Rouge, LA: Louisiana State University Press; 1953.

30. Benenson A, ed. *Control of Communicable Diseases in Man*. Washington, DC: American Public Health Association; 1990.

31. Ellis J. Businessmen and public health in the urban south during the nineteenth century: New Orleans, Memphis, and Atlanta. *Bull Hist Med*. 1970;44(4):346–71.

32. Porter E. The history of public health and the modern state, introduction [editorial]. *Clio Medica*. 1994;26:1–44.

33. Shattuck L. *General Plan for the Promotion of Public and Personal Health*. Boston: Dutton & Wentworth, State Printers; 1850.

34. Kramer H. Agitation for public health reform in the 1870s. *J Hist Med Allied Sci*. 1948;III(4):473–88.

35. Winslow CEA. *The Untilled Fields of Public Health*. New York: Health Service, New York County Chapter of the American Red Cross; 1920.

36. Jeckel J. Health departments in the US 1920–1988: statements of mission with special reference to the role of C.E.A. Winslow. *Yale J Biol Med*. 1991;64:467–79.

37. Kivlahan C. Public health in the next century. *Mo Med*. 1994;91(1):19–23.

38. Winslow C. Public health at the crossroads. *Am J Public Health*. 1926;16:1075–85.

39. U.S. Department of Health and Human Services, Public Health Service. *For a Healthy Nation: Returns on Investment in Public Health. Executive Summary*. Washington, DC: US Government Printing Office; 1994.

40. Young Q. Public health: a powerful guide. *J Health Care Finance*. 1998;25(1):1–4.

41. Jones W, Johnson J. *AIDS Programs and Initiatives in Education and Prevention*. Freeman, SD: Pine Hill Press; 1994

42. Valdiserri R. Thirty years of AIDS in America: a story of infinite hope. *AIDS Education and Prevention*. 2011;23(6):479–94.

43. NACCHO. Local health department job losses and program cuts: findings from the January 2012 Survey. Available at: http://www.naccho.org/topics/infrastructure/lhdbudget/upload/Research-Brief-Final.pdf. Accessed December 3, 2012.

44. Jarris P. Challenging times for the government public health enterprise. *J Public Health Management Practice*. 2012;18(4):372–4.

45. Olshansky S, Antonucci T, Berkman L, et al. Differences in life expectancy due to race and educational differences are widening, and may not catch up. *Health Affairs*. 2012;31(8):1803–13.

46. Frieden TR. A framework for public health action: the health impact pyramid. *Am J Public Health*. 2010;100(4):590–5.

47. Institute of Medicine. *For the Public's Health: The Role of Measurement in Action and Accountability*. Washington, DC: National Academy of Sciences; 2010.

48. Institute of Medicine. *For the Public's Health: Revitalizing Law and Policy to Meet New Challenges*. Washington, DC: National Academy of Sciences; 2011.

49. Institute of Medicine. *For the Public's Health: Investing in a Healthier Future*. Washington, DC: National Academy of Sciences; 2012.

50. Institute of Medicine. *Primary Care and Public Health: Exploring Integration to Improve Population Health*. Washington, DC: National Academy of Sciences; 2012.

51. NACCHO. Public Health and Prevention Provisions of the Affordable Care Act. Available at: http://www.naccho.org/advocacy/upload/PH-and-Prevention-Provisions-in-the-ACA-Revised.pdf. Accessed November 29, 2012.

52. Centers for Disease Control and Prevention. Community Transformation Grants. Available at: http://www.cdc.gov/communitytransformation/. Accessed December 4, 2012.

53. National Prevention Council. National Prevention Council Action Plan. June 2012. Available at: http://www.healthcare.gov/prevention/nphpphc/2012-npc-action-plan.pdf. Accessed December 4, 2012.

54. Johnson J. *Introduction to Public Health Management, Organizations, and Policy*. Clifton Park, NY: Delmar-Cengage; 2013.

Additional Resources

Institute of Medicine. *The Future of Public Health*. Washington, DC: National Academies Press; 1988.

Bunker J. Improving health: measuring effects of medical care. *Milbank Q. 1994*;72:225–258.

Cameron GO. *A Treatise on the Cannon of Avicenna, Incorporating a Translation of the First Book*. London: Luzac; 1930.

Siraisi NG. *Avicena in Renaissance Italy. The Canon and Medical Teaching in Italian Universities after 1500*. Princeton: Princeton University Press; 1987.

Amundsen DW. Medicine and surgery as art or craft: the role of schematic literature in the separation of medicine and surgery in the late Middle Ages. *Trans Stud Coll Physicians Phila*. 1979;1:43–57.

Allbutt CT. *The Relations of Medicine and Surgery to the End of the Sixteenth Century*. London: Macmillan; 1905.

Brody SN. *The Disease of the Soul: Leprosy in Medieval Literature*. Ithaca: Cornell University Press; 1974.

Gilman S. *Disease and Representation: Images of Illness from Madness to AIDS*. Ithaca: Cornell University Press; 1988.

Pelling M. Contagion, Germ Theory/Specificity. In: Bynum WF, Porter R. eds. *Companion Encyclopedia of the History of Medicine, 2 vols*. London: Routledge; 1993: 309–334.

The Iliad of Homer. Translated by Alexander Pope. Connecticut: Easton Press; 1998.

At the Gates: Our Safety Depends Upon Official Vigilance. Wood engraving from Harper's Weekly 29 (September 5, 1885); 592. In: George R. *A History of Public Health*; 1993.

Public Health and Social Determinants of Health

Leiyu Shi

LEARNING OBJECTIVES

- To define such key terms as population health, public health, social determinants of health, and public policy
- To assess the impact of public health on population health
- To understand the relationship between public health and social determinants of health
- To enumerate instances where public health influences social determinants of health
- To describe the relationship between public health and public policy
- To appreciate the *Healthy People* initiative
- To discuss the challenges facing the U.S. public health system infrastructure

---

Introduction

The growing importance of public health is evidenced by its expanding responsibilities. Public health has been known for its contribution to the reduction and control of infectious diseases through such efforts as increasing environmental sanitation (by securing safe air and water), advocating for hygienic practices (such as food pasteurization and sterile surgery), spurring the elimination of smallpox and polio (through immunization), and reducing overcrowding (through birth control methods). Now, as chronic diseases replace infectious diseases as the leading causes of death, public health must shift its focus toward health-promotion programs focused on lifestyle changes in diet, tobacco, and exercise to prevent contemporary health threats, including cardiovascular disease, type 2 diabetes, and obesity. In recent years, as a result of a series of natural calamities such as Hurricanes Katrina and Rita and the spread of swine flu and West Nile virus and human-created disasters such as the possibility of terrorist attacks involving chemical, biological, radiological, or nuclear weapons, public health has again assumed center stage as it has been called upon to handle these emerging threats.

However, little is known about how the public health system can be organized to effectively and efficiently handle the modern-day threats of infectious and chronic diseases, and natural and human-created environmental disruptions. Moreover, public health remains a marginalized field in many countries' healthcare systems; the United States in particular has rarely used public policy to emphasize public health. Worldwide, there remains a deep lack of appreciation of what public health can accomplish toward improving population health.

Chapter Overview

This chapter addresses the relationships between public health and social determinants of health and public policy. Sorting out these relationships will help clarify the role of public health in improving population health and identify key determinants of public health system performance, including public policy. A broad understanding of these relationships will benefit priority setting in public health research and improve public health performance. The chapter is not intended to be a literature review. Rather, it serves to bring our attention to the importance of public health and the role public policy plays in advancing it.

This chapter is organized into two parts. In the first part, "The Relationship Between Public Health and Social Determinants of Health," we summarize the major contributions of public health to population health (including the role of public health entities as preventative agents of and responders to health threats). Then, we illustrate the pathways (aspects of social determinants) through which public health influences population health in order to highlight the major contributions of public health practice to population health. In the second part, "The Relationship Between Public Health and Public Policy," we summarize this relationship to point out the interconnectedness of these areas, while analyzing the deficiencies within the United States in this area.

The Relationship Between Public Health and Social Determinants of Health

When discussing the relationship between public health and the social determinants of health, a specialized vocabulary is often used. The key terms we use in our discussion are summarized in **Table 3.1**. These include population health, public health, social determinants of health, and public policy. Since the chapter will use these terms extensively, a clear understanding of their meanings is essential.

Table 3.1   Definitions of Key Terms Related to Public Health Systems Research

- **Population health** refers to the physical, mental, and social wellbeing of defined groups of individuals and the differences (disparities) in health between population groups.
- **Public health** reflects society's desire and specific efforts to improve the health and wellbeing of the total population, relying on the government, the private sector, and the public, and by focusing on the determinants of population health.
- **Social determinants of health** represent nonmedical factors that affect both the average and distribution of health within populations, including distal determinants (political, legal, institutional, and cultural factors) and proximal determinants (socioeconomic status, physical environment, living and working conditions, family and social network, lifestyle or behavior, and demographics).
- **Public policy** encompasses the intentional actions or inactions by government to address a problem affecting the public.

Figure 3.1 shows the relationship among public health, social determinants, and population health. As depicted in the figure, public health has both direct and indirect (through social determinants) impacts on population health. In this section, we summarize the major contributions of public health to population health and illustrate the pathways (i.e., aspects of social determination) for these accomplishments.

The Impact of Public Health on Population Health

At the turn of the new millennium, the Centers for Disease Control and Prevention (CDC) summarized 10 major achievements of public health in the United States since 1900.[1] Their list included:

- Vaccination, which has resulted in the control or eradication of smallpox, poliomyelitis, measles, rubella, tetanus, diphtheria, *Haemophilus influenzae* type b, and other infectious diseases
- Motor-vehicle safety (through safer vehicles and highways; use of safety belts, child safety seats, and motorcycle helmets; and decreased drinking and driving), which has resulted in significant reductions in motor vehicle–related deaths
- Safer workplaces (particularly in mining, manufacturing, construction, and transportation), which has resulted in significant reductions in fatal occupational injuries

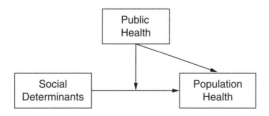

Figure 3.1   The Relationship Between Public Health, Social Determinants, and Population Health

- Control of infectious diseases (from clean water and improved sanitation, and antimicrobial therapy), which has resulted in the reduction of typhoid, cholera, tuberculosis, and sexually transmitted diseases
- Decline in deaths from coronary heart disease and stroke (through risk factor modification such as smoking cessation, blood pressure control, and early detection)
- Safer and healthier foods (from decreases in microbial contamination and increases in nutritional content), which has eliminated nutritional deficiency diseases such as rickets, goiter, and pellagra
- Healthier mothers and babies (through better hygiene and nutrition), which has resulted in significant infant and maternal mortality reductions
- Access to family planning and contraceptives, which has resulted in smaller family size, fewer infant, child, and maternal deaths, and fewer HIV and STDs
- Fluoridation of drinking water, which has reduced tooth decay and tooth loss
- Recognition of tobacco use as a health hazard, which has reduced smoking-related deaths

In 2011, the CDC updated the list to reflect the new "advances in public health during the first 10 years of the 21st century."[2] The list still includes several of the previous achievements, including the continued decline of vaccine-preventable diseases, the overall prevention and control of infectious disease, better maternal and infant health, improved motor vehicle safety, cardiovascular disease (CVD) prevention, and increased occupational safety. However, several new additions were also included:

- Tobacco control, which by 2009, had led to a large reduction in the number of adults and youths who smoke. The reduction in youth smoking between 1999 and 2009 was 15.3%. Additionally, 25 states had passed comprehensive smoking bans by 2010, whereas no state had implemented such policy as recently as 2000. The fight against tobacco continues with increasing cigarette excise taxes, stricter laws against youth access to tobacco, and new, graphic warning labels and anti-smoking campaigns.
- Cancer prevention, especially though the increased knowledge of and adherence to screening recommendations, plus simultaneous increases in testing quality. Cooperation among federal, state, and local actors, both public and private, has led to increased use of these services at lower costs to the patients, reducing disparities in screening rates and reducing cancer deaths in several notable categories (e.g., decreasing colorectal cancer mortality by approximately 2.7% per year, each year from 1998–2007).
- Childhood lead poisoning prevention, which has improved dramatically since the year 2000. As of 2012, 23 states have comprehensive preventive laws, whereas only five had such legislation in 1990. Today, high blood lead levels (> 10 micrograms/deciliter) are detected in only 0.9% of children age 1–5 years, a more than 85% reduction from the levels found in testing between 1976 and 1980, and the disparities felt by minority children have also been reduced.
- Public health preparedness and emergency response, which came to the forefront of public concern after the 9/11 terrorist attacks. This has led to an increased focus on preparation, such as improved performance by state-level public health laboratories, which has in turn improved responses to recent outbreaks of pathogens like H1N1 (i.e., "swine flu").

From these achievements, it is clear that the major contribution of public health has been to prolong life and improve its quality. In the 20th century, public health efforts resulted in the reduction and prevention of mortality due to infectious diseases, infant and maternal mortality, and accidents and injuries. Later, public health's focus shifted to the reduction of morbidity and mortality due to selected chronic diseases. The dramatic decline in mortality from infectious diseases took place between 1850 and 1950, as life expectancy at birth improved from about 40 to 68 years. Between 1950 and 2000, when chronic diseases replaced infectious diseases as the leading causes of death, life expectancy further improved from 68 to 77 years. Even from 1999–2009, "the age-adjusted death rate in the United States declined from 881.9 per 100,000 population to 741.0, a record low and a continuation of a steady downward trend that began during the last century."[2] Much of this decline can be contributed to improved public health.

Historically, the major public health strategy to control infectious diseases has been to improve the living environment through efforts such as ensuring the availability of clean water, nutritious food, adequate sewage disposal, and adequate housing with minimal crowding. The major public health strategies to lower infant and maternal mortality have included immunization, family planning, and provision of accessible pre- and postnatal care. The major public health strategy to reduce accidents and injuries has been legislation and regulations that reduce risks that contributed to occupational, home, and automobile injuries. The major public health strategy to contain chronic diseases has been the use of population-based prevention programs aimed at reducing individual risk through eliminating tobacco use, controlling blood pressure, reducing obesity and dietary fat, and adhering to preventive screening regimens. The next section illustrates how public health has influenced these social determinants of population health.

Public Health and Social Determinants of Population Health

As defined previously, social determinants represent nonmedical factors that affect both the average and distribution of health within populations. These determinants include the distal political, legal, institutional, and cultural factors that affect health, and the more proximate elements of socioeconomic status, physical environment, living and working conditions, family and social network, lifestyle or behavior, and demographics. In order to ultimately improve population health, public health interventions must take social determinants into consideration. In the sections that follow, we examine how these concepts have been applied in the United States.

Political Considerations

Political will is a key determinant of a nation's public health orientation, reflected in a nation's public policy regarding population health. As discussed in the next part on public policy, population health–oriented public policy is more prevalent in other industrialized countries than in the United States. In the United States, political and policy consideration of population health has taken place only in recent years, marked noticeably by the *Healthy People* (*2000*, *2010*, and *2020*) initiative which acknowledges that macro-level social and economic forces are at play in shaping population health and that a broader policy agenda is needed to successfully improve population health. However, strong political will remains lacking among elected officials and concrete policies have not been implemented.

Legal Considerations

Properly constructed, laws and regulations could have a positive impact on population health. Over the decades, there have been numerous instances where public health advocates have relied on laws and regulations to create conditions conducive to better health. For example, the formulation and enforcement of sanitation laws and regulations were critical in the reduction of agents causing infectious diseases. Through regulation, the Environmental Protection Agency (EPA) banned the addition of lead from gasoline in the mid-1970s, resulting in a significant decline in blood lead levels. Federal legislation such as requiring standard safety belts for all automobile occupants and the National Highway Traffic Safety Administration have been important in reducing motor vehicle injuries. Public health advocates have also worked with the school system to establish immunization standards that all school-age children must meet, thus increasing prevention and decreasing transmission of many childhood diseases. They have also worked with city councils to create ordinances regulating cigarettes sales to youth and to establish smoking bans in bars and restaurants. Overall, the legal system has been used effectively by public health advocates to improve population health, but more could certainly be done.

Institutional Considerations

Because of its multiple responsibilities, the public health system is complex and includes a wide variety of institutions. Although the U.S. Department of Health and Human Services (HHS) and the CDC are considered federal lead agencies on public health, charged with providing guidance to state and local health departments that carry out the essential public health services, many other agencies are also involved. For example, the U.S. Department of Agriculture plays a significant role in meat and poultry inspection, food safety (along with the Food and Drug Administration, or FDA), the school lunch program, and federal food stamp program. Other government involvement in public health includes: the U.S. Department of Labor (on occupational health and safety matters), the Department of Energy (on nuclear waste cleanup), the Environmental Protection Agency (EPA) (on water and air pollution), and the U.S. Department of Transportation (on highway safety). On the surface, these institutions appear to share a widespread agreement on the overall mission of public health. However, when it comes to action, there is a lack of consensus as to what constitutes necessary public health services and coordination both among and within agencies providing public health services. The results are that both the breadth and the depth of public health services vary widely from place to place and neither providers nor beneficiaries know what to expect.[3]

Cultural Considerations

The United States is a "melting pot" of differences, including populations from various cultural origins. Due to the society's dominant Western cultural values, some "non-Western-origin"/ minority persons or groups may face additional health risks that contribute to health disparities. Some issues in minority health include marginalization, stigmatization, loss or devaluation of language and culture, and lack of access to culturally appropriate health care and services. The public health community increasingly recognizes these barriers and has begun to incorporate cultural considerations in designing and delivering public health services. For example, the community health center program provides essential primary care services to vulnerable populations; today, most community health center patients have low incomes and are racial or ethnic minorities. This may be due, at least in part, to the community health centers' emphasis on cultural and linguistic competency in rendering essential primary healthcare services.

Socioeconomic Status Considerations

An unfortunate truth in the United States, and in nearly every developed country in the world, is that individuals with the greatest financial resources also have the best health. Although socioeconomic status (SES) has perhaps the greatest impact on population health, in the United States there has been very limited public health effort that focuses on improving SES among the general population and reducing SES disparities in particular. For example, among racial and ethnic groups, in 2010, the median household income of Asians and whites reached $64,308 and $51,846 respectively, compared to $37,759 and $32,068 for Hispanic and black households.[4] In 2010, 27.4% of blacks and 26.6% of Hispanics were living in poverty, compared to only 13.0% of whites. Likewise, educational attainment is not equally distributed across racial/ethnic groups. In 2010, 5.1% of whites and 2.8% of Asian Americans dropped out of high school, but 9.1% of blacks and 16.3% of Hispanics had done so.[5] Even greater disparities exist in college education, with rates of bachelor's degree or higher completion ranging from 56% for Asian Americans and 39% for whites, to 20% for blacks and 13% for Hispanics.[5] As with income and education, there are differences in unemployment rates across racial/ethnic groups. In general, minorities have higher rates of unemployment than whites, and these disparities have remained relatively consistent over the years. In 2010, in the recession, the rate of unemployment was 16.0% for blacks, 12.5% for Hispanics, and only 8.7% for whites.[6]

Physical Environment and Living Condition Considerations

One of the major achievements of public health is our ability to prevent or control disease and death resulting from interactions between people and their environment. The sanitary revolution launched in the 1850s addressed overcrowded housing, inadequate sewage and solid waste disposal, lack of safe water, and insufficient and unsafe food. These factors directly led to high total and infant mortality and contributed to infectious diseases. Specific public health interventions included housing improvement, sewage system construction, garbage collection, chlorinated water supply, pasteurized milk, and access to vaccines and antitoxins. Environmental intervention has hugely contributed to the control of infectious diseases, leading to their significant reduction in the United States. Today, public health professionals at all levels are continually working on such environmental issues as indoor and outdoor air quality (and thus addressing related health issues such as asthma, allergies, carbon monoxide poisoning, chronic obstructive pulmonary disease, tobacco/smoking, asbestos, and mold), bioterror agents, chemical agents, environmental hazards and exposure, food safety, hazardous substances, hazardous waste sites, herbicides, hydrocarbons, lead, natural disasters, pesticides, smoking and tobacco use, urban planning for healthy places, vessel sanitation and health, and water quality.

Working Condition Considerations

Not only is unemployment related to health, conditions at work (both physical and psychosocial) can also have a profound effect on people's health and wellbeing. The physical and psychosocial effects of work conditions on health are manifest in the National Institute for Occupational Safety and Health's (NIOSH) Worker Health Chartbook.[7] The NIOSH chartbook presents data on workplace injury and illness caused by exposure to toxins and other sources of physical harm, but it also pays close attention to morbidity and mortality caused by work-induced anxiety, stress, and neurotic disorders. NIOSH found workers affected by anxiety, stress, and neurotic disorders experienced a much greater work loss (i.e., a median of 25 days away from work in 2001) than those with all nonfatal injuries or illnesses (i.e., a median of 6 days away from work in 2001). People who have more control over their work circumstances and fewer stressful job demands are healthier and often live longer than those in more tense or riskier work and activities. NIOSH interventions to reduce stress and increase safety and wellbeing in the workplace range from improving safety and evacuation training for coal miners to improving the ergonomics of the desks and computers of office workers.[8] Another recent public health campaign to improve workplace conditions has been the joint effort of federal and state governments and maternal and child health advocates to establish progressive breastfeeding policies for new mothers in the workforce.[9]

Family and Social Network Considerations

Support from family and other close relations is associated with better health. The caring and respect that occurs in familial relationships, and the resulting sense of satisfaction and wellbeing, seem to act as a buffer against health problems. Adequate family support can be very important in helping people solve problems and deal with adversity, as well as in maintaining a sense of mastery and control over life circumstances. On the other hand, intrapersonal violence has a devastating effect on the health of victims in both the short and long term. Women who are assaulted often suffer severe physical and psychological health problems. The importance of social support also extends to the broader community. **Civic vitality** refers to the strength of social networks within a community, region, province or country. It is reflected in the institutions, organizations, and informal social practices that people create to share resources and build attachments with others. In the United States, high levels of trust and group membership have been found to be associated with reduced mortality rates. Both family and community support can add resources to an individual's repertoire of strategies to cope with changes and can help foster better health. Recognizing the importance of family and community support in promoting health, the American Cancer Society sponsors several types of support groups for people with cancer and their families and friends.[10] Groups such as the Family Caregiver Alliance offer support for those caring for an ailing family member or friend. Caregivers often suffer an increased burden of stress and illness, but may benefit from support from other caregivers, their families, and their communities.[11] Some communities are mobilized to build coalitions that can change prevalent behaviors; for example, coalitions at the community level have changed local tolerance about underage drinking, especially when facilitated by adults, and campaigns have been organized in support of screening school-age children for vision and hearing issues.

Lifestyle or Behavior Considerations

Influencing the behavioral determinant of health has been another major achievement of public health. The risk-reduction campaign launched with the *Healthy People* initiative was in response to the growing burden of chronic diseases, which are now the leading causes of death, and their correlation with such behavioral risks as tobacco use, alcohol abuse, high-fat diets, and sedentary lifestyles. Specific public health interventions aim to affect lifestyle/behavioral changes, including smoking cessation, alcohol consumption reduction, drug control, and increasing the use of screening or preventive services. These ongoing interventions have been attributed to delaying the onset of disease, increasing the chances for early detection and treatment of disease, and prolonging life in the general population. As nutrition is a major modifiable determinant of chronic disease, public health professionals are working on strategies that reduce nutrition-related risk factors (e.g., high total blood cholesterol, high systolic blood pressure, high body mass index, and inadequate vegetable and fruit intake) and offer dietary adjustments that may reduce such diseases as cancer, cardiovascular disease, and diabetes.

Demographics Considerations

Demographic determinants of population health include consideration of individual biology, gender, age, and race/ethnicity. The basic biology and organic makeup of the human body are fundamental determinants of personal health. For example, genetic makeup appears to predispose certain individuals to particular diseases or health problems. Regarding gender, men are more likely to die prematurely than women, largely as a result of heart disease, fatal unintentional injuries, cancer, and suicide, but women are more likely to suffer depression, stress overload (often due to efforts to balance work and family life), chronic conditions such as arthritis and allergies, and injuries and death resulting from family violence. People of young or old age are particularly vulnerable to health risks. Infants and children who are neglected or abused are at higher risk for injuries; a number of behavioral, social, and cognitive problems later in life; and death. A low weight at birth is linked with problems not just during childhood, but also in adulthood. At the other end of the lifespan, the elderly experience greater chronic health problems and disabilities, and require significant monetary expenditures on health care. Public health interventions targeting special populations include the U.S. Department of Agriculture's Women, Infants, and Children (WIC) program, which provides nutritious foods, nutrition education and counseling, and screening and referrals to other health, welfare, and social services to low-income pregnant and postpartum women, infants, and children. Fifty-three percent of all infants born in the United States are served by WIC.[12] The federal government supports the health of the elderly population through its comprehensive Senior Citizens' Resources website, which includes links to numerous programs and resources to help seniors facing issues with health, housing, and end-of-life concerns.[13] Racial and ethnic minorities are another special population in the United States. Public health interventions targeting racial disparities in health include the CDC's Office of Minority Health and Health Equity, which aims to "eliminate health disparities for vulnerable populations as defined by race/ethnicity, socioeconomic status, geography, gender, age, disability status, risk status related to sex and gender, and among other populations identified to be at-risk for health disparities" through programs like Racial and

Ethnic Approaches to Community Health (REACH), which administers grants for innovative approaches designed to reduce disparities and a variety of training programs designed to increase the percentage of minority healthcare professionals.[14]

The Relationship Between Public Health and Public Policy

This section summarizes the relationship between public health and public policy. To illustrate, **Figure 3.2** presents a framework of the public health system (adapted from Handler et al. and described earlier).[15] The outcome or performance of the system can be measured in terms of effectiveness (e.g., improving population health status), efficiency (i.e., cost-beneficial), or ability to achieve equity (e.g., reducing disparities) among populations. As underlined, public policy, while acting as a distal component, exerts direct impact on both the configuration of the public health system and greatly influences health outcomes. Knowledge of the interconnections between public health performance and public policy will help guide future improvement and research directions.

Public Health System Performance and Public Policy

The development of public policy is influenced by the political, economic, and social environments within which governments and public health activities must operate. The interplay of policy with these environments dictates the type of health model espoused and the ensuing public policy that reflects these beliefs. If the dominant health model values an individualized approach and focuses on biological dispositions and the effects of risk factors, the ensuing public policy will likely direct efforts to managing risk factors and treating illness on an individual basis.

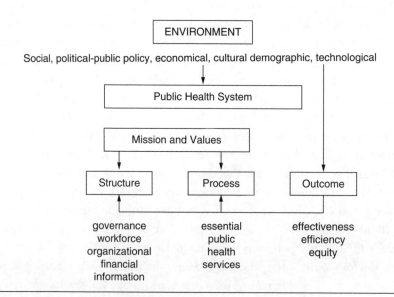

Figure 3.2   A Framework of Public Health System

If the dominant health model values a collective approach and focuses on structural factors such as organization of society and resource distribution, the corresponding public policy will likely be directed at the social determinants of health such as income, education, employment, housing, and healthcare services.

Among industrialized countries, the broad public policy goal of improving population health is quite common. In Europe, for example, many countries consider improving population health to depend on addressing "basic determinants" and root causes of socioeconomic inequities.[16] Sweden has perhaps the most comprehensive and upstream public policies related to population health. The National Institute of Public Health has the role of monitoring Sweden's national objectives for public health, designed to address the determinants deemed most important by the Swedish government. Examples of these objectives include: participation and influence in society, economic and social security, secure and favorable conditions during childhood and adolescence, healthier working life, healthy and safe environments and products, and health and medical care that more actively promote good health.[17] The overarching public policy aim is to create the conditions for good health on equal terms for the entire population.

Great Britain also follows a population-oriented public policy with the ultimate aim of improving the health and wellbeing of all people in England. The nation's top objectives of public health reflect this orientation: to lead sustained improvements in public health and wellbeing, with specific attention to the needs of disadvantaged and vulnerable people; to enhance the quality and safety of health and social care services, providing faster access and better patient and user choice and control; and to improve the capacity, capability, and efficiency of the health and social care system.[18]

Outside Europe, Canada has long embraced a population health perspective. This is evidenced in a series of noteworthy policy documents including the Lalonde report, which recognized the importance of social, political, and physical environments in improving population health;[19] the Ottawa Charter for Health Promotion, which focused on social and economic determinants of health such as income and education; and the report by the Federal, Provincial, and Territorial Advisory Committee on Population Health of 1974 that demonstrates a national commitment to population health and provides a framework to guide population health efforts. The public policy goal is to promote and protect the health of Canadians through leadership, partnership, innovation, and action in public health. Core values include leadership, healthy work environment, ethical behavior, commitment to excellence, and dedication to service.[20] Guided by these principles, the public health system's programs, services, and institutions emphasize the prevention of disease, the promotion of health, and the health needs of the population as a whole. The public health and healthcare systems share the same goal of maximizing the health of Canadians and work in conjunction, for it is just as critical to have a well functioning public health system as it is to have a strong healthcare delivery system. Furthermore, both systems must work well together to respond effectively to threats to the public's health.[21]

Current public health practice in Australia also reflects an upstream, population health–focused use of public policy. Basic to their current public health practice is the understanding that many of the determinants of health lie outside the healthcare system itself, requiring interdisciplinary approaches. There is also a commitment to meeting the health needs of the community through policy and programs that combine a "top-down" philosophy with a process that encourages community consultation and input.[22] Government plays an instrumental role in Australian public health. The national government is an important source of policy initiatives and funds a large portion of public health programs throughout the continent, operating through the Australian Health Protection Committee (AHPC) and the Australian Population Health Development Principal Committee (APHDPC). State government has typically been the main source of population-based preventive services and health service delivery. The resources available to governments in achieving public health objectives are considerable and include universities, nongovernment and community organizations, the workforce, and programs and institutions of the primary healthcare system.[22] Successful public health activities are carried out through multidisciplinary teams, often with highly specialized expertise, using the range of regulatory powers available to the states with cooperation of the national-level agencies.

The situation in the United States is an altogether different story. For the most part, the United States has not embraced the population health perspective. There is lack of a clear and consistent vision for government involvement in public health. Rather, health is narrowly seen as the absence of disease and illness and an individual-level responsibility. This is evidenced by the conspicuous lack of a coherent public policy that focuses on preventive population health. The United States spends the bulk of its resources on treating people who are already sick. Most developed countries have national health insurance programs run by the government and financed through general taxes. Almost all the citizens in such countries are entitled to receive healthcare services. Such is not the case in the United States, where not all Americans are automatically covered by health insurance, and many go uninsured for extended periods of time.

In the United States, the public sector assumes a secondary role in health care. The market-oriented economy in the United States attracts a variety of private entrepreneurs who are driven by the pursuit of profits in carrying out the key functions of healthcare delivery. There is little standardization in a system that is functionally fragmented. This system is not subject to long-range planning, direction, and coordination from a central agency or government. Due to this missing dimension of system-wide planning, direction, and coordination, there is duplication, overlap, inadequacy, inconsistency, and waste, which lead to a complex and inefficient system.

Some changes in public health policy have occurred with the advent of the *Healthy People* initiative. Since 1980, the Unites States has undertaken 10-year plans outlining certain key national health objectives to be accomplished during each period of time. These initiatives have focused on the integration of medical care with preventive services, health promotion, and education; integration of personal and community health care; and increased access to these integrated services. Accordingly, the objectives are developed by a consortium of national and state organizations under the leadership of the U.S. Surgeon General. The first of these programs, with objectives for 1990, provided national goals for reducing premature deaths and for preserving the independence of older adults. Next, *Healthy People 2000: National Health Promotion and Disease Prevention Objectives*, released in 1990, identified health improvement goals and objectives to be reached by the year 2000. As part of this process, standardized health status indicators (HSIs) were developed to facilitate the comparison of health status measures at national, state, and local levels over time. According to the final review published by the National Center for

Health Statistics, the major accomplishments of *Healthy People 2000* included surpassing the targets for reducing deaths from coronary heart disease and cancer; meeting the targets for incidence rates for AIDS and syphilis, mammography exams, violent deaths, and tobacco-related deaths; nearly meeting the targets for infant mortality and number of children with elevated levels of lead in blood; and making progress in reducing health disparities among special populations.[23]

Healthy People 2010: Understanding and Improving Health, launched in January 2000, continued in the earlier traditions as an instrument to improve the health of the American people in the first decade of the 21st century. However, the national objectives for *Healthy People 2010* were developed in a different context from their predecessors. Advanced preventive therapies, vaccines, and pharmaceuticals, and improved surveillance and data systems were widely available. Demographic changes in the United States had led to an older and more racially and ethnically diverse population. Global forces, such as fluctuating food supply, emerging infectious diseases, and environmental interdependence presented novel public health challenges. The objectives also defined new relationships between public health departments and healthcare delivery organizations.[24] *Healthy People 2010* specifically emphasized the role of community partners—such as businesses, local governments, and civic, professional, and religious organizations—as effective agents for improving health in their local communities.

Healthy People 2010 was designed to achieve two overarching goals: to increase quality and years of healthy life and to eliminate health disparities.[25] The first goal was to help individuals of all ages increase life expectancy and improve their quality of life. The second goal of *Healthy People 2010* was to eliminate health disparities among different segments of the population. These include differences that occur by gender, race or ethnicity, education, income, disability, living in rural localities, and sexual orientation.

Using data gathered through January 2005, the HHS released a midcourse review of progress toward achieving the *Healthy People 2010* goals, and the feedback from this review was used to fine-tune the objectives and strategies of the program. Regarding the first overarching goal (increase quality and years of healthy life), the final review reported that while life expectancy continues to increase, significant gender and racial/ethnic differences remain. In addition, the United States continues to have lower life expectancy than many other developed nations, even with these improvements. Two quality of life measures (i.e., expected years in good or better health and expected years free of activity limitations) improved slightly, while a third quality of life measure (i.e., expected years free of selected chronic diseases) declined slightly.[26]

With regard to the second overarching goal of *Healthy People 2010* (eliminate health disparities), the final review reported very little progress was made. While there were reductions in several health areas with disparities, there were increases in disparities in other health areas, and many more stayed fairly consistent. The final review noted that the lack of data on education, income, and other socioeconomic factors for many *Healthy People 2010* objectives has limited the capabilities to plan programs that are effective in reducing and eliminating disparities.[26]

One of the reasons for the slow progress in meeting these goals might be the lack of evidence-based strategies that improve population health, especially in a market-dominated society that still considers health and health care to be primarily individual responsibilities. Indeed, the

Healthy People initiatives are typically strong on goals and objectives but weak on solutions and strategies.

The current initiative, *Healthy People 2020*, was launched in December 2010. *Healthy People 2020* takes into account some of the achievements over the last decade, such as increased life expectancy and a decreased death rate from coronary heart disease and stroke, and identifies other areas for improvement over the next decade. *Healthy People 2020*'s objectives include: identifying nationwide health improvement priorities; increasing public awareness and under-standing of the determinants of health, disability, and disease; providing measurable objectives and goals that are applicable at all levels; engaging multiple sectors to take action to strengthen policies and improve practices that are driven by the best available evidence and knowledge; and identifying critical research, evaluation, and data collection methods. *Healthy People 2020* will measure progress through measures of general health status, health-related quality of life and wellbeing, determinants of health, and disparities.[27]

Public Health System Performance and Governance Structure

Although the HHS and CDC provide guidance and major funding to state (and sometimes local) health departments, the authority for public health matters constitutionally resides with state governments. State health departments craft policy and entrust the operational compo-nents to local health departments.

Based on a 2010 survey conducted by the Association of State and Territorial Health Officials (ASTHO), total per capita state health spending for 2009 was $98.[28] State health departments employ a total of 107,000 full-time equivalent (FTE) workers, with 27,778 employees working in local health departments and 17,333 working in regional or district offices.

At the state level, 55% of state public health agencies were free-standing, independent departments and 45% were part of an umbrella agency.[28] In terms of organizational control between state and local public health agencies, the decentralized configuration was most com-mon (54%), followed by mixed/shared (20%), and centralized (26%). The lead state health officer was appointed by the state governor in 63% of the states surveyed and by the secretary of health and human services 18% of the time; the appointed official reports directly to the governor in 53% of arrangements and the secretary of health and human services in 29% of arrangements. State public health agencies administer a huge variety of programs and initiatives (state health departments are responsible for 96% of Maternal, Infant, and Child Health services prenatal care, receive 94% of CDC preparedness grants, and collect 90% of the National Center for Health Statistics [NCHS] Vital Statistics). Eighty-four percent of departments have health disparities/minority health initiatives, 63% of states also report resource sharing with local pub-lic health departments.[28]

The National Association of County and City Health Officials (NACCHO) also conducted a survey in 2010 to determine the effect of local health organizations on public health. There were 2,565 local health departments in the country, with a median annual expenditure of $1.5 million, employing 160,000 FTE workers. The top programs and functions of local public health agencies included: adult immunization (92%); communicable disease epidemiology and surveillance (92%); child immunization (92%); tuberculosis screening (85%); food service inspection (78%); tobacco control (69%); WIC program (64%); septic tanks (64%); HIV/AIDS screening (62%); sexually transmitted disease (STD) screening (64%); obesity (55%); family planning (55%); early and periodic screening, diagnosis, and treatment (EPSDT, 40%); school health (38%); injury prevention (39%); prenatal care (30%); syndromic surveillance (45%); public water supply monitoring (35%); oral health (27%); home health (25%); hazardous materials handling and disposal (17%); comprehensive primary care (13%); and mental health services (10%).[29] While the goals of state and local public health agencies are broad and important to maintaining population health, there also exists a series of challenges facing the nation's public health system infrastructure.

Discrepancies Between Missions and Funding Level

In the wake of the 9/11 terrorist attacks and Hurricane Katrina, public health assumed the new responsibility of preparing for and responding to bioterrorism and natural disasters. At the same time, the original responsibilities of health protection, health promotion, and disease prevention remain. Meanwhile, population-based core public health activities such as disease monitoring, surveillance, outbreak investigation, and response receive little funding. Funding for public health remains dismally low at less than $150 per capita (less than 2.5% of the overall healthcare spending), causing severe resource constraints. In contrast, Canada spent 6.3% of its total health expenditure on public health in 2011, more than a percentage increase since 2005.[30] In the United States, public health is an undervalued sector: Little investment is made in technology, workforce training and recruitment, or facility construction or renovation.

Within the United States, spending on public health also varies widely across communities, raising concerns about how these differences may affect the availability of essential public health services. May and colleagues examined the association between public health spending and the performance of essential public health services and noted that performance of essential public health services is significantly associated with public health spending levels (particularly local funds), and that higher levels of spending could prevent more deaths.[31]

Categorical Funding

In addition to inadequate funding, the categorical nature of public health funding also presents a challenge. Public health funding is typically distributed through programs and must be spent in specific ways, thereby reducing flexibility and efficiency. Categorical funding at the federal and state levels may limit the ability of local agencies to maintain core public health infrastructure and activities that fall outside of these categories.

Lack of Leadership and Shared Vision

In the United States, there is no single entity that has overall authority and responsibility for creation, maintenance, and oversight of the nation's public health infrastructure. Policymakers across jurisdictions and levels of government have not developed a shared, realistic vision of what public health should accomplish and who in the public health hierarchy should be held accountable for achieving these results.

This is not the case in other industrialized countries. For example, in Sweden, the National Institute of Public Health has the role of monitoring Sweden's national objectives for public health activities, formulating interim targets, and developing indicators of how well objectives are being met.[17]

In Canada, the creation of the Public Health Agency of Canada (PHAC) marked the beginning of a new approach to federal leadership and collaboration with provinces and territories on efforts to renew the public health system in Canada and support a sustainable healthcare system. Focusing on more effective efforts to prevent chronic diseases and injuries, and respond to public health emergencies and infectious disease outbreaks, PHAC works closely with provinces and territories to keep Canadians healthy and help reduce pressures on the healthcare system.[20] PHAC serves as the nerve center for Canada's expertise and research in public health, effectively coordinating efforts with other partners to identify, reduce, and respond to public health risks and threats.[32]

Discrepancies Between Expanding Roles and Old Infrastructure

The organizational infrastructure that supports public health services is largely a remnant of the previous century when infectious diseases were the main target. Systematic failure of this infrastructure due to conflicting priorities, diffuse responsibilities, and inadequate resources are made readily apparent in numerous live tests of public health capabilities (such as Hurricane Katrina, the outbreak of severe acute respiratory syndrome [SARS], and the anthrax attacks). Even though recent preparedness funding may be used to update and strengthen certain aspects of public health infrastructure, the funding is widely believed to be inadequate. In addition to the expanded preparedness role, public health, especially at the local levels, is increasingly depended on as a medical service provider of last resort. The need to serve as a safety net for medical services otherwise unobtainable by some populations (particularly the medically disenfranchised) has been a major impediment to investing in a stronger public health protection role.

Structural Variability

There are significant variations in the structure of health departments across the country. The result of the current, decentralized system is a nationally fragmented public health enterprise characterized by diverse practices across about 3,000 local agencies charged with meeting varying missions under 50 state health departments. The absence of nationally consistent systems leads to profound operational disconnects between public health authorities and hampers public health efforts to coordinate among different responder sectors, especially during disasters that cross geopolitical borders.

Inadequate Workforce

The public health workforce is faced with a shortage and competence challenge. On the one hand, there is a shortage of public health workers. The ratio of public health workers to U.S. residents fell from 1:457 to 1:635 between 1970 and 2000.[33] A recent survey by ASTHO revealed a rapidly aging state agency workforce, high retirement eligibility rates, high vacancy rates, and high annual staff turnover rates.[34] The average tenure of a state health department's chief executive is 2 years. Nurses represent the largest professional group among public health workers, but they are rapidly retiring and already in short supply. Given the rising challenge of treating long-term chronic diseases and preparing for emerging threats, the decline in workforce represents a serious erosion of public health system capacity.

On the other hand, the current public health workforce may not have the competency to handle today's challenges that require new expertise for preparedness such as informatics, epidemiology, logistics, and risk communications.[34] Self-assessment of public health competency by public health workers consistently shows gaps between mastery and what is needed for effective practice. Only 44% of public health workers have had any formal, academic training in public health. Moreover, a sizable proportion of current public health workforce obtains higher paying positions in hospitals, private laboratories, industry, and academia. The graduates of schools and programs of public health tend to find employment in academic and research careers, rather than in relatively low-paying state and local public health agencies. The current compensation packages for public health cannot ensure the hiring of the brightest and best trained workforce.

Inconsistent Information Technology

Throughout the country, there is a lack of a comprehensive electronic health intelligence and information system, which would be necessary to detect unusual disease events, trace vulnerable populations, monitor cases of diseases, catalog adverse event reports, track the course of outbreaks, resupply critical resources, deploy personnel during an epidemic, and scrutinize spending. States also vary in their infrastructure for information and data systems.[33]

Future Outlook

This chapter summarizes current knowledge regarding the relationships between public health, social determinants of health, and public policy; identifies the priority areas for further research and knowledge development; and recommends a course of action to carry them out. The next step is for the public health practice and research community to deliberate and reach consensus on these and work out concrete plans to implement research. With public health gaining attention and importance, there is going to be increasing demand for public health research to guide the development of public health services and improvement of public health performance. A shared understanding on the priority research areas and strategies for implementing research is paramount to advancing the field of public health research.

Discussion Questions

1. Provide a critical assessment of the impact of public health on population health.
2. What is the relationship between public health and social determinants of health?
3. Provide examples to illustrate the influences of public health on the social determinants of health.

4. What is the relationship between public health and public policy?
5. What is the purpose of the *Healthy People* initiative? How does the *Healthy People* initiative advance population health and reduce health disparities?
6. What are the challenges facing the U.S. public health system infrastructure? How can these challenges be overcome?

References

1. Centers for Disease Control and Prevention. Ten great public health achievements—United States, 1900–1999. *MMWR.* 1999;281:1481.
2. Centers for Disease Control and Prevention. Ten great public health achievements—United States, 2001–2010. *MMWR.* 2011;60(19):619–23.
3. Lee PR, Estes CL. *The Nation's Health.* 6th ed. Sudbury, MA: Jones and Bartlett Publishers; 2003.
4. DeNavas-Walt C, Proctor BD, Smith JC, U.S. Census Bureau. *Current Population Reports: Income, Poverty, and Health Insurance Coverage in the United States: 2010.* Washington, DC: U.S. Government Printing Office; 2011.
5. Aud S, Hussar W, Johnson F, et al. *The Condition of Education 2012* (National Center for Education Statistics 2012-045). Washington, DC: U.S. Department of Education; 2012.
6. U.S. Census Bureau. *Labor Force, Employment, and Earnings: Unemployed Persons. Statistical Abstract of the United States: 2012.* Rockville, MD: U.S. Census Bureau; 2012.
7. National Institute for Occupational Safety and Health. Worker health chartbook, 2004. Available at: http://www.cdc.gov/niosh/docs/2004-146/pdfs/2004-146.pdf. Accessed February 7, 2013.
8. National Institute for Occupational Safety and Health. Safety and prevention. Available at: http://www.cdc.gov/niosh/topics/safety.html. Accessed February 8, 2013.
9. Shealy KR, Li R, Benton-Davis S, et al. *The CDC Guide to Breastfeeding Interventions.* Atlanta: U.S. Department of Health and Human Services, Centers for Disease Control and Prevention; 2005.
10. American Cancer Society. Find support programs and services in your area. Available at: http://www.cancer.org/Treatment/SupportProgramsServices/index. Accessed February 8, 2013.
11. Family Caregiver Alliance. A population at risk. Available at: http://caregiver.org/caregiver/jsp/content_node.jsp?nodeid=1822. Accessed February 8, 2013.
12. U.S. Department of Agriculture. WIC at a glance. Available at: http://www.fns.usda.gov/wic/aboutwic/wicataglance.htm. Accessed February 8, 2013.
13. U.S. Government. Senior citizens' resources. Available at: http://www.usa.gov/Topics/Seniors.shtml. Accessed February 8, 2013.
14. Office of Minority Health and Health Equity. Executive orders & initiatives. Available at: http://www.cdc.gov/minorityhealth/ExecutiveOrders.html. Accessed February 8, 2013.
15. Handler A, Issel M, Turnock B. A conceptual framework to measure performance of the public health system. *Am J Public Health.* 2001;91:1235–9.
16. World Health Organization Regional Office for Europe. *Health21: The health for all policy framework for the WHO European region.* Copenhagen: WHO regional office for Europe; 1999.
17. Swedish National Institute of Public Health. Public health policy—11 objectives. Available at: http://www.fhi.se/en/About-FHI/Public-health-policy/. Accessed February 8, 2013.
18. U.K. Department of Health. Public health. Available at: http://www.dh.gov.uk/health/category/policy-areas/public-health/. Accessed February 8, 2013.
19. Lalonde M. *A New Perspective on the Health of Canadians: A Working Document.* Ottawa: Minister of Supply and Services Canada; 1974.
20. Public Health Agency of Canada. About the agency. Available at: http://www.phac-aspc.gc.ca/about_apropos/index.html. Accessed February 8, 2013.
21. Institute of Population and Public Health. The future of public health in Canada: developing a public health system for the 21st century. Available at: http://www.cihr-irsc.gc.ca/e/19573.html. Accessed February 8, 2013.

22. National Public Health Partnership. Public health in Australia: the public health landscape. Available at: http://www.nphp.gov.au/publications/broch/contents.htm. Accessed February 8, 2013.

23. National Center for Health Statistics. *Healthy People 2000: Final Review*. Hyattsville, MD: Department of Health and Human Services; 2001.

24. Department of Health and Human Services. *Healthy People 2010 Objectives: Draft for Public Comment*. Washington, DC: U.S. Government Printing Office; 1998.

25. Department of Health and Human Services. *Healthy People 2010: Understanding and Improving Health*. 2nd ed. Washington, DC: U.S. Government Printing Office; 2000.

26. Department of Health and Human Services. *Healthy People 2010: Final Review*. Available at: http://www.cdc.gov/nchs/data/hpdata2010/hp2010_final_review_executive_summary.pdf. Accessed February 8, 2013.

27. U.S. Department of Health and Human Services. About healthy people. Available at: http://www.healthypeople.gov/2020/about/default.aspx. Accessed February 8, 2013.

28. Association of State and Territorial Health Officials. ASTHO profile of state public health, volume two. Available at: http://astho.org/uploadedFiles/_Publications/Files/Survey_Research/ASTHO_State_Profiles_Single%5B1%5D%20lo%20res.pdf. Accessed February 8, 2013.

29. National Association of County and City Health Officials. 2010 national profile of local health departments. Available at: http://www.naccho.org/topics/infrastructure/profile/resources/2010report/upload/2010_Profile_main_report-web.pdf. Accessed February 8, 2013.

30. Canadian Institute for Health Information. National health expenditure trends, 1975 to 2011. Figure 12. Available at: https://secure.cihi.ca/free_products/nhex_trends_report_2011_en.pdf. Accessed February 8, 2013.

31. Mays GP, Smith SA. Evidence links increases in public health spending to declines in preventable deaths. *Health Affairs*. 2011;30(8):1–9.

32. Evans R, Law M. The Canadian health care system: where are we and how did we get there. In: Dunlop DW, Martins JM, eds. *An International Assessment of Health Care Financing. Lessons for Developing Countries*. Washington, DC: World Bank Publications; 1995:79–114.

33. Baker EL, Potter MA, Jones DL, et al. The public health infrastructure and our nation's health. *Annual Review Public Health*. 2005;26:303–18.

34. Association of State and Territorial Health Officials. *State public health employee worker shortage report: A civil service recruitment and retention crisis*. Available at: http://www.heartlandcenters.slu.edu/ephli/envHealthScan/ReadingList11/6Workforce.pdf. Accessed February 8, 2013.

Public Health Administration and Practice Framework

Cynthia B. Morrow and James A. Johnson

LEARNING OBJECTIVES

- To gain perspective from an overall framework for public health
- To better understand key developments in forming this framework
- To know about major influences currently shaping public health
- To realize the importance of a community perspective in public health
- To know the core functions and essential services of public health

Chapter Overview

Activities performed under the auspices of public health have evolved throughout the centuries. One change in the focus of public health in the United States was the Institute of Medicine's (IOM) pivotal report, *The Future of Public Health*,[1] which established recommendations for a new way of organizing public health activities that emphasize population-based efforts rather than personal healthcare delivery. Three core public health functions were identified: assessment, policy development, and assurance. Several years later, a federally sponsored task force developed another taxonomy of public health activity that centered around the

"Ten Essential Public Health Services."[2] In 2003, the IOM published a follow-up report, *The Future of the Public's Health in the 21st Century*,[3] focusing on the need to strengthen the government's public health infrastructure while recognizing the need to establish and maintain partnerships to further enhance the public health system. The latest IOM report, *Primary Care and Public Health: Exploring Integration to Improve Population Health*,[4] published in 2012, further deals with the challenges and opportunities in addressing population health outcomes through partnerships with an emphasis on delivery of primary care health services through the lens of public health. Contemporary public health activities have been shaped not only by efforts to redefine the conceptual basis of public health practice but also by efforts to redefine specific national public health goals, as most recently outlined and promoted by the U.S. Department of Health and Human Services (HHS) in the 2010 report, *Healthy People 2020: Improving the Health of Americans*.[5]

Core Public Health Functions

The monumental IOM report, *The Future of Public Health*, set out recommendations for a new categorization of public health functions.[1] These functions were recommended to counter the attrition of public health vigilance in protecting the public. Lack of agreement concerning mission, politicized decision making, and unsatisfactory linkages with private medicine were cited as underlying difficulties. Little attention to management and the lack of development of leaders were also described as root causes of ineffective public health action. Recommendations included designating central responsibility to state health departments and grouping all primarily health-related functions there. State delegation of this responsibility to local government was foreseen. The IOM report provided a new categorization of public health functions, which has become widely adopted. **Core functions** were denoted as assessment, policy development, and assurance.[1] See **Figure 4.1**.

Assessment

The committee recommended every public health agency regularly and systematically collect, assemble, analyze, and make available information on the health needs of the community, including statistics on health status, community health needs, and epidemiologic and other studies of health problems.[1]

Policy Development

The committee recommended that every public health agency exercise its responsibility to serve the public interest in the development of comprehensive public health policies by promoting the use of the scientific knowledge base in decision making about public health and by developing public health policy.

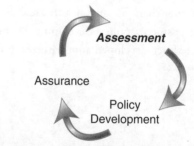

Figure 4.1   Core Functions of Public Health
Source: State of Florida, Department of Health.

Agencies must take a strategic approach, developed on the basis of a positive appreciation for the democratic political process.[1]

Assurance

The committee recommended that public health agencies assure their constituents that services necessary to achieve agreed-upon goals are provided, either by encouraging actions by other entities (private or public sector), by requiring such action through regulation, or by providing services directly.

The committee further recommended that each public health agency involve lay policy makers and the general public in determining a set of high-priority personal and community-wide health services, including subsidization or direct provision of high-priority personal health services that governments guarantee to every member of the community, even those unable to afford them.[1, pp. 8–9]

The categorization of assessment, policy development, and assurance has become a commonly used rubric to describe public health activities. By grouping public health functions into overall population-based health improvement plans, communities can address specific activities to improve community health status.[6]

In response to the question of whether a health department should provide assurance of care, acting as a guarantor versus actually engaging in the delivery of medical care, the IOM strongly recommended the assurance role rather than actual delivery. The responsibility of providing medical care to the poor was seen as draining resources and attention away from disease prevention and health promotion activities that benefit the entire community. It was believed that government had the responsibility to provide access and services, but by another mechanism.[1]

Other mechanisms to provide access to health care and to assure a safety net within the healthcare delivery system itself have developed over the past few decades. In 1991, the Federally Qualified Health Center Medicare benefit was added with the primary purpose of assuring a safety net by enhancing the provision of primary care services in underserved urban and rural communities.[7]

The Health Security Act, introduced to Congress in 1993, was designed to provide universal access to health services by providing entry to all individuals and their families to a healthcare plan. These plans were to integrate a schedule of clinical preventive services such as immunization, serum cholesterol measurement every 5 years, and screening for cervical cancer and mammography for women as part of comprehensive provision of health care.[8] Furthermore, this legislation was to provide resources ($750 million by year 2000) to address the recommendations of a core functions group of the U.S. Public Health Service, chaired by the Assistant Secretary for Health and the Surgeon General. This group vigorously supported the necessary role of public health and population-based programs for a reformed healthcare insurance system in the United States and emphasized the need to address health priorities and conditions of populations, as distinct from individuals.[9]

Although the Health Security Act ultimately failed to pass, the prospect of this legislation raised a number of questions for public health practice. With the requirements for managed care plans to provide clinical prevention and medical care, these activities would no longer be required of public health agencies. While there were ongoing questions concerning a need for public health services under a reformed system of health care, it became clear that the provision of population-based preventive functions was essential. The public health system was identified to assume this responsibility.

Important exceptions or variations to this theme of distancing the public health system from delivery of personal health services still exist. According to the National Association of County and City Health Officials (NACCHO), in 2010, 13% of health departments still functioned as the comprehensive primary medical care safety net, 36% directly provided well child care, and 30% provided prenatal medical care (not including home visitation services). More commonly though, local health departments (LHDs) provided personal health services only in the context of communicable diseases. For example, more than 90% of LHDs provided immunizations and most provided limited screening and treatment of communicable diseases. With respect to screening, 85% of LHDs provided screening for tuberculosis and between 60% and 65% provided screening for sexually transmitted diseases and HIV/AIDS. With respect to treatment, 75% of LHDs provided treatment for TB, 59% for STDs, and 21% for HIV/AIDS.[10]

Development of the 10 Essential Public Health Services

Although the core functions described the role of public health activities in broad terms, more specific delineation of public health functions was needed. In 1989, the Centers for Disease Control and Prevention (CDC) convened a meeting with public health practice organizations. This brainstorming session resulted in the identification of more than 140 essential activities or functions. At additional meetings, 10 groups of organizational practices were determined.[11] These 10 practices provided a basis for both implementing and measuring the performance of the three core functions. Studies determining the allocation of effort among these functions by local health agencies showed that the assurance function received the majority of time and resources, with few resources being devoted to assessment and policy development.[12]

Although the concept of core functions became more widespread in the public health field after 1993, there was inconsistency in the terminology and expectations. In the spring of 1994, Dr. David Satcher and Dr. J. Michael McGinnis chaired a committee to unify the public health community around these core functions. This led to the development of a uniform set of essential services representing the further development of the previously established core functions and organization practices. In the fall of 1994, the Core Public Health Functions Steering Committee issued a vision and mission statement listing the "Ten Essential Public Health Services" (**Exhibit 4.1**). This structure has since become the commonly accepted taxonomy for public health functions.[13]

Exhibit 4.1   Public Health in America

Vision

Healthy people in healthy communities

Mission

Promote physical and mental health and prevent disease, injury, and disability

Public Health:

- Prevents epidemics and the spread of disease
- Protects against environmental hazards
- Prevents injuries
- Promotes and encourages healthy behaviors
- Responds to disasters and assists communities in recovery
- Assures the quality and accessibility of health services

Essential Public Health Services:

1. Monitor health status to identify community health problems.
2. Diagnose and investigate health problems and health hazards in the community.
3. Inform, educate, and empower people about health issues.
4. Mobilize community partnerships to identify and solve health problems.
5. Develop policies and plans that support individual and community health efforts.
6. Enforce laws and regulations that protect health and ensure safety.
7. Link people to needed personal health services, and assure the provision of health care when otherwise unavailable.
8. Assure a competent public health and personal healthcare workforce.
9. Evaluate effectiveness, accessibility, and quality of personal and population-based health services.
10. Research for new insights and innovative solutions to health problems.

Source: Data from Core Public Health Functions Steering Committee Members: American Public Health Association; Association of Schools of Public Health; Association of State and Territorial Health Officials; Environmental Council of the States; National Association of County and City Health Officials; National Association of State Alcohol and Drug Abuse Directors; National Association of State Mental Health Program Directors; Public Health Foundation; U.S. Public Health Service—Agency for Health Care Policy and Research; CDC; Food and Drug Administration (FDA); Health Resources and Services Administration (HRSA); Indian Health Service; National Institutes of Health; Office of the Assistant Secretary for Health; Substance Abuse and Mental Health Services Administration.

This functional framework has gained momentum. It is commonly used by public health practitioners and policymakers. Cost studies by the Public Health Foundation have been performed to determine expenditures by function for state and local departments of health.[14] Furthermore, this format provides a common vocabulary and expresses the mission of public health in terms of community-wide health improvement and now constitutes the framework of public health accreditation, with the first 10 of 12 domains of accreditation addressing the 10 essential services.

Although widely accepted, the essential service framework groups public health activities into categories that may not be immediately recognizable to budget officers, legislators, or the public, all of whom expect more concrete service activities. A similar difficulty had been previously described with the core public health functions. To address these challenges, the Public Health Foundation prepared a crosswalk matching essential public health services with specific service activities (**Table 4.1**).

Table 4.1   State/Local Health Department Crosswalk of Program Activities to Essential Services

Essential Service	Includes but Is Not Limited to	Does Not Include
1. Monitor health status to identify community health problems.	• Disease and injury registries • Epidemiology (surveillance, disease reporting, sentinel events), including injury epidemiology, mental health epidemiology, and substance abuse epidemiology • Population-based/community health needs assessments • State/community report cards/development of health status indicators • Vital statistics • Environmental epidemiology • Immunization status tracking • Public Health Laboratory Information System (PHLIS) • Linkages of data sets for population-based applications • Population-based health interview surveys (e.g., BRFSS or other state surveys)	• Management of client-based data systems should be included under #7b. • Cost of accessing client-based data systems to evaluate accessibility and quality of care should be included under #9.

2. Diagnose and investigate health problems and health hazards in the community.	• Communicable disease detection (case finding)
	• Chronic disease detection (case finding)
	• Injury detection
	• HIV/AIDS prevention:
	  – Counseling and testing
	  – Partner notification
	• Outbreak investigation and control (including immunizations as part of outbreak control)
	• Early periodic screening detection or treatment (EPSDT)
	• Population-based screening services (e.g., cholesterol), including follow-up counseling (e.g., nutrition and exercise)
	• Contact tracing (e.g., STDs or TB)
	• Environmental risk assessment
	• Environmental sampling
	• Lead investigation
	• Radon detection
	• Asbestos detection
	• Diagnostic laboratory services (e.g., bacteriology, parasitology, virology, immunology, clinical chemistry) in support of population-based health activities
	• Environmental laboratory services (e.g., environmental microbiology samples, environmental chemistry samples, and occupational safety and health samples)
		• Primary care services
		• Treatment of STDs, TB, and other communicable diseases
		• Dental health services (including topical fluoride treatments in schools)
		• Treatment of diabetes, lupus, hemophilia, sickle cell anemia, epilepsy, Alzheimer's disease, and other chronic diseases
		• Genetic disease services
		• Home healthcare services
		• Purchase and provision of AZT/other drugs
		• Prenatal/perinatal care
		• Services for premature and newborn infants and preschool-aged children
		• Services to children with special healthcare needs
		• Immunizations, except as part of outbreak control
		(Note: All the above activities should be included under #7b.)

3. Inform, educate, and empower people about health issues.

- Comprehensive school health education
- Population-wide health promotion/risk reduction programs:
  - Injury prevention education and promotion
  - Parenting education
  - Physical activity and fitness
  - Population-based risk reduction programs
  - Seat-belt education/promotion
  - Sexuality education
  - Tobacco use prevention and cessation
- Nutrition education (e.g., Five-A-Day programs)
- Nutrition education as part of WIC
- School campaigns (e.g., "Say No To Drugs Day")
- Substance abuse prevention
- Public education campaigns
- Worksite health promotion
- HIV education/information
- Educational activities as part of outreach
- Educational activities related to enforcement of laws and regulations (i.e., education of tobacco vendors)

- Counseling and education as part of personal health services (e.g., nutrition counseling as part of prenatal care [include under #7b])

4. Mobilize community partnerships and action to identify and solve health problems. (See #5 for planning and policy development activities.)

- Coalition building
- Collaboration with outside agencies/organizations
- Forming community partnerships to solve health problems (e.g., task forces, multidisciplinary advisory groups)
- Advocacy and budget justification (e.g., testifying at hearings)
- Technical assistance to facilitate mobilization of local health agencies or community groups
- HIV community planning (include portion, if any, that involves building community partnerships; planning portion should be included under #5)

- Development of legislation, policies, or plans (include under #5)

- Form partnerships to solve health problems (include under #4).

5. Develop policies and plans that support individual and community health efforts. (See #4 for collaborative activities.)

- Agenda setting
- Development of policies and guidelines
- Legislative activities (e.g., drafting legislation, developing agency budgets)
- Planning (including certificate of need)
- *Healthy People 2000* objective-setting activities
- APEX PH Parts I and II/Healthy Communities/ PATCH/other planning models
- HIV community planning (include portion related to planning; portion supporting community partnerships should be included under #4)

(*continues*)

Table 4.1   State/Local Health Department Crosswalk of Program Activities to Essential Services (continued)

Essential Service	Includes but Is Not Limited to	Does Not Include
6. Enforce laws and regulations that protect health and ensure safety.	• Air quality (indoor and outdoor) • Asbestos control • Consumer protection and sanitation • Food sanitation • General sanitation • Housing • Public lodging • Recreational sanitation • Shellfish sanitation • Substance control/product safety • Vector/rodent control • Fluoridation services • Hazardous materials management (accidents, transportation spill, etc.) • Occupational health and safety • Radiation control • Lead abatement • Radon mitigation • Waste management—sewage, solid, and toxic • Water quality control (public/private drinking water, groundwater protection, etc.) • Emergency response teams to toxic spills, product recalls, and response to natural disasters (including the maintenance and development of emergency systems) • Medical examiner, toxicology, and other forensic medicine • Enforcement activities related to compliance with youth access to tobacco regulations • Enforcement activities related to the agency's police authority (e.g., quarantine, forcing patients to take medications)	• Construction of facilities and physical plans (this is generally funded through special capital accounts)

7a. Link people to needed personal health services.	• Case management/care coordination services • Information and referral hotlines • Outreach services related to linking individuals to personal health services • School health outreach, case finding, and referral services • Transportation and other enabling services • Development of primary care services in underserved communities	• Direct healthcare services • School-based clinical services (include under #7b)

7b. Ensure the provision of care when otherwise unavailable.	• Personal health services, including:
	  – Primary care services
	  – Treatment of STDs, TB, and other communicable diseases
	  – CD4-testing
	  – Dental health services (including topical fluoride treatments in schools)
	  – Treatment of diabetes, lupus, hemophilia, sickle cell anemia, epilepsy, Alzheimer's disease, and other chronic diseases
	  – Genetic disease services
	  – Home health care
	  – Hospitals
	  – Purchase and provision of AZT/other drugs
	  – Prenatal/perinatal care
	  – Services for premature and newborn infants and preschool-aged children
	  – Services to children with special healthcare needs
	• Clinical preventive services (e.g., routine immunizations, family planning)
	• School-based clinical services
	• Management of client-based data systems that support the services above
		• Population-based health services

8. Ensure a competent public health and personal healthcare workforce.	• Required continuing education • Recruitment and retention of health professionals • Professional education and training • Health and environmental professionals licensing • Leadership training/programs	• Facilities licensing (include under #9) • Quality improvement (include under #9)

(continues)

Table 4.1 State/Local Health Department Crosswalk of Program Activities to Essential Services (continued)

Essential Service	Includes but Is Not Limited to	Does Not Include
9. Evaluate effectiveness, accessibility, and quality of personal and population-based health services.	• Facilities licensing • Healthcare systems monitoring • Hospital outcomes data • Personal health services monitoring (including analysis and use of client-based data) • Program evaluation • Data systems related to service availability, utilization, cost, and outcome • Laboratory regulation and quality control services • Regulation of EMS personnel/services • Quality assurance/quality improvement activities (implementation)	• Management of client-based data systems (include under #7b) • Development (vs. implementation) of a quality improvement plan/policy (see #5)
10. Research for new insights and innovative solutions to health problems.	• Biomedical, preventive, and clinical investigations • Health services research • Research and monitoring about the effects of the changing healthcare environment and unique strategies employed by public health agencies • Demonstration programs • Methods development • Research grants to others • Innovative technologies	
General administration	• Stand-alone administration activities (e.g., accounting, legal, or personnel activities) • Office of the health director • Computer support • Maintenance of buildings and grounds • Reporting requirements	

Source: The Public Health Expenditures Project Team, 1998; Public Health Foundation; National Association of County and City Health Officials; National Association of Local Boards of Health; Association of State and Territorial Health Officials; with funding from the Office of Disease Prevention and Health Promotion, Department of Health and Human Services. Dr. James Johnson UNC Kenan-Flagler School of Business.

Core Functions and Essential Public Health Services: Implementation

Surveys of state public health agencies reveal virtually all respondents adopting and agreeing with the importance of the three core functions described in the first IOM report on public health.[15,16] A high proportion indicate that their operations include performance of these functions: assessment (80%), policy development (49%), and assurance (42%).[15] As recommended earlier by the same IOM report, there is evidence of outreach by state health agencies with increasing legislative activity and relationships with voluntary health agencies.[15]

The World Health Organization (WHO) decided to **employ essential public health functions** (EPHFs) as a tool for implementing "Health for All in the 21st Century."[17] This initiative began when WHO members agreed to pursue health gains for their countries.[18] In the late 1990s, an international Delphi survey (a validated process for attaining anonymous consensus) of 145 public health leaders, managers, professors, and practitioners was performed.[17] The essential public health categories and functions that resulted from this process are similar to those developed by the Core Public Health Functions Steering Committee.

It was strongly agreed by the survey participants that public health functions may be performed by nongovernmental entities, including the private sector. The rationale advanced was that because the determinants of health status are not confined to the health sector, essential health services can be carried out in other areas, although it identified that the implementation of EPHFs did need to be monitored by government agencies.[17]

The extent to which nongovernmental entities can provide public health is expanding. Private-sector healthcare providers, previously involved with inpatient care, are evolving into consolidated and integrated healthcare systems. These changes in the healthcare marketplace potentially could lead to interest in providing essential public health services.[19] The current emphasis on accountable care organizations reflects these changes.

The Future of the Public's Health

In the United States, the concept of partnerships as a means to improve population health was addressed in a follow-up report by the Institute of Medicine, *The Future of the Public's Health in the 21st Century*.[3] This report explored the public health infrastructure and the potential challenges within the public health system that could jeopardize the health of the public. The report outlines the concept of population health and the government's fundamental duty to protect it. Further, it "describes the rationale for multisector engagement in partnership with the government and the roles different actors can play to support a healthy future for the American people."[3, p. 1] An illustration of the intersectoral public health system is shown in **Figure 4.2**. The IOM report, in seeking to address the health challenges facing the American public currently and in the future, identified six areas of change and actions, including the following:[3, p. 4]

- Using a population health approach
- Strengthening public health infrastructure

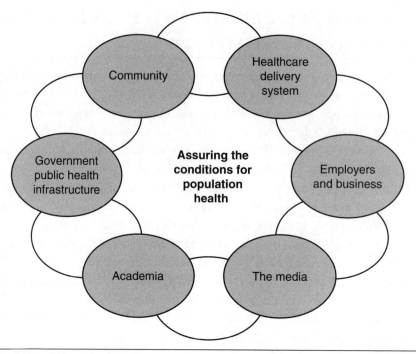

Figure 4.2   The Public Health System
Source: Reprinted with permission from National Academies Press. Institute of Medicine. *Future of the Public's Health in the 21st Century.* Washington, DC: National Academies Press; 2003; 30.

- Supporting and promoting intersector partnerships, as shown in Figure 4.2, paying special consideration to meeting the needs of diverse populations
- Developing a systematic approach to ensure the quality and availability of public health services
- Supporting and promoting evidence-based public health
- Improving communication within the public health system

The focus on the intersectoral approach was supported in *Healthy People 2010,* which, when referring to essential public health services, stated, "the totality of the public health infrastructure includes all governmental and nongovernmental entities that provide any of these services."[20]

National Health Objectives

National health objectives remain an important component of public health administration. Prior to the IOM's 1988 pivotal report, national health objectives for the United States grew out of a health strategy initiated with the publication in 1979 of *Healthy People: The Surgeon General's Report on Health Promotion and Disease Prevention.*[21] After preliminary work by U.S.

Public Health Service agencies, 167 nongovernmental experts were convened at a conference in 1979 and organized into 15 working groups that developed the draft objectives for the priority areas.[21] This resulted in the 1980 publication of *Promoting Health/Preventing Disease: Objectives for the Nation*, which set 226 goals in 15 priority areas (based on the risk factors most closely associated with the most common causes of morbidity and mortality) across three categories: preventive health services, health protection, and health promotion.[22] The report was organized into five broad health status goals keyed to the various stages of the lifecycle, from healthy infants, healthy children, healthy adolescents and young adults, and healthy adults, to healthy older adults. The health promotion effort behind this was based on the theory of multiple determinants of health involving biologic, social, environmental, and behavioral factors. Prevention and risk reduction strategies were aimed at individuals' susceptibilities and behaviors, agents of disease, environmental factors, and particularly the interaction between these determinations. *Healthy People* emphasized the importance of personal behaviors of the individual in determining health status and also recognized the role of environmental factors.[21]

By 1987, measurement tools showed that nearly half of the objectives had been reached. An additional one-quarter of the objectives were not achieved, and data were not available for monitoring the objectives in the remaining quarter. Considerable progress was documented in the priority areas, including the control of high blood pressure; immunization; control of infectious diseases; unintentional injury prevention; and control of smoking, alcohol, and drugs. Areas where progress lagged included pregnancy and infant health, nutrition, physical fitness, family planning, STDs, and occupational safety and health.[23] Major declines in the death rates for heart disease, stroke, and unintentional injury during this 1980–1990 period gave hope for progress in succeeding decades, spurring the next installment of objectives, *Healthy People 2000: National Health Promotion and Disease Prevention Objectives*.[23]

Healthy People 2000

Healthy People 2000, based on regional hearings with testimony from more than 750 individuals and organizations, presented a new national prevention strategy, identifying three broad goals: increasing the span of life, reducing health disparities, and achieving access to preventive services. The 21 areas were in three broad categories: health promotion, health protection, and preventive services.[23]

Health promotion strategies focused on lifestyle and personal behaviors including physical activity, nutrition, and tobacco and alcohol consumption. **Health protection** strategies included environmental and regulatory activities. **Preventive services** included counseling, screening, and immunization. A special category was established in *Healthy People 2000* for data and surveillance activities. Each priority area was assigned to a government lead agency such as the CDC, the National Institutes of Health, or the Health Resources and Services Agency.

Healthy People 2000 was designed to offer a vision for the new century based on achieving reductions in preventable disability and death. For example, when work on this report began in 1987, a new health threat, human immunodeficiency virus (HIV) infection, had appeared. The devastating impact it had on the nation's health was evident. Given the importance of this new threat, an entire priority area (priority area 18) was devoted to the disease.

Healthy People 2010 *Objectives*

In 2000, *Healthy People 2010* was released by the HHS. The comprehensive health promotion and disease prevention agenda was "designed to identify the most significant preventable threats to health and to establish national goals to reduce these threats."[24] The final report had two overarching goals: to increase quality and years of life and to eliminate health disparities.

Increase Quality and Years of Healthy Life

This first goal of *Healthy People 2010* was to increase the quality in addition to the years of healthy life. A healthy life means a full range of functional capacity throughout each life stage. A range of measures was used for this goal, including morbidity, mortality, and quality. With success in extending life expectancy, more attention was focused toward improving the quality of life (QOL). Health-related quality of life (HRQOL) includes both physical and mental health and their determinants.[25] HRQOL has a relationship to individual perception and ability to function. On a community basis, HRQOL includes all aspects that have an influence on health (**Table 4.2**).

Eliminate Health Disparities

Eliminating disparities was a goal of *Healthy People 2000*, which had special population targets for some objectives. These targets did not aim at eliminating health disparities by the year 2000. In February 1998, President Clinton called for eliminating disparities between racial and minority groups in six areas: infant mortality, cancer, cardiovascular disease, diabetes, HIV/acquired immune deficiency syndrome (AIDS), and immunizations.

Public Health Infrastructure

For the first time, *Healthy People 2010* included a focus area in public health infrastructure, with the goal of ensuring capacity to provide the essential public health services at federal, state, and local levels. Objectives for this area are shown in **Exhibit 4.2**.

Table 4.2   Health-Related Quality of Life (HRQOL)

"Health"	vs. HRQOL	vs. QOL
Individual level		
Death	Functional status	Happiness
Disease	Wellbeing	Life satisfaction
Community level		
Life expectancy	Environment	Participation
	Livability	Sustainability

Source: Reprinted from *Healthy People 2010* Objectives, U.S. Department of Health and Human Services, Office of Public Health and Science.

Exhibit 4.2   Public Health Infrastructure

Number	Objective
1.	Competencies for public health workers
2.	Training in essential public health services
3.	Continuing education and training by public health agencies
4.	Use of the Standard Occupational Classification System
5.	Onsite access to data
6.	Access to public health information and surveillance data
7.	Tracking *Healthy People 2010* objectives for select populations
8.	Data collection for *Healthy People 2010* objectives
9.	Use of geocoding in health data systems
10.	Performance standards for essential public health services
11.	Health improvement plans
12.	Access to laboratory services
13.	Access to comprehensive epidemiology services
14.	Model statutes related to essential public health services
15.	Data on public health expenditures
16.	Collaboration and cooperation in prevention research efforts
17.	Summary measures of population health and the public health infrastructure

Source: Reprinted from *Healthy People 2010* Objectives, U.S. Department of Health and Human Services, Office of Public Health and Science.

Infrastructure has been described as the basic support for the delivery of public health activities. Five components of infrastructure are skilled workforce, integrated electronic information systems, public health organizations, resources, and research. The need for infrastructure was pointed out by the IOM reports as well. Keeping pace with information technology, availability of a trained workforce, and availability of resources for local public health problems are infrastructure priorities. This new focus area did not target health outcomes but rather addressed the need to increase capacity to deliver public health services. Apart from building workforce competency and increasing training and continuing education opportunities, the majority of infrastructure objectives directly addressed the capacity of state and local health agencies by calling for increases in the use of technology, scientific disciplines, planning, and improved organization of services. For example, a target of 90% was set for the proportion of state and local public health agencies that use electronic data and online information for data to improve their operations. Another objective targeted the availability of individuals with epidemiology skills for local and state public health agencies. In addition to these objectives, state and local public health jurisdictions were expected to develop health improvement plans to monitor and meet performance standards for the essential public health services.

Inclusion of the infrastructure objectives in *Healthy People 2010* signified the importance of a core capacity for population-based activities as provided by local, state, and federal public health agencies in collaboration with communities and other providers in the public and private sectors. Public health departments responsible for the health of communities need the basic tools: a skilled workforce and the resources necessary for it to perform its tasks. This noncategorical approach focused on the skills, manpower, and technology available to these agencies for the array of public health functions, rather than for specific programmatic use.

Creating infrastructure objectives does not lead to their realization without the necessary resources and the commitment to implement them. Requests for infrastructure funding from federal, state, or local governments may suffer because they can appear generic or not directly relevant to activities addressing more visible health issues such as infectious disease, maternal and child health, and environmental hazards. Various approaches to this difficulty can be used, such as attaching and integrating infrastructure needs with program budgets.

Healthy People 2020 *Objectives*

As described by the HHS, *Healthy People 2020: Improving the Health of Americans* has continued in the tradition of the previous national health plans with its ambitious 10-year agenda for improving the nation's health. *Healthy People 2020* is the result of a multiyear process that reflects input from a diverse group of individuals and organizations through an extensive stakeholder feedback involving more than 2,000 organizations and the general public. More than 8,000 comments were considered in drafting a comprehensive set of objectives. This new national health plan, consistent with those in the past, articulates its vision and goals via their website and distribution throughout the public health community. This helps focus and organize efforts across all sectors and levels of government. **Exhibits 4.3** and **4.4** list the mission, vision, and goals of *Healthy People 2020*. It is also useful to visit the *Healthy People 2020* website: http://www.healthypeople.gov/2020/about/.

Exhibit 4.3   Vision and Mission of *Healthy People 2020*

Vision

A society in which all people live long, healthy lives

Mission

Healthy People 2020 strives to:

- Identify nationwide health improvement priorities.
- Increase public awareness and understanding of the determinants of health, disease, and disability and the opportunities for progress.
- Provide measurable objectives and goals that are applicable at the national, state, and local levels.
- Engage multiple sectors to take actions to strengthen policies and improve practices that are driven by the best available evidence and knowledge.
- Identify critical research, evaluation, and data collection needs.

Source: Reproduced from U.S. Department of Health and Human Services. *Healthy People 2020*. Available at: http://www.healthypeople.gov/2020/. Accessed February 7, 2013.

Exhibit 4.4   Goals of *Healthy People 2020* Overarching Goals

Goal 1: Attain high-quality, longer lives free of preventable disease, disability, injury, and premature death.

Goal 2: Achieve health equity, eliminate disparities, and improve the health of all groups.

Goal 3: Create social and physical environments that promote good health for all.

Goal 4: Promote quality of life, healthy development, and healthy behaviors across all life stages.

Source: Reproduced from U.S. Department of Health and Human Services. *Healthy People 2020.* Available at: http://www.healthypeople.gov/2020/. Accessed February 7, 2013.

Based on the input from the public and other stakeholders, a number of new focus areas are included in the initiative as well:

- Adolescent health
- Blood disorders and blood safety
- Dementias, Alzheimer's disease
- Early and middle childhood
- Genomics
- Global health
- Health-related quality of life and wellbeing
- Healthcare-associated infections
- Lesbian, gay, bisexual, and transgender health
- Older adults
- Preparedness
- Sleep health
- Social determinants of health

As the public health community moves forward in working on these goals and objectives, the public will face economic and demographic challenges. The national health plan should help organize the needed focus and resources during the second decade of the 21st century. As in the past, a review of achievements and mid-range goal accomplishments will be measured.

Governmental and Nongovernmental Aspects of Public Health

Historically, the government's role has been central to the provision of health protection for the community because the genesis of public health activities was in addressing imminent environmental and disease threats, especially with respect to infectious diseases. Countering these hazards to health required a governmental presence as manifested by statutory protection, regulation, inspection, and enforcement. As described earlier, public health practice evolved with a broader definition of scope, extending well beyond infectious disease. Private-sector involvement in communities' preventive activities has grown more important with business, media, community-based organizations, and others partners taking on more responsibility. For example, in its 2009 report, "Tobacco Use: Targeting the Nation's Leading Killer," the CDC recognizes the numerous community agencies, including the American Cancer Society and the American Heart Association, as important partners in national efforts to promote tobacco prevention and control initiatives.[26]

The role of governmental activity in public health varies with larger political and social trends and is shaped by community priorities that often originate in nongovernmental sectors. Federal activities in public health experienced growth from the 1930s through the 1970s as part of President Franklin Roosevelt's New Deal and President Johnson's Great Society. However, a dominant element of public policy with respect to public health activities has been devolution since then with the shift of responsibilities from the federal government to the states and then to the localities, and now often to private vendors.[27]

There are essentially four limitations of government in the public health arena, including a reduced probability of success for interventions, management by crisis, fragmentation, and competing governmental agencies.[28] These limitations heighten the importance of community partnerships, including the private sector, in population health improvement. The first limitation is that many current public health issues and interventions do not necessarily inspire governmental action as did the 19th-century threats from infectious diseases, where the proposed actions had high probabilities of success at limited costs. In contrast, 21st-century threats associated with chronic diseases are often considered low yield and high cost given the complexities of the associated determinants of health. A second limitation is that public health crises have been associated with short-term public management of the problem but not long-term policy changes. A third limitation is the fragmentation of health responsibilities among a number of different public agencies using separate approaches to public health problems.[28] Fourth, competition for resources between governmental agencies, including welfare, corrections, and police, leaves public health agencies at a disadvantage, particularly because their activities are not perceived as being of similar critical importance to their counterparts.

Contemporary relationships that support core public health functions can be described in four categories:

1. Between different health agencies at various levels of government
2. Between health agencies and other public agencies
3. Between health agencies and the private sector
4. Between private and voluntary organizations[1]

All of these interactions occur regularly in practice so that public health cannot be categorized as a strictly governmental or nongovernmental activity. Instead, the public health system is best conceptualized as a network of functions involving both sectors. Relationships between health agencies occur at multiple levels, including, for example, funding and guidance offered by state public health agencies to local health departments. Information and recommendations involve exchanges between these levels, with possible involvement of federal health agencies including the CDC, HRSA, and the FDA.

Relationships between governmental public health agencies and the private and/or voluntary sector are also manifold. Local health departments work with both nonprofit and investor-owned organizations, including hospitals and businesses interested in promotion of health activities. Voluntary associations such as the American Heart Association and the American Diabetes Association act in the private sector, often in cooperation with governmental activities. In the late 1990s, the Turning Point collaborative, initially sponsored by the W. K. Kellogg and the Robert Wood Johnson foundations, demonstrated that the private sector was committed to public health systems improvement with its mission "to transform and strengthen the public health system in the United States to make the system more effective, more community-based, and more collaborative."[29]

The 2012 IOM report, *Primary Care and Public Health: Exploring Integration to Improve Population Health*,[4] addresses the intersection between personal healthcare delivery and the public health system with particular attention to the governmental and nongovernmental aspects of public health. For example, a table in the report (**Table 4.3**) addresses how provisions in the Patient Protection and Affordable Care Act (ACA) can transform population health. These examples show how the ACA has the potential to help public health agencies tackle the leading causes of death and root causes of costly, preventable chronic disease; detect and respond rapidly to health security threats; and prevent accidents and injuries all while working side by side with community partners. With this investment, the ACA helps states and the nation as a whole focus on fighting disease and illness before they happen.

Table 4.3   Selected Provisions of the Patient Protection and Affordable Care Act That Offer Opportunities for HRSA and CDC

Essential Public Health Service (EPHS)	Number of Activities Addressing EPHSs	
	Predominantly	Total
Assessment	-	-
Monitor	6	18
Investigate	2	6
Policy development	-	-
Inform	7	15
Mobilize	4	9
Plan	—	6
Assurance	-	-
Enforce	—	—
Link	21	27
Competent workforce	3	6
Evaluate	1	5
Research and development	—	2
Total	44	94*

*Each of the 44 activities could address more than one essential public health service.

Source: Reprinted with permission from National Academies Press. Institute of Medicine. *Future of the Public's Health in the 21st century*. Washington, DC: National Academies Press; 2003; 30.

Community Perspective

As discussed, the domain of public health extends beyond the range of governmental activities. Many individuals, organizations, and other entities are directly or indirectly involved with community health.[30] In addition to public health agencies, stakeholders include individual health providers, purchasers of care, and voluntary and community organizations.[31] Even agencies without an explicit health designation, including schools, businesses, and the media, can have important health-related roles. This broad net of entities serving public health purposes is warranted but makes a single definition of public health practice or designation of the public health workforce complex. Edward Baker, former Director of the Public Health Practice Office at the CDC and current Director of the North Carolina Institute for Public Health has emphasized this broader approach:

> We present a redefinition of public health practice that extends well beyond the usual government efforts and aggressively seeks out and embraces the skills and resources of many new nontraditional players. While in no way diminishing the importance of public health agencies, we foresee a significantly greater participation by the private sector, particularly the personal medical care system in the future.[32, p. 1276]

The interaction between governmental public health agencies and the private sector is currently in flux. The increase in the number of organized healthcare delivery systems, including health plans, is making it possible for governmental health agencies to *ensure* access to care rather than to *deliver* personal health services. As reported in the 1996 IOM report, *Healthy Communities: New Partnerships for the Future of Public Health*, there is a question of how many elements of public health can or should be subsumed by the private sector.[31] The number could be considerable. An earlier study described nonprofit organizations performing essential public health services.[19] The 2003 follow-up IOM report further addressed the need of nongovernmental agencies to carry out the three fundamental functions. Although maintaining that governmental public health agencies have a special duty as "the backbone of the public health system," the report provides recommendations for community partners including the healthcare delivery system, employers and businesses, media, and academia.[3] There are many provisions in the ACA that further support partnerships. One example is the creation of the Prevention and Public Health Fund (PPHF), which provides for an unprecedented investment in promoting wellness, preventing disease, and protecting against public health emergencies. As described by the HHS, the Community Transformation Grants, which are funded by the PPHF, support

> State and local governmental agencies and community-based organizations in the implementation, evaluation, and dissemination of evidence-based community health activities in order to reduce chronic disease rates, prevent the development of secondary conditions, address health disparities, and develop a stronger evidence base of effective prevention programming.[33]

A range of for-profit and nonprofit organizations are already involved in activities that incorporate public health practices using any definition. Two notable examples include the Henry Ford Health System and Parkland Health and Hospital System.

The Henry Ford Health System (HFHS) is a major comprehensive nonprofit organization serving seven counties in southeastern Michigan. Based in Detroit, the system provides care to the insured and uninsured in areas with high rates of poverty, unemployment, and violence. Principles used in operation include a definition of health as more than the absence of disease, participation in community prevention, and use of the *Healthy People* goals.[34] In 2004, the system provided the community with $127 million in uncompensated care. The system has won numerous prestigious awards for the services it provides in improving the health of the community it serves.[35] In 2011, it was awarded the Malcolm Baldrige National Quality Award by the National Institutes of Standards and Technology.[36]

The Parkland Health and Hospital System (PHHS) is one of the nation's largest teaching hospitals and has served as a safety net for Dallas for more than 100 years, serving primarily Medicare, Medicaid, or uninsured clients. With a mission and vision beyond healthcare delivery, PHHS describes itself as "redefining public health care."[37] Health care is also provided in nontraditional settings, including care for the homeless. Measurements of health outcomes are used to evaluate the program's effectiveness. Health outcomes are calculated using preexisting morbidity based on morbidity and mortality rate data in the served community. The assumption is that the delivery of preventive care will improve the health of the community.[38]

Medicine and Public Health

For far too long, medicine and public health have operated separately in the United States, pursuing different approaches to health improvement. However, several factors have emerged that may improve the once dysfunctional relationship between medicine and public health. The increased recognition of the value of partnerships and collaboration by public health entities has led to efforts by both sectors to bridge this historical separation. Leaders within both the American Medical Association (AMA) and the American Public Health Association (APHA) have met for this purpose, and a working partnership was established with support of the Josiah Macy, Jr., and the W. K. Kellogg foundations.[39] A historic congress brought together nearly 400 leaders of the professional organizations representing those in practice, education, and research in public health and medicine.[39] The following seven elements were agreed on:[39]

1. Engage the community.
2. Change the educational process.
3. Create joint research efforts.
4. Devise a shared view of health and illness.
5. Work together in healthcare provision.
6. Develop healthcare assessment measures.
7. Create local and national networks.

The AMA and the APHA have made a long-term commitment to this medicine–public health initiative. As previously described, to fully realize improvement in health outcomes at both the individual and population levels, however, public health and the medical community must work in concert to improve health outcomes. Successful integration of the two disciplines has not yet fully occurred. However, the 2012 publication of the IOM's report on *Primary Care and Public Health: Exploring Integration to Improve Population Health* is another resource for public health administrators and, as such, has the potential to improve the relationship between these currently distinct communities.[4]

Future Outlook

A variety of administrative and policy frameworks now exist to assist public health institutions in defining, organizing, managing, and evaluating their core activities. Nonetheless, important differences remain in how institutions conceptualize and practice public health. A key point of contention involves the role of public health organizations in delivering personal health services. Despite differences of opinion in certain process-related issues, public health organizations appear to be reaching consensus about the larger public health mission, goals, and objectives. A key area of consensus involves core functions that should be performed by public health organizations in both governmental and private settings. Another area of consensus concerns the importance of cooperation between public and private organizations and between medical practice and public health practice. Accreditation and the growing acceptance of these shared goals promise to improve performance among individual public health organizations and within the public health system as a whole.

Discussion Questions

1. Describe the *Healthy People* reports initiative by the HHS and discuss its evolution over time.
2. Do you feel *Healthy People 2020* is adequate for the challenges currently faced by public health? What might you add? Explore the website to become more familiar.
3. Discuss the core functions of public health.
4. Identify the 10 essential public health services. How might they be utilized by a public health agency?
5. Why is a community perspective so important in public health administration and practice?

References

1. Institute of Medicine. *The Future of Public Health*. Washington, DC: National Academies Press; 1988.
2. Centers for Disease Control and Prevention. Ten essential public health services. Available at: http://www.cdc.gov/nphpsp/essentialservices.html. Accessed February 7, 2013.
3. Institute of Medicine. *The Future of the Public's Health in the 21st Century*. Washington, DC: National Academies Press; 2003.
4. Institute of Medicine. *Primary Care and Public Health: Exploring Integration to Improve Population Health*. Washington, DC: National Academy of Sciences; 2012.
5. U.S. Department of Health and Human Services. *Healthy People 2020: Improving the Health of Americans*. Available at: http://www.healthypeople.gov/2020/. Accessed December 1, 2012.
6. National Association of County and City Health Officials. *1992–1993 National Profile of Local Health Departments*. Washington, DC: NACCHO; 1995.

7. U.S. Department of Health and Human Services. Federally qualified health center. Available at: http://www.cms.gov/Outreach-and-Education/Medicare-Learning-Network-MLN/MLNProducts/downloads/fqhcfactsheet.pdf. Accessed February 7, 2013.

8. Health Security Act of 1993, 103rd Cong., 1st sess.

9. Core Functions Project, U.S. Public Health Service. Health care reform and public health: a paper on population-based core functions. *J Public Health Policy*. 1998;19(4):394–419.

10. National Association of County and City Health Officials. Statement of policy: provision of clinical services by local health departments. Available at: http://www.naccho.org/advocacy/positions/upload/12-17-Provision-of-Clinical-Services.pdf. Accessed February 7, 2013.

11. Dyal W. Ten organizational practices of public health: a historical perspective. *Am J Prev Med*. 1995;6(Suppl):6–8.

12. Studnicki J, Steverson B, Blais H, et al. Analyzing organizational practices in local health departments. *Public Health Rep*. 1994;109(4):485–90.

13. Harrell JA, Baker EL. The essential services of public health. *Leadership Public Health*. 1994;3(3):27–30.

14. Eilbert K, Barry M, Bailek R, et al. Public health expenditures: developing estimates for improved policy making. *J Public Health Manage Pract*. 1997;3(3):1–9.

15. Scott H. The future of public health: a survey of states. *J Public Health Policy*. 1990;11(3):296–304.

16. Scutchfield F, Beversdof C, Hiltabiddle S, et al. A survey of state health department compliance with the recommendations of the Institute of Medicine report, The Future of Public Health. *J Public Health Policy*. 1997;18(2):13–29.

17. Bettcher D, Sapirie S, Goon E, et al. Essential public health functions: results of the international Delphi Study. *World Health Stat Q*. 1998;51:44–55.

18. McGinnis J. Objectives-based strategies for disease-prevention. In: Holland W, Detels R, Knox G, eds. 2nd ed. *Oxford Textbook of Public Health*. New York: Oxford University Press; 1991:127–144.

19. Chapel T. Private sector health care organizations and essential public health services: potential effects on the practice of local public health. *J Public Health Manage Pract*. 1999;4(1):36–44.

20. U.S. Department of Health and Human Services, Office of Disease Prevention and Health Promotion. *Healthy People 2010*, focus area 23, public health infrastructure. Available at: http://www.cdc.gov/nchs/healthy_people/hp2010/focus_areas/fa23_phi2.htm. Accessed February 11, 2013.

21. U.S. Department of Health, Education, and Welfare. *Healthy People: The Surgeon General's Report on Health Promotion and Disease Prevention*. Washington, DC: U.S. Government Printing Office (PHS) 79-55071; 1979.

22. U.S. Department of Health and Human Services. *Promoting Health/Preventing Disease: Objectives for the Nation*. Washington, DC: U.S. Government Printing Office; 1980.

23. U.S. Department of Health and Human Services, Public Health Service. *Healthy People 2000: National Health Promotion and Disease Prevention Objectives*. Washington, DC: U.S. Government Printing Office (PHS) 91-50212; 1991.

24. U.S. Department of Health and Human Services, Office of Disease Prevention and Health Promotion. *Healthy People 2010*. Available at: http://www.healthypeople.gov/2010/Implementation/slides/HP_Steps_03262004_files/frame.htm. Accessed January 13, 2012.

25. U.S. Department of Health and Human Services, Office of Public Health and Science. *Healthy People 2010 Objectives, Draft for Public Comment*. Washington, DC: U.S. Government Printing Office; 1998.

26. Centers for Disease Control and Prevention. Tobacco use: targeting the nation's leading killer. Available at: http://www.cdc.gov/chronicdisease/resources/publications/aag/pdf/tobacco.pdf. Accessed February 7, 2013.

27. Baxter R. The roles and responsibilities of local public health systems in urban health. *J Urban Health*. 1998;75(2):322–9.

28. Fox D. Accretion, reform, and crisis: a theory of public health politics in New York City. *Yale J Biol Med*. 1991;64:455–66.

29. Turning Point. Mission statement. Available at: http://www.turningpointprogram.org/Pages/about.html. Accessed January 31, 2013.

30. Patrick D, Wickizer T. Community and health. In: Amick B, Levine S, Tarlov A, et al., eds. *Society and Health*. New York: Oxford Press; 1995:46–92.

31. Stoto M, Abel C, Dievler A, eds. *Healthy Communities: New Partnerships for the Future of Public Health*. Washington, DC: Institute of Medicine; 1996.

32. Baker E, Melton R, Stange P, et al. Health reform and the health of the public. *JAMA*. 1994;272(16): 1276–82.

33. U.S. Department of Health and Human Services. PPHF 2012 Community Transformation Grant. Available at: http://www.hhs.gov/open/recordsandreports/prevention/solicitations/ppfh_2012_com_trans_grnt.html. Accessed February 7, 2013.

34. Whitelaw N, Warden G, Wenzler M. Current efforts toward implementation of an urban health strategy: the Henry Ford Health System. *J Urban Health*. 1998;75(2):356–66.

35. The Henry Ford Health System. Facts and figures. Available at: http://www.henryfordhealth.org/body.cfm?id=38768. Accessed February 7, 2013.

36. NIST Baldrige Performance Excellence Program. Four U.S. organizations honored with the 2011 Baldrige National Quality Award. Available at: http://www.nist.gov/baldrige/baldrige_recipients2011.cfm. Accessed February 7, 2013.

37. Parkland Health and Hospital System. Who we are. Available at: http://www.parklandhospital.com/whoweare/at_a_glance/index.html. Accessed February 7, 2013.

38. Anderson R, Pickens S, Boumbulian P. Toward a new urban health model: moving beyond the safety net to save the safety net—resetting priorities for health communities. *J Urban Health*. 1998;75(2):367–78.

39. Reiser S. Medicine and public health. *JAMA*. 1996;276(17):1429–30.

Additional Resources

Emerson H. *Local Health Units for the Nation*. New York: The Commonwealth Fund; 1945.

Jekel J. Health departments in the US, 1920–1988: statements of mission with special reference to the role of C. E. A. Winslow. *Yale J Biol Med*. 1991;64:467–479.

American Public Health Association. An official declaration of attitude of the American Public Health Association on desirable standard minimum functions and suitable organization of health activities. *Am J Public Health Yearbook*. 1933:6–11.

Mountin JW. Distribution of health services in the structure of state government. *Public Health Rep*. 1941;34:1674–1698.

Terris M, Kramer N. Medical care activities of full-time health departments. *Am J Public Health*. 1949;39:1129–1135.

Miller A, Moos MK. *Local Health Departments: Fifteen Case Studies*. Washington, DC: American Public Health Association; 1981.

Meyers B, Steinhardt BJ, Mosley ML, et al. The medical care activities of local health units. *Public Health Rep*. 1968;83:757–769.

Grason HA, Guyer B. *Public MCH Program Functions Framework: Essential Public Health Services to Promote Maternal and Child Health in America*. Baltimore, MD: Johns Hopkins University; 1995.

Grason HA. Use of MCH functions framework as a tool for strengthening public health practice. *J Public Health Manage Pract*. 1997;3(5):14–15.

Wilcox L. Important directions in public health surveillance and community-based research in maternal and child health: a CDC perspective. *J Public Health Manage Pract*. 1997;3(5):17–19.

Gerzoff R. Comparisons: the basis for measuring public health performance. *J Public Health Manage Pract*. 1997;3(5):20–21.

Scutchfield F. Compliance with the recommendations of the Institute of Medicine report, The Future of Public Health: a survey of local health departments. *J Public Health Policy*. 1997;18(2):155–166.

US Department of Health and Human Services, Centers for Disease Control and Prevention. *Healthy People 2000 Review*. Washington, DC: US Government Printing Office (PHS) 99-1256; 1998–1999.

Keppel KG, Percy JN, Klein RJ. *Measuring progress in Healthy People 2010*. In: Statistical Notes 25. Hyattsville, MA: National Center for Health Statistics; 2004.

US Department of Health and Human Services. *Healthy People 2010.* Available at: http://www.healthypeople .gov/2010/Implementation/slides/HP_Steps_03262004_files/frame.htm. Accessed October 10, 2012.

US Department of Health and Human Services. *Healthy People 2010.* Progress review, nutrition and over-weight. Public Health Service, 2004. Available at: http://www.healthypeople.gov/2010/Implementation /slides/HP_Steps_03262004_files/frame.htm.

US Department of Health and Human Services. *Healthy People 2010.* Progress review, public health infra-structure. Public Health Service, 2004. Available at: http://www.healthypeople.gov/Data/2010prog /focus23/.

Omenn G. What's behind those block grants in health? *N Engl J Med.* 1982;306(17):1057–1060.

Wall S. Transformations in public health systems. *Health Affair.* 1998;17(3):64–80.

Lumpkin J. Impact of Medicaid resources on core public health responsibilities of local health depart-ments in Illinois. *J Public Health Manage Pract.* 1998;4(6):69–78.

Parkland Health and Hospital System. Who we are. Available at: http://www.parklandhospital.com /index.html. Accessed November 5, 2012.

Fee E. *The origins and development of public health in the US.* In: Holland W, Detels R, Knox G, et al., eds. *Oxford Textbook of Public Health.* New York: Oxford University Press; 1991:3–22.

Viseltear A. The ethos of public health. *J Public Health Policy.* 1990;11(2):146–150.

Fee E. Public health and the state: the United States. *Clio Medica.* 1994;26:224–275.

Lasker R. *Medicine & Public Health: The Power of Collaboration.* New York: New York Academy of Medi-cine; 1997.

Duffy J. The American medical profession and public health: from support to ambivalence. *Bull Hist Med.* 1979;53:1–22.

Council on Scientific Affairs. The IOM report and public health. *JAMA.* 1990;264(4):508–509.

Organization of the Public Health System

Glen P. Mays and Alene Kennedy-Hendricks[*]

LEARNING OBJECTIVES

- To distinguish the major roles of federal, state, and local governmental entities, as well as nongovernmental organizations, in creating and implementing public health policies and programs
- To identify the responsibilities of the major federal agencies composing the public health infrastructure
- To recognize new trends in oversight of public health programs
- To be familiar with the different types of administrative relationships that states have with local health departments
- To define a local health department and its key functions and responsibilities

---

Chapter Overview

A complex array of institutions supports the delivery of public health services in the United States. Both governmental and private organizations factor prominently in the nation's public health system, yet there is no definitive division of labor among the institutions that make up this system. This chapter examines the defining organizational and structural characteristics of the public health delivery system in the United States. Effective management of public health services in any setting requires a thorough understanding of these basic structural elements.

---

[*]Glen P. Mays is the author of the original chapter, published in 2008. Revisions to the text were contributed by Alene Kennedy Hendricks in 2012.

The practice of public health in the United States encompasses a broad and evolving scope of activities. Governmental agencies often play leading roles in the public health system, and their responsibilities flow in part from the federalist system of government that defines federal, state, and local governmental authority. Additionally, in many communities, nongovernmental organizations contribute substantially to public health activities, including private physicians, hospitals, and other healthcare providers; professional and civic associations; educational institutions; philanthropic and charitable organizations; health insurers; and private businesses. In fact, many public health activities are implemented through the cooperative efforts of multiple organizations. The organizational landscape of public health activities varies widely across communities and is shaped by the confluence of public priorities and values, available health resources and financing mechanisms, specific political processes and interest groups, and unique historical and environmental conditions.

This chapter examines the defining organizational and structural characteristics of public health activities in the United States. We define a public health system as the constellation of organizations, both governmental and private, that contribute to the delivery of core public health services for a defined population. In some communities these systems are well defined and coordinated, but in other communities the systems are fragmented and diffused. The effective management of public health programs, services, and organizations in any setting requires a thorough understanding of these systems and their structural characteristics.

Governmental Public Health Organizations

Governmental responsibilities in public health evolve in response to public needs and demands as well as political will. Economic theory has long provided a rationale for decisions concerning the most appropriate governmental roles in public health service delivery. Those services that represent public goods or that generate positive externalities are likely to be underproduced by the private marketplace despite the fact that such services are beneficial to society at large. Governmental involvement in the provision of these types of services is therefore essential for social wellbeing.[1] Public health services that promote clean air and water and safe food produce health benefits for large segments of the community, and it is difficult if not impossible to exclude individuals from benefiting from these services. Services are regarded as having positive externalities when they produce benefits that can be enjoyed even by those individuals not directly involved in producing or using the services.

The organization of governmental public health activities in the United States flows directly from the limited federalist system of government based on national, state, and local levels of authority. States occupy pivotal positions within this system because they maintain governmental authority that is not expressly reserved for the federal government through constitutional provisions and legislative power. States, in turn, choose whether to exercise this authority directly or delegate it to local governmental bodies in accordance with state constitutional and legislative provisions. In the domain of public health, the federal government exercises authority primarily through its constitutional powers to tax, spend, and regulate interstate commerce.[2] By comparison, state government agencies typically play even larger roles in public health regulatory activities while also carrying out substantial responsibilities in public health program administration and **resource allocation**. States often delegate to local governmental agencies the primary responsibilities for implementing public health programs within communities. States vary markedly in the scope of public health activities that they delegate to local governmental control.[3,4] Specific organizational structures used to support public health activities at federal, state, and local levels are examined in the following sections.

Federal Agencies Contributing to Public Health

Federal agencies are important actors in the public health arena because of their ability to formulate and implement a national health policy agenda and to allocate health resources across broad public priorities.[5] Both executive agencies and legislative institutions engage in federal health policy and resource-allocation activities. As part of the policy development and administration process, many federal health agencies provide information and technical assistance to state and local agencies as well as nongovernmental organizations.[6] In some cases, federal agencies also engage directly in implementing public health activities within specific communities or populations. Direct federal involvement in public health practice typically occurs only for narrowly defined public health activities such as the investigation and control of major health threats, the study of new interventions, or the response to major disasters and emergencies. A 2006 study found that federal agencies were directly involved in implementing public health activities in 61% of the largest local public health jurisdictions, an increase from 44% in 1998.[7] However, in those jurisdictions, federal agencies contributed to only 12% of the core public health activities. Increased federal involvement may be related to rising alarm about bioterrorist threats, emerging infectious diseases, and escalating rates of obesity.[7]

Federal agencies undertake public health activities using a variety of policy and administrative instruments. Agencies that are part of the executive branch of federal government use instruments that include regulatory development and enforcement, resource allocation, information production and dissemination, and policy advocacy and agenda setting. The specific set of policy instruments used by a given agency for a given public health issue depends on the authority granted to the agency by Congress, as well as the administrative and political environment in which the agency operates.

Federal Policy and Administrative Instruments for Public Health

Regulatory Development and Enforcement

Federal agencies receive their regulatory power either through congressional legislation or, less frequently, through presidential executive order. Often their authority involves a directive to establish the administrative procedures and infrastructure necessary to enforce a specific regulatory provision enacted by Congress. For example, the Patient Protection and Affordable Care Act (ACA) of 2010 charges the U.S. Department of Health and Human Services (HHS) with enforcing new provisions related to governmental insurance plans, as well as overseeing states' enforcement of the new regulations that apply to private plans.[8] Alternatively, federal agencies may be empowered to develop standards and regulations within a broad domain of activity, subject to a public review and evaluation process. Many of the environmental health regulations enforced by the U.S. Environmental Protection Agency (EPA), for example, are developed by the agency itself under broad regulatory authority established by federal laws such as the National Environmental Policy Act of 1970 and the Clean Water Act of 1972.

In the domain of public health, federal health agencies make relatively limited use of regulatory powers. The most active federal regulatory activities occur in the areas of food protection, drug and device development, occupational health and safety, and environmental health protection. For example, federal regulations concerning the manufacture, processing, and labeling of food products are carried out as consumer protection activities through agencies such as the U.S. Food and Drug Administration (FDA) and the U.S. Department of Agriculture (USDA).

By comparison, the federal government historically has been reluctant to engage in regulatory activities in the field of medical practice and healthcare financing—preferring to delegate these tasks to state agencies and to the health professions themselves. However, federal involvement in this area has increased in recent years as concern has grown regarding the quality and cost of medical care and health insurance.[9,10] In 2010, President Barack Obama signed the ACA, arguably the most significant reform of the U.S. healthcare system since the establishment of the Medicare and Medicaid programs in 1965. This law requires insurance plans to cover children on their parents' plans up to the age of 26, prohibits denial of coverage for preexisting conditions, specifies the minimum percentage of premiums that insurance plans must spend on health care (rather than on marketing or profits), as well as a number of other new regulations of the insurance market and healthcare system.[11]

Health Resource Allocation

Another powerful public health instrument wielded by federal agencies derives from the federal government's power to tax and to spend. Most federal public health programs are carried out through financial and technical support provided to state and local public health organizations. Federal agencies allocate financial resources through two principal avenues: **categorical grants-in-aid** and **block granting**. Categorical grant programs are targeted at specific public health services and population groups; block grants allocate financial resources to broad domains of activity that are largely determined by the grant recipients. All block grants and many categorical grants are allocated exclusively to state governments, which are charged with disbursing funds appropriately to specific programs and providers. Categorical grants allow federal agencies to exercise more control over how public health funds are spent than do block grants, which allow greater levels of state discretion in resource use.

Categorical and Block Grant Programs.   Categorical grants are often criticized as a resource-allocation vehicle for their tendency to encourage public health organizations to operate in accordance with federal funding streams rather than in accordance with needs and priorities in the populations served. Block grants are often viewed as a strategy for preventing poorly targeted resource allocation. Critics of block grant strategies argue, however, that these funding vehicles may allow important but low-visibility programs and health needs—including many public health services—to be deemphasized in times of financial crisis. Nevertheless, block grants remain important components of federal health financing and include the Preventive Health and Health

Services Block Grant, the Maternal and Child Health Block Grant, the Community Mental Health Services Block Grant, and the Substance Abuse Prevention and Treatment Block Grant.

Entitlement and Discretionary Programs.   Several of the largest federal categorical grant-in-aid programs in the domain of public health confer program benefits to broad classes of individuals and therefore constitute **entitlement programs**. Two of these programs—Medicaid and the State Children's Health Insurance Program (SCHIP)—provide funds to states for the purchase of healthcare services for low-income families and children. Although most of the outlays for these programs fund the delivery of medical care, these programs are also important sources of financing for public health services. The **Medicaid** program, for example, finances the delivery of clinical preventive services, prenatal care, case management services, communicable disease screening and treatment services, family planning services, and childhood developmental screening services. These programs function as entitlements because funds are allocated to states in amounts based on a proportion of the expenditures incurred by states in serving eligible recipients. Funding levels are therefore determined by program eligibility and utilization, rather than by explicit policy decisions concerning the allocation of federal resources to specific program areas.

Most other grant-in-aid programs that support public health activities are **discretionary programs** that operate through a fixed appropriation of federal revenue that is subject to periodic updates, adjustments, and revisions. Discretionary programs are generally much more sensitive to political bargaining and governmental financing obligations than are entitlement programs. As a result, many of these programs experience periodic fluctuations in funding levels and scope of authority as they come due for reauthorization and appropriation decisions in Congress. A prominent example of a federal discretionary program in public health is the Preventive Health and Health Services Block Grant, administered by the U.S. Centers for Disease Control and Prevention (CDC). Through grants to state health agencies, the CDC supports programs in heart disease and stroke prevention, cancer early detection, nutrition, physical fitness, and other areas.

Matching Requirements.   Many federal grant-in-aid programs include a requirement that grantees contribute a specified amount of nonfederal funds in order to secure federal funding under the program. **Matching requirements** enable federal agencies to secure larger investments in priority areas and also require grantees to share the financial risks associated with investments in public programs—an arrangement that potentially creates additional incentives for the grantee to achieve desirable program performance. Both the Medicaid and the SCHIP entitlement programs include a federal matching component that requires the state grantees to contribute a specified amount of state funds in order to secure federal funds through the program. In Medicaid, the proportion of funds that derive from the federal government varies across states. Under the ACA-mandated Medicaid expansions, the federal government will increase its proportion of funding in order to support the costs of expanding state Medicaid programs to all adults with incomes up to 133% of the federal poverty level.[11]

Competitive and Performance-Based Allocation.   Increasingly, federal agencies are adopting competitive systems for allocating resources to public health activities, including performance-based funding strategies. In one example of this approach, research and demonstration grants are used by federal agencies to develop and test innovative models for public health service delivery that may eventually be suitable for widespread dissemination and use. Under these types of grants, federal agencies solicit competitive proposals from prospective grantees and select those proposals that hold the greatest potential for success while also meeting budgetary and programmatic requirements. If successful program models are identified through the initial set of funded projects, federal agencies may allocate resources to additional grantees for replication and expansion of successful program features.

A good example of this resource allocation approach can be found in the Healthy Start Initiative administered by the Bureau of Maternal and Child Health (MCH) Services within the Health Resources and Services Administration (HRSA). Through a competitive proposal process, the HRSA initially funded 15 community-based projects designed to reduce infant mortality and improve MCH outcomes in communities with high rates of infant mortality and morbidity. After an initial demonstration period, the HRSA awarded additional grants to replicate successful program features in other communities.[12] Many other federal agencies that support public health programs also include competitive features as part of their resource-allocation processes.

More recently, many federal agencies have moved to adopt performance-based resource-allocation systems for public health programs. Under the Government Performance and Results Act (GPRA) of 1993, federal agencies are now required to routinely measure the performance and outcomes of the programs they administer and to demonstrate accountability for the federal funds they use to support these programs. In response, federal funds for public health programs are increasingly allocated on the basis of objective performance measures rather than simply on the basis of need or program potential. For example, states that receive funds under the Maternal and Child Health Services Block Grant report on a number of performance and outcome measures. Each state also develops and reports on additional measures that are unique to their priorities and not otherwise captured by the standardized federal reporting measures.[13,14] This initiative places additional emphasis on the ability of state health agencies to measure public health performance at state and local levels and to demonstrate accountability for federal funds.

In a similar vein, efforts to incentivize greater quality and efficiency on the part of providers caring for Medicare and Medicaid patients have expanded under the ACA. For example, the federal **Medicare** program that provides healthcare coverage for the elderly and disabled populations, instituted a value-based purchasing program in 2011.[15] This program rewards hospitals with higher payments if they perform well on objective measures of quality of care. Conversely, hospitals receive no payment if certain so-called "never events" occur, such as some hospital-acquired infections or foreign objects left in the patient's body postoperatively.

Taxation Authority. The federal government's power to tax not only generates the revenue to fund federal public health programs, but it also provides an instrument for influencing the health-related activities of individuals and corporations. Tax policy can be used to discourage unhealthy activities by raising the effective "price" of engaging in these activities, such as through federal taxes on tobacco, firearms, and products that degrade air and water quality. Similarly, tax policy can be used to encourage beneficial activities such as tax exemptions for employers that provide workers with subsidized health insurance. State and local governments similarly can use their taxation powers to encourage or discourage health-related activities in the private sector, such as exemptions for housing developers that build sidewalks and designate land for recreational use.

Information Production and Dissemination

A third type of policy instrument used by federal agencies involves the production and dissemination of information. In the domain of public health, this information is often produced through federally financed research efforts, surveillance systems, and policy studies. All of the major federal health agencies maintain units devoted to research activities, but the dominant federal agencies for health-related research include the National Institutes of Health (NIH), the Agency for Healthcare Research and Quality (AHRQ), and the CDC. Agencies carry out data collection and research efforts through internal activities and through extramural relationships with universities, professional associations, and contract research organizations. The public health impact of these federal research activities is substantial. For example, biomedical research supported by the NIH leads to the development of new clinical technologies and practices that can be used for health promotion and disease prevention. Likewise, health services research supported through the AHRQ and the CDC produces information about effective strategies for encouraging physicians to deliver clinical preventive services and for encouraging healthcare consumers to comply with screening recommendations. Other federal research efforts produce valuable information regarding the cost-effectiveness of public health interventions in areas such as nutrition, physical activity, and environmental conditions.

The public health impact of federal activities in health information production often hinges on the effectiveness of federal efforts to disseminate this information appropriately. Federal agencies pursue an array of dissemination strategies that includes making data resources available to outside organizations for further analysis and application and informing health professionals and consumers about the implications of new research findings. This first approach is actively used by the CDC, because many state and local public health organizations use data from its surveillance systems to identify public health needs and evaluate the impact of public health interventions at state and community levels. Similarly, many health researchers and policy analysts make use of data from the CDC's numerous national health surveys for scientific investigations of health status, health behavior, and healthcare delivery.

Several federal health agencies also actively engage in educating relevant organizations and individuals about the public health implications of new health information. In some cases, this approach serves as an alternative to the use of regulatory power by federal agencies. Agencies use the quality of the available information, together with the visibility and authority of their federal office, to educate and influence behavior. The EPA, for example, maintains an array of "industry partnerships" through which it encourages voluntary compliance with strategies to reduce the production and release of harmful pollutants. In some cases, it may be the implicit threat of federal regulation or resource reallocation, rather than the influential power of information and education, that encourages voluntary compliance with such strategies. Nevertheless, federal agencies often are able to use the visibility and authority of their offices to draw public attention to important public health issues.

Policy Advocacy and Agenda Setting

A final policy instrument used by federal health agencies in the public health arena involves policy advocacy and agenda setting in the legislative process. The U.S. Constitution's separation of powers doctrine ensures that agencies in the executive branch of the federal government have no formal legislative authority. Nonetheless, these agencies often play important roles in placing public health issues on Congress's legislative agenda and in garnering support for public health legislative proposals at the federal level.[16] These roles are perhaps carried out most frequently by informing members of Congress and their staff about important public health issues using tools such as legislative briefings, testimony, and conferences. Additionally, federal health agencies often participate in the design of model legislation and recruit legislators to sponsor these proposals. Finally, federal health agencies may play roles in garnering legislative support (or opposition) for proposals under consideration in Congress through informal lobbying efforts and direct appeals to professional associations, political interest groups, and members of the public. Through these types of activities, federal health agencies can exert a strong voice in legislative decisions that have implications for public health.

Congress also has its own internal structures for acquiring information about public health programs, policies, and resource needs. These federal legislative agencies play important roles in public health policy development and implementation at the federal level. The U.S. Government Accountability Office (GAO) is known as the investigative arm of Congress, and it conducts policy analysis, program evaluation, and financial auditing activities for all federal agencies and federally funded programs. Most often, these activities are initiated in response to requests from specific congressional bodies or members of Congress. Other federal legislative agencies that perform important functions in the policy development process include the Congressional Budget Office, which examines the effects of current and proposed policies on federal spending, and the Congressional Research Service, which produces summaries and policy briefs on a wide range of policy issues of interest to Congress.

Overview of Federal Agencies with Public Health Responsibilities

Many of the federal agencies that contribute to public health activities are organized within the HHS (**Figure 5.1**). This cabinet-level department in the executive branch of federal government administers programs involving public health services, medical care financing and delivery, mental health and substance abuse services, and social services, including income support and child welfare programs. Several of these agencies within HHS that perform core public health activities are described in the following sections.

The CDC

As the federal government's lead public health agency, the CDC administers a range of programs designed to prevent and control specific disease, injury, and disability risks on a national level

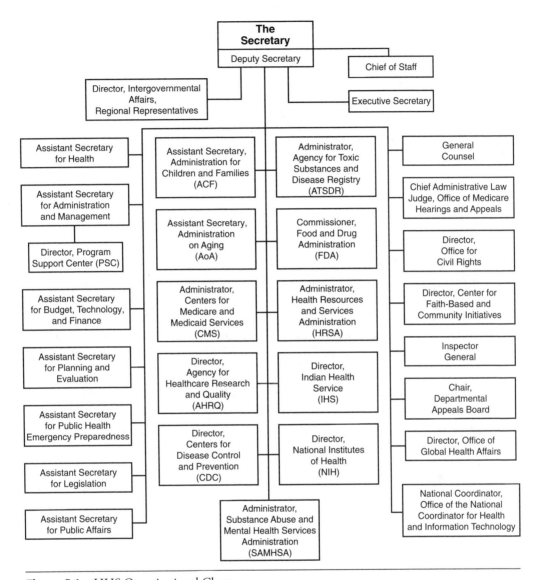

Figure 5.1   HHS Organizational Chart
Source: Reproduced from the U.S. Department of Health and Human Services. (2012). U.S.
Department of Health and Human Services Organizational Chart. US DHHS website. [Online]
Available at: http://www.hhs.gov/about/orgchart/.

through epidemiologic surveillance and investigation, research, and program development and
dissemination activities. The CDC carries out this mission with a full-time staff of more than
9,000 and an annual budget that totals $6 billion (fiscal year [FY] 2012). The CDC maintains
a strong intramural research program that uses state-of-the-art laboratory and field resources to
examine a wide range of public health threats. Additionally, the CDC maintains an extensive
extramural research program that involves a broad network of university-based research centers.

Historically, the CDC's research and development initiatives have emphasized laboratory and epidemiologic methods for investigating disease transmission, control, and prevention mechanisms. In recent decades, the CDC's scientific agenda in public health has grown to include an expanded emphasis on the behavioral and social sciences in studying public health issues such as the adoption and diffusion of prevention practices among healthcare providers and populations at risk, the cost-effectiveness of community-level interventions such as health education campaigns, and the adequacy of state and local public health infrastructure.

The CDC underwent significant structural changes in 2005 and 2009. Currently, three coordinating offices at the CDC oversee many of the individual centers and institutes that are organized around specific disease processes and intervention opportunities (**Figure 5.2**).[17] The Office of Surveillance, Epidemiology, and Laboratory Services houses the following centers:

- The National Center for Health Statistics functions as the nation's public health data repository by fielding national surveys of health status, health behavior, and healthcare practices and by maintaining vital and health statistics databases. Among the periodic national surveys and surveillance systems fielded by the center are the National Health Care Survey, the National Immunization Survey, the National Health Interview Survey, and the National Health and Nutrition Examination Survey. The center also maintains efforts for tracking national statistics on prenatal care, births, and deaths through the National Vital Statistics System.
- The Office of Public Health Genomics supports an improved understanding of human genomic discoveries and how they can be used to improve public health and prevent disease.
- The Public Health Surveillance and Informatics Program Office supports public health surveillance programs and the use of informatics and IT tools in sharing information relevant to public health and preparedness.
- The Epidemiology and Analysis Program Office promotes the use of epidemiologic methods, systematic literature reviews, and other analytic methods in public health practice and decision making. It also oversees the publication of the *Morbidity and Mortality Weekly Report (MMWR)*, a major avenue through which the CDC disseminates up-to-date information to public health professionals.

The Office of Noncommunicable Diseases, Injury and Environmental Health oversees the following centers:

- The National Center for Injury Prevention and Control designs and fields research and intervention programs that focus on the prevention of both unintentional and intentional injuries occurring outside the workplace.
- The National Center for Environmental Health/Agency for Toxic Substances and Disease Registry fields research and intervention efforts designed to forestall illness, disability, and death due to human interaction with harmful environmental substances.
- The National Center for Chronic Disease Prevention and Health Promotion fields research and development activities involving chronic disease prevention and early intervention for health issues such as cancer, cardiovascular disease, diabetes, and the special health

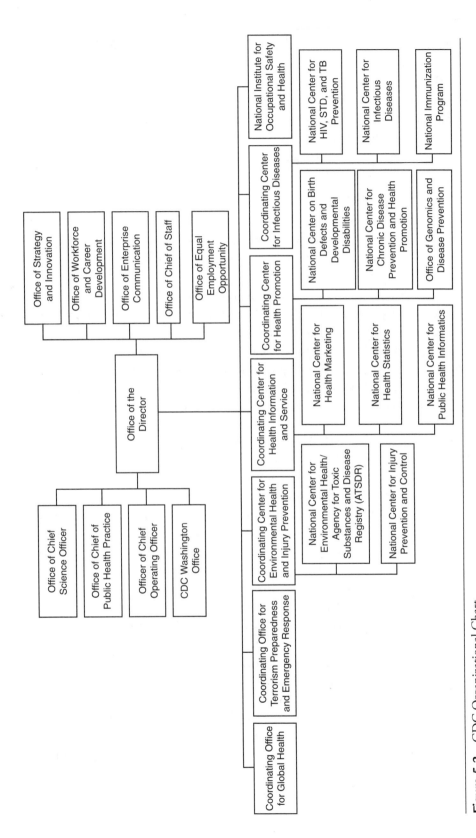

Figure 5.2 CDC Organizational Chart

Source: Reproduced from the Centers for Disease Control and Prevention. (2013). Department of Health and Human Services Centers for Disease Control and Prevention (CDC) Chart. [Online] Available at: http://www.cdc.gov/maso/pdf/CDC_Chart_wNames.pdf.

concerns of maternal and child populations. This center also fields the Behavioral Risk Factor Surveillance System, which collects periodic national and state-level data on adult health risk factors.

- The National Center on Birth Defects and Developmental Disabilities provides national leadership for preventing birth defects and developmental disabilities and for improving the wellbeing of people with disabilities.

The Office of Infectious Diseases includes the following centers:

- The National Center for HIV/AIDS, Viral Hepatitis, STD, and TB Prevention administers surveillance and disease prevention and control programs that target the transmission of the serious and often interrelated communicable diseases of human immunodeficiency virus (HIV), viral hepatitis, other sexually transmitted diseases (STDs), and tuberculosis (TB).
- The National Center for Emerging and Zoonotic Infectious Diseases sponsors research and program development activities designed to prevent and control a wide array of existing, emerging, zoonotic, and resurgent infectious diseases.
- The National Centers for Immunization and Respiratory Diseases oversees national and state-based efforts to expand age-appropriate vaccination coverage rates for children, adolescents, and adults. This agency has been heavily involved in the development of immunization registries and tracking systems at the provider, community, and state levels.

In addition, the National Institute for Occupational Safety and Health (NIOSH) supports scientific investigations of workplace health threats and designs prevention and control programs to improve safety and wellness and reduce health risks within occupational settings.[17] While many of the aforementioned entities address significant domestic public health priorities, the Center for Global Health supports the role of the CDC in global health activities, collaborating with international organizations and national ministries of health.

Among all of the federal health agencies, the CDC is the most heavily invested in intergovernmental relationships with state and local public health organizations. Many of the CDC's initiatives in disease surveillance and control depend on activities carried out by state public health agencies and their affiliated local health departments. For example, the National Notifiable Diseases Surveillance System and the Behavioral Risk Factor Surveillance System depend on data that are collected and reported by state and local agencies. Likewise, state and local agencies frequently depend on the specialized expertise and technology maintained at the CDC for activities such as laboratory analysis of newly detected unknown pathogens and control of particularly potent infectious disease outbreaks. To address these mutual dependencies, the CDC maintains a series of efforts to equip state and local public health workforces with the necessary expertise and technology to carry out public health activities of national importance. For example, the CDC assigns trained staff to work in each of the nation's state public health agencies, as well as many local health departments, carrying out disease surveillance and control activities as well as special research and demonstration initiatives. Perhaps the oldest and largest of these initiatives, the CDC's Epidemiologic Intelligence Service (EIS), has placed health professionals in state health departments around the nation since 1951 to carry out 2-year fellowships devoted to epidemiologic investigation. The CDC also maintains a number of workforce development initiatives designed to strengthen state and local public health agency capacities for implementing core public health activities.

Finally, the CDC routinely develops cooperative agreements with state and local agencies as well as professional associations for the development of specific programs and tools to enhance public health capacity. For example, the CDC has worked collaboratively with the National Association for County and City Health Officials (NACCHO), the Association of State and Territorial Health Officials (ASTHO), and other professional associations for more than a decade in developing self-assessment tools for local and state public health organizations, including the widely used National Public Health Performance Standards Program.

Other Agencies of the U.S. Department of Health and Human Services

The CDC effectively functions as the federal government's lead agency for both scientific and practice-based public health activities. Nevertheless, a number of other federal agencies within the HHS carry out critical public health functions that largely complement those of the CDC. These agencies are discussed in the following sections.

Health Resources and Services Administration (HRSA).   The HRSA administers approximately $9 billion (FY 2012) in federal programs designed to expand public access to healthcare professionals and facilities, particularly in underserved areas. The Maternal and Child Health Bureau within the HRSA oversees an array of services and programs designed to increase the timely delivery and uptake of prenatal, infant, and child health services in order to ensure the health of children and their families.

Bureau of Primary Health Care.   The Bureau of Primary Health Care within the HRSA provides funding and technical assistance to agencies that provide comprehensive primary care services in medically underserved areas, including local health departments as well as nonprofit community health centers. The ACA has authorized additional funding for the community health center program to expand existing centers and to construct new centers. The HRSA's Bureau of Health Professions maintains programs for monitoring and improving the accessibility of health professionals within the United States, including the National Health Services Corps, which sponsors professionals to practice in medically underserved communities. The HIV/AIDS Bureau administers funding and technical assistance to programs that provide primary medical care and support services to individuals with HIV and AIDS, and to programs that conduct clinical research on HIV services. Finally, the Healthcare Systems Bureau manages a variety of health resource programs, such as: 1) the Hill-Burton Program to ensure that health facilities funded through the federal Hill-Burton Act meet their obligations to provide adequate levels of free and reduced-fee care to low-income populations, and 2) the federal Organ Procurement and Transplantation Network that coordinates organ and tissue donation activities.

National Institutes of Health (NIH).   The nation's leading agency for funding and administering health research and demonstration initiatives is the NIH. The institutes that compose the NIH conduct intramural as well as extramural research activities in areas of public health importance. The NIH contributes to local public health practice by leading investigations of public health threats, conducting demonstrations of public health interventions, and supporting the public health research interests of local health departments and other community organizations. Consisting of 27 separate research institutes and centers, the NIH is the lead federal agency for biomedical research, and therefore emphasizes both laboratory research and, to a lesser but growing extent, clinical and behavioral research. Medical schools and academic health centers across the country depend on the NIH for most of their research funding because the NIH operates with a total budget of close to $30.9 billion (FY 2012). NIH units with a particular public health focus include the National Cancer Institute; the National Institute of Allergy and Infectious Diseases; the National Institute of Child Health and Human Development; the National Heart, Lung, and Blood Institute; and the National Institute of Environmental Health Sciences. In recent years, the NIH has placed greater emphasis on health equity. In 2008, the NIH held its first health disparities summit and under the ACA reforms, elevated its National Center on Minority Health and Health Disparities to an institute.[18]

Agency for Healthcare Research and Quality (AHRQ).   AHRQ administers a much smaller research enterprise in comparison to the NIH. The agency's sponsored research generally focuses on the organization, delivery, and financing of health services—which includes prevention and public health services but often emphasizes medical care services. Issues of healthcare quality and accessibility are additional research areas with particular relevance to public health activities. The agency is especially active in the development of clinical practice guidelines and strategies for evidence-based clinical practice grounded in sound scientific research. Through its information dissemination activities, the agency maintains strong relationships with major health profession organizations and healthcare financing organizations.

Food and Drug Administration (FDA).   The FDA functions as the nation's largest consumer protection agency by administering regulatory programs to ensure the safety of food, cosmetics, medicines, medical devices, and radiation-emitting products. As specified in the Federal Food, Drug, and Cosmetics Act of 1962 and the FDA Modernization Act of 1997, the FDA's responsibility in drug and device regulation involves ensuring the safety as well as the efficacy of these products. For all of the products monitored by the FDA, the agency ensures accurate labeling, marketing, and consumer information. In carrying out these activities, the FDA inspects manufacturing facilities, tests products, reviews scientific evidence, and monitors labeling and marketing practices. The FDA enforces its regulatory authority through both governmental influence and legal sanction. In addition to encouraging voluntary corrections or voluntary product recalls when problems are identified, the agency can obtain court orders to prohibit the manufacture and sale of products or to seize and destroy products. The agency can also pursue criminal penalties against manufacturers and distributors.

Indian Health Service (IHS).   The IHS administers programs that provide health services to federally recognized American Indian and Alaska Native tribes. This public health service agency provides health services directly and by contract with tribal organizations. As of 2012, federally operated facilities consisted of 29 hospitals, 68 health centers, and 41 health stations. These health organizations provide both medical and public health services to nearly 2 million American Indians and Alaska Natives.

Substance Abuse and Mental Health Services Administration (SAMHSA).   SAMHSA administers programs for the prevention, treatment, and rehabilitation of substance abuse and mental illness. The agency manages two large federal block grant programs that provide states with funds to implement an array of prevention and treatment programs: the Community Mental Health Services Block Grant and the Substance Abuse Prevention and Treatment Block Grant. The agency also maintains an extensive surveillance and research portfolio concerning the quality, cost, accessibility, and outcomes of mental health and substance abuse services for prevention, treatment, and rehabilitation. Finally, the agency is actively involved in providing technical assistance and consultation to mental health and substance abuse service providers as well as promoting public awareness of these health issues.

Several other agencies within the HHS play important roles in public health activities, although their primary area of operation lies outside the functional domain of public health. Prime among these agencies is the Centers for Medicare and Medicaid Services (CMS), which administers medical care financing programs that include the Medicare program for disabled and elderly individuals, and the Medicaid and SCHIP programs for low-income families and children. The ACA expands Medicaid by broadening eligibility to all those under age 65 (and thus, not eligible for Medicare) who also have incomes at or below 133% of the federal poverty level. The CMS programs are important financing systems not only for medical care, but also for public health services needed by vulnerable and underserved populations. CMS exercises only partial control over the design and operation of these programs because individual states have flexibility to modify eligibility standards, program benefits, and delivery and payment mechanisms under these programs.

Because it controls a substantial proportion of the nation's healthcare financing resources, CMS often uses its influence and its purchasing power to effect changes in clinical and administrative practice across the entire U.S. health system. For example, CMS increasingly uses its payment policies to create incentives for hospitals, physicians, managed care plans, and other organizations to engage in quality measurement and reporting activities designed to improve adherence to evidence-based standards of healthcare delivery. The ACA, for instance, contains provisions that encourage hospitals and providers to organize as accountable care organizations (ACOs) that can share with CMS in cost savings if participating providers meet specified quality of care thresholds.[11] CMS also requires healthcare facilities that participate in the Medicare and Medicaid programs to undergo periodic accreditation processes and inspections in order to ensure quality of care in these facilities.

Other agencies within the HHS that contribute to public health activities include the Administration on Aging, which administers social and health services programs for older Americans, and the Administration for Children and Families, which operates programs for the social and economic support of children and families. The Administration on Aging offers programs that address the elderly's health information and education needs; nutritional, social support, and long-term care needs; and safety, injury prevention, and violence prevention needs. By comparison, the Administration for Children and Families' programs that are relevant to public health include the federal Head Start program that provides early educational opportunities and nutritional support to young impoverished children; the Family and Youth Services program that, among other activities, provides health education and counseling services to homeless and runaway youth; programs to prevent and treat sexual abuse among children; and programs that provide health and support services to children and adults with developmental disabilities and mental retardation.

Finally, the HHS maintains several offices at the department level that are designed to coordinate public health activities across the major agencies and units within the department. These offices help the department as a whole to realize opportunities for cross-agency collaboration in addressing major public health issues that span multiple areas of operation and expertise. These offices also help the department to achieve a unified voice in communicating public health issues to the public and other major constituencies in health. The Office of the Surgeon General, perhaps the most widely known departmental office, serves as the nation's leading spokesperson for public health issues. The surgeon general also oversees the U.S. Public Health Service Commissioned Corps, a collection of more than 6,500 federal health professionals who provide first-response intervention in the event of national public health emergencies. The Office of Disease Prevention and Health Promotion works to coordinate federal preventive health programs across the department, including the effort to develop and monitor national health promotion and disease prevention objectives for the nation through the *Healthy People* initiative.[19,20] Several other department-level offices develop policy, public awareness strategies, and research initiatives for major national health priorities, including the Office of HIV/AIDS and Infectious Disease Policy, the Office of Minority Health, the Office on Women's Health, and the President's Council on Fitness, Sports and Nutrition.

Other Federal Agencies with Public Health Responsibilities

A number of other federal agencies are not a part of the HHS but nonetheless contribute to public health activities on a national level. These agencies include the following:

- The USDA sponsors an array of health-related programs involving nutritional support (such as Women, Infants, and Children [WIC]), migrant health, food safety, and the prevention of occupational exposure to pesticides.
- The EPA develops and enforces a wide array of environmental health and safety programs.
- The Department of Housing and Urban Development administers programs to address the health and social problems of populations residing in public housing facilities, homeless shelters, and economically disadvantaged communities.
- The Department of Education maintains programs to address the health education and health services needs of students.
- The Department of Labor administers programs to promote health and safety in the workplace.

These agencies make important contributions to public health activities through the programs and services they administer independently and in cooperation with other federal agencies.

Federal Oversight, Governance, and Advisory Organizations

To understand the organization and operation of federal agencies in the domain of public health, it is necessary to examine the intricate systems for governance, oversight, and advice under which these agencies function. These oversight systems help to shape the policy and programmatic agendas of federal agencies while also ensuring that the agencies remain accountable to the executive and legislative branches of federal government and responsive to the needs of constituents and the public at large. Among agencies organized within the HHS, all programs and services fall under the jurisdiction of the Office of the Inspector General (OIG) for investigations of potential fraud and abuse cases. The OIG also reviews for inappropriate and inadequate financial management practices among state agencies and other recipients of federal public health and health services grant funds.

Programs and services maintained by the HHS agencies also fall under the purview of the Office for Civil Rights for ensuring equal access to programs and services for all eligible population groups. This office is also involved in ensuring that health facilities funded under the federal Hill-Burton Act provide adequate access to free and reduced-fee health services for uninsured and underinsured individuals. Agencies outside the HHS are not subject to these specific oversight mechanisms, but many of these agencies fall under similar review processes maintained by other cabinet-level executive departments.

All agencies in the executive branch of the federal government are subject to the oversight responsibilities of the president. The Office of Management and Budget serves as the president's lead agency for overseeing the programs and activities of the executive branch and for evaluating the effectiveness of agency programs, policies, and administrative procedures. All federal public health research studies and surveillance systems involving human subjects come under the scrutiny of this office, including a review of data-collection instruments. This office is also the lead agency for making funding-allocation decisions within the executive branch and for preparing the president's federal budget requests to Congress. The Office of Management and Budget is also the lead agency for the administration of the Government Performance and Results Act of 1993. In compliance with this program, all federal agencies must submit periodic performance plans, program performance measures, and progress reports to demonstrate the effectiveness and efficiency of federal programs and services. In addition to the oversight provided in the executive branch, federal public health agencies are also subject to legislative oversight carried out by the GAO, described previously.

Federal agencies also make use of a wide array of external advisory committees to help shape their programs and policies in public health as well as in other spheres of activity. Scientific advisory committees consisting of leading researchers and scholars are maintained by agencies such as the NIH, the AHRQ, and the CDC, and carry out a broad mission in public health research and surveillance. Although an independent body, the U.S. Preventive Services Task Force (USPSTF) relies on administrative and technical support from AHRQ to make evidence-based recommendations regarding appropriate provision of clinical preventive services.[21] In addition, scientific review committees are assembled by these agencies to review and evaluate specific proposals for research funding. Review committees are often empowered to go beyond simple advisory activities and play a substantial role in making decisions concerning awards of funding.

Advisory committees made up of healthcare industry representatives and healthcare consumer groups are often empaneled to oversee the regulatory and rule-making activities carried out by federal health agencies. Appointments to these committees are most commonly made by senior officials within the agencies themselves. Although often invisible to external observers, these types of committees can have substantial influence over the organization and operation of federal agencies. These committees often reflect political relationships within the executive branch or between the executive and legislative branches of federal government. For these reasons, knowledge concerning the structure and composition of external governance and advisory committees may be relevant for understanding the roles that federal health agencies play in public health activities.

One final advisory body that provides important assistance in formulating and evaluating federal public health policy is the **Institute of Medicine** (IOM) within the National Academy of Sciences. Congress established the National Academy of Sciences in 1863 to serve as an external source of research, investigation, and advice for any federal agency requesting assistance. The IOM is an independent nonprofit organization that empanels committees of the nation's top scholars and practitioners to study health policy issues and to report findings and recommendations to policy makers, health professionals, and the public at large. The institute has produced many influential studies of public health issues on topics such as emerging infectious diseases, vaccine safety, bioterrorism, and public health performance measurement.

Between 2009 and 2012, the IOM produced a series of three reports exploring ways in which the U.S. public health infrastructure could be strengthened. The first report, focusing on measurement, warned that the U.S. system for gathering and disseminating population health information is not coordinated or coherent, and recommended changes to support information gathering and accountability.[22] Embracing a "health in all policies" approach, the second report recommended updates to current law and policies to promote public health more effectively.[23] The final report in the series described inadequate levels of funding for public health—and population health–oriented activities, and a comparative overemphasis in spending on the clinical system.[24] The work that Congress and numerous federal agencies perform in the domain of public health is aided immeasurably by the independent analysis and expertise contributed by the IOM.

State Agencies Contributing to Public Health

Whereas federal roles in public health consist primarily of national policy development and resource-allocation activities, state public health agencies are responsible for administering specific public health programs and services on a statewide basis. Part of this responsibility requires agencies to carry out the regulatory and policy objectives outlined in federal public health policies, and part of this responsibility requires the development and implementation of new policies and programs tailored to the specific health needs, resources, and priorities within the state governments. State public health agencies are operational in all 50 states, the District of Columbia, and eight U.S. territories. Federal agencies and the programs they administer have a substantial influence on the structure and function of state health agencies; nonetheless, state agencies exhibit marked diversity in their organization and operation due to the historical and contemporary effects of state-specific political, economic, social, and environmental forces. Understanding this variation is requisite for understanding the larger architecture of public health practice in the United States, because state agencies play a pivotal role in shaping the public health activities of local health departments and nongovernmental organizations.

State Health Agencies

The organization of state public health agencies generally follows one of two basic models: a free-standing agency structure headed by an administrator who reports directly to the state's governor, or an organizational unit within a larger superagency structure that includes other functions such as medical care and social services programs.[25] Slightly more than half of the states in the United States employ the free-standing agency model for their public health agency, in which the state agency is a cabinet-level unit within the executive branch of state government.[25] For example, the state of Washington employs the free-standing structural model for its public health agency (**Figure 5.3**). Its Department of Health contains administrative units for core public health functions and is distinct from the state departments that administer medical assistance (Medicaid) and social services programs.

In the remaining 45% of states, the health agency is located within a superagency structure that also includes agencies that administer medical assistance, social services, and sometimes environmental programs.[25] In these states, the public health agency does not occupy a cabinet-level position within the executive branch of government, but rather the superagency provides cabinet-level representation for public health issues along with other issues within its purview. An example of this organizational model is found in North Carolina's Department of Health and Human Services (**Figure 5.4**). In addition to its public health division, this agency contains administrative divisions for medical assistance (Medicaid) and a variety of social services. A cabinet-level secretary of health administers the entire department, and the state's public health director reports directly to the secretary. These two alternative models of state health agency organization offer clear trade-offs in terms of institutional complexity, governmental authority and power, and visibility within the state government bureaucracy.

Regardless of the organizational model used, most states do not consolidate all public health responsibilities within a single governmental agency. Rather, these functions are typically distributed across an array of separate departments and agencies. For example, although most state health agencies take the lead in overseeing environmental health epidemiology and food safety promotion, most do not function as the lead environmental agency.[25,26,27] Rather, typically, a separate environmental agency carries out this authority, often in coordination with the state public health agency. On the other hand, most state health agencies are empowered with the authority to collect health data and manage vital statistics, declare public health emergencies, oversee health professions and health facilities licensing, and maintain programs for children

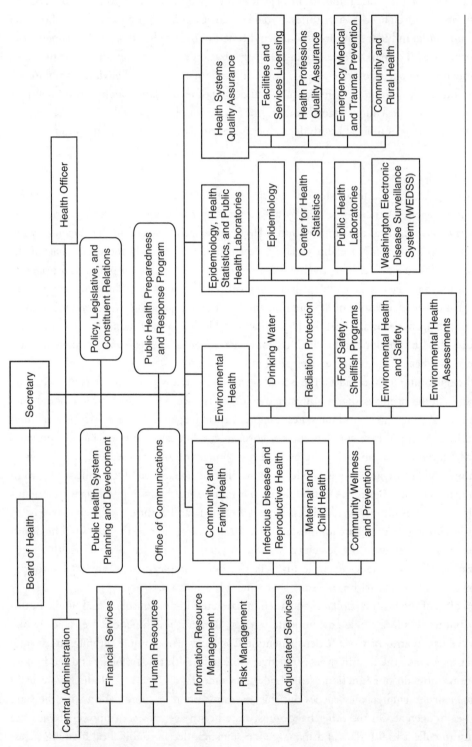

Figure 5.3   Washington State Department of Health Organizational Chart
Source: Washington State Department of Health. Available at: www.doh.wa.gov/AboutUs/ProgramsandServices/OrganizationChart.aspx.

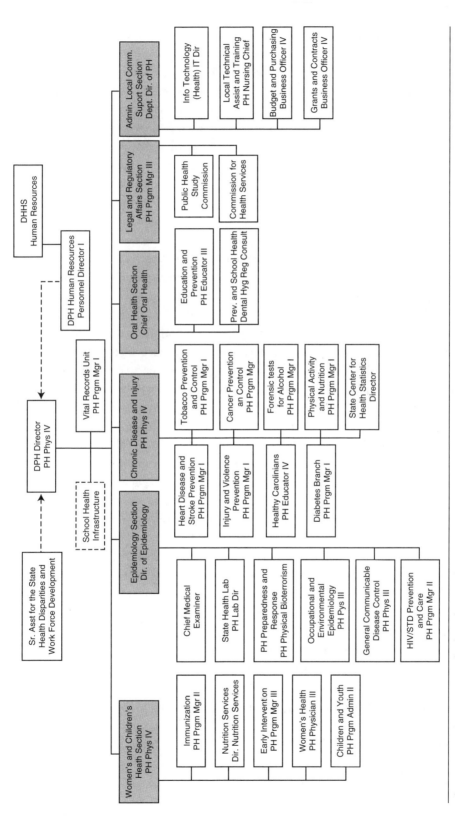

Figure 5.4 Organizational Chart for North Carolina's Department of Health and Human Services Division of Public Health

Source: Reprinted from North Carolina Department of Health and Human Services.

with special healthcare needs. States that distribute public health functions across multiple governmental agencies often rely on interagency mechanisms to achieve coordination among health-related activities that cannot be consolidated within a single agency's authority.[28] Consensus has yet to be reached concerning the optimal organizational structure for a state health agency, as states aggregate and disaggregate their state health agencies continually—usually in response to leadership changes at the governor or cabinet levels.

Over half of states statutorily require the senior health official in the state to have a medical degree.[25] This administrator is appointed by the governor in most states, although a state board of health appoints this official in four states and a superagency administrator appoints this official in nine states.[29] States vary in requirements that appointees be confirmed by the state legislature.[29] State boards of health exist in 26 states, allowing health professionals and often private citizens to participate in the governance of their agency.[29] Nearly half of the 26 states with boards of health allow the boards to have some level of adjudication powers.[29]

A key feature in the organization and operation of state health agencies is the administrative relationship between the state agency and the local public health agencies that operate within the state.[30] This relationship varies substantially from state to state, depending largely on the governmental powers that are delegated to local governments under state constitutions and legislation. State health agencies rely heavily on local public health agencies to implement health policies and programs at the local level, but all state agencies do not have strong and direct administrative authority over the operation of these local agencies. Forty-eight states have statutorily established home rule law in which local governments have some amount of legal authority to address public health issues.[31] With this authority, local governments may adopt their own local constitutions and exercise a broad range of governmental powers usually reserved for states, such as the levying and collection of taxes to support local programs and services.

State health agencies may have less administrative control over the operation of local health agencies that function under home rule authority; in these cases, states rely on other means such as resource allocation and regulatory authority to influence the operations of local agencies.[30] Such decentralized or mostly decentralized administrative relationships between state and local health agencies exist in 27 of the states.[25] In other states and localities where home rule authority does not exist, state health agencies may directly control and operate local health agencies as centralized administrative units of the state, making key decisions regarding agency staffing, financing, and organization.[30] Such centralized administrative relationships exist in 14 states. Several of these states, such as Delaware and Rhode Island, do not contain any local public health agencies and are therefore served only by the state health agency. In other states, like Vermont and Hawaii, the state agency operates regional offices that function as local public health agencies.[29]

Other states operate with a third type of administrative relationship in which local health agencies are subject to the shared authority of both the state agency and the local government.[27] This shared authority model exists in five states.[29] Finally, in the remaining states, state health agencies maintain decentralized relationships with local health agencies in some jurisdictions while exercising centralized administrative control over agencies in other jurisdictions.[29] This mixed authority model predominates among states that extend home rule authority to some local governments but not others.[32]

State health agencies in 28 states organize their jurisdictions into subunits such as districts or regions for the purposes of program administration.[29] In these states, district offices often maintain close working relationships with the local public health agencies that fall within their catchment area. In states without such districts, public health programs are administered centrally. In most states, a county system of government operates at the local level, with state governments relying heavily on this system for the implementation of state programs and services.[25,27] Some state health agencies interact not only with county public health agencies but also with public health agencies organized by other forms of local government such as cities, towns, or special districts.

Other State Agencies Contributing to Public Health

Because of the diversity of ways in which the official public health agency is organized and empowered at the state level, many state agencies other than this official agency may contribute substantially to public health activities. These contributions may be carried out in concert with the official state agency through an array of interagency relationships, or they may be produced quite independently of the official agency. The predominant public health contributors include the following types of agencies:

- Environmental protection—These state agencies are often charged with enforcing federal environmental health regulations in addition to state-specific policies. Jurisdiction over water, air, soil, and waste disposal issues are commonly granted to these agencies, whereas food protection enforcement authority may be retained within the state public health agency.
- Human services—In states without superagencies, the human services department often serves as the single-point-of-contact state Medicaid agency. The administrative separation between Medicaid authority and public health authority is disconcerting to some because Medicaid programs and public health programs serve many of the same population groups and because of the powerful effects that Medicaid financing policies have on public health programs and services. State human services agencies also often administer state programs for mental health, substance abuse, and developmental disabilities services.
- Labor—State departments of labor often administer programs for workforce safety and wellness. These departments may also have jurisdiction over workers' compensation insurance funds.
- Insurance—State departments of insurance maintain regulatory authority over managed care plans and other types of health-insuring organizations. Increasingly, these agencies are called on to establish systems for monitoring the quality, cost, and accessibility of care provided by these types of organizations.
- Transportation—State transportation agencies are substantively involved in traffic safety campaigns as well as policy initiatives designed to reduce mortality and morbidity due to automobile crashes.
- Housing—State housing departments often contribute to public health activities that address the health needs of public housing clients and homeless individuals. For example,

programs to detect and control the incidence of tuberculosis and other communicable diseases among homeless shelter residents have become important state agency functions.

- Agriculture—Agriculture agencies are increasingly involved in public health activities including health interventions for migrant and seasonal farm workers, programs to ensure the safety of agricultural products, and nutritional assistance for vulnerable populations.

- Governor's office—In addition to cabinet-level state agencies, a variety of state offices focusing on public health issues are often organized within state governors' offices. These offices typically serve to attract public and legislative attention to high-priority health issues and to attract external resources to the state for use in addressing these issues.

State Intergovernmental Relationships

A diverse collection of governmental agencies forms the public health infrastructure at the state level. State agency involvement in public health activities tends to focus on statewide program administration and policy development; nevertheless, these agencies are also substantively involved in program implementation at the community level. One survey of the nation's largest local public health jurisdictions found that state agencies were involved in direct program implementation at the community level in nearly all local jurisdictions with at least 100,000 residents.[7] In these jurisdictions, local public health administrators reported that state agencies were directly involved in performing nearly half of the core public health services undertaken within the jurisdictions.[7] The official state public health agency provides leadership and direction for many of these activities, but other state agencies are often key contributors as well.

One increasingly important vehicle of interaction between state and local public health agencies exists in the form of performance measurement activities. State health agencies face both internal and external pressures to measure the products and outcomes of public health activities undertaken within their jurisdictions. In 2011, the Public Health Accreditation Board (PHAB) launched a national voluntary public health accreditation initiative that aims to have 60% of the U.S. population served by an accredited health department by 2015.[33] Accreditation standards are grouped into 12 domains that cover the 10 Essential Public Health Services (defined by the CDC National Public Health Performance Standards Program), management and administration, and governance.[34] The specific measures for these standards and their applicability vary by the health agency's level of jurisdiction (i.e., state, local, or tribal). In addition to PHAB's accreditation initiative, the Association of State and Territorial Health Officials is funding five state health agencies as part of the National Demonstration Initiative on Quality Improvement Practices; this program is intended to help states prepare for accreditation, improve quality of public health services, and manage limited budgets more effectively.[35] These initiatives represent important vehicles for intergovernmental interaction and information sharing in public health.

Increasingly, state legislatures are demanding greater accountability for funds spent on public health and other publicly funded services. Similarly, the federal effort to develop "performance partnerships" with state health agencies as a condition of continued grant funding places additional emphasis on the ability of state health agencies to measure the performance of public health activities at state and local levels and to demonstrate accountability for federal funds.[36]

State agencies also use performance measurement activities to monitor progress toward their own internal objectives for organizational effectiveness and efficiency.

An additional forum for state and federal intergovernmental relations is the professional organization for state health officials, the Association of State and Territorial Health Officials. Consisting of senior administrators from each state and territorial public health agency, this organization serves not only as a forum for professional exchange among the state health agencies, but also as a powerful voice for state public health issues in the nation's capital. The association develops consensus statements, policy positions on a broad array of issues, and model state legislation to assist members in the policy development process. The association also serves as a vehicle for developing and implementing multistate responses to specific public health issues having a regional impact. Through forums such as this association, state agencies obtain a voice in national public health policy development and maintain mechanisms for intergovernmental coordination.

Local Governmental Agencies in Public Health

Local governmental public health agencies retain the most direct and immediate responsibility for performing public health activities at the community level. Their prevalence across the nation varies with the definition used to describe them, but recent studies estimate that about 3,000 local agencies are operational across the United States when defined as "an administrative or service unit of local or state government, concerned with health, and carrying some responsibility for the health of a jurisdiction smaller than a state."[37] The organizational structures and operational characteristics found among local public health agencies are more diverse even than those observed at state and federal levels. Several explanations for this variation are readily apparent. First, the local governmental entities that sponsor these agencies vary widely in their political authority and jurisdiction—including counties, cities, rural townships, special districts, and state governments. Second, local public health agencies vary widely in the size and composition of the populations they serve. Finally, these agencies show marked diversity in the political, economic, social, and intergovernmental environments in which they operate. The structure and function of local public health agencies are in many ways tailored to these community characteristics.

Operational Definition of a Local Health Department

"Governmental public health departments are responsible for creating and maintaining conditions that keep people healthy."[38] The National Association for County and City Health Officials (NACCHO) has defined a **local health department** (LHD) as the public health government entity at a local level, including a locally governed health department, state-created district, department serving a multicounty area, or any other arrangement with governmental authority and responsibility for public health functions at this local level. The functions of an LHD are shown in **Exhibit 5.1**.

There is currently wide variation from community to community in the degree to which the public's health is protected. Standards were set forth by NACCHO to guide the fundamental

Exhibit 5.1   NACCHO: A Functional Local Health Department

A Functional Local Health Department:
- Understands the specific health issues confronting the community and how physical, behavioral, environmental, social, and economic conditions affect them
- Investigates health problems and health threats
- Prevents, minimizes, and contains adverse health effects from communicable diseases, disease outbreaks from unsafe food and water, chronic diseases, environmental hazards, injuries, and risky health behaviors
- Leads planning and response activities for public health emergencies
- Collaborates with other local responders and with state and federal agencies to intervene in other emergencies with public health significance (e.g., natural disasters)
- Implements health promotion programs
- Engages the community to address public health issues
- Develops partnerships with public and private healthcare providers and institutions, community-based organizations, and other government agencies (e.g., housing authority, criminal justice, education) engaged in services that affect health to collectively identify, alleviate, and act on the sources of public health problems
- Coordinates the public health system's efforts in an intentional noncompetitive, and non-duplicative manner
- Addresses health disparities
- Serves as an essential resource for local governing bodies and policymakers on up-to-date public health laws and policies
- Provides science-based, timely, and culturally competent health information and health alerts to the media and to the community
- Provides its expertise to others who treat or address issues of public health significance
- Ensures compliance with public health laws and ordinances, using enforcement authority when appropriate
- Employs well trained staff members who have the necessary resources to implement best practices and evidence-based programs and interventions
- Facilitates research efforts, when approached by researchers, that benefit the community
- Uses and contributes to the evidence base of public health
- Strategically plans its services and activities, evaluates performance and outcomes, and makes adjustments as needed to continually improve its effectiveness, enhance the community's health status, and meet the community's expectations

Source: Reprinted from the National Association of County and City Health Officials. "Operational Definition of a Functional Local Health Department." November, 2005.

responsibilities of LHDs (based on governance, staffing patterns, size) recognizing that each LHD may have specific duties related to the needs of the community it serves. The standards include the following:[37]

1. Monitor health status and understand health issues facing the community.
2. Protect people from health problems and health hazards.
3. Give people information they need to make healthy choices.
4. Engage the community to identify and solve health problems.
5. Develop public health policies and plans.
6. Enforce public health laws and regulations.

7. Help people receive health services.

8. Maintain a competent public health workforce.

9. Evaluate and improve programs and interventions.

10. Contribute to and apply the evidence base for public health.

Organizational Structure

Most local public health agencies are units of county government. A 2010 survey of these agencies indicates that 68% are county departments and 21% are city based.[37] Eight percent of the departments are organized as district or multicounty departments—a strategy used by some small and rural local governments to realize economies of scale by combining their health operations. The remaining departments may serve several cities or serve both a county and a city not lying within that county's boundaries.[37] (Refer to **Figure 5.5**.)

The vast majority of local public health agencies (75%) operate in tandem with a local board of health.[37] These boards vary widely in their structure and function. Most boards contain appointed members only, but nearly one-third includes elected officials as members.[39] In some cases, a preexisting elected body such as a board of county commissioners or a city council serves as the local board of health. Local boards of health are more common among departments serving smaller jurisdictions (less than 75,000 residents). More than half of the local boards perform both advisory and policy-making functions, such as approving the departmental budget or appointing senior administrative officials in the department, for their local public health

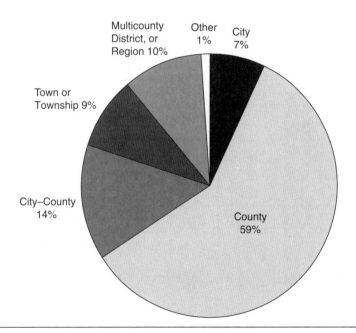

Figure 5.5   Percentage Distribution of LHDs, by Type of Geographic Jurisdiction
Source: Adapted from the National Association of County and City Health Officials. (2010). National Profile of Local Health Departments, Washington, DC: NACCHO, 2011.

agency.[39] In the remainder of cases, boards provide advice to local health departments but wield no policy-making authority.

Nearly two-thirds of the nation's local health departments serve jurisdictions of less than 50,000 residents.[37] However, collectively, these departments serve only 11% of the total U.S. population. By comparison, departments serving the nation's largest jurisdictions—those with more than 500,000 residents—make up only 5% of all local health departments but they serve 49% of the U.S. population. (Refer to **Figure 5.6**.) The remaining departments operate in jurisdictions of between 50,000 and 500,000 residents and collectively serve 32% of the U.S. population.[37]

Scope of Local Public Health Services

The scope of public health services performed by local public health agencies varies markedly across regions and states. These agencies typically adapt their service offerings in order to complement the breadth and accessibility of public health services delivered by other community providers. Nearly all local agencies are involved in communicable disease control activities. A 2010 survey of the nation's local health departments revealed that 92% offered immunizations for children and adults.[37] Nearly two-thirds of the departments offer testing for STDs, and 59% provide treatment services for these diseases.

The delivery of primary care services by local public health agencies has been subject to much debate. While some observe that these agencies fill the needs of vulnerable populations facing financial, linguistic, and other barriers to accessing care,[1,4] others have argued that the delivery of personal health services detracts local public health agencies from their primary mission in

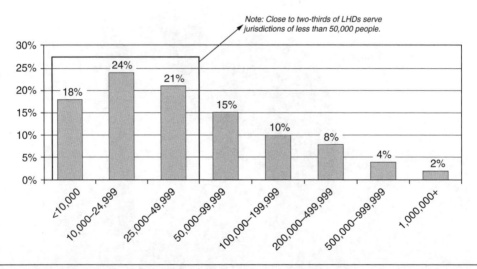

Figure 5.6   Percentage Distribution of LHDs, by Size of Population Served
Source: Adapted from the National Association of County and City Health Officials. (2010). National Profile of Local Health Departments, Washington, DC: NACCHO, 2011.

performing population-based public health services.[40] Nevertheless, the momentum seems to be moving toward establishing a way to coordinate the efforts of primary care and public health, as evidenced by a 2012 IOM report exploring collaboration between these two sectors.[41] Currently, 36% of local health departments are actively involved in delivering well-child care, 30% offer prenatal services, 25% offer home health services, and 13% deliver comprehensive primary care services.[4,37] In the area of health promotion and disease prevention activities, 69% of the nation's local health departments are engaged in tobacco prevention programs.[4,37] Close to 70% of the local departments provide blood pressure screening, 44% provide screening for diabetes, 39% provide cancer screening services, and 39% maintain injury prevention programs.[4,37]

The vast majority of health departments maintain capacities for epidemiologic surveillance and assessment activities. Ninety-two percent of local departments conduct surveillance activities for communicable diseases, while 77% perform these activities for environmental health conditions, 41% for chronic diseases, and 26% for injury.[37] The majority of local health departments are also involved in some type of environmental health protection activity, such as septic system regulation (68%) and lead inspection (48%).[37] Since the late 1990s, some local public health agencies have chosen to privatize the delivery of certain public health activities.[42] Nearly three-quarters of local health departments contract out at least one public health service that traditionally had been provided by the health department.[43] Contracting has become increasingly prevalent for more clinically oriented services, although contracting with outside organizations to provide environmental health services, health education, and community outreach services is becoming increasingly common.[44] The growth of Medicaid managed care initiatives has encouraged this activity in some states because these programs have encouraged larger numbers of private healthcare providers to serve Medicaid recipients and other population groups who historically obtained care from public health agencies.[45]

Staffing and Financing

Local public health agencies are sparsely staffed in comparison to many other types of organizations having a comparable scope and scale of activity.[4,46] Half of the nation's local health departments employ fewer than 18 full-time equivalent staff, and 15% of health departments employ fewer than 5 full-time equivalent staff members.[37] Furthermore, health departments are vulnerable to cuts during economic downturns. From 2008 to 2010, the estimated number of full-time equivalent staff at local health departments fell by around 6,000 nationwide.[37]

Correspondingly, local health departments operate with relatively modest levels of financial resources. The median annual local department expenditures totaled $1.5 million in 2010, and nearly one-quarter of the nation's departments operated on less than $833,000 during that year.[37] On a per capita basis, the median local health department spends $41 per resident per year. Analysis of longitudinal data has shown significant variation in spending by local public health departments across the country.[47] The 20% of health departments with the highest levels of spending have expenditures that are 13 times those of health departments with the lowest levels of expenditures. Varying mechanisms for obtaining revenue may play a role in contributing to these disparities.[46]

The largest share of revenue for local public health agency activities derives from local governmental appropriations, which accounted for 26% of the average agency's budget in 2010.[37] By comparison, these agencies receive 21% of their funding from state government appropriations (excluding Medicaid) and 20% from federal sources (excluding Medicare). More than half of the federal funding received by local agencies comes in the form of pass-through funding controlled by the state government (14%). The Medicaid and Medicare programs account for another 13% and 3% of local agency budgets, respectively.[37] Local health departments obtain the remaining funds from private grants and fees assessed for clinical services, permits, and licenses. (Refer to **Figure 5.7**.) A 15-year longitudinal study of a diverse group of local health departments indicated that fee-based revenue sources have become increasingly important components of local public health financing as direct federal grants have declined precipitously since the early 1990s.[48]

The mechanisms through which local health departments obtain state and local revenue vary considerably.[1,47] In some states, local health departments receive a dedicated share of revenue from a specific financing vehicle collected within their jurisdiction. In other states, most of the state revenue is transferred to local agencies via contracts and grants that are subject to periodic reauthorizations and renegotiations. At the local level, departments may also receive dedicated shares of revenue streams such as property or sales taxes, or they may receive funds through the legislative appropriations processes.

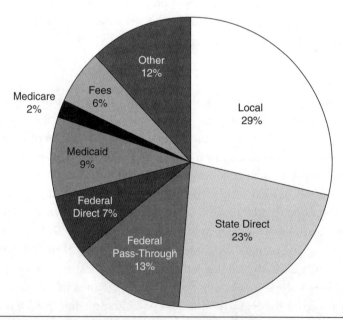

Figure 5.7   Percentage of Total Annual LHD Revenues, by Revenue Source
Source: Adapted from the National Association of County and City Health Officials. (2010). National Profile of Local Health Departments, Washington, DC: NACCHO, 2011.

Regionalization

A major trend since the 1990s has been the increasing regionalization of local health departments. This has been a functional regionalization rather than one accomplished through statutory change. The impetus for this regionalization is that small health departments serving limited populations do not have enough capacity for many specialized public health functions. The momentum toward regionalization has been encouraged by funding of grant programs and bioterrorism preparedness resources in particular. Small counties, by themselves, would only receive a limited disbursement of bioterrorism funds and would not be able to mount many of the necessary components for preparedness alone.

Other Local Governmental Agencies Contributing to Public Health

The official local health department is not the only unit of local government that contributes to public health agencies in a given jurisdiction. A study of public health activities in the nation's largest local jurisdictions (those with 100,000 or more residents) indicated that the average local public health agency directly provides about 40% of the public health activities performed within the jurisdiction.[7] Other units of local government participate in public health activities in 97% of these large jurisdictions, and these other agencies are involved in an average of 51% of all essential public health activities performed within these jurisdictions.

Frequent contributors to public health activities include local social service agencies, elementary and secondary public schools, housing departments, fire and police departments, planning offices, parks and recreation departments, public libraries, public transit authorities, waste management agencies, and water and sewer authorities.[47] These organizations often maintain valuable resources for developing and implementing community-wide public health initiatives such as support staff, specialized expertise, building space and equipment, information and communications infrastructure, and public outreach mechanisms.[7,47]

Nongovernmental Public Health Organizations

Governmental public health agencies are in many cases the dominant institutions within public health delivery systems. These organizations control much of the human capital and financial resources that are dedicated specifically for public health activities within the United States. Nonetheless, nongovernmental organizations play instrumental roles in the production of public health services, both independently and in concert with governmental health agencies. Collaborative activities in medical practice and public health practice became more prevalent during the 1990s as the growth of managed health care encouraged hospitals and physician practices to consider the healthcare needs of defined populations rather than only the needs of individual patients.[49] Other types of nongovernmental organizations maintain a long history of involvement in public health activities such as voluntary associations, philanthropic institutions, and some health professions schools. Some of the most frequent nongovernmental contributors to public health activities are described in the following sections.

Community Hospitals and Health Systems

Community hospitals have long been important contributors to local public health activities. The federal Hill-Burton Program, which financed many hospital construction and capital improvement projects from 1946–1997, required hospitals that used this funding to provide charitable services. As providers of uncompensated acute care services, hospitals continue to play invaluable roles in ensuring access to health care for vulnerable and underserved populations.[50] More recently, hospitals have faced pressures from policymakers and regulators to demonstrate the production of community benefits in order to retain their tax-exempt status. Additionally, the growth of managed care and other cost-containment approaches has created financial incentives for hospitals to engage in public health activities as strategies to encourage greater efficiency in hospital utilization.[47]

Hospitals contribute to local public health activities in a variety of ways. In some communities, hospitals participate in directly providing community health services through such efforts as operating primary care clinics for underserved populations, sponsoring health education programs, and conducting health screening fairs. Hospitals are also major contributors to community health assessment efforts. These contributions are motivated in part by the Joint Commission's decision to require its accredited hospitals to engage in community health assessment processes.[49] In many communities, hospitals wield significant political power through the substantial human and capital resources that they control. Consequently, hospitals can be powerful agents for mobilizing communities around public health issues and for organizing collaborative efforts to address these issues.

Ambulatory Care Providers

Ambulatory care providers also make important contributions to public health in many communities. These providers include private physician practices, community health centers supported by federal, state, and local government subsidies, and community health workers operating out of a variety of care settings. Private physicians often engage in public health activities through local and state medical societies.[47] Medical societies vary widely in the extent of their involvement in public health activities. Some societies maintain only minimal involvement while others are actively involved in designing and operating community health interventions such as free medical clinics, health fairs, and community health assessments. Private physicians may also contribute to public health activities independently, through such diverse efforts as volunteering in community health clinics, serving on local boards of health, or developing service agreements with local health departments for providing reduced-fee care to the uninsured. Additionally, ambulatory care providers often participate in public health surveillance activities by reporting diagnoses of various communicable diseases to the state or local public health agency, which transmits this information to the CDC's National Notifiable Disease Surveillance System.

Community **health centers** provide access to primary care services for vulnerable and underserved populations, and also serve as important sources for health education, counseling, and social support services.[51] These centers include those that receive grants through one of the five federal health center programs administered by the HRSA (community health centers, migrant health centers, homeless health centers, public housing health centers, and school-based health centers), as well as those look-alike health centers that receive support through state, local, or private funding. In many communities, health centers and local health departments develop reciprocal referral agreements and other collaborative arrangements for targeting health services to vulnerable populations.[49]

Community health workers (CHWs) have been defined by the American Public Health Association as "frontline public health workers who are trusted members of and/or have an unusually close understanding of the community served."[52] CHWs serve as liaisons between the medical and public health worlds and the communities in which they work. They conduct outreach, impart health information in more accessible formats, support community members in navigating the health system, and facilitate access to important health-enabling resources.[53]

Health Insurers and Managed Care Plans

Health insurers and **managed care** plans make important contributions to local public health practice in some communities. For some insurers, these contributions are motivated by altruistic missions of community service; other insurers hope to reduce medical care costs or attract new members through their contributions to public health.[54] Insurers are able to communicate with large numbers of community residents and healthcare providers through their extensive membership networks. Some insurers use this capacity to encourage health promotion and disease prevention practices among their members and to create incentives for affiliated providers to deliver appropriate clinical preventive services to their patients. Insurers also participate in public health activities as strategies for obtaining information about community health risks and disease patterns.[55] Other insurers conduct surveillance activities within their own populations of members and contribute this information to public health assessment efforts maintained by other community organizations.

Nonprofit Agencies

A range of other nonprofit organizations engages in public health activities at local, state, and national levels. Prime among these agencies are the local, state, and national chapters of voluntary health associations such as the American Heart Association, American Cancer Society, American Diabetes Association, and the American Lung Association. These organizations implement public awareness campaigns and health education initiatives concerning disease risks and advocate for the public and private support of prevention, treatment, and control interventions. Similarly, social service organizations such as the United Way, the Urban League, and Rotary International are often active in sustaining community-level efforts to identify health risks and to implement community health interventions. Through their active fundraising efforts, these organizations often serve as important sources of local, nongovernmental revenues to fund public health interventions carried out through a variety of organizations. In addition to these national affiliates, many communities are served by locally developed organizations, such as neighborhood associations, parent–teacher associations, church groups and other faith-based organizations, and local environmental coalitions.

Philanthropic Foundations

Important public health functions are also supported by an expanding array of philanthropic foundations and charities. Several large and well established health foundations maintain a distinguished history of supporting research and demonstration initiatives in public health. These initiatives have helped to develop the public health infrastructure at state and local levels, while also building the public knowledge base. Two of the largest and most active national foundations in public health are the Robert Wood Johnson Foundation and the W. K. Kellogg Foundation.

Another type of foundation, which has seen marked growth over the last decade, is the community foundation. Many of these foundations were formed with the proceeds from acquisitions, mergers, and ownership conversions among local hospitals and health insurers.[56] In some communities, these foundations play important roles in developing and financing health interventions, such as health assessment activities and the delivery of uncompensated health care to uninsured and underinsured community residents.

Universities

Universities and other institutions of higher education also make important contributions to local public health practice in many communities. Health professions schools such as schools of public health, medicine, and nursing are perhaps the most common contributors. Faculty from schools of public health often provide technical assistance to local health departments and other community organizations for activities such as conducting disease investigations, community health assessments, and community health planning activities. Additionally, universities may contribute to local public health practice by developing specialized training and continuing education opportunities for local health professionals.

Health professions schools are not the only institutions of higher education that contribute to local public health practice. Other types of institutions—including liberal arts colleges, community colleges, and technical schools—also play important roles in contributing technical assistance, training, and educational expertise to community health interventions.

Other Organizations

A range of other organizations may contribute to public health activities in local communities. In some localities, employers are becoming active in promoting health within their workforces. Employer activities include efforts to reduce worksite health risks, promote healthy lifestyles and behaviors among employees and their families, and assist in the early identification and treatment of diseases. Employers face compelling incentives for engaging in these types of activities given their potential effects on employee productivity and costs incurred for health insurance and workers' compensation benefits.

Other organizations contributing to public health activities include elementary and secondary schools, faith-based organizations, professional associations, labor unions, and other community-based organizations. A national survey found that 83% of local public health departments engaged in partnerships with local faith communities.[57] These organizations vary widely in their involvement in public health issues and in their motivations for doing so. None-theless, their potential for making meaningful contributions should not be overlooked within individual communities.

Interorganizational Efforts in Public Health

Interorganizational relationships have become a widely prevalent approach for improving qual-ity, efficiency, and accessibility in public health as in other fields of practice.[58] Much of the collaborative activity occurring to date among health-related organizations has focused on enhancing performance within individual organizations. More recently, health organizations have begun to expand the scope of their collaborative efforts to address health issues that exist beyond the boundaries of individual organizations.[59] The diversity of organizations contributing to public health activities has also increased since 2000.[60] These collective efforts strive for health improvement within broad segments of the community population, although they also may offer opportunities for individual organizational gain as well. Examples range from coordinated efforts to increase childhood immunization rates within a neighborhood to jointly sponsored programs that provide health care to uninsured populations.[49] These initiatives, termed **public health partnerships** because of their loose and flexible structures, are defined here as coordi-nated efforts among public health organizations to address health problems and risks faced by broad segments of a community's population. The term *partnership* indicates that coordination is achieved through loosely structured agreements between organizations that fall somewhere between the two extremes of ad hoc exchange and a consolidated bureaucracy.[61,62]

The organizational motivations for engaging in public health partnerships are varied and range from economic gain to community health improvement.[59] Consequently, a broad array of organizations—public and private, proprietary and nonprofit—participate in these arrange-ments. For organizations with an overriding mission of public service and community benefit, partnerships offer strategies for achieving an enhanced impact on community health through pooled resources and expertise. Organizations may also face individual economic incentives for participating in public health partnerships. Partnerships may offer opportunities for addressing community health issues that impose substantial financial or administrative burdens on health-care organizations, such as the costs of such preventable diseases as type 2 diabetes and obesity that are faced by health insurers. The financial incentives for collaboration may be particularly powerful for organizations that operate under payment systems that reward efficiency and qual-ity in health services delivery, or that serve significant portions of the population and thus stand to gain from improvements in the public's health.[59]

In its 2011 report on the role of law and policy in public health,[23] the IOM urged a "health in all policies" approach, which envisions health as an important consideration in decision mak-ing by diverse governmental and private actors, not just by those entities considered part of the traditional public health system. This integration of health into other realms of policy may translate into more significant advances in population health than segregated policies that ignore the role other realms play in contributing to population health.[63] This type of approach requires considerable interorganizational and interagency cooperation and collaboration.

Future Outlook

As recent IOM reports have suggested, the U.S. public health infrastructure can be improved upon with additional financial investment,[24] a broadened view of what constitutes public health–promoting policies,[23] and by expanding data-collection capabilities and measurement efforts.[22] For a country with considerable economic and human resources, the United States consistently fares poorly on many important population health indicators in comparison to other industrialized countries.[64] In a time of fiscal belt tightening, our nation's policymakers will have to determine how best to distribute limited resources. The IOM suggests that our expenditures on medical care grossly outweigh what we spend on public health efforts and that increased investment in population-based prevention efforts may avoid some of the need for additional spending on clinical care.[24] Understanding the structure and functions of the key entities forming the public health infrastructure in the United States is imperative to making informed decisions about the direction our country takes in protecting Americans' health.

• • •

This examination of the public health delivery system in the United States reveals the enormous complexity of the system. No clear division of labor emerges among different types of organizations involved; nonetheless, the scale and scope of activity that is produced by the system is considerable. Governmental health agencies factor prominently in this mix of institutions, reflecting the federalist system of government from which they derive. Nongovernmental organizations are also active participants and often leaders in public health delivery at local, state, and national levels. Many public health activities are now carried out not within institutions but between them, through interorganizational and intergovernmental partnerships. The number and variety of organizations that participate in these relationships is encouraging. By pooling the resources and skills of multiple organizations within the community, these efforts offer promising strategies for improving the public health delivery system in the United States.

Discussion Questions

1. Discuss the concept of public health as a public good. What does this suggest about the responsibility for funding and overseeing public health programs?
2. How has governmental oversight of public health programs changed in the last several decades?
3. What are some of the mechanisms through which the federal government funds and oversees state and local public health efforts?
4. How has the CDC's scientific agenda changed in recent years? Discuss what factors you think may be driving this change.
5. What might be some of the benefits and disadvantages of the two major types of state health agency organizational structures?
6. How does home rule authority affect a state health agency's ability to direct public health activities in local jurisdictions?

7. Do you think clinical primary care functions should be distinguished from more traditional public health agency responsibilities?

8. How do nongovernmental organizations contribute to public health efforts?

9. What might be some of the challenges in pursuing a "health in all policies" approach?

10. How do you think maintenance of the U.S. public health infrastructure might be achieved in an era of fiscal restraint?

References

1. Arrow KJ. The organization of economic activity: issues pertinent to the choice of market versus non-market allocation. In: Arrow KJ, ed. *Collected Papers of K.J. Arrow*. Vol. 2. Cambridge, MA: Harvard University Press; 1969:147–85.

2. Gostin LA. *Public Health Law: Power, Duty, Restraint*. Berkeley, CA: University of California Press; 2000.

3. Turnock BJ. *Public Health: What It Is and How It Works*. Gaithersburg, MD: Aspen Publishers; 1996.

4. Rawding N, Brown C. An overview of local health departments. In: Mays GP, Miller CA, Halverson PK, eds. *Local Public Health Practice: Trends and Models*. Washington, DC: American Public Health Association; 2000.

5. Lee PR, Benjamin AE. Health policy and the politics of health care. In: Lee PR, Estes CL, eds. *The Nation's Health*. 4th ed. Boston: Jones and Bartlett; 1994:121–37.

6. Litman TJ. The politics of health: establishing policies and setting priorities. In: Lee PR, Estes CL, eds. *The Nation's Health*. 4th ed. Boston: Jones and Bartlett; 1994:107–20.

7. Mays GP, Scutchfield FD, Bhandari MW, et al. Understanding the organization of public health delivery systems: an empirical typology. *Milbank Q*. 2010;88(1):81–111.

8. U.S. Congressional Research Service, Statman J. Enforcement of private health insurance market reforms under the Patient Protection and Affordable Care Act. Available at: http://www.ppsv.com/assets/attachments/crsreport.pdf. Accessed February 11, 2013.

9. Roper WL. Regulating quality and clinical practice. In: Altman SH, Reinhardt VE, Shactman D, eds. *Regulating Managed Care: Theory, Practice, and Future Options*. San Francisco: Jossey-Bass; 1999:145–159.

10. Moran DW. Federal regulation of managed care: an impulse in search of a theory. *Health Affairs*. 1997;16(6):7–33.

11. Patient Protection and Affordable Care Act, Pub. L. No. 111-148, §2702, 124 Stat. 119, 318–319 (2010).

12. National Healthy Start Association. Healthy Start initiative. Available at: http://www.nationalhealthy start.org/healthy_start_initiative. Accessed February 11, 2013.

13. U.S. General Accounting Office. *Performance Budgeting: Past Initiatives Offer Insights for GPRA*. Washington, DC: GAO; 1997.

14. U.S. Health Resources and Services Administration. Title V Maternal and Child Health Services Block Grant Program. Available at: http://mchb.hrsa.gov/programs/titlevgrants/index.html. Accessed February 11, 2013.

15. U.S. Department of Health and Human Services. Administration implements Affordable Care Act provision to improve care, lower costs. Available at: http://www.hhs.gov/news/press/2011pres/04/20110429a.html. Accessed February 11, 2013.

16. Rochefort DA, Cobb RW. *The Politics of Problem Definition: Shaping the Policy Agenda*. Lawrence, KS: University of Kansas Press; 1997.

17. Centers for Disease Control and Prevention. About CDC: CDC organization. Available at: http://www.cdc.gov/about. Accessed October 1, 2012.

18. National Institutes of Health. Chronology of Events, NIH Almanac. Available at: http://www.nih.gov/about/almanac/historical/chronology_of_events.htm#year2010. Accessed February 11, 2013.

19. U.S. Department of Health and Human Services. *Healthy People 2010.* Conference ed. Washington, DC: US Government Printing Office; 2000.

20. U.S. Department of Health and Human Services. *Healthy People 2020.* Available at: http://www .healthypeople.gov. Accessed February 11, 2013.

21. U.S. Agency for Healthcare Research and Quality. U.S. Preventive Services Task Force. Available at: http://www.ahrq.gov/clinic/uspstfix.htm. Accessed February 11, 2013.

22. Institute of Medicine. *For the Public's Health: The Role of Measurement in Action and Accountability.* Washington, DC: National Academies Press; 2010.

23. Institute of Medicine. *For the Public's Health: Revitalizing Law and Policy to Meet New Challenges.* Washington, DC: National Academies Press; 2011.

24. Institute of Medicine. *For the Public's Health: Investing in a Healthier Future.* Washington, DC: National Academies Press; 2012.

25. Association of State and Territorial Health Officials. ASTHO profile of state public health. Vol. 1. Available at: http://www.astho.org/Research/Major-Publications/Profile-of-State-Public-Health-Vol-1/. Accessed February 11, 2013.

26. Beitsch LM, Brooks RG, Grigg M, et al. Structure and functions of state public health agencies. *Am J Public Health.* 2006;96(1):167–72.

27. Maralit M, Orloff TM, Desonia RA. *Transforming State Health Agencies to Meet Current and Future Challenges.* Washington, DC: National Governors Association; 1997.

28. Kaluzny AD, Zuckerman HS, Ricketts TC. *Partners for the Dance: Forming Strategic Alliances in Health Care.* Ann Arbor, MI: Health Administration Press; 1995.

29. Association of State and Territorial Health Officials. ASTHO profile of state public health. Vol. 2. September 2011. Available at: http://www.astho.org/uploadedFiles/_Publications/Files/Survey_ Research/ASTHO_State_Profiles_Single%5B1%5D%20lo%20res.pdf. Accessed February 11, 2013.

30. DeFriese GH, Hetherington JS, Brooks EF, et al. The program implications of administrative relationships between local health departments and state and local government. *Am J Public Health.* 1981;71(10):1109–15.

31. McCarty KL, Nelson GD, Hodge JG, et al. Major components and themes of local public health laws in select U.S. jurisdictions. *Public Health Reports.* 2009;124:458–62.

32. Beitsch LM, Brooks RG, Grigg M, et al. Structure and functions of state public health agencies. *Am J Public Health.* 2006;96(1):167–72.

33. Riley WJ, Bender K, Lownik E. Public health department accreditation implementation: Transforming public health department performance. *Am J Public Health.* 2012;102(2):237–42.

34. Public Health Accreditation Board. PHAB Standards and Measures Version 1.0. Available at: http:// www.phaboard.org/accreditation-process/public-health-department-standards-and-measures/. Accessed February 11, 2013.

35. Association of State and Territorial Health Officials. Quality improvement. Available at: http://www .astho.org/Programs/Accreditation-and-Performance/Quality-Improvement/. Accessed February 11, 2013.

36. Office of the Inspector General. *Results-based systems for public health programs. Volume 1: Lessons from state initiatives Department of Health and Human Services.* Washinton, DC: Department of Health and Human Services; 1997.

37. National Association of County and City Health Officials. *2010 National Profile of Local Health Departments.* Washington, DC: NACCHO; 2011.

38. National Association of County and City Health Officials. *Operational definition of a local health department.* Washington, DC: NACCHO; 2005:1–9. Available at: http://www.naccho.org/topics /infrastructure/accreditation/OpDef.cfm. Accessed February 11, 2013.

39. National Association of Local Boards of Health. *National Profile of Local Boards of Health, Centers for Disease Control and Prevention.* Washington, DC: NALBOH; 2011.

40. Institute of Medicine. *The Future of Public Health.* Washington, DC: National Academies Press; 1988.

41. Institute of Medicine. *Primary Care and Public Health: Exploring Integration to Improve Population Health.* Washington, DC: National Academies Press; 2012.

42. Halverson PK, Kaluzny AD, Mays GP, et al. Privatizing health services: alternative models and emerging issues for public health and quality management. *Qual Manage Health Care*. 1997;5(2):1–18.

43. Keane C, Marx J, Ricci E, et al. The perceived impact of privatization on local health departments. *Am J Public Health*. 2002;92(7):1178–80.

44. Keane C, Marx J, Ricci E. Privatization and the scope of public health: a national survey of local health department directors. *Am J Public Health*. 2001;91:611–7.

45. Wall S. Transformation in public health systems. *Health Affairs*. 1998;17(3):64–80.

46. Gerzoff RB, Brown CK, Baker EL. Full-time employees of the US local health departments, 1992–1993. *J Public Health Manage Pract*. 1999;5(3):1–9.

47. Mays GP, Smith SA. Geographic variation in public health spending: correlates and consequences. *Health Services Research*. 2009;44(5):1796–817.

48. Mays GP, Miller CA, Halverson PK. *Local Public Health Practice: Trends and Models*. Washington, DC: American Public Health Association; 1999.

49. Roper WL, Mays GP. The changing managed care–public health interface. *JAMA*. 1998;280(20): 1739–40.

50. Nelson H. *Nonprofit and For-Profit HMOs: Converging Practices but Different Goals?* New York: Milbank Memorial Fund; 1996.

51. U.S. Health Resources and Services Administration. What is a health center? Available at: http://bphc .hrsa.gov/about/index.html. Accessed February 11, 2013.

52. American Public Health Association. *Support for community health workers to increase health access and to reduce health inequities*. Washington, DC: American Public Health Association; 2009. Available at: http://www.apha.org/advocacy/policy/policysearch/default.htm?id=1393/. Accessed February 11, 2013.

53. Balcazar H, Rosenthal EL, Brownstein JN, et al. Community health workers can be a public health force for change in the United States: Three actions for a new paradigm. *Am J Public Health*. 2011;101(12):2199–202.

54. Halverson PK, Mays GP, Kaluzny AD, et al. Not-so-strange bedfellows: models of interaction between managed care plans and public health agencies. *Milbank Q*. 1997;75(1):1–26

55. Mays GP, Halverson PK, Stevens R. The contributions of managed care plans to public health practice: evidence from the nation's largest local health departments. *Public Health Rep*. 2001;116 (suppl 1):50–67.

56. Lewin T, Gottlieb M. In hospital sales, an overlooked side effect. *New York Times*. April 27, 1997:1

57. Barnes PA, Curtis AB. A national examination of partnerships among local health departments and faith communities in the United States. *J Public Health Manag Pract*. 2009;15(3):253–63.

58. Kanter RM. Collaborative advantage: the art of alliances. *Harvard Bus Rev*. 1994;72:96–108.

59. Kanter RM. Becoming PALs: pooling, allying, and linking across companies. *Acad Manage Exec*. 1989;3:183–93.

60. Mays GP, Scutchfield FD. Improving public health system performance through multiorganizational partnerships. *Prev Chronic Dis*. 2010;7(6):A116. Available at: http://www.cdc.gov/pcd/issues/2010/ nov/10_0088.htm. Accessed February 11, 2013.

61. Mays GP, Halverson PK, Kaluzny AD, et al. Managed care, public health, and privatization: a typology of interorganizational arrangements. In: Halverson PK, Kaluzny AD, McLaughlin CP, eds. *Managed Care and Public Health*. Gaithersburg, MD: Aspen Publishers; 1998:185–200.

62. Scott WR. Innovation in medical care organizations: a synthetic review. *Med Care Rev*. 1990;47(2): 165–192.

63. Terris M. A social policy for health. *Am J Public Health*. 2011;101(2):250–2.

64. Institute of Medicine. *US Health in International Perspective: Shorter Lives, Poorer Health*. Washington, DC: National Academies Press; 2013.

Professionalism and Ethics in Public Health Practice and Management

Ruth Gaare Bernheim and Elizabeth Fenton

LEARNING OBJECTIVES

- To understand ethics in public health practice as a way to analyze the moral dimensions of and provide justifications for public health interventions and policies
- To gain competence in the use of ethical principles, including public health
- Code of Ethics, and vocabulary relevant to the practice of public health
- To explore public health case scenarios using a framework to analyze ethical issues

Chapter Overview

In their roles as leaders and managers in public health systems and organizations, public health professionals must address increasingly complex ethical conflicts in day-to-day practice. Ethical questions arise not only about the appropriate scope of public health (e.g., whether the focus of public health should include socioeconomic conditions, such as homelessness, and unhealthy behaviors, such as smoking or unhealthy eating) but also about the justification for particular public health interventions (e.g., whether it is ethical to take actions that infringe on the interests of one or some individuals for the benefit of others). Although law provides the foundation for public health authority to act, it is often broadly framed, leaving much room for administrative discretion about when and how to use public health authority. Ethics plays an important complementary role in helping public health officials determine and justify the appropriate course of action.[1]

Adding to the challenge of managing the ethical tensions in public health is the expansion of the concept of the public health system and of the stakeholders who should be involved in the decision-making process. Although the landmark 1988 Institute of Medicine (IOM) report on public health focused on strengthening federal, state, and local government agencies (as they had primary responsibility to protect and promote the health of the public),[2] the 2003 IOM report, *The Future of the Public's Health in the 21st Century*, describes the public health system as a "complex network of individuals and organizations that have the potential to play critical roles in creating the conditions for health."[3] The actors in the public health system include community groups, businesses, and the media, as well as academics, healthcare providers, and many others. This means that public health professionals not only often work in large organizations or agencies, but also are expected to work in partnerships[4] and collaboratively with communities, stakeholder groups, and citizens—who have widely varying values that often shift over time as the political and social context evolves. These complex relationships can give rise to ethical tensions and conflicts as public health managers navigate their obligations to different stakeholders.

Public health ethics is a field of study that can enrich and support real-world public health decision making and management of ethical conflict. It is receiving increasing professional and scholarly attention as public health agencies struggle with issues such as increasingly limited budgets and the allocation of scarce resources in practice, biopreparedness planning, increasing rates of morbidity and mortality due to chronic diseases, and growing evidence of the impact of socioeconomic conditions on health. Recent reports from national public health associations highlight the need for public health officials to develop competencies in public health ethics,[5] and public health leaders have developed a code of ethics for professional practice.[6] Integration of ethics principles and codes into public health leadership and at all levels of decision making within health organizations can contribute to the efforts of health departments to gain accreditation, and will ultimately enhance both the practice of public health professionals and the health of their communities.[7]

The goals of this chapter are to provide an overview of ethics in public health and to present ethics tools, including a framework to guide deliberation about ethical dimensions of public health decisions. Public health managers can use these tools to integrate ethics into the public health agency's regular management activities and to facilitate deliberation about particular cases. A brief introduction to ethics is provided first.

Ethics and the Foundations of Public Health

Ethics as a discipline is the study of right and wrong actions. Ethical theories offer norms or principles of good conduct that aim to guide us about how to live our lives, how to treat one another, and how, all things considered, we should act. In the most basic sense, ethics is concerned with providing guidance on how to live life well, or how to live a *good* life.

Different ethical theories ground these norms and principles in different ideas of what is central to human morality, such as the consequences of actions, the rights and liberties of individuals, or the notion of virtue or good character. The first of these, the set of theories known as **consequentialism** or **utilitarianism**, plays a prominent role in many areas of public and professional life. Consequentialist theories claim that whether an action is right or wrong depends on its consequences—for example, whether it produces a net amount of benefit or utility, whether it benefits more people than it harms, or whether it produces, to use a famous phrase, the "greatest good for the greatest number."

These utilitarian or consequentialist theories are often criticized for focusing on the overall or total amount of benefit produced by an action, rather than paying attention to how particular individuals are benefited or harmed, or how the benefits are distributed among the population. Critics of utilitarianism argue that this view is *unjust*, because it does not respect the individual persons who may be harmed when we act to produce the greatest amount of utility or benefit. Moreover, its focus on the *quantity* rather than *distribution* of benefits may result in distributions that are unfair—because they worsen existing inequities between groups, for example—or they violate other moral principles, such as those based on the rights of individuals.

Because of its focus on populations and its goal of increasing the health of populations as a whole, public health is often viewed as reflecting a utilitarian ethic of maximizing welfare. Many public health interventions are designed to create the greatest health benefit for the greatest number of people, and where there are costs to individuals of those actions, they are considered justifiable by the amount of benefit generated. A good example of this argument is the use of quarantine in a disease outbreak. Although this intervention is a significant cost for the quarantined individuals, that cost is justified by the fact that it will protect the health of many more individuals in the population as a whole. A less dramatic example is mandatory vaccination, where individuals are required to participate in vaccination programs in order for the population as a whole to achieve immunity against infectious disease. Although the law sometimes permits individuals to opt out of vaccination in order to respect the rights of those individuals, it is generally assumed that the majority of people will agree to bear the (very small) risks associated with vaccination in order to serve the greater good of population protection from infectious disease.

These examples are paradigmatic cases of public health interventions in which the goal of maximizing the health of the population is used to justify the inconvenience or limited risk imposed on individuals. Many of the issues in public health ethics concern this fundamental tension between improving population health and respecting individual rights and liberties. But public health also serves another important goal: ensuring that the benefits of interventions are distributed fairly and justly within the population. An alternative view of the moral foundations of public health emphasizes the extent to which public health is concerned with *social justice*—that is, with ensuring that everyone in the population has a sufficient level of health, and with minimizing unjust inequalities in health between different groups.[8] According to this view, what matters in public health is not simply that we produce the most health possible for the population, but that we focus our efforts particularly on those groups who, through poverty and other forms of unjust disadvantage, are less healthy than others. There are many examples of the principles of social justice at work in public health, such as the development of urban green space, efficient public transport, and strategies to address food deserts in low-income neighborhoods, to name just a few. Public health practitioners are increasingly motivated by social justice and the reduction of unjust health inequalities as core values underlying public health activities.[9]

Ethics in Public Health Practice

Public health professionals face numerous ethical challenges in their profession and in their daily public health activities.[7, p. 358] These challenges can arise from at least two aspects of public health practice. First, in their dual role as government officials and health professionals, public health professionals are often confronted with ethical tensions and conflicts that arise from their obligations to a wide range of stakeholders, including individual community members, other health professionals (e.g., physicians), public and private organizations, and the public at large. As government officials, for example, they have obligations to the public they serve and under the police powers authorized to them by state and federal law. The exercise of those powers in the interests of the health of the community as a whole may place them in conflict with other stakeholders in that community.

Second, public health professionals face the challenge of an evolving understanding of the scope of public health and rapid changes in the social and political landscape in which they act. In its mission to protect and promote the health of populations contemporary public health focuses not only on preventing the transmission of infectious disease but on the social environment and upstream social and economic conditions that influence human health. This broader focus is captured in the "healthy people in healthy communities" vision of the U.S. government's *Healthy People* strategy, which aims to improve health and enhance quality of life by exploring the social, behavioral, and political determinants of health in different communities.[10] Public health has also evolved to place a stronger emphasis on chronic diseases, reflecting the fact that in much of the world chronic disease has overtaken infectious disease as the leading cause of death and disability, accounting for 60% of all deaths and 43% of the global burden of disease.[11]

The growing emphasis on the social determinants of health and chronic diseases raises significant ethical challenges for public health officials and for the formation of public health policy. One reason for this is that while the law provides strong authority to public health agents to act to protect the population from direct harm as is the case in an infectious disease outbreak, for example, their authority is more controversial when it comes to protecting people from the causes of ill health related to individual choices and behaviors or social conditions that may be only indirectly related to health. Whereas restrictions on individual liberty and other exercises of state power may be acceptable in the face of infectious diseases, in the case of individual lifestyle choices or broader social and economic policy, these restrictions may be perceived as heavy handed, paternalistic, unjustified, or simply outside the appropriate scope of public health practice.

Moreover, public health interventions aimed at individual behaviors may undermine public health's role in achieving social justice. In the debate over outdoor smoking bans, for example, it has been pointed out that since a much larger proportion of people on low incomes are smokers than is the case in the general population, thus policies that ban smoking in parks and other public meeting places will have a disproportionate effect on the poor, who may be more dependent on public spaces for recreation and social contact.[12]

Addressing these ethical tensions between improving population health, respecting individual liberties, and addressing social inequities requires public health leaders to foster strong relationships with the communities they serve. Ethical decision making can provide an important way to develop and strengthen these relationships, as it is a process that involves not only reflection and analysis by public health officials themselves, but also engagement and deliberation with community stakeholders. An *imaginative* engagement with community members about options for public health interventions, given a shared risk of harm and vulnerability and shared interests in protecting and benefiting health, can help to forge strong community bonds.[13] This is particularly important for activities such as emergency preparedness management, in which effective public health leadership relies not on force but on persuasion and collaboration.[7, p. 359, 14]

Another important strand of ethical decision making in public health is the need to provide the public with justifications for interventions and policies. For many issues and cases in public health there is no "right" answer, and the goal of ethical deliberation is to arrive at what seems to be the most ethically justifiable decision, all things considered, at that time and in a particular context. Even in cases in which public health law authorizes a particular intervention, such as quarantine, those implementing that action are accountable to the public to explain and provide reasons for the decision to implement that action. By providing reasons and justifications for their actions public health officials *express* rather than *impose* community—that is, they do not simply demand compliance, but rather treat the public as partners in a common endeavor.[14, p. 354] Moreover, providing the reasons for a public health decision is an important aspect of transparency, which is crucial for building trust and a willingness to cooperate within the community.[14, p. 357]

Given the religious and moral pluralism in our society, it is inevitable that ethical tensions arise in public health that cannot be resolved without some controversy and without policy justifications. Ethical analysis and justification occur in the "gap" between our knowledge about which actions will improve population health, and the implementation of those actions (**Figure 6.1**). In this gap are the social values, norms, and competing claims of stakeholders that create the context in which public health actions must be assessed and justified. Implementation of publicly acceptable programs and policies requires understanding the competing moral claims in this gap and developing counter claims and policy rationales that resonate ethically with the public at any given time.

Public health ethics provides those in the practice of public health with vocabulary, concepts, and frameworks to analyze the ethical dimensions of cases and policies when they arise in practice, and to provide public justifications for their actions in those cases that are morally challenging and on which there may be widespread disagreement. A deeper understanding of the ethical underpinnings of public health can enrich the work of public health practitioners, encouraging greater transparency about the values implicit in decisions and policies, and helping to define the priorities and boundaries of their work.[15]

In the remainder of this chapter we discuss different approaches to ethics in public health, and a framework designed to guide public health mangers and leaders in ethical analysis.

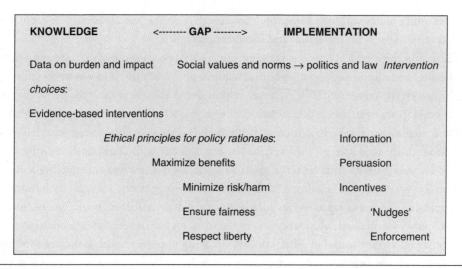

Figure 6.1   The Knowledge-Implementation Gap

Approaches to Ethics in Public Health

There are at least three ways to approach ethics in the practice of public health. These include focusing on: 1) the agent or public health professional, 2) the organization or public health agency, and 3) the action or public health intervention (i.e., reasoning about the right action to take).

An approach to ethics that focuses on the character of the agent, in this case the public health manager, can be traced back to Aristotle, who emphasized the cultivation of virtues. In a contemporary **virtue ethics** approach to business management, Robert Soloman suggests that the list of important virtues includes honesty, loyalty, sincerity, courage, reliability, trustworthiness, and benevolence.[16] He emphasizes that important considerations for management, among others, are the cultivation in managers and executives of excellence (expertise), integrity (the integration of one's roles, responsibilities, and values), and judgment (practical wisdom).

In addition to cultivating individual virtues, public health managers and leaders must nurture complex professional relationships with the communities or "clients" they serve. These relationships are instrumental to the success of public health interventions, particularly as the focus of public health shifts to include the socioeconomic determinants of health. **Professional ethics** focuses on this important relationship between the individual officials and the community.[7, p. 359]

Organizational ethics, on the other hand, focuses on the mission, values, and systems within an agency that create a climate for ethical behavior, practices, and policies. It has received attention in health care since 1995 when the Joint Commission promulgated standards that explicitly require healthcare organizations to have programs and practices that address institutional ethics.[17] The current initiative to accredit public health agencies through the Public Health Accreditation Board (PHAB) creates a similar new opportunity to integrate ethics into organizational accreditation standards.

Public health professionals have recognized the importance of organizational ethics for the practice of public health and have developed a code of ethics to guide public health professionals and agencies that addresses the relationship between public health institutions and the populations they serve. The Public Health Leadership Society (PHLS), in consultation with public health practitioners from across the United States, promulgated the "Principles of the Ethical Practice of Public Health,"[18] which was formally adopted by the American Public Health Association executive board in 2002 and has subsequently been either adopted or endorsed by at least six other national organizations. The current principles are broad statements that will be updated over time to incorporate lessons learned from practitioners. The code is provided as a reference for practitioners in clarifying among themselves and with the public the values and purposes of the public health profession (**Exhibit 6.1**).

The consideration and adoption of a statement of broad ethical principles, like the PHLS code of ethics, is only a first step for organizations in developing an ethics program. Public health agencies must also encourage managers and their staffs to integrate ethics into training, management, and decision-making processes. This process requires both a bottom-up and top-down process of active participation and discussion by professionals throughout the agency. For public health agencies, this code of ethics can provide important guidance and a foundation

---

Exhibit 6.1   The Principles of the Ethical Practice of Public Health

1. Public health should address principally the fundamental causes of disease and requirements for health, aiming to prevent adverse health outcomes.
2. Public health should achieve community health in a way that respects the rights of individuals in the community.
3. Public health policies, programs, and priorities should be developed and evaluated through processes that ensure an opportunity for input from community members.
4. Public health should advocate for, or work for the empowerment of, disenfranchised community members, ensuring that the basic resources and conditions necessary for health are accessible to all people in the community.
5. Public health should seek the information needed to implement effective policies and programs that protect and promote health.
6. Public health institutions should provide communities with the information they have that is needed for decisions on policies or programs and should obtain the community's consent for their implementation.
7. Public health institutions should act in a timely manner on the information they have within the resources and the mandate given to them by the public.
8. Public health programs and policies should incorporate a variety of approaches that anticipate and respect diverse values, beliefs, and cultures in the community.
9. Public health programs and policies should be implemented in a manner that most enhances the physical and social environment.
10. Public health institutions should protect the confidentiality of information that can bring harm to an individual or community if made public. Exceptions must be justified on the basis of the high likelihood of significant harm to the individual or others.
11. Public health institutions should ensure the professional competence of their employees.
12. Public health institutions and their employees should engage in collaborations and affiliations in ways that build the public's trust and the institution's effectiveness.

for ethics discussions about all public health activities, from disease surveillance and outbreak investigations to determining appropriate interventions to conducting research and program evaluation. The most important impact of adopting this code may be that it can serve as a catalyst for management and staff reflection and deliberation about the ethical dimensions of their day-to-day activities in public health and about ways they can continually improve their practices and policies to reflect ethical values.

A third way to approach ethics in public health is **public policy ethics**, which examines the ethical dimensions of particular government actions or decisions and provides a framework for deliberation and public justification. As noted earlier, public officials must provide justifications of their decisions to the public they serve; moral justifications, based on analysis of the benefits and burdens of different options and on the interests and values of relevant stakeholders, are as critical as scientific and legal justifications for public health interventions.[7, p. 365]

Public health ethics can provide a systematic approach to balancing competing moral considerations and stakeholder interests so that public health officials can explore the ethical dimensions of a range of possible options and explain or justify decisions. It prompts ethical decision making by asking: All things considered, what is the right action to take in this situation, and why? Balancing the competing moral claims in a situation is similar to the process officials use in understanding and making public health cost-benefit tradeoffs. The difference is that instead of weighing and balancing "quantifiable" health gains or losses, public health ethics focuses on identifying, weighing, and balancing moral interests and values at stake in a particular situation.[19]

A Framework for Ethical Analysis

Public health decisions generally are made in public health agencies and are reached as a result of group deliberation and reflection. There are a number of different frameworks for guiding ethical analysis in public health practice, all of which attempt to target the goals and functions of public health that make it distinct from other professional domains, particularly clinical medicine. These different frameworks may emphasize particular values or principles over others, but certain core values, such as fairness and equity, minimization of harm, respect for individual liberty and autonomy, trust, accountability, and community are common denominators.[20] The framework outlined in this chapter is not intended to be a simple formula for decision making, but is rather a series of questions designed to provoke rigorous deliberation in public health agencies or ethics advisory groups, and with community stakeholders. (See **Exhibit 6.2**.) The goal is to facilitate ethical reflection and deliberation in order to reach the best possible resolution, all things considered.

1. Analyze the Ethical Issues in the Situation

As a first step, public health officials need to explore the particular context and identify the goals and potential harms of the public health action. Consider the case of a fast food restaurant partnering with a dental practice (see **Case Study 6.1** for details) from the perspective of the health department officials: What are the key public health goals in this situation? To provide care for vulnerable populations, to maintain community relationships and trust, and so on? What is the

---

Exhibit 6.2   Framework for Analysis and Deliberation About Ethical Issues in Public Health

1. Analyze the ethical issues in the situation.
   a. What are the public health risks and harms of concern in this particular context?
   b. What are the public health goals?
   c. Who are the stakeholders, and what are their moral claims?
   d. Is the source or scope of legal authority in question?
   e. Are precedent cases or the historical context relevant?
   f. Do professional codes of ethics provide guidance?
2. Identify the various public health options and evaluate the ethical dimensions of those options.
   a. Utility—Does a particular public health action produce a balance of benefits over harms?
   b. Justice—Are the benefits and burdens distributed fairly (distributive justice), and do legitimate representatives of affected groups have the opportunity to participate in making decisions (procedural justice)?
   c. Respect for individual interests—Does the public health action respect individual choices and interests (autonomy, liberty, privacy)?
   d. Respect for legitimate public institutions—Does the public health action respect professional and civic roles and values, such as transparency, honesty, trustworthiness, keeping promises, protecting confidentiality, and protecting vulnerable individuals and communities from undue stigmatization?
3. Provide justification for one particular public health action.
   a. Effectiveness—Is the public health goal likely to be accomplished with this option?
   b. Proportionality—Will the probable benefits of the action outweigh the infringed moral considerations?
   c. Necessity—Is it necessary to override the conflicting ethical claims in order to achieve the public health goal?
   d. Least infringement—Is the action the least restrictive and least intrusive?
   e. Public justification—Can public health agents offer public justification for the action or policy that citizens, particularly those most affected, can find acceptable?

Adapted from Lee LM. Public Health Ethics Theory: Review and Path to Convergence. *J Law Med Ethics.* 2012;40:85-98. Courtesy of James A. Johnson.

---

harm or potential risk of harm and the ethical issues of concern? Is there a professional conflict of obligations, given that the health department regulates and inspects restaurants? A focus for this case discussion is the range of stakeholders, which is defined as those in the community who are in any way affected by the decisions. For each stakeholder, the ethical analysis should identify the stakeholder's interests, goals, and concerns; power and reputation in the community; and likely preferred outcome. In addition, the framework invites consideration of previous cases, because an analysis of the situation's relevant similarities and differences from precedent cases often provides an important starting point or presumption in case deliberation.

2. Evaluate the Ethical Dimensions of the Various Public Health Options

Ethical deliberation first involves an exploration of the various options for public health action in the situation. When all of the possible scenarios or options are on the table, decision makers can begin to analyze the ethical dimensions of the options. This imaginative and analytic process can facilitate social learning about building consensus and making decisions collectively. Take, for example, the options available for HIV prevention among adolescents and young adults. Some reports suggest that half of all new HIV infections in the United States are among those between the ages of 10 and 24, and approximately 50% of those infected have not been tested.[21] Options range from routine HIV screening for all young adults who visit physician offices to targeted testing for those among the young adult population at highest risk. Ethical deliberation might focus on the following questions: Does the option of testing only those at high risk produce a balance of benefits over harms? Are the benefits and burdens distributed fairly? These are complex questions given the 25-year history of the AIDS epidemic that includes discrimination, stigma, and socioeconomic harms for those diagnosed with the disease. It may be that both options are ethically defensible, meaning that ethical justifications can be made for both options, and then the question becomes how does one choose and justify one option over another? Part 3 of the framework poses questions to help public health decision makers justify a particular option.

3. Provide Justification for a Particular Public Health Action

As noted earlier, justification of actions to the public is a central element of public health practice. Six justificatory conditions provided in the form of questions guide deliberation and decisions about whether choosing one option that promotes one value (e.g., utility or public health benefit) warrants overriding other values (e.g., individual liberty or justice). The justificatory conditions require public health officials to consider whether any proposed program will likely realize the public health goal that is sought (effectiveness), whether its probable benefits will outweigh the infringed general moral considerations (proportionality), whether the policy is essential to realize the end (necessity), whether it involves the least infringement possible consistent with realizing the goal that is sought (least infringement), and whether it can be justified.

Consider the issue of screening for HIV. A comparison of different HIV screening programs illustrates ways that screening programs can meet or fail to meet some of the justificatory conditions. Mandatory screening of donated blood clearly meets all of the justificatory conditions, as does the screening of individuals in some settings where they can expose others who cannot protect themselves. For each of these circumstances, screening is effective and necessary to achieve the public health goal. In contrast, mandatory screening programs for all those seeking a marriage license do not meet the justificatory conditions, given that mandatory screening in this case is neither necessary, impartial, nor the least intrusive means to identify and protect sexually active individuals in the larger population.

Ethical justifications for public health interventions can evolve over time as scientific evidence, treatment options, and social norms and values also evolve. HIV screening programs for pregnant women are a useful example of this evolution. In the mid-1980s the Centers for Disease Control and Prevention (CDC) recommended that pregnant women in high-risk groups be "offered" the HIV test, despite some calls for mandatory screening of pregnant women in high-risk groups. Voluntary, selective (high-risk) screening, rather than mandatory or routine screening, was justified because no treatment was available for HIV infection at the time. Mandatory screening of high-risk women would have been an unjustifiable violation of autonomy and justice. In 1995, after treatment by zidovudine (ZDV) was shown to reduce perinatal HIV transmission, the CDC and the American Academy of Pediatrics (AAP) recommended universal voluntary counseling and HIV testing for pregnant women to allow for prophylactic use of

ZDV. The shift from targeted to universal, voluntary counseling and screening, however, did not eliminate perinatal transmission. Given the subsequent continuing perinatal transmission, an Institute of Medicine report in 1999 recommended universal HIV screening of pregnant women, with patient notification and the option for patients to opt out of testing.[22] In subsequent years, a universal opt-out approach was endorsed by health professional organizations and the CDC. The shift from universal voluntary screening to a routine, opt-out approach was justified given the evidence demonstrating that it was necessary in order to achieve the goal of eliminating perinatal transmission.

Given evidence that HIV transmission occurs during pregnancy in women who tested negative for HIV early in pregnancy, the CDC now recommends a routine second HIV test during the third trimester for women known to have elevated risk for HIV infection and in areas with elevated HIV prevalence among women of childbearing age.[23] Again, this targeted second screening of pregnant women is justified because of the potential significant harm to the neonate that can be avoided through medical interventions before and during birth.

The following case studies provide further examples of how ethical deliberation, guided by an ethics framework, might enrich public health decision making.

CASE STUDY 6.1   With Whom to Partner?

The health department in a poor community with major dental healthcare needs is invited by a local fast-food restaurant to be a partner on a dental health project. The restaurant, with support from its soda vendor, proposes to donate $100,000 a year toward a free dental clinic at the health department. In exchange, the restaurant wants only to have its name and the name of the soda listed in very small print on health department educational material on dental health distributed to the community. Two health department officials, including the nutritionist directing the obesity program, believe such a partnership is unethical. What should the health commissioner do?

In a study of ethical issues in public health,[24] public health officials identified public–private partnerships (PPPs) like the one described in this case as examples of the challenges arising in day-to-day practice, given increasingly limited public resources, the opportunities that collaborations and partnerships create for additional resources, and the funding requirements of many grantors and policymakers for multidisciplinary, community collaborations. Public health practitioners felt the need to address and understand potential ethical issues arising from the different cultures, different values, and different governance structures of potential partners in the private sphere. Some practitioners felt that the potential partners were more powerful, in a sense, than their public health organizations, and that this created ethical tension.

In approaching a case about public–private partnerships, one health director suggested consideration of the following factors:

1. Congruency of goals for the project and mission of the different partners and collaborations—Are the missions and goals of the partners consistent with that of the local public health agency?

2. Conflicts of interest—Is there a perceived or real conflict of interest in the partnership?

3. Conflicts of obligation or accountability—To whom and to what are local public health agencies accountable?

4. Ethical values and moral claims—What values are local public health agencies balancing in the decision? Who are the stakeholders involved in this case, and what are their moral claims? What values should public health officials protect? What is the role of the public health professional?[25]

(continues)

CASE STUDY 6.1   With Whom to Partner? (continued)

This case illustrates that ethical analysis for a public health decision involves weighing the ethical considerations at stake in the particular context, such as what the goals and potential benefits of this partnership are, what the harm or perceived harm of such collaboration is; whether the partners have a history of working together for the public good, what the moral claims of the vulnerable populations who may not have other options for dental care are, how involved in the decision making those most affected are, and so on.

CASE STUDY 6.2   Mandatory Vaccination of Healthcare Workers

Each year, influenza causes 200,000 hospitalizations and 36,000 deaths in the United States. Although the CDC recommends that all healthcare workers should be vaccinated annually against influenza, national vaccination rates for this group remain low, and voluntary programs have been largely unsuccessful at increasing these rates.[26,27]

A skilled nursing facility in your public health area is developing a mandatory influenza vaccination policy for its employees in an effort to increase vaccination uptake. The director of the facility has approached your department for advice on the development of this policy. What ethical issues might arise in this policy that you should discuss with the nursing home director?

In analyzing this policy some of the important points to consider include:

- Who are the stakeholders, and what are their interests and values?
- How might the interests and values of different stakeholders be in tension?
- Are the benefits of the policy likely to outweigh its risks or burdens?

The central interests at stake in this case are those of the patients, who want to minimize their risk of contracting influenza, and those of healthcare workers, who may wish to make their own decisions about whether to receive an influenza vaccine, and who may have objections to the vaccine that they believe ought to be respected by their employers.

An ethical analysis must take into account these different interests and balance them against relevant ethical principles, such as the first principle in the public health code of ethics, which states that public health actions must aim to avoid adverse health outcomes. Protecting patients from influenza would fall under this aim.

In this case it may be determined that the burdens of mandatory vaccination borne by healthcare workers are outweighed by the potential of this policy to reduce influenza infections.[28] Alternatively, it may be argued that mandatory vaccination programs are acceptable only if they allow individuals to opt out for medical or religious reasons, thus respecting the values held by individual healthcare workers. Whether such opt-out provisions undermine the effectiveness of vaccination programs is a further ethical question to consider.

CASE STUDY 6.3   Vaccination for Human Papillomavirus (HPV)

You are a public health director in a state with a high incidence of cervical cancer and low rates of HPV vaccination. The state health department has been asked to explore options for increasing HPV vaccination rates. The two options on the table are: 1) to make HPV vaccination mandatory for school entry for girls aged 11–12 years, or 2) to provide the vaccine at significantly reduced cost for high-risk groups in the population. Which of these two options do you think is most ethically justifiable?

Mandatory vaccination programs are typically justified by appealing to the notion of harm to others: Because vaccination prevents significant harm to others, individuals can justifiably be required to participate in the program. But unlike most vaccine-preventable diseases, HPV is not spread by casual contact, so vaccination against it is not needed to protect, for example, a classroom of children. Some argue that this makes school-based mandates for HPV vaccination ethically unjustifiable.

Recent debate in the literature has emphasized the extent to which disparities in cervical cancer rates may be attributable to disparities in access to preventive measures, such as screening.[29] Current evidence suggests that HPV vaccine uptake is lowest among those girls and women who are at highest risk for developing cervical cancer and who, because of lack of access to other preventive measures, are likely to benefit most from vaccination.[30]

These disparities highlight a second ethical issue surrounding mandatory vaccination programs: Is mandatory vaccination the most equitable way to distribute vaccines and protect against disease? School-entry vaccine requirements are an effective and efficient method of sustaining high vaccination rates, in part because they ensure that almost all children have been immunized by the time they reach school age, regardless of race, ethnicity, geographic location, or socioeconomic status.[31] Vaccines that are consistently required for school entry across the states show much smaller disparities based on race/ethnicity or poverty.[32]

In analyzing this policy option some of the important questions to consider include:

- What considerations might count against mandatory HPV vaccination for all girls aged 11–12?
- Would public health be overstepping its authority by requiring vaccination for a sexually transmitted disease?
- How should the financial costs of mandatory vaccination be factored into this decision?

The second option for increasing HPV vaccination rates is targeted distribution of the vaccine to at-risk groups. While this strategy avoids the ethical difficulties of a vaccine mandate, it raises other ethical concerns:

- Would targeted groups be vulnerable to stigmatization?
- Would uptake of the vaccine be sufficient to justify the costs of a targeted program?

This case illustrates the complexities of isolating the central ethical issues in a public health decision and determining which of a set of actions is most defensible from an ethical point of view. Since both of the options in this case have pros and cons in terms of their ability to achieve public health goals, analysis of the ethical issues they raise concerning health inequities, the just distribution of resources, and respect for individual liberty is key to the decision-making process.

CASE STUDY 6.4   Smoking on the Beach

A member of the city council of your community is considering introducing new legislation that would ban smoking in all beaches and parks. The council member has contacted you, the local health director, for your input on whether and how an outdoor smoking ban should be enacted. How should you respond to the councilor?

Arguments in favor of outdoor smoking bans focus on the potential harms of public smoking. The harms of environmental tobacco smoke (ETS, or "secondhand smoke") are substantial: ETS causes an estimated 46,000 premature deaths from heart disease and 3,400 deaths from lung disease each year among nonsmokers in the United States.[33] Supporters of outdoor smoking bans argue that no level of ETS is risk free. As is documented in a report by the U.S. Surgeon General, even brief exposures to ETS can cause health harms, particularly for vulnerable populations, triggering asthma attacks in children and adverse events for individuals with heart disease.[34] In addition, smoking in public spaces may encourage or influence smoking habits among children, who tend to mimic the behaviors they observe and perceive as normal. The bans are also part of a larger anti-tobacco strategy that aims to change social norms associated with smoking and tobacco use.

Arguments against outdoor smoking bans claim that the evidence of harm from ETS in outdoor settings is insufficient to warrant a ban, and question whether individual choices can be restricted based on potential indirect harms, such as the risk of children mimicking smoking

(continues)

CASE STUDY 6.4   Smoking on the Beach (continued)

behavior. It is also argued that such bans are excessively paternalistic, as they aim to restrict the practice of smoking itself, and so may negatively affect the public's perception of and support for public health activities more broadly.

In analyzing this case several ethical issues are particularly relevant. First is the question of harms. It is important in this case to consider not only the harms of the status quo (i.e., the harms that the proposed ban aims to eliminate), but also the harms of the proposed policy. Antitobacco policies tend disproportionately to affect lower socioeconomic groups, among whom smoking is more prevalent. Bans on smoking in parks and beaches may have negative consequences for communities in which smoking is more popular, for example by discouraging socializing in outdoor spaces, leading to social isolation and decreased opportunities for enjoyment and recreation. These harms must be weighed against the potential benefits of the proposed ban. Are these benefits significant enough to warrant imposing these costs on affected communities? Is the policy just if its burdens are felt primarily among lower socioeconomic groups and communities?

This case also raises the issue of public trust and respect for public health. It is important to note that unlike bans on indoor smoking, in which the harms to nonsmokers are well established, the risk of harm to others posed by smoking in outdoor settings is much lower. Bans on outdoor smoking may therefore be perceived as attempts to further stigmatize smokers and pressure them to quit rather than as attempts to protect the health of the nonsmoking public. These perceptions may undermine trust in public health agencies and in the public health agenda more broadly. Whether public health officials can adequately justify outdoor smoking bans to their communities is an important ethical consideration in the development of such policies.

This case illustrates the appropriateness of ethical analysis when the questions are: Should there be a law, and, if so, what should the law be? The goal of ethical deliberation is to analyze and provide reasons for a public health decision that are grounded in moral norms and that take into account the ethical dimensions of the issues at stake for various stakeholders.

Key questions in such cases are:

- Who are the stakeholders, and what are their positions?
- Are precedent cases and the historical context relevant?
- What are the available policy options?

Conclusion

This chapter presents an introduction to the ways ethics can be incorporated into public health practice and management. It offers two resources, the code of ethics for public health practice and a framework for decision making, that can be deployed by public health officials as they navigate the challenging ethical issues that confront them in their daily practice and in their strategic planning for the future direction of public health.

Ethics in public health has at least three dimensions: the character and virtues of the agent or decision maker and the profession of which they are members, the integration of ethics throughout an organization, and a systematic process for deliberation about particular cases or ethical dilemmas. For each of these dimensions, ethics in public health requires an ongoing process of reflection about such ethical questions as: What are the virtues of a public health professional? What are the goals and ethical responsibilities of the public health agency? What, all things considered, is the ethical action in a particular case, given the stakeholders' interests and moral claims and the responsibilities of the public health professional? This process of reflection is both imaginative and analytical, and provides an opportunity for public health leaders to engage and build relationships with their communities.

This chapter highlights some of the moral values that underpin the practice of public health, such as fairness and justice, respect for individual rights and freedoms, community solidarity, and trust. It also emphasizes the importance of certain principles in public health, such as maximizing benefits and minimizing harms, reducing health inequalities, and providing justifications for decisions that are morally acceptable to the public. These values and principles and their role in public health practice evolve as our understanding evolves in response to new situations, innovations in science and technology, and a deeper understanding of human health and the many factors that influence it. They are not fixed, but rather are important focus points for debate and discussion among those who work in public health and the communities they serve.

Future Outlook

The social, economic, and political context in which public health officials practice continues to generate complex ethical issues like those outlined in the cases presented in this chapter. However, some features of the contemporary public health landscape present particular ethical challenges for future practice:

1. As chronic diseases are increasingly the leading causes of death worldwide, public health's focus is shifting toward individual behavior and choices and the upstream social conditions that influence health. In addition to protecting the population from the threat of infectious disease, public health now looks to the way people live their lives—the choices they make, the risks they take, and the social conditions that make certain choices or risks inevitable or unavoidable. Justifying policies and interventions that address these issues requires public health officials to be alert and sensitive to questions of social justice, individual liberty, and responsibility. Should individuals be held responsible for the choices they make that influence their health? How might assigning personal responsibility for health affect efforts at health promotion?[35] Do governmental agencies like the CDC or state health departments have a role to play in changing the social conditions that influence human health?

2. As the United States grapples with the challenges of health reform, health systems the world over are confronting resource limitations that make priority setting increasingly urgent and difficult. As members of the health profession, public health officials play a role in determining where health resources may be most necessary or most beneficial for the communities they serve. Ethical deliberation is essential for deciding where cuts in services can be justified and where services must be preserved or extended, both in terms of promoting the health of the community as a whole and reducing health inequities within the community. Together with their communities, public health leaders must ask: Which factors are ethically relevant in deciding how to set priorities in public health? Which underlying public health values justify cuts to services?

3. Despite growing mortality rates from chronic diseases, infectious diseases such as HIV/AIDS, severe acute respiratory syndrome (SARS), and influenza continue to pose challenges for public health officials in terms of control, monitoring, and community protection. In addition, threats of bioterrorism and natural disasters loom large for public health

officials responsible for biopreparedness and emergency planning in their communities. Significant ethical questions arise in planning for these events—for example, what sacrifices in terms of individual liberty the community is prepared to bear for protecting health, how to distribute preventative and treatment measures fairly and efficiently, and how to maintain the public's trust and cooperation in the face of widespread fear and panic. Leaders in public health play a crucial role in guiding the community through the deliberative process of making ethical decisions for these eventualities.

Discussion Questions

1. What are the central ethical values underlying the practice of public health?
2. How can public health leaders engage their communities in deliberation on ethical issues?
3. How can public health agencies and institutions incorporate ethics into their day-to-day practice?
4. Why is justification so crucial for ethical decision making in public health?
5. How can public health leaders build and strengthen relationships with their communities and stakeholders? What elements are particularly important in these relationships?

References

1. Childress JF, Faden RR, Gaare RD, et al. Public health ethics: mapping the terrain. *J Law Med Ethics.* 2002;30:170–8.
2. Institute of Medicine. *The Future of Public Health*. Washington, DC: National Academies Press; 1988:28.
3. Institute of Medicine. *The Future of the Public's Health in the 21st Century*. Washington, DC: National Academies Press; 2003.
4. Reich MR. Public private partnerships for public health. *Nature Medicine.* 2000;6(6):617–20.
5. Institute of Medicine. *Who Will Keep the Public Healthy? Educating Public Health Professionals for the 21st Century*. Washington, DC: National Academies Press; 2003.
6. Thomas JC, Sage M, Dillenberg J, et al. A code of ethics for public health. *Am J Public Health.* 2002;92:1057–1059.
7. Bernheim RG, Melnick A. Principled leadership in public health: integrating ethics into practice and management. *J Public Health Manag Pract.* 2008;14:358–66.
8. Powers M, Faden R. *Social Justice: The Moral Foundations of Public Health and Health Policy*. Oxford: Oxford University Press; 2006.
9. Nuffield Council on Bioethics. *Public Health: Ethical Issues*. London: Nuffield Council on Bioethics; 2007.
10. U.S. Deparment of Health and Human Services. *Healthy People 2020*: Determinants of health. Available at: http://www.healthypeople.gov/2020/about/DOHAbout.aspx. Accessed April 4, 2012.
11. World Health Organization. *The World Health Report 2002—Reducing Risks, Promoting Healthy Life*. Geneva: World Health Organization; 2002.
12. Colgrove J. Nowhere left to hide? The banishment of smoking from public spaces. *N Engl J Med.* 2011;364:2375–7.
13. Childress JF, Bernheim RG. Beyond the liberal and communitarian impasse: a framework and vision for public health. *Fla L Rev.* 2003;55:1191–219.
14. Swain GR, Burns KA, Etkind P. Preparedness: Medical ethics versus public health ethics. *J Public Health Manag Pract.* 2008;14(4):354–7.

15. Baum NM, Gollust SE, Goold SD, et al. Looking ahead: addressing ethical challenges in public health practice. *J Law Med Ethics.* 2007;35(4):657–67.

16. Solomon RC. Corporate roles, personal virtues: an Aristotelean approach to business ethics. *Bus Ethics Q J Soc Bus Ethics.* 1992;2(3):317–39.

17. Spencer E, Mills AE, Rorty MV, et al. *Organization Ethics in Health Care.* Oxford: Oxford University Press; 2000:6.

18. Public Health Leadership Society. Principles of the ethical practice of public health. Available at: http://www.phls.org/home/section/3-26/. Accessed April 4, 2012.

19. Bernheim RG, Nieburg P, Bonnie RJ. Ethics and the practice of public health. In: Goodman RA, Hoffman RE, Lopez W, et al., eds. *Law in Public Health Practice.* 2nd ed. Oxford: Oxford University Press; 2007.

20. Lee LM. Public health ethics theory: review and path to convergence. *J Law Med Ethics.* 2012;40:85–98.

21. Nguyen TQ, Ford CA, Kaufman JS, et al. HIV testing among young adults in the United States: associations with financial resources and geography. *Am J Public Health.* 2006;96:1031–4.

22. Institute of Medicine, National Research Council. *Reducing the Odds: Preventing Perinatal Transmission of HIV in the United States.* Washington, DC: National Academies Press; 1999.

23. Centers for Disease Control and Prevention. Achievements in public health: reduction in perinatal transmission of HIV infection—United States, 1985–2005. *MMWR.* 2006;55(21):592–7.

24. Bernheim RG. Public health ethics: the voices of practitioners. *J Law Med Ethics.* 2003;31:S104–7.

25. Reich MR, Hershey JH, Hardy GE, et al. Workshop on public health law and ethics, I & II: the challenge of public/private partnerships (PPPs). *J Law Med Ethics.* 2003;31(4, suppl):90–3.

26. Poland GA, Tosh P, Jacobson RM. Requiring influenza vaccination for health care workers—seven truths we must accept. *Vaccine.* 2005;23(17-18):2251–5.

27. Babcock HM, Gemeinhart N, Jones M, et al. Mandatory influenza vaccination of health care workers: translating policy to practice. *Clin Infect Dis.* 2010;50(4):459–64.

28. Van Delden JJM, Ashcroft R, Dawson A, et al. The ethics of mandatory vaccination against influenza for health care workers. *Vaccine.* 2008;26(44):5562–6.

29. Watson M, Saraiya M, Benard V, et al. Burden of cervical cancer in the United States, 1998–2003. *Cancer* 2008;113(Suppl):2855–64.

30. Bach PB. Gardasil: from bench, to bedside, to blunder. *Lancet.* 2010;375:963–4.

31. Orenstein WA, Hinman AR. The immunization system in the United States—the role of school immunization laws. *Vaccine.* 1999;17:S19–S24.

32. Centers for Disease Control and Prevention. National and state vaccination coverage among adolescents aged 13 through 17 years—United States 2010. *MMWR.* 2011;60:1117–23.

33. Centers for Disease Control and Prevention. Smoking-Attributable mortality, years of potential life lost, and productivity losses—united states, 2000–2004. *MMWR.* 2008;57(45):1226–8.

34. U.S. Department of Health and Human Services. *The Health Consequences of Involuntary Exposure to Tobacco Smoke: A Report of the Surgeon General.* Atlanta: U.S. Department of Health and Human Services, Centers for Disease Control and Prevention; 2006.

35. Wikler D, Brock DW. Population-level bioethics: mapping a new agenda. In: Dawson A, Verweij M, eds., *Ethics, Prevention, and Public Health.* New York: Oxford University Press; 2007.

Public Health Law

Lawrence O. Gostin

LEARNING OBJECTIVES

- To better understand the role and purpose of law in public health
- To be familiar with key laws and regulations pertaining to public health
- To understand local versus federal powers in the public health domain
- To gain perspective on the complexity of the legal system and public health
- To be familiar with public health law reform

Chapter Overview

Laws are enacted to influence healthy behavior, respond to health threats, and enforce health and safety standards. Public health law is principally concerned with government's assurance of the conditions for the population's health—what government may, and must, do to safeguard human health. Federal, state, tribal, and local governments exercise public health powers derived from the complex legal relationships among these levels of government. Protecting and preserving community health is not possible without an effective legal framework to guide a wide range of public and private endeavors.

Preservation of the public's health is among the most important purposes of government. The enactment and enforcement of law, moreover, is a primary means by which government creates the conditions for people to lead healthier and safer lives. Law creates a mission for public health agencies, assigns their functions, and specifies the manner in which they may exercise their authority. The law is a tool for public health practice, which is used to influence norms for healthy behavior, identify and respond to health threats, and set and enforce health and safety standards. The most important social debates concerning public health take place in legal forums—legislatures, courts, and administrative agencies—and in the law's language of rights, duties, and justice.[1] It is no exaggeration to say, "the field of public health . . . could not long exist in the manner in which we know it today except for its sound legal basis."[2, p. 4]

The Institute of Medicine (IOM), in its foundational 1988 report, *The Future of Public Health*, acknowledged that law was essential to public health, but cast serious doubt on the soundness of public health's legal basis. Concluding that "this nation has lost sight of its public health goals and has allowed the system of public health activities to fall into disarray," the IOM placed some of the blame on an obsolete and inadequate body of enabling laws and regulations.[3, p. 19] The IOM recommended:

> states review their public health statutes and make revisions necessary to accomplish the following two objectives: (1) clearly delineate the basic authority and responsibility entrusted to public health agencies, boards, and officials at the state and local levels and the relationship between them; and (2) support a set of modern disease control measures that address contemporary health problems such as AIDS, cancer, and heart disease, and incorporate due process safeguards (notice, hearings, administrative review, right to counsel, standards of evidence).

> Reproduced from Institute of Medicine. *The Future of Public Health*. Washington, DC: National Academies Press; 1988, p. 10.

The IOM reiterated its call for public health law reform in its 2003 report, *The Future of the Public's Health in the 21st Century*: "Public health law at the federal, state, and local levels is often outdated and internally inconsistent. This leads to inefficiency and a lack of coordination and may even pose a danger in a crisis."[4, p. 4] The IOM commended the "pioneering work" of two model public health statutes: 1) the Model State Emergency Health Powers Act, drafted at the request of the Centers for Disease Control and Prevention (CDC) following the terrorist attacks of 2001, which provides public health agencies with powers in a declared emergency; and 2) the Turning Point Model State Public Health Act, a Robert Wood Johnson Foundation project, which provides a comprehensive structure for the mission, powers, and duties of public health agencies. Both model laws are considered in more detail later in this chapter.

In a 2012 report, the IOM again recommended that states should systematically review and revise their public health statutes, many of which were enacted in different eras when communicable disease was the primary population health threat. The Committee sought a "health in all policies" approach whereby all government departments place health closer to the center of their mission.[5]

This chapter reviews the state of public health law in the United States. First, a theory and definition of public health law are offered. Second, public health powers within the constitutional design are explained. Third, the current structure of federal, state, and local health agencies is examined. Finally, the future of public health law is considered, explaining the deficiencies in state public health statutes and proposing guidelines for law reform.

A Theory and Definition of Public Health Law

Public health law is often used interchangeably with other terms that signify a connection between law and health, such as health law, law and medicine, and forensic medicine. Despite the similarity of these names, public health law is a distinct discipline capable of definition. Public health law can be defined as:

> the study of the legal powers and duties of the state, in collaboration with its partners (e.g., health care, business, the community, the media, and academe), to assure the conditions for people to be healthy (e.g., to identify, prevent, and ameliorate risks to health in the population) and the limitations on the power of the state to constrain the autonomy, privacy, liberty, proprietary, or other legally protected interests of individuals for the common good. The prime objective of public health law is to pursue the highest possible level of physical and mental health in the population, consistent with the values of social justice.

> Reproduced from Gostin LO. *Public Health Law: Power, Duty, Restraint.* 2nd ed. Berkeley, CA: University of California Press; 2008; Gostin LO. *Public Health Law and Ethics: A Reader.* 2nd ed. Berkeley, CA: University California Press; 2010.

Public health law has at least five characteristics that help separate it from other fields at the intersection of law and health: government, populations, relationships, services, and coercion.

Government's Essential Role in Public Health Law

Public health activities are primarily (but not exclusively) the responsibility of government. The importance of government in ensuring the conditions for the population's health is demonstrated by its constitutional powers and its role in a democracy. The Preamble to the Constitution reveals the ideals of government as the wellspring of communal life and mutual security: "We the People of the United States, in Order to form a more perfect Union, establish Justice, insure domestic Tranquility, provide for the common defense, promote the general Welfare, and secure the Blessings of Liberty to ourselves and our Posterity, do ordain and establish this Constitution. . . ." The constitutional design reveals a plain intent to vest power in government at every level to protect community health and safety. Government is empowered to collect taxes and expend public resources, and only government can require members of the community to submit to regulation.

The role of government in a democracy also helps explain its importance in advancing the public's health. People form governments precisely to provide a means of communal support and security. Acting alone, individuals cannot ensure even minimum levels of health. Individuals may procure personal medical services and many of the necessities of life; any person of means can purchase a home, clothing, food, and the services of a physician or hospital. Yet, no single individual, or group of individuals, can ensure his or her health. Meaningful protection and assurance of the population's health requires communal effort. The community as a whole has a stake in environmental protection, hygiene and sanitation, clean air and surface water, uncontaminated food and drinking water, safe roads and products, and the control of infectious disease. Each of these collective goods, and many more, are essential conditions for health. Yet, these goods can be secured only through organized action on behalf of the population.

This discussion does not suggest that the private and voluntary sectors are not important in public health. Manifestly, private (e.g., health insurers), charitable (e.g., the Red Cross), and community (e.g., AIDS support groups) organizations play roles that are critical to the public's health. Nevertheless, communal efforts to protect and promote the population's health are primarily a responsibility of government, which is why government action represents a central theoretical tenet of what we call public health law.

Serving the Health Needs of Populations

Public health focuses on the health of populations rather than on the clinical improvement of individual patients. Generally, public health focuses on prevention and communal health, whereas medicine focuses on the health of individuals. Clearly, there is an overlap between the two,[6] as President Obama's Patient Protection and Affordable Care Act demonstrates.[7] However, classic definitions of public health emphasize this population-based perspective:

> As one of the objects of the police power of the state, the "public health" means the prevailingly healthful or sanitary condition of the general body of people or the community in mass, and the absence of any general or widespread disease or cause of mortality.[8, p. 721]

Public health services are those that are shared by all members of the community and are organized and supported by, and for, the benefit of the people as a whole. Thus, whereas the art or science of medicine seeks to identify and ameliorate ill health in the individual patient, public health seeks to improve the health of the population.

Relationships Between Government and the Public

Public health contemplates the relationship between the state and the population (or between the state and individuals who place themselves or the community at risk) rather than the relationship between the physician and the patient. Public health practitioners and scholars are interested in organized community efforts to improve the health of populations. Accordingly, public health law observes collective action—principally through government—and its effects on various populations. The field of public health law similarly examines the benefits and burdens placed by government on legally protected interests. This is in direct contrast to the field of healthcare law, which concerns the micro relationships between healthcare providers and patients as well as the organization, finance, and provision of personal medical services.

Population-Based Services

Public health deals primarily with the provision of population-based health services rather than personal medical services. The core functions of public health agencies are those fundamental activities that are carried out to protect the population's health:

- Assessment—the collection, assembly, and analysis of community health needs
- Policy development—the development of public health policies informed through scientific knowledge
- Assurance—assurance of the services necessary for community health

Activities regarded as essential public health services include efforts to monitor community health status and investigate health risks; inform, educate, and empower people about health; mobilize community partnerships; regulate individual and organizational behavior; evaluate effectiveness, accessibility, and quality of personal health services; and pursue innovative solutions to health problems. Moreover, the public health community is increasingly interested in scientific methodologies to monitor the efficacy of services.

Demand Conformance with Health and Safety Standards

Public health possesses the power to coerce individuals for the protection of the community and thus does not rely on a near-universal ethic of voluntarism. Although government can do much to promote the public's health that does not require the exercise of compulsory powers, it alone is authorized to require conformance with publicly established standards of behavior. The degree of compulsory measures necessary to safeguard the public's health is, of course, subject to political and judicial resolution. Yet, protecting and preserving community health is not possible without the constraint of a wide range of private activities. Absent an inherent governmental authority and ability to coerce individual and community behaviors, threats to public health and safety could not be reduced easily.

Having defined public health law and distinguished it from other fields, it will be helpful to examine public health law in our constitutional system of government.

Public Health in the Constitutional Design

No inquiry is more important to public health law than understanding the role of government in the constitutional design. If public health law is principally about government's assurance of the conditions necessary for the population's health, what must government do to safeguard human health? Analyzing this question requires an assessment of duty (what government must do), authority (what government can, but is not required to, do), limits (what government cannot do), and responsibility (which government—whether federal, state, or local—is to act).

The U.S. Constitution is the starting point for any analysis concerning the distribution of governmental powers. Although the Constitution is said to impose no affirmative obligation on governments to act, provide services, or protect individuals and populations, it does serve three primary functions: 1) it allocates power among the federal government and the states (federalism), 2) it divides power among the three branches of government (separation of powers), and 3) it limits government power (to protect individual liberties). In the realm of public health, then, the Constitution acts as both a fountain and a levee; it originates the flow of power—to preserve the public health—and it curbs that power—to protect individual freedoms.

If the Constitution is a fountain from which government powers flow, **federalism** represents a partition in the fountain that separates federal and state powers. By separating the pool of legislative authority into these two tiers of government, federalism preserves the balance of power among national and state authorities. Theoretically, the division of government powers is distinct and clear. The federal government is a government of limited power whose acts must be authorized by the Constitution. The states, by contrast, retain the powers they possessed as sovereign governments before ratification of the Constitution. The most important state authority is the power to protect the health, safety, morals, and general welfare of the population. In practice, however, the powers of the federal and state governments intersect in innumerable areas, particularly in areas of traditional state concern, like public health.

Federalism functions as a sorting device for determining which government (federal, state, or local) may respond legitimately to a public health threat. Often, federal, state, and local governments exercise public health powers concurrently. Where conflicts among the various levels of government arise, however, federal laws likely preempt state or local actions pursuant to the supremacy clause: the "Constitution, and the Laws of the United States . . . and all Treaties made . . . shall be the supreme law of the Land."[9]

In addition to establishing a federalist system, the Constitution separates governmental powers into three branches: 1) the legislative branch, which has the power to create laws; 2) the executive branch, which has the power to enforce the laws; and 3) the judicial branch, which has the power to interpret the laws. States have similar schemes of governance pursuant to their own constitutions. By separating the powers of government, the Constitution provides a system of checks and balances that is thought to reduce the possibility of governmental oppression.

The **separation of powers doctrine** is essential to public health. Each branch of government possesses a unique constitutional authority to create, enforce, or interpret health policy. The legislative branch creates health policy and allocates the necessary resources to effectuate that policy. Some believe that legislators are ill equipped to make complex public health decisions. Yet, as the only "purely" elected branch of government, members of federal or state legislatures ultimately are politically accountable to the people.

The executive branch, which enforces health policy, has an equally significant role in public health. Most public health agencies reside in the executive branch and are responsible for implementing legislation that may often require establishing and enforcing complex health regulations. The executive branch and its agencies are uniquely positioned to govern public health. Public health agencies are designed and created for the purpose of advancing community health. They have sufficient expertise and resources to focus on health problems for extended periods of time. Agencies, however, may occasionally suffer from stale thinking, complicity with the subjects of regulation, and the inability to balance competing values and claims for resources.

The judicial branch, which interprets the law and resolves legal disputes, also has an important role concerning public health. Courts can exert substantial control over public health policy by determining the boundaries of government power and the zone of autonomy, privacy, and liberty to be afforded individuals. Courts decide whether a public health statute or policy is constitutional, whether agency action is authorized legislatively, whether agency officials have sufficient evidence to support their actions, and whether governmental officials or private parties have acted negligently. Although the exercise of judicial power may serve public health, courts may fail to review the substance of health policy choices critically. Federal judges, once appointed, are politically less accountable (though state judges may be elected). Courts, bound by the facts of a particular case or controversy, may be overly influenced by disfavored expert opinions and may focus too intently on individual rights at the expense of public health protections.

The separation of powers doctrine is not a model of efficiency. Dividing broad powers among branches of governments significantly burdens governmental operations, which may actually thwart public health. The constitutional design appears to value restraint in policy making: legislative representatives reconcile demands for public health funding with competing claims for societal resources; the executive branch straddles the line between congressional authorization and judicial restrictions on that authority; and the judiciary tempers public health measures with individual rights. As a result, the possibility of strong public health governance by any given branch is compromised in exchange for constitutional checks and balances that prevent overreaching and foster political accountability.

A third constitutional function is to limit governmental power to protect individual liberties. Governmental actions to promote the communal good often infringe on individual freedoms. Public health regulation and individual rights may directly conflict. Resolving the tension between population-based regulations and individual rights requires a tradeoff. Thus, although the Constitution grants extensive powers to governments, it also limits that power by protecting individual rights and freedoms. The Bill of Rights (the first 10 amendments to the Constitution), together with the Reconstruction Amendments (13th, 14th, and 15th Amendments) and other constitutional provisions, create a zone of individual liberty, autonomy, privacy, and economic freedom that exists beyond the reach of the government. Public health law struggles to determine the point at which governmental authority to promote the population's health must yield to individual rights and freedoms.

Understanding and defining the limits of public health powers by the federal, state, tribal, and local governments is an integral part of our constitutional system of government. In the following sections, the constitutional authority and exercise of public health powers by each of these levels of government are explored.

Federal Public Health Powers

The federal government must draw its authority to act from specific, enumerated powers. Before an act of Congress is deemed constitutional, two questions must be asked: 1) does the Constitution affirmatively authorize Congress to act, and 2) does the exercise of that power improperly interfere with any constitutionally protected interest?

In theory, the United States is a government of limited, defined powers. In reality, political and judicial expansion of federal powers through the doctrine of implied powers allows the federal government considerable authority to act in the interests of public health and safety. Under the doctrine of implied powers, the federal government may employ all means "necessary and proper" to achieve the objectives of constitutionally enumerated national powers.[10] For public health purposes, the chief powers are the powers to tax, to spend, and to regulate interstate commerce. These powers provide Congress with independent authority to raise revenue for public health services and to regulate, both directly and indirectly, private activities that endanger human health.

The taxing power is a primary means for achieving public health objectives by influencing, directly and indirectly, health-related behavior through tax relief and tax burdens. Tax relief encourages private, health-promoting activity; tax burdens discourage risky behavior. Through various forms of tax relief, government provides incentives for private activities that it views as advantageous to community health (e.g., tax benefits for self-insured healthcare plans).

Public health taxation also regulates private behavior by economically penalizing risk-taking activities. Tax policy discourages a number of activities that the government regards as unhealthy, dangerous, immoral, or adverse to human health. Thus, the government imposes significant excise or manufacturing taxes on tobacco, alcoholic beverages, and firearms; penalizes certain behaviors such as gambling; and influences individual and business decisions through taxes on gasoline or ozone-depleting chemicals that contribute to environmental degradation.

The spending power provides Congress with independent authority to allocate resources for the public good or general welfare without the need to justify its spending by reference to a specific enumerated power. Closely connected to the power to tax, the spending power authorizes expenditures expressly for the public's health. The grant of such expenditures can be conditioned on a number of terms or requirements. The conditional spending power is thus like a private contract: In return for federal funds, the states agree to comply with federally imposed conditions. Such conditions are constitutionally allowed provided the conditions are clearly authorized by statute and do not coerce the funding recipient, and a reasonable relationship exists between the condition imposed and the program's purposes.[10]

The need for federal public health funds effectively induces state conformance with federal regulatory standards. Congress and federal agencies use conditional spending to induce states to conform to federal standards in numerous public health contexts, including direct health care, prevention services, biomedical and health services research, public health regulation and safety inspection, and workplace safety and health.

The commerce power, more than any other enumerated power, affords Congress potent regulatory authority. Congress has the power to regulate: 1) all commerce among foreign nations and Indian tribes, and 2) interstate commerce among the states. Although the scope of the interstate commerce power has been judicially limited during the course of our constitutional history, the current conception of Congress's commerce powers is extensive, although not unlimited.

The Supreme Court's modern construction of the interstate commerce power has been described as "plenary" or all embracing, and has been exerted to affect virtually every aspect of social life. The expansive interpretation of the commerce clause has enabled the national government to invade traditional realms of state public health power, including the fields of environmental protection, food and drug purity, occupational health and safety, and other public health matters. Thus, the commerce clause gives national authorities the power to regulate throughout the public health spectrum.

Any legitimate exercise of federal taxing, spending, or commerce power in the interests of public health may be determined to trump state public health regulation. By authority of the supremacy clause, Congress may preempt state public health regulation, even if the state is acting squarely within its police powers. Federal preemption occurs in many areas of public health law, such as with cigarette labeling and advertising regulations and occupational health and safety.

As a result of broad interpretations of its supreme, enumerated powers, the federal government has a vast presence in public health. It is nearly impossible to find a field of public health that is not heavily influenced by U.S. governmental policy. Public health functions, including public funding for health care, safe food, effective drugs, clean water, a beneficial environment, and prevention services, can be found in an array of federal agencies.

Although the courts have normally afforded the federal government broad authority in the realm of health, the division of state and federal health powers can be highly contentious—both politically and legally. Perhaps the best illustration is *Florida v. HHS*, currently being considered by the Supreme Court at the time of writing.[11] The two crucial issues in that case are Medicaid expansion and the individual mandate to purchase health insurance, both under President Obama's Patient Protection and Affordable Care Act. On the Medicaid expansion issue, the Court is considering whether the broad responsibilities placed on states as a condition of federal Medicaid funding is "unduly coercive." The states' argument is that they could not realistically turn down such substantial federal funding for indigent health care. On the individual mandate issue, the Court is considering whether Congress can compel an individual to purchase a private product, such as health insurance. The key question is whether forcing someone to buy health insurance is an appropriate regulation of interstate commerce.[12]

State Police Powers

Despite the broad federal presence in modern public health regulation, historically, states have had a predominant role in providing population-based health services. States still account for the majority of traditional public health spending for public health services (not including personal medical services or the environment). The 10th Amendment of the Constitution reserves to the states all powers that are neither given to the federal government nor prohibited by the Constitution. These reserved powers, known as the **police powers**, support a dominant role in protecting the public's health.[13]

The police powers represent the state's authority to further the goal of all government, which is to promote the general welfare of society. Police powers can be defined as:

> the inherent authority of the state (and, through delegation, local government) to enact laws and promulgate regulations to protect, preserve, and promote the health, safety, morals, and general welfare of the people. To achieve these communal benefits, the state retains the power to restrict, within federal and state constitutional limits, private interests—personal interests in liberty, autonomy, privacy, and association, as well as economic interests in freedom of contract and uses of property.[14]

This definition of police power reflects three principal characteristics: 1) the government's purpose is to promote the public good, 2) the state authority to act permits the restriction of private interests, and (3) the scope of state powers is pervasive. States exercise police powers for the common good—that is, to ensure that communities live in safety and security, in conditions that are conducive to good health, with moral standards, and, generally speaking, without unreasonable interference with human wellbeing.

Government, in order to achieve common goods, is empowered to enact legislation, regulate, and adjudicate in ways that necessarily limit, or even eliminate, private interests. Thus, government has inherent power to interfere with personal interests in autonomy, liberty, privacy, and association, as well as economic interests in ownership and uses of private property. The police power affords state government the authority to keep society free from noxious exercises of private rights. The state retains discretion to determine what is considered injurious or unhealthful and the manner in which to regulate, consistent with constitutional protections of personal interests.

Police powers in the context of public health include all laws and regulations directly or indirectly intended to reduce morbidity and premature mortality in the population. The police powers have enabled states and local governments to promote and preserve the public health in areas ranging from injury and disease prevention to sanitation, waste disposal, and water and air pollution. Police powers exercised by the states include vaccination, isolation and quarantine, inspection of commercial and residential premises, abatement of unsanitary conditions or other nuisances, and regulation of air and surface water contaminants, as well as restriction on the public's access to polluted areas, standards for pure food and drinking water, extermination of vermin, fluoridation of municipal water supplies, and licensure of physicians and other health-care professionals.

Local Public Health Powers

In addition to the significant roles that federal and state governments have concerning public health law in the constitutional system, local governments also have important public health powers. Public health officials in local governments, including counties, cities, municipalities, and special districts, are often on the front line of public health. They may be directly responsible for assembling public health surveillance data, implementing federal and state programs, administering federal or state public health laws, operating public health clinics, and setting public health policies for their specific populations.

Although states have inherent powers as sovereign governments, localities have delegated power. Local governments in the constitutional system are subsidiaries of their states. As a result, any powers that local governments have to enact public health law or policies must be granted either in the state constitution or in state statutes. Sometimes state grants of power are so broad and generic that they afford cities home rule. For example, if the state constitution expressly affords a city the power to protect the health, safety, and welfare of local inhabitants, this is an important guarantee of home rule. Absent constitutionally protected delegations of power to local governments, however, states may modify, clarify, preempt, or remove "home rule" powers of local government.

New Federalism

Since the founding of the United States, the division of federal and state governmental powers has been an important and highly controversial part of our federalist system of government. The Supreme Court, at least since Franklin Delano Roosevelt's New Deal, has liberally interpreted the federal government's enumerated powers, leading to an unprecedented expansion of national public health authority. More recently, however, the Rehnquist Court had emphasized that there exist enforceable limits on Congress's powers. Known as **new federalism**, federal courts have begun to hold that federal police powers should be circumscribed, with more authority returned to the states.

The Supreme Court has narrowed the scope of the commerce power, holding that the federal government cannot regulate purely intrastate police power matters. In *United States v. Lopez*, the Court held that Congress exceeded its commerce clause authority by making gun possession within a school zone a federal offense. Concluding that possessing a gun within a school zone did not "substantially affect" interstate commerce, the Court declared the statute unconstitutional.[15] The Court continued to narrow the scope of the commerce power in *United States v. Morrison* when it struck down the private civil remedy in the Violence Against Women Act.[16] The act created a civil rights remedy, permitting survivors to bring federal lawsuits against perpetrators of sexually motivated crimes of violence. Congress proclaimed that violence impairs women's abilities to work, harms businesses, and increases national healthcare costs. But the Court, reiterating its arguments from *Lopez*, found no national effects.

In addition to *Lopez* and *Morrison*, the Supreme Court has held in a series of recent cases that Congress, even if empowered to act for the public good, must exert its authority in ways that do not excessively intrude on state sovereignty. In *New York v. the United States*, the Supreme Court struck down a federal statute providing for the disposal of radioactive waste as violating the 10th Amendment. The Constitution, stated the Court, does not confer upon Congress the ability to "commandeer the legislative processes of the States by directly compelling them to enact and enforce a federal regulatory program."[17, p. 175] The Supreme Court used the same reasoning to overturn provisions in the Brady Handgun Violence Prevention Act, which directed state and local law enforcement officers to conduct background checks on prospective handgun purchasers.[18]

In this era of new federalism, some federal public health laws may be vulnerable to state challenges. National environmental regulations are particularly at risk because they invade core state concerns and are being challenged in the court system.

In summary, a highly complex, politically charged relationship exists between various levels of government regulating for the public's health—federal, state, tribal, and local. The Constitution ostensibly grants the federal government limited powers, but these powers have been construed in ways that have facilitated an enormous growth of national public health authority. The Constitution does not grant states any power because, as sovereign governments that predated the Republic, the states already had broad powers. Known as the police powers, states may act to protect the health, safety, and wellbeing of the population. Local governments, as subsidiary entities of states, possess only those public health powers delegated by the state. In an era of new federalism, the Supreme Court has gradually limited federal public health powers and returned them to the states. Even so, the vast majority of public health functions currently exercised by the federal government are likely to survive constitutional scrutiny.

The Modern Public Health Agency

The deep-seated problems of modern society caused by industrialization and urbanization pose complex, highly technical challenges that require expertise, flexibility, and deliberative study over the long term. Solutions cannot be found within traditional governmental structures such as representative assemblies or governors' offices. As a result, governments have formed specialized entities within the executive branch to pursue the goals of population health and safety.

These administrative agencies form the bulwark for public health activities in the United States. Public health agencies are found at all levels of government—federal, state, tribal, and local.

Federal Public Health Agencies

The modern role of the federal government in public health is broad and complex. Public health functions, which include public funding for health care, safe food, effective drugs, clean water, a beneficial environment, and prevention services, can be found in an array of agencies. The U.S. Department of Health and Human Services (HHS) is the umbrella agency under which most public health functions are located. Under the aegis of the HHS, various programs promote and protect health. The Health Care Financing Administration (now the Centers for Medicare and Medicaid Services) was created in 1977 to administer the Medicare and Medicaid programs. The Centers for Disease Control and Prevention (CDC) provides technical and financial support to states in monitoring, controlling, and preventing disease. The CDC's efforts include initiatives such as childhood vaccination and emergency response to infectious disease outbreaks. The National Institutes of Health (NIH) conducts and supports research, trains investigators, and disseminates scientific information. The Food and Drug Administration (FDA) ensures that food is pure and safe and that drugs, biologicals, medical devices, cosmetics, and products that emit radiation are safe and effective.

The Department of Labor (DOL) administers a variety of federal labor laws, some of which pertain to workers' rights to safe and healthy working conditions. Specifically, the Occupational Safety and Health Administration (OSHA) develops occupational safety and health standards and monitors compliance. In 1970, the Environmental Protection Agency (EPA) was created to control and reduce pollution in the air, water, and ground. The EPA develops national standards, provides technical assistance, and enforces environmental regulations. In 2002, Congress established the Department of Homeland Security (DHS), which consolidated 22 agencies, unifying a variety of security functions in a single agency.

State Public Health Agencies

The state's plenary power to safeguard citizens' health includes the authority to create administrative agencies devoted to that task. State legislation determines the administrative organization, mission, and functions of public health agencies. Contemporary state public health agencies take many different forms that defy simple classification. Before 1960, state public health functions were located in health departments with policy-making functions residing in a board of health (e.g., issuing and enforcing regulations). As programs expanded (e.g., increased federal funding for categorical programs and block grants), certain public health functions were assigned to other state agencies (e.g., mental health, medical care financing for the indigent, and environmental protection). Currently, 55 state-level health agencies (including the District of Columbia, American Samoa, Guam, Puerto Rico, and the U.S. Virgin Islands) exist, each of which may be a free-standing, independent department or a component of a larger state agency.

The trend since the 1960s has been to merge state health departments with other departments—often social services, Medicaid, mental health, and/or substance abuse—to form superagencies. Under this framework, the public health unit is often called a division of health or public health. Another common framework is to assign public health functions to a cabinet-level agency. Under this framework, the public health unit is often called a department of health or public health.

The Institute of Medicine has called for greater consolidation of state and local public health agencies, so that all public health authorities have the capacity to carry out the essential public health functions.[19]

The trend has also been to eliminate or reduce the influence of boards of health. These boards, once ubiquitous and highly influential, are now often replaced or supplemented with specialized boards or committees established by state statute to oversee technical or politically controversial programs (e.g., genetics, rural health, expansion of healthcare facilities). The chief executive officer of the public health agency—the commissioner or, less often, the secretary—is usually politically appointed by the governor, but may be appointed by the head of a superagency or, rarely, the board of health. Qualification standards may include medical and public health expertise, but increasingly, chief executives with political or administrative experience are appointed.

Local Public Health Agencies

Local government exercises voluminous public health functions derived from the state, such as air, water, and noise pollution; sanitation and sewage; cigarette sales and smoking in public accommodations; drinking water fluoridation; drug paraphernalia sales; firearm registration and prohibition; infectious diseases; rodents and infestations; housing codes; sanitary food and beverages; trash disposal; and animal control. Local government also often regulates (or owns and operates) hospitals or nursing homes.

Municipalities, like the states, have created public health agencies to carry out their functions. Local public health agencies have varied forms and structures: centralized (directly operated by the state), decentralized (formed and managed by local government), or mixed. Local boards of health, or less often, governmental councils, still exist in most local public health agencies with responsibility for health regulation and policy. The courts usually permit local agencies to exercise broad discretion in matters of public health, sometimes even beyond the geographic area if necessary to protect the city's inhabitants (e.g., during a waterborne disease outbreak).

Local public health agencies serve a political subdivision of the state such as a city (a municipality or municipal corporation), town, township, county, or borough. Some local public health functions are undertaken by special districts that are limited governmental structures that serve special purposes (e.g., drinking water, sewerage, sanitation, or mosquito abatement).

Rule Making, Enforcement, and Quasi-Judicial Powers

Public health agencies are part of the executive branch of government but wield considerable authority to make rules to control private behavior, interpret statutes and regulations, and adjudicate disputes about whether an individual or company has conformed to health and safety standards. Under the separation of powers doctrine, the executive branch is supposed to enforce law, but not enact or interpret it. Nevertheless, the lines between law making, enforcement, and adjudication have become blurred with the rise of the administrative state.

The courts, at least theoretically, can carefully scrutinize legislative grants of power to public health agencies. Conventionally, representative assemblies may not delegate legislative or judicial functions to the executive branch. Known as **nondelegation**, this doctrine holds that the legislative branch of government should undertake policy-making functions (because assemblies are politically accountable), whereas the judicial branch should undertake adjudicative functions (because courts are independent).

The nondelegation doctrine is rarely used by federal courts to limit agency powers. The doctrine, however, has received varying interpretations at the state level—some jurisdictions liberally permit delegations whereas others are more restrictive. In 1987, New York State's highest court, for example, found unconstitutional a health department prohibition on smoking in public places because the legislature, not the health department, should decide the "tradeoffs" between health and freedom. "Manifestly," the court said, "it is the province of the people's elected representatives, rather than appointed administrators, to resolve difficult social problems by making choices among competing ends."[20, p. 1356] By 2003 however, the people's elected representatives did resolve this issue when the New York Clean Indoor Air Act (Public Health Law, Article 13-E) was passed prohibiting smoking in virtually every workplace, including bars and restaurants. The law also allowed that "localities may continue to adopt and enforce local laws regulating smoking. However, these regulations must be at least as strict as the Clean Indoor Air Act."[21]

Rule Making

Although public health agencies possess considerable power to issue detailed rules, they must do so fairly and publicly. Federal and state administrative procedure acts (as well as agency-enabling acts) govern the deliberative processes that agencies must undertake in issuing rules. (Unless specified by statute, state administrative procedure acts generally have been held not to apply to local governmental agencies.) Administrative procedure acts often require two different forms: 1) informal, simple and flexible procedures often consisting of prior notice (e.g., publication in federal or state register), written comments by interested persons, and a statement of basis and purpose for the rule; and 2) formal, more elaborate procedures often requiring a hearing.

Enforcement

Health departments do not possess only legislative power. They also have the executive power to enforce the regulations that they have promulgated. Enforcement of laws and regulations is squarely within the constitutional powers of executive agencies. Although legislatures set the penalty for violations of health and safety standards, the executive branch monitors compliance and seeks redress against those who fail to conform. Pursuant to their enforcement power, health departments may inspect premises and businesses, investigate complaints, and generally monitor the activities of those who come within the orbit of health and safety statutes and administrative rules.

Quasi-Judicial Powers

Modern administrative agencies do not simply issue and enforce health and safety standards. They also interpret statutes and rules as well as adjudicate disputes about whether standards are violated. Federal and state administrative procedure acts and agency-enabling legislation often enumerate the procedures that agencies must follow in adjudicating disputes. Rarely, these laws require formal adjudications. Formal adjudications typically are conducted by an administrative law judge (ALJ), followed by an appeal to the agency head. Formal adjudications usually include notice, the right to present evidence, and agency findings of fact and law as well as reasons for the decision. Even in the absence of statutory requirements, federal and state constitutions require procedural due process if the regulation deprives an individual of property or liberty interests.

In summary, modern administrative agencies exercise legislative power to issue rules that carry heavy penalties, executive power to investigate potential violations of health and safety standards and prosecute offenders, and judicial power to interpret law and adjudicate disputes over violations of governing standards. Agency powers have developed for reasons of expediency (because of agency expertise) and politics (because specialists are presumed to act according to disinterested scientific judgments).

Although ample agency power is critically important for achieving public health purposes, it is also troubling and perplexing in a constitutional democracy. One important problem is that commercial regulation may simply transfer wealth from one private interest group to another, rather than promote a public good. For example, licenses can exclude competitors from the market, or regulation of one industry may benefit another providing comparable services (e.g., coal, electrical, or nuclear energy). A related problem is that agencies may be unduly influenced, or "captured," by powerful constituencies or interest groups. Agencies, over the long term, may come to defend the economic interests of regulatory subjects. Finally, agencies may operate in ways that appear unfair or arbitrary, inefficient or bureaucratic, or unacceptable to the public. The very strengths of public health authorities (e.g., neutrality, expertise, and broad powers) can become liabilities if they appear politically unaccountable and aloof from the real concerns and needs of the governed. This is why governors' offices, representative assemblies, and courts struggle over the political and constitutional limits that should be placed on agency action that is nominally intended for the public's health and safety.

Public Health Law Reform

Effective public health protection is technically and politically difficult. Law cannot solve all, or even most, of the challenges facing public health authorities. Yet, law can become an important part of the ongoing work of creating the conditions necessary for people to live healthier and safer lives. A public health law that contributes to health will, of course, be up to date in the methods of assessment and intervention it authorizes. It should also conform to modern standards of law and prevailing social norms. It should be designed to enhance the reality and the public perception of the health department's rationality, fairness, and responsibility. It should help health agencies overcome the defects of their limited jurisdiction over health threats facing the population. Finally, both a new law and the process of its enactment should provide an opportunity for the health department to challenge the apathy about public health that is all too common within both the government and the population at large.

The law relating to public health is scattered across countless statutes and regulations at the state and local levels. Problems of antiquity, inconsistency, redundancy, and ambiguity render these laws ineffective, or even counterproductive, in advancing the population's health. In particular, health codes frequently are outdated, built up in layers over different periods of time, and highly fragmented among the 50 states and territories.

Problem of Antiquity

The most striking characteristic of state public health law and the one that underlies many of its defects is its overall antiquity. Certainly, some statutes are relatively recent in origin, such as those relating to health threats that became salient in the latter part of the 1900s (e.g., environmental law). However, a great deal of public health law was framed in the late 1800s and early to mid-1900s and contains elements that are 40–100 years old (e.g., infectious disease law). Certainly, old laws are not necessarily bad laws. A well written statute may remain useful, effective, and constitutional for many decades.

Nevertheless, old public health statutes that have not been altered substantially since their enactment are often outmoded in ways that directly reduce both their effectiveness and their conformity with modern standards. These laws often do not reflect contemporary scientific understandings of injury and disease (e.g., surveillance, prevention, and response) or legal norms for the protection of individual rights. Rather, public health laws use scientific and legal standards that prevailed at the time they were enacted. Society faces different sorts of risks today and deploys different methods of assessment and intervention. When many of these statutes were written, public health (e.g., epidemiology and biostatistics) and behavioral (e.g., client-centered counseling) sciences were in their infancy. Modern prevention and treatment methods did not exist.

At the same time, many public health laws predate the vast changes in constitutional (e.g., tighter scrutiny and procedural safeguards) and statutory (e.g., disability discrimination) law that have transformed social and legal conceptions of individual rights. Failure to reform these laws may leave public health authorities vulnerable to legal challenge on grounds that they are unconstitutional or that they are preempted by modern federal statutes such as the Americans with Disabilities Act. Even if state public health law is not challenged in court, public health authorities may feel unsure about applying old legal remedies to new health problems within a very different social milieu.

Problem of Multiple Layers of Law

Related to the problem of antiquity is the problem of multiple layers of law. The law in most states consists of successive layers of statutes and amendments—built up in some cases over 100 years or more in response to existing or perceived health threats. This is particularly troublesome in the area of infectious diseases, which forms a substantial part of state health codes. Because communicable disease laws have been passed piecemeal in response to specific epidemics—for example, smallpox, yellow fever, cholera, tuberculosis, venereal diseases, polio, and acquired immune deficiency syndrome (AIDS)—they tell the history of disease control in the United States. Through a process of accretion, the majority of states have come to have several classes of communicable disease law, each with different powers and protections of individual rights: those aimed at traditional sexually transmitted diseases (or venereal diseases), including

gonorrhea, syphilis, chlamydia, herpes; those targeted at specific currently or historically pressing diseases, such as tuberculosis and HIV; and those applicable to "communicable" or "contagious" diseases, a residual class of conditions ranging from measles to malaria whose control does
not usually seem to raise problematic political or social issues. There are, of course, legitimate
reasons to treat some diseases separately. Nevertheless, affording health officials substantially different powers, under different criteria and procedures, for different diseases is more an accident
of history than a rational approach to prevention and control.

The disparate legal structure of state public health laws can significantly undermine their
effectiveness. Laws enacted piecemeal over time are inconsistent, redundant, and ambiguous.
Even the most astute lawyers in departments of health or offices of the attorneys general have
difficulty understanding these arcane laws and applying them to contemporary health threats.

Problem of Inconsistency Among the States and Territories

Public health laws remain fragmented not only within states but also among them. Health codes
within the 50 states and the U.S. territories have evolved independently, leading to profound
variation in the structure, substance, and procedures for detecting, controlling, and preventing injury and disease. In fact, statutes and regulations among American jurisdictions vary so
significantly in definitions, methods, age, and scope that they defy orderly categorization. Ordi-
narily, a different approach among the states is not a problem and is often perceived as a virtue;
an important value of federalism is that states can become laboratories for innovative solutions
to challenging health problems. Nevertheless, there may be good reason for greater uniformity
among the states in matters of public health. Health threats are rarely confined to single jurisdictions, but pose risks within whole regions or the entire nation. For example, geographic
boundaries are largely irrelevant to issues of air or water pollution, disposal of toxic waste, or the
spread of infectious diseases.

Public health law, therefore, should be reformed so that it conforms to modern scientific and
legal standards, is more consistent within and among states, and is more uniform in its approach
to different health threats. Rather than making artificial distinctions among diseases, public
health interventions should be based primarily on the degree of risk, the cost and efficacy of the
response, and the burdens on human rights. A single set of standards and procedures would add
needed clarity and coherence to legal regulation and would reduce the opportunity for politically motivated disputes about how to classify newly emergent health threats.

The Model State Emergency Health Powers Act

Following the anthrax attacks in October 2001, the CDC asked the Center for Law and the
Public's Health (CLPH) to draft the **Model State Emergency Health Powers Act (MSEHPA)**.[22]
The MSEHPA has been adopted in whole or part by the majority of states and the District of
Columbia. MSEHPA is structured to reflect five basic public health functions to be facilitated
by law: preparedness, surveillance, management of property, protection of persons, and public information and communication. The preparedness and surveillance functions took effect
immediately upon passage of MSEHPA. However, the compulsory powers over property and

persons take effect only once the governor has declared a public health emergency, defined as the occurrence of imminent threat of an illness or health condition caused by bioterrorism or a novel or previously controlled or eradicated infectious agent or biological toxin. The health threat must pose a high probability of a large number of deaths or serious disabilities in the population.

MSEHPA facilitates systematic planning for a public health emergency. The state Public Health Emergency Plan must include: coordination of services; procurement of vaccines and pharmaceuticals; housing, feeding, and caring for affected populations (with appropriate regard for their physical and cultural/social needs); and the proper vaccination and treatment of individuals in the event of a public health emergency.

The act provides authority for surveillance of health threats and continuing power to follow a developing public health emergency. For example, the act requires prompt reporting for healthcare providers, pharmacists, veterinarians, and laboratories. MSEHPA also provides for the exchange of relevant data among lead agencies such as public health, emergency management, and public safety.

MSEHPA provides comprehensive powers to manage property and protect persons to safeguard the public's health and security. Public health authorities may close, decontaminate, or procure facilities and materials to respond to a public health emergency; safely dispose of infectious waste; and obtain and deploy healthcare supplies. Similarly, MSEHPA permits public health authorities to physically examine or test individuals as necessary to diagnose or to treat illness, vaccinate or treat individuals to prevent or ameliorate an infectious disease, and isolate or quarantine individuals to prevent or limit the transmission of a contagious disease. The public health authority also may waive licensing requirements for healthcare professionals and direct them to assist in vaccination, testing, examination, and treatment of patients.

Finally, MSEHPA provides for a set of postdeclaration powers and duties to ensure appropriate public information and communication. The public health authority must provide information to the public regarding the emergency, including protective measures to be taken and information regarding access to mental health support.

The Turning Point Model State Public Health Act

The Turning Point National Collaborative on Public Health Statute Modernization seeks to transform and strengthen the legal framework to better protect and promote the public's health. Funded by the Robert Wood Johnson Foundation as part of its Turning Point Initiative, the collaborative is a multidisciplinary group comprising representatives from five states, nine national organizations and government agencies, and experts in specialty areas of public health.

Released on September 16, 2003, after 3 years of development and a national commentary period, the **Turning Point Model State Public Health Act (MSPHA)** is designed to serve as a tool for state, local, and tribal governments to use to revise or update public health statutes and administrative regulations.

Consistent with findings from the IOM's report, *The Future of the Public's Health in the 21st Century*,[4] the act adopts a systematic approach to public health powers and duties. It focuses on the provision of essential public health services and functions. The act presents a broad mission for state and local public health agencies to be carried out in collaboration with public and private entities within the public health system. Much of the substance of the act concerns traditional powers of state or local public health agencies (e.g., contagious disease control, nuisance abatement, and inspections). These powers are articulated within a framework of modern jurisprudence and public health science that balances the protection of the public's health with respect for the rights of individuals and groups.

Guidelines for Public Health Law Reform

Based on the MSEHPA and the MSPHA, the following should guide the process for public health law reform:

1. Define a mission and essential functions and take responsibility for ensuring the conditions of health: State public health statutes should define a cogent mission for the health department and identify a full set of essential public health functions that it should, or must, perform. Broad, well considered mission statements in state public health statutes are important because they establish the purposes or goals of public health agencies. By doing so, they inform and influence the activities of government and, perhaps ultimately, the expectations of society about the scope of public health.

2. Provide a full range of public health powers: Voluntary cooperation is the primary way to obtain compliance with public health measures. However, where voluntary strategies fail, public health officials need a full range of powers to ensure compliance with health and safety standards. At present, public health officials in many states have a sterile choice of either exercising draconian authority, such as deprivation of liberty, or refraining from coercion at all. The temptation is either to exercise no statutory power or to reach for measures that are too restrictive of individual liberty to be acceptable in a modern democratic society. As a result, authorities may make wrong choices in two opposite directions: failing to react in the face of a real threat to health or overreacting by exercising powers that are more intrusive than necessary. Public health authorities need a more flexible set of tools, ranging from incentives and minimally coercive interventions to highly restrictive measures.

3. Impose substantive limits on powers (a demonstrated threat of significant risk): Whereas public health authorities should have all the powers they need to safeguard the public's health, statutes should place substantive limits on the exercise of those powers. The legislature should clearly state the circumstances under which authorities may curtail liberty, autonomy, privacy, and property interests. At present, a few state statutes articulate clear criteria for the exercise of public health powers; others provide vague or incomplete standards; still others leave their use partly or wholly within the discretion of public health officials. Although public health authorities may prefer an unfettered decision-making process, the lack of criteria does not serve their interests or the interests of regulatory subjects. Effective and constitutionally sound public health statutes should set out a rational and reliable way to assess risk to ensure that the health measure is necessary for public protection. Most importantly, public health authorities should be empowered to employ a compulsory intervention only to avert a significant risk based on objective and reliable scientific evidence and made on an individualized (case-by-case) basis.

4. Impose procedural limits on powers (procedural due process): There are good reasons, both constitutional and normative, for legislatures to require health authorities to use a fair process whenever their decisions seriously infringe on liberty, autonomy, proprietary, or other important interests. For example, if health authorities seek to close a restaurant, withdraw a professional (e.g., physician) or institutional (e.g., restaurant) license, or restrict personal freedom (e.g., civil confinement), they should provide procedural due process. Procedural protections help to ensure that health officials make fair and impartial decisions and to reduce community perceptions that public health agencies arbitrarily employ coercive measures. Where few formal procedures exist, public health officials risk rendering biased or inconsistent decisions and erroneously depriving persons and businesses of their rights and freedoms. Although public health authorities may feel that procedural due process is burdensome and an impediment to expeditious action, it can actually facilitate deliberative and accurate decision making.

5. Provide strong protection against discrimination: Throughout the modern history of disease control, the stigma associated with serious diseases and the social hostility that is often directed at those with, or at risk of, disease has interfered with the effective operation of public health programs. The field of public health has always had to consider issues of race, gender, sexual orientation, and socioeconomic status carefully. Persons who fear social repercussions may resist testing or fail to seek needed services. As part of any effort to safeguard the public's health, legislators must find ways to address both the reality and the perception of social risk. Public health statutes should have strong non-discrimination provisions.

6. Provide strong protection for the privacy and security of public health information: Privacy and security of public health data are highly important from the perspective of both the individual and the public at large. Individuals seek protection of privacy so that they can control intimate health information. They have an interest in avoiding the embarrassment and stigma of unauthorized disclosures to family or friends. They similarly have an interest in avoiding discrimination that could result from unauthorized disclosures to employers, insurers, or landlords. At the same time, privacy and security protection can advance the public's health. Privacy assurances can facilitate individual participation in public health programs and promote trust between health authorities and the community. Public health laws, therefore, should have strong safeguards of privacy to protect these individual and societal interests.

Future Outlook

This chapter explores the varied roles of law in advancing the public's health. The field of public health is purposive and interventionist. It does not settle for existing conditions of health, but actively seeks effective techniques for identifying and reducing health threats. Law is a critically important but perennially neglected tool in furthering the public's health. To achieve improvements in public health, law must not be seen as an arcane, indecipherable set of technical rules buried deep within state health codes. Rather, public health law must be seen broadly as the authority and responsibility of government to ensure the conditions for the population's health. As such, public health law has transcending importance in how we think about government, politics, and health policy in the United States.

Discussion Questions

1. Discuss the importance of understanding public health law.
2. Identify two examples of key legislation pertaining to public health and describe them.
3. What is the purpose of public health law reform?
4. What are the guidelines for public health law reform? Describe and discuss.
5. What role do federal agencies have in public health law?
6. What is the role of state health agencies? How does this differ from the federal?
7. Interview a law professor at your university to assess their understanding of public health law or their perspective on health reform.

References

1. Gostin LO, Burris S, Lazzarini Z. The law and the public's health: a study of infectious disease law in the United States. *Columbia Law Rev.* 1999;99(1):59–128.
2. Grad FP. *Public Health Law Manual.* 3rd ed. Washington, DC: American Public Health Association; 2005.
3. Institute of Medicine. *The Future of Public Health.* Washington, DC: National Academies Press; 1988.
4. Institute of Medicine. *The Future of Public's Health in the 21st Century.* Washington, DC: National Academies Press; 2003.
5. Institute of Medicine. *For the Public's Health: Revitalizing Law and Policy to Meet New Challenges.* Washington, DC: National Academies Press; 2011.
6. Institute of Medicine. *Primary Care and Public Health: Exploring Integration to Improve Population Health.* Washington, DC: National Academies Press; 2012.
7. Gostin LO, Jacobson PD, Record KL, et al. Restoring health to health reform: integrating medicine and public health to advance the population's wellbeing. *Penn L Rev.* 2011;159:1777–823. Available at: http://papers.ssrn.com/abstract=1780267. Accessed February 16, 2013.
8. Garner BA, ed. *Black's Law Dictionary.* 7th ed. New York: West Group; 1999.
9. U.S. Constitution, art. 6, cl. 2.
10. *South Dakota v. Dole*, 483 US 203 (1987).
11. *Florida v. HHS*, 567 (2012).
12. Gostin LO, Garcia KK. Affordable Care Act litigation: the Supreme Court and the future of health care reform. *JAMA.* 2012;307(4):369–70.
13. *Jacobson v. Massachusetts*, 197 US 11 (1905).
14. Gostin LO. *Public Health Law: Power, Duty, Restraint.* 2nd ed. Berkeley, CA: University of California Press; 2008.
15. *United States v. Lopez*, 514 US 549 (1995).
16. *United States v. Morrison*, 529 US 598 (2000).
17. *New York v. United States*, 505 US 144 (1992).
18. *Printz v. United States*, 521 US 898 (1997).
19. Institute of Medicine. *For the Public's Health: Investing in a Healthier Future.* Washington, DC: National Academies Press; 2012.
20. *Boreali v. Axelrod*, 517 N.E. 2d 1350 (1987).
21. New York State Department of Health. A guide to the New York State Clean Indoor Air Act. Available at: http://www.health.ny.gov/publications/3402/index.htm. Accessed February 16, 2013.
22. Gostin LO, Sapsin JW, Teret JP, et al. The Model State Emergency Health Powers Act: planning and response to bioterrorism and naturally occurring infectious diseases. *JAMA.* 2002;288:622–8.

Public Health Policy

Walter J. Jones

LEARNING OBJECTIVES

- To understand the relationships between public health and community/population health, and how these sectors of health involve the production of "public goods"
- To appreciate the cyclical nature of health policymaking, and the extent to which problems and issues are addressed but not finally "solved"
- To comprehend how U.S. government structure limits system-wide policymaking due to constitutional features such as federalism and separation of powers
- To learn how to analyze public health policymaking by using the "micro" (marketplace) and "macro" (systems) models, as shown in the chapter examples
- To understand why public health professionals will need both technical and political skills if public health is to be effectively reformed in the 21st century

---

Chapter Overview

Public health has a unique (and uniquely important) place in health policy. Unlike most other areas of health care, public health, often combined with community health, is most concerned about community and population (not individual) health status and outcomes. According to the U.S. Department of Health and Human Services (HHS) and the Centers for Disease Control and Prevention (CDC), essential public health services include community health status monitoring, investigation and diagnosis of health problems and hazards, community health education, community health partnership development, public health law enforcement, provision of access to health services to those who otherwise could not obtain them, public health professional education, and public health research (see **Figure 8.1**).[1]

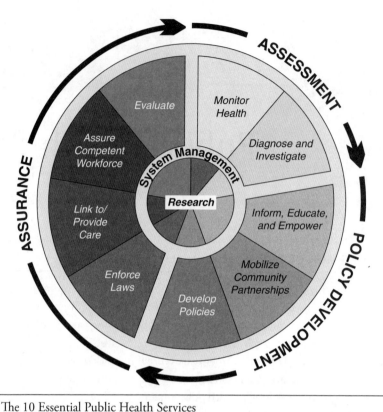

Figure 8.1   The 10 Essential Public Health Services
Source: Reprinted from Centers for Disease Control and Prevention, National Public Health
Performance Standards Program: Orientation to the Essential Public Health Services. Available at:
http://www.cdc.gov/nphpsp/essentialServices.html. Accessed on March 25, 2012.

The public health system is more distinctive and integrated than most of the other health
"systems" in the United States, which are often systems in name only. Working together, local
and state public health agencies, supported by federal government agencies, particularly the
CDC, have a range of overarching responsibilities. As with other areas of government, these
responsibilities do ultimately require policy direction, both from public health administrators
and entities outside of public health. This determination of policies inevitably entails value and
ideological judgments, which in turn involves politics.

Community/population health is inherently a public good.[2] Attaining and maintaining a
public good is challenging, since goods such as community/population health cannot be individually marketed through a supply and demand pricing system. Everyone benefits from public
health goods such as required public health immunization that prevents epidemic diseases, but
since individuals do not have to (in fact, cannot) purchase such a good by themselves, there is
the constant threat of a "tragedy of the commons."[3] Without vigilant government regulation, the
"commons" may deteriorate—parents begin to avoid having their children immunized, overall
immunization rates decline, and the risk of epidemic disease correspondingly rises. Public health

policies therefore require government action. They also touch upon the relationships between individual freedom and social obligation, making them often politically controversial.

Consequently, if one is to understand public health policymaking and policies, it is important to comprehend when, where, and how public health politics is conducted. The exact forms and substance of public health policies, the behavior of individual and institutional actors within the policy process, and policy outcomes vary through time and by location. However, it is always important to understand that politics, whatever the form, is ubiquitous. The simplest definition of **politics** is "who gets what, when, how."[4] Politics is always about the use of political power to get and use resources for the benefit of individual and group interests. This chapter discusses the particular nature of public health and how its objectives create a distinctive politics within policymaking at both the micro (individual actor) and macro (society and its institutions) levels.

Public Health and the Policy Process: Micro and Macro Dimensions

Public health policymaking, like economics, can be usefully analyzed using a **micro** and a **macro** framework. These policy frameworks are roughly analogous to microeconomics (the study of economic interactions at the level of individual producers and consumers) and macroeconomics (the analysis of economic activity at the sector, regional, national, and international levels). For the purposes of policy analysis, they are interrelated and should both be used if the dynamics, substance, and outcomes of public health policymaking are to be fully understood.

Micro Policymaking: The Policy Marketplace Model

The **marketplace model** of policymaking is outlined most completely in Feldstein.[5] As the term indicates, it is adapted from economic theory, with suppliers and demanders, as in the economic marketplace. The policy marketplace model has the following characteristics:

- Like its economic counterpart, the policy marketplace model assumes that individuals and groups are constantly interacting to satisfy their needs. All policy actors are both suppliers and demanders, since they must *exchange* some commodity in the marketplace to "purchase" the other goods that they want. For example, politicians supply favorable policies. In democratic states, these usually include financial subsidies, regulations, and additional health-related services for constituency groups such as senior citizens, hospitals, and medical schools. In exchange, the politicians receive political support, which could include financial contributions, votes, and other desirable commodities.[5]
- As in the economic marketplace, the policy marketplace features disparities in power.[5] Individuals and groups that can supply more can demand more in exchange. In the United States, physicians, senior citizens, hospitals, pharmaceutical and insurance companies, and academic health centers are among the "haves," since they are politically organized, particularly through interest groups and professional associations such as the American Hospital Association (AHA), the American Medical Association (AMA), and the American

Association of Retired Persons (AARP). Members of these groups receive relatively generous government services and legal protections. On the other hand, politically unorganized groups are often less educated, politically powerful, and geographically well situated, and as a consequence receive substandard or no medical services.[6,7]

- In the policy marketplace, the currency used in exchanges can be money and other financial resources, but it can also include superior leadership, more effective organization, more and higher quality information, access to and greater articulation through communications media, and greater group member "intensity," or willingness to exert great efforts in order to advance the interests of the group.[5,6] The latter is evident in U.S. health policymaking with disease-specific and vulnerable groups, such as people with HIV/AIDS and family members with mental illness.[8,9,10] Money matters, but power in the policy marketplace involves much more than money alone.

- To gain control over their relevant areas of the marketplace, nongovernmental groups attempt to forge enduring alliances with governmental agencies. For example, disease-specific groups in the United States lobby for more federal funding for research via the National Institutes of Health (NIH) in their area of disease. More politically powerful groups will be generally more successful at this than the "have-nots." Often, these groups engage in their activities via enduring "iron triangles" or more transient "issue networks" of power and influence.[7,11]

Macro Policymaking: The Policy Systems Model

In contrast to the marketplace of micro policymaking, the macro level of policymaking can be best conceived of as the continual evolution of a complex system. Systems theory was developed in the disciplines of engineering and ecology. It was first applied to political systems by Easton[12] and has been modified for use to describe health policymaking by Longest.[7] As applied to policy systems, it has the following characteristics:

- *Complexity.* Numerous influences interact to produce a system that is continually in flux while generally attaining some level of equilibrium or stability. Individuals, social groups, and organizations are all actors in the policy process.
- *Interrelatedness.* Most significant activities are connected to one another by feedback loops, with direct and indirect impacts. All policy actions create reactions within the system, some perhaps modifying the system itself.
- *Cyclical processes.* With complexity and interrelatedness, the policy process does not have a definite beginning or end, but continues on as long as organized society continues to exist. There are no permanent policy successes or failures.

As noted, the **systems model** is cyclical, so strictly speaking, there is no start or finish—just a continual cycle in which any beginning is arbitrary. In Longest's model,[7] the policy process has the following stages:

1. Recognition of inputs. There are numerous elements of feedback from previous policy decisions (health outcomes, budgets, programs, elections, etc.). These include support and

opposition to current policies, and demands for modifications of these policies. These inputs are recognized by policy actors (including elected officials, interest group leaders, and regulators), and lead to the reactive efforts by policy actors to engage in further policy activities.

2. Policy formulation. Significant policy actors attempt to develop new policies to address these new inputs. In advanced nations, these efforts usually center on formal policymaking structures, such as executive, legislative, judicial, and regulatory institutions. Executive orders are issued, legislation passes through Congress or a similar assembly, lawyers bring cases for consideration before judicial bodies, or regulatory agencies take up issues brought before them. As with the other stages of policymaking, the actions of policy formulation cannot be separated from politics and political considerations.

3. Policy outputs. Efforts at formulation can result in a variety of policy outputs. The most obvious and conventional include statutory laws and regulatory directives (passed by legislatures but subsequently implemented by regulatory agencies). These actions can also contain subsidy and taxation provisions, thus redistributing wealth from one area of society to another. One output can in fact be a **nondecision**—a phenomenon first described by Crenson,[13] defined as a decision to do nothing, which itself has political and policy impacts. An example of this occurred when the U.S. Congress blocked President Bill Clinton's Health Security Act in 1994 without holding any formal hearings or votes.[14,15]

   Many policy outputs also intentionally provide some element of *political symbolism*. As described by Edelman,[16] symbolic politics is virtually inseparable from policymaking, since it provides both policymakers and the mass public with threatening and/or reassuring images that emotionally "condense" often complex arguments into easily accessible reactions. Often these symbols include evocative legislative titles, such as the Medicare Modernization Act of 2003, which not only added a prescription drug benefit for seniors in the United States, but also multibillion dollar subsidies for the U.S. health insurance and pharmaceuticals industries. Who could oppose "modernization"? Symbols can often be used in policymaking to distract the public from policy details that powerful and focused interest groups have worked out for their own benefit (if not the general public's).[16]

4. Implementation. Any policy output which is not a nondecision has to be implemented to have a social impact, and that implementation can be highly variable.[17,18] Government agencies must often work through nongovernmental elements of society to implement policies, and the values and political skills and preferences of leaders in these organizations often determine whether or not (and, if so, how) a new governmental policy is realized through implementation.[7] Due to the vagaries of implementation, the actual impacts of policies are often unanticipated.[19,20]

5. Outcomes. Policies create individual, group, and social impacts. In health policy, the most obvious outcome may involve changes in individual, group, and social health resource consumption and health status. Usually, however, health policies have nonhealth outcomes that may be equally important politically. There are always "winners" and "losers." Some individuals and groups get more resources; others pay. Some have their needs attended to; others are neglected. Policy outcomes may also have profound long-range impacts that were unanticipated, such as the creation of new ethical issues (e.g., in the case

of new technological development resulting from the Human Genome Project) and the need for explicit resource rationing (when government research funding leads to useful but costly new medical technologies and procedures).[21,22]

6. Feedback and subsequent modification. As in previous policy cycles, outputs and outcomes create the reactions in society mentioned earlier and related further efforts at policy development. The policy agenda is refreshed, and the cycle continues on. Often the success of a previous cycle (e.g., the enactment of Medicare and Medicaid to address the lack of healthcare access for seniors and some categories of the "poor") leads to the challenges faced in a subsequent cycle (e.g., how to cope with the unsustainable healthcare demands and cost inflation triggered by events such as the introduction of large government health insurance programs such as Medicare and Medicaid).[23,24] Health policymaking does result in great benefits for individuals and society, but it also seems like "one thing after another" when viewed in terms of day-to-day activities. Problems and issues are addressed during the policy cycle, but are almost never completely solved, since the byproducts of policymaking usually create side effects and other associated changes that themselves lead to new challenges and problems.

The Impact of Government Structure on Policymaking

Those who would like sweeping and innovative government reforms and policy initiatives are often disappointed that such things seldom happen in U.S. health policymaking (or *any* area of U.S. policymaking, for that matter). They should realize that the primary reason for less expansive health reforms in the United States than in other democracies stems from the U.S. Constitution, and the structure of government that it sets forth. As was famously noted by James Madison when arguing for its adoption in *The Federalist Papers*, one of the central aims of the U.S. Constitution was to minimize the likelihood of government tyranny through the establishment of divided government (separate executive, legislative, and judicial branches) and federalism (distinct national and state governments with differing powers and prerogatives).[25] Major political change could not and would not take place without a strong national consensus—a consensus beyond mere majority support. Finally, even if there is a social/political consensus for change, any national and/or state government initiatives can be struck down if declared unconstitutional in a judicial review by (usually) unelected and life-appointed judges.

Examined from this perspective, the U.S. system of government and the Constitution have been very successful. The United States has remained a political democracy since the Constitution was adopted in 1787 (albeit with enormous flaws in that democracy when it came to slavery and the rights of women and racial and ethnic minority groups). We have not had a government where democracy collapsed into totalitarian dictatorship under economic, social, and political pressures (as Germany, Japan, and Italy did). The great 20th-century rival to limited democracy ("bourgeois democracy," as they would denigrate it), Marxism/Leninism, promised true social revolution and equality, but instead produced political absolutism, social misery, economic dislocation and mass imprisonment, and murder in most nations that adopted it.[26]

However, at least in the United States, that system of government has also historically been a strong force against major social change. No other democracy has been so slow to adopt the belief that all of its citizens deserve some minimum level of health care. None of the other democracies are questioning such a belief under the notion that such a universal benefit is somehow an unconstitutional "power grab" by the national government against its citizens.[27]

The U.S. political system is designed to slow or stop most major policy initiatives, in health care as elsewhere. Because of this, elected representatives, along with dominant interest groups and individuals already receiving significant benefits from the system, usually adopt a supportive attitude toward the policy status quo. For example, whatever the range of attitudes toward health reform among senior citizens and AARP members, the overwhelming majority of these individuals oppose any major program cutbacks in "their" programs, especially Medicare. For most involved individuals and groups, the operational definition of "good health reform" often becomes "a reform that helps others *and does not have an adverse impact on my own situation.*"

In practice, this leads to most major policy actors agreeing to oppose major changes, since such changes are more likely to disrupt long-standing configurations of power and resource distribution. Most policymaking is incremental—modest changes on accepted laws and programs. Even the Patient Protection and Affordable Care Act (ACA), which can be considered a major system reform, was only enacted after being significantly redesigned to meet the objections (and possible vetoes) by influential groups such as senior citizens (no changes in the structure of Medicare), pharmaceutical companies (no national government price controls or formularies on drugs), trial lawyers (no changes in existing tort and liability laws), and health insurance companies (no universal insurance coverage without a requirement that all individuals must purchase health insurance—the "individual mandate").[28] In contrast, individuals and groups clearly not receiving adequate health care through the current system are disproportionately poor, uneducated, and (most importantly) unorganized. They undoubtedly would support nonincremental health reform, but in reality do not have enough political power to get their preferences enacted into law.[5]

One final, fundamental impact of U.S. government structure is to discourage systems thinking—concern for the entire system, as opposed to one part of it. All but one elected policymaker (the U.S. president) gain power through the support of a smaller, nonnational constituency—a statewide or local district. Since the policy process is incremental, to have a significant impact on policy, an elected policymaker has to specialize and focus on a small subset of policy issues especially important to her or his constituency. In addition, he or she has to stay in office for multiple terms. As has been said, the first rule of politics is to get elected. The second rule is to get reelected. Because of this, veteran lawmakers always, first and foremost, focus on taking care of "the folks back home"—individuals, communities, and interest groups.

As a consequence, the concept of national, system-wide health reform is not really politically useful. No one gains popularity and reelection by reforming the system. Rather, they get into and stay in office through efforts to modify the healthcare system in a way that "the folks back home" support—usually through higher benefit levels, subsidies, and/or rights (and usually without simultaneous tax increases to cover the costs of these initiatives). Like it or not, for policymakers the U.S. political system features a constant focus on one's own constituency groups and interests. In reality, the question is almost never, "What would best benefit the nation?"

Instead, the constituents ask their elected policymakers, "What have you done for me lately?" The elected policymaker, if he or she wishes to survive politically, needs to respond with convincing evidence of the benefits provided to those constituents. While the nation's citizens and policymakers pay solemn lip service to reforming the system, in fact it is never the primary concern of anyone who really matters in health policymaking.

Public Health Policy Issues

Public health is not as visible or publicized as many other aspects of health care. When polled, the public generally approves of public health measures, but most of the time pays little attention to what it feels is (in the absence of a general crisis, such as a pandemic) an obscure and somewhat boring area of health care. There have been exciting and popular TV series about individual physicians (*Ben Casey, Dr. Kildare, Trapper John, MD, House,* and *Private Practice,* to name a few) and areas of health care such as the emergency room (*ER*) and combat military medicine (*MASH*). It is hard to imagine such a phenomenon taking place with public health—restaurant inspection, disease control (unless it involves a pandemic that kills millions worldwide, which can then become a movie like *Outbreak* or *Contagion*), and health education are just not as dramatic and glamorous.

However little the public really thinks about public health, it is clear that public health agencies at the national and state levels do face determined skepticism and often outright opposition from influential organizations and industries whose perceived economic wellbeing and/or freedom of choice face regulation or curtailment due to public health concerns. Thus, however invisible public health is to the public itself, what it does in terms of policy clearly has political dimensions. Public health organizations and leaders have no choice other than to become involved in health policymaking and the political arena.

Many of the most important current public health policy issues feature active political conflict at multiple levels of government and society. By using the marketplace (micro) and system (macro) models presented earlier, one can analyze public health policy activities and issues on these multiple levels. The sections that follow describe two examples of public health issues, viewed using these models.

Vaccines and Autism: Public Activism Against Science and Public Health

Context
One of the central tenets of public health, verified through centuries of experience, is that infectious disease is best kept at bay through the maintenance of "herd immunity" through mass vaccination (with at least an 80% vaccination rate). Vaccination programs in the United States (and elsewhere) have generally been successful. Vaccine-preventable diseases have declined such that annual totals are at or near record lows in the United States.[29] There are still some problems in getting people vaccinated, particularly in poor and minority communities. Consequently, public health programs try to target vulnerable populations to increase vaccination rates and reduce disparities.

However, the imperative to maximize vaccination rates has come into increasing conflict with highly motivated individuals and groups asserting their right to choose whether or not they (or often, their children) need to or should be vaccinated. These groups have become increasingly well organized and assert their opposition to public health vaccination laws through the mass media, state and local elections, and the judicial system. In the early 21st century, one of the most visible examples of this has been the controversy over the alleged relationship between autism and vaccines.

The "scientific" cornerstone of the case that vaccines cause autism has been a single study published in *The Lancet* by Wakefield et al. in 1998.[30] The study was seized upon by understandably concerned parents of autistic children, and Dr. Wakefield himself became active in the effort to mobilize opposition to vaccination. Some public health officials supporting vaccination efforts in testimony before legislative bodies had to face angry, demonstrating groups of parents who claimed that they had severely harmed their children through vaccination. *The Lancet* study was eventually discredited by subsequent investigations, and the publishing journal retracted it. However, a small group of scientists continue to produce studies asserting the vaccine–autism link in what has been termed "a tale of shifting hypotheses."[31]

The policy marketplace

The marketplace in the vaccine–autism controversy has featured a variety of participants, with differing demands and resource levels. The most important participants include:

- *Public health officials.* As would be expected, their primary demand is active enforcement of public health laws, including immunization of all children. This requires cooperation from elected officials and the judiciary. Their resources include health scientific information and expertise, and a general respect from and credibility with most American policymakers, health professionals, and the public.

- *Elected policymakers.* As noted earlier, whatever their public service and ideological commitments and professions, first and foremost, they want to be reelected. That means showing sympathy and support for groups and causes that appear to be generally favored by the public, most certainly including anguished parents with autistic children who believe that vaccination caused the disorder. Most elected officials respect and appreciate public health professionals and their efforts, but do not want to lose political support by too strongly supporting public health imperatives against the affected parents and children.

- *Judicial policymakers.* One particular characteristic of U.S. policymaking in general is that it is likely to involve litigation at some point. In this case, activist parents have engaged lawyers to launch several highly publicized lawsuits.[32] The primary resource that judges have is substantial legal independence—the ability to make independent rulings on the cases before them. However, most judges do not have a substantial amount of medical scientific knowledge, so they need others to supply expertise in those areas. Both sides on the vaccine–autism conflict have attempted to provide scientific documentation in their court briefs (with the provaccination side being much more successful in doing this, given the nature of current scientific knowledge).

- *Parents of children with autism.* As the catalysts for the antivaccination efforts, their most important resources include general public sympathy and support, and a high degree of intensity. For many of them, getting support for their plight and changing vaccination policies has become their life mission. Their primary spokespersons are sometimes highly visible celebrities such as Jenny McCarthy, who has an autistic child and has founded the Generation Rescue organization to help parents with autism.[33]
- *Vaccine manufacturers.* Certainly manufacturers want to make profits, but the pharmaceutical industry has entered a turbulent economic period, with questions about the viability of their basic business model.[34] Companies are always wary of the expenses and bad publicity that may result from litigation. Consequently, when sued they will defend themselves, but they are also likely to attempt to avoid the risk of litigation for any particular problem by threatening to stop manufacturing the vaccine in question unless they can get special government legislation that protects them from such litigation.[35]

The Policy System

The process of drug approval and marketing has been modified over time, but is fairly mature, with established procedures and experienced institutions.[36] While there are significant issues with post-market safety, drug approval and marketing practices are accepted by all of the policy participants mentioned earlier (except, in their particular situation, parents with autistic children). This means that changes in drug and vaccination policies are usually incremental in nature. Because of this, the odds of the parents with autistic children (and their lawyers) winning a lawsuit against current policies have always been slight. As with other parent groups concerned about vaccine safety, they have been able to reduce *de facto* compliance, but not the laws requiring compliance.

Some time ago, the established policy players were able to overcome the lack of expertise concerning vaccines in the judicial system—and the fear of runaway costs through frequent and large lawsuits—through the enactment of the National Childhood Vaccine Injury Act of 1986. As the U.S. Court of Federal Claims has noted, "Congress intended that the Vaccine Program provide individuals a swift, flexible and less adversarial alternative to the often costly and lengthy civil arena of traditional tort litigation."[37] The program established the Office of Special Masters in the Court of Federal Claims. Special Masters are judicial personnel who have special training and powers to deal with the complex scientific issues surrounding vaccine safety. The entire legal process is streamlined and fact based. There is no jury selected from average citizens (most having little understanding of science); instead, the cases are decided by specialists. This tends to provide a strong advantage to drug manufacturers and other health professionals, and hampers the maneuvers of trial lawyers. As shown in **Table 8.1**, this advantage has been clearly present in the legal conflicts over vaccines and autism through the Vaccine Court since 1989.

One family did receive a $1.5 million court award in 2010, but without any admission of a vaccine–autism link. However, in March 2010, the Special Masters of the U.S. Court of Federal Claims examined three test cases, and ruled that the evidence of such a link was "scientifically

Table 8.1 Vaccine Court Adjudications of Autism Claims Under the National Childhood Vaccine Injury Act of 1986

| Fiscal Year | Omnibus Autism Proceeding (OAP) | | |
	Compensable*	Dismissed	Total
FY 1989	0	0	0
FY 1990	0	0	0
FY 1991	0	0	0
FY 1992	0	0	0
FY 1993	0	0	0
FY 1994	0	0	0
FY 1995	0	0	0
FY 1996	0	0	0
FY 1997	0	0	0
FY 1998	0	0	0
FY 1999	0	0	0
FY 2000	0	0	0
FY 2001	0	0	0
FY 2002	0	4	4
FY 2003	0	21	21
FY 2004	0	112	112
FY 2005	0	51	51
FY 2006	0	110	110
FY 2007	0	34	34
FY 2008	0	56	56
FY 2009	0	187	187
FY 2010	1**	215	216
FY 2011	0	1,263	1,263
FY 2012	0	1,650	1,650
Totals	1	3,703	3,704

*May include case(s) that were originally filed and processed as OAP cases but in which the final adjudication does not include a finding of vaccine-related autism.

**HHS has never concluded in any case that autism was caused by vaccination.

Source: Health Resources and Services Administration. Statistics Reports. Available at: http://www.hrsa.gov/vaccinecompensation/statisticsreports.html#Stats. Accessed March 17, 2012.

unsupportable."[38] In early 2011, the U.S. Supreme Court issued a major decision that prevented parents with autistic children from continuing to sue drug makers through the regular court system. They declared that any legal action would have to go through the U.S. Court of Federal Claims.[39] Given the general back-and-forth indecisiveness in other areas of health litigation such as medical malpractice, this was a stunningly complete victory for the drug industry and associated medical professionals, precluding almost all possible avenues for further legal action. The prevailing health legal policies concerning vaccination liability were maintained more or less intact, as was the specific protection from litigation gained by the pharmaceutical industry through the health policy process.

Global Public Health and Infectious Disease: National Political Imperatives Against International Disease Prevention

Context

The effectiveness (or lack thereof) of public health in monitoring, controlling, and responding to infectious disease not only affects the health status of millions of people around the world, but also affects the national security, economy, and society of the United States and the rest of the world in numerous and often unpredictable ways.[40] At the highest level, global public health problems such as infectious disease and air, water, and land pollution can create national security problems for the United States. The Department of Defense is engaged in active monitoring of public health efforts in many areas of Africa, South America, and Asia, since health problems in other nations can create governmental instability that in turn endanger U.S. security interests.[40] Poorly controlled infectious diseases can threaten the readiness of military units, as has already been seen in nations such as South Africa.[40]

The U.S economy has become increasingly integrated with the rest of the world, with the rise of global supply chains and international product markets. Because American businesses depend on foreign production and consumption for their economic viability, health problem such as pandemics can disrupt commercial activities. One striking example of this occurred in 2003, when the severe acute respiratory syndrome (SARS) epidemic spread throughout East Asia. Americans were not directly affected by the disease, but the East Asian nation of Taiwan had many citizens who contracted the disease. As a public health response, it temporarily shut down many of its businesses to slow the transmission of SARS, including factories manufacturing computer chips and motherboards. Since Taiwan is one of the largest producers of these and other electronic components for the world market, the production and distribution of computers dropped sharply. Given the importance of computers in almost every aspect of production, worldwide (and U.S.) economic activity was significantly slowed during that year.[41]

The growth of HIV/AIDS provides a dramatic example of the relationship between the spread of infectious disease and worldwide economic change. The disease apparently originated in Africa in the 1920s. Its diffusion steadily increased as world travel and commerce grew during the rest of the 20th century. As recounted in the seminal history of AIDS in the United States by Randy Shilts, the spread of AIDS was accelerated by the sexual promiscuity of already HIV-infected individuals such as Patient Zero, Gaetan Dugas, who was a Canadian airline attendant who had sexual partners all over the world.[42] Unsafe sexual practices (and the growth of industries such as sex tourism in many nations) create public health problems that are especially dangerous with increasing population mobility across national borders.

The policy marketplace

The global health policy marketplace is, of course, global. It is distinguished from the previous case involving autism and vaccines by involving a broader range of public and private sector national and international health-relevant institutions.

- At the international level, there are a number of significant health organizations concerned with infectious disease. The most important of them is undoubtedly the *World*

Health Organization (WHO). It is generally accepted and respected, with most nations actively participating. WHO engages in vitally important data collection on health and disease, and provides some health services within national borders. It also places a good deal of emphasis on health education and prevention, which work to reduce the danger and impact of infectious disease.[43] However, as an international organization, the WHO can get caught up in global political controversies, such as the conflicts between public health imperatives and Catholic Church doctrine and practice opposing the use of condoms to reduce HIV transmission.[44]

- At the national level, most countries have one or more public health agencies. With respect to infectious disease, the most important U.S. agency is the *Centers for Disease Control and Prevention*. The CDC is the leading policy actor with respect to U.S. infectious disease surveillance and research, and works globally with the WHO and its national counterparts.[45] However, the CDC does not have any authority over ongoing U.S. public health provision—that is a state and local responsibility. It can inform and advise state and local public health agencies, but it cannot compel any action in response to an epidemic. Questions about the future course of the CDC—along with doubts about the effectiveness of its leaders—have led to serious employee morale problems and attracted the critical scrutiny of the U.S. Congress.[46] As might be expected, the authority and resource levels of public health agencies in other nations vary widely.

- At the national level, the United States has additional organizations involved in various activities that relate to infectious disease monitoring and control. The *Department of Defense (DoD)* is well equipped to detect and respond to infectious disease as part of its military preparedness, but its authority to act domestically is limited (it has to be invited in by a state government unless a national emergency is declared), and it is usually cautious and reluctant to engage in such domestic activities, feeling that they might interfere with its international response capabilities.[47] The *Department of Agriculture (DoA)* handles inspection and surveillance for food-borne disease, including imported products. The *Federal Emergency Management Agency (FEMA)* focuses on disaster response and relief, which could include a pandemic. The *Department of Homeland Security (DHS)* can coordinate the activities of relevant federal government agencies with respect to a disease outbreak, but it is primarily oriented toward a response to terrorist threats such as bioterrorism, rather than "natural" epidemics. The *Food and Drug Administration (FDA)* works with other U.S. and foreign agencies on food and drug safety issues, but does not concentrate on disease aspects. Taken as a whole, the United States has a multiplicity of national government organizations concerned with infectious disease, but *none* of these organizations has the legal authority and mission to respond without coordinating its efforts with the other involved agencies and/or levels of government. Voluntary cooperation is usually needed for joint activities, as shown in **Figure 8.2**.

- *State Health Agencies*, responsible for state public health policies and activities, exist in each of the 50 American states, along with the District of Columbia and each American territory and commonwealth. Their umbrella professional organization is the Association of State and Territorial Health Officials (ASTHO). Within each state, the health agency

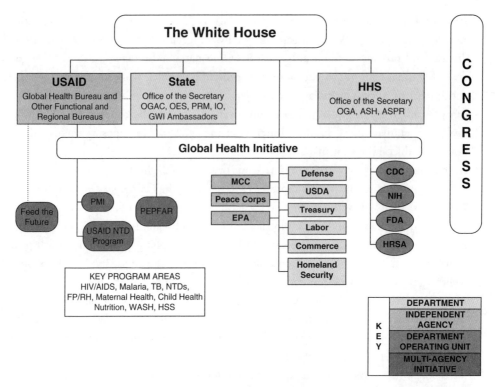

Figure 8.2   The U.S. Government's Global Health Architecture
Source: From: Kaiser Family Foundation. The U.S. government's global health policy architecture: Structure, programs and funding. Available at: http://www.kff.org/globalhealth/7881.cfm. Accessed on March 15, 2012.

usually dominates infectious disease policymaking, but obviously has no legal interstate power. As with the multiple federal agencies, they are generally limited to information sharing and other voluntary activities.

- *National policymakers (elected or otherwise)* have the ultimate responsibility for setting policies and initiating activities regarding infectious disease. As in the example of vaccines and autism, whatever public health professionals and their organizations decide, in the U.S. nonroutine activity in response to infectious disease usually requires the assent of elected executives (state governors and/or the president). Whatever the formal governmental differences, the same is true in other nations. That means that infectious disease decision making will not just involve public health considerations. Other state and national imperatives (national security, legal precedent, and issues of political impact) will also figure into deliberations.

- *Nongovernmental Organizations (NGOs)* play an increasing role in providing public health services, particularly in less developed and conflict-ridden nations. Public and international public health–oriented NGOs include such groups as the International Committee of the Red Cross, Doctors Without Borders, Oxfam, Save the Children, and Project HOPE. Their nongovernmental status often permits them great operational flexibility and the ability to successfully provide innovative services. However, their nongovernmental status also limits their abilities, since they have to get the permission (or at least the tolerance) of national governments in order to carry out their work.[48]

The Policy System

In contrast to the situation with vaccines and autism, the lack of a central governmental mechanism inherently limits the effectiveness of efforts to combat infectious disease at the global level. As was noted at the beginning of this chapter, public health is ultimately a public good, in that the primary benefits cannot be parceled out using a market system. In the case of infectious disease, this means that if the United States is going to best protect itself, it must become proactively involved in public health and disease prevention efforts in other countries, especially those nations in Africa and Asia that are most likely to be the sites for initial disease development.

Since the early 1990s, the United States has indeed followed this strategy of proactive involvement. The Department of Health and Human Services now has an Office of Global Health Affairs. President George W. Bush committed significant U.S. resources to worldwide efforts to combat AIDS, and the Obama administration has followed up with a Global Health Initiative to expand efforts against such pandemic diseases as AIDS and malaria.[49] These efforts are certainly laudable and have had significant impacts. But the president (and any other national leader) faces fundamental obstacles to any effort to address global infectious disease problems.

To begin with, the attempt of any nation to work with another nation entails inevitable political considerations. In the abstract, all nations want to reduce infectious disease, but in practice differing political ideologies can keep them apart. Arab nations will almost never work directly with Israel on public health concerns, for example. Any U.S. international health effort will be viewed with suspicion by nations that feel threatened by the United States—Iran and North Korea, for example. And *no* nation will permit international health concerns to limit its sovereignty and prerogatives, if it can help it. This can hamper cooperative public health efforts to reduce infectious disease.

International infectious disease efforts are also hampered by a combination of the "tragedy of the commons" and localized political representation factors mentioned earlier in the chapter. Every nation does benefit from controlling infectious disease, whether or not they actually contribute to the effort; it is a true public good. As with individuals, there is always the "free rider" temptation. The actual global efforts to control infectious disease usually have disproportionate contributions of resources from a small number of wealthier nations. Even if the other nations are not willing to contribute, they will reap some of the benefits.

There are also political issues surrounding the payment for and control of international infectious disease programs. As was just discussed, no nation wants to be openly dictated to, so national leaders' jealously might control political sovereignty. This is true whether or not the national government in question has the competence to effectively administer public health policies, or whether the government is a democracy or a dictatorship, or whether it is administratively honest or corrupt. The nations that actually pay for these policies may have different attitudes, however. Their policymakers are elected or otherwise answer to their own citizens, not the world community. In the United States, there is a general perception that the nation spends far more on foreign assistance of all types than it actually does. Public opinion surveys show that Americans believe that the United States devotes up to 20% of the federal government budget to foreign aid; the real figure is closer to 2%.[50]

The U.S. public also believes that much of this aid is worthless and/or futile—"a waste of our tax dollars." Elected U.S. representatives pick up quickly on such attitudes, and make sure that their policy behavior reflects them. Everyone benefits from global public health efforts to control disease, but the most immediate beneficiaries—the people living in the (often Third World Asian, Latin American, or African) nations where infectious diseases like HIV and influenza begin their initial growth and movement due to poor environments and inadequate education, nutrition, and health care—do not vote in U.S. elections. In contrast, cynical and skeptical U.S. taxpayers do vote in sizable numbers. Following the political imperative noted earlier (get elected, and then get reelected), U.S. politicians agree with their constituents and do what they say they want—cut foreign aid budgets, including funding for international public health agencies such as WHO.

International public health agencies (including NGOs as well as governments) therefore operate in a perennial world of inadequate funding and scope. Despite the fact that more global health spending on infectious disease would probably be highly cost effective from a *global* standpoint, policymaking structures that are inherently *national* in orientation ensure that global infectious disease policies will always be circumscribed in authority, underfunded, and always reliant on voluntary cooperation. Sooner or later, nationalism always seems to trump international health—even if the individual nations and their citizens ultimately suffer from the resulting public health failures.

Future Outlook

In an era of national economic difficulties, ever-tightening budgets, and considerable public skepticism about the effectiveness (or even the utility) of government, it is a considerable challenge to "sell" public health. As the Institute of Medicine noted in a 2002 report, Americans often seem unenthusiastic about the longer term health improvements brought forth through public health and environmental programs. Rather, they appear to be more interested in (and willing to provide resources for) the development of individually oriented, "silver bullet" health solutions that can address poor personal health once it develops.[51] As noted earlier, public health is not "sexy" or "dramatic" to the general public. It therefore must usually be "sold" to policymakers more directly, on the basis of the considerable benefits it provides at relatively modest costs.

The world is becoming more complex, interrelated, and (as *New York Times* columnist Thomas Friedman would say) "flat."[52] To meet the needs of the 21st century, public health policymakers must devise reforms to address a number of critical issues, including those that follow.

Coordination of Public Health Activities

As was discussed earlier, the U.S. constitutional features of federalism and separation of powers, along with the multiplication of federal government agencies with some public health responsibility, has meant that it is difficult to coordinate activities. As with homeland security, it may be necessary to set up an umbrella agency or some combined national/state government entity to ensure that public health efforts are working together to maximize operational and cost effectiveness.[53]

Improving Public Health Preparedness

According to RAND Corporation testimony before Congress, the United States must continue to invest in interoperable information technology for routine and enhanced surveillance, provider notification, outbreak investigation, and event management by public health. However, RAND also cautions that these investments must come with improved linkages between public health and other organizations with responsibilities for shared situational awareness and emergency response to public health crises such as the 9/11 terrorist attacks and Hurricane Katrina.[54] For such situations, lawmakers need to more clearly define public health responsibilities, and how these responsibilities can be harmonized with those held by law enforcement, military, social service, and emergency medical and other emergency-response entities.

Improvement of Public Health Outcomes Research and Financial Management Methodologies and Tools

To consider the state of public health outcomes research, the U.S Department of Health and Human Services, Office of Minority Health, assisted by the Robert Wood Johnson Foundation, convened a Public Health Systems Research expert panel. In their summary and recommendations report in February 2008, they concluded that as a professional subfield, public health is considerably behind many other areas of health care in being able to define, measure, and assess related health outcomes. Their suggestions for improvement included more interaction with outcomes researchers in other fields to develop distinctive public health outcomes research methodologies, and to develop means by which research can be integrated with the reform of public health management practices.[55]

Public health organizations also need improved financial management methods and tools. A 2012 Institute of Medicine report concluded that "the public health financing structure is broken.... Each funder has its own rules of accounting, performance, monitoring and evaluation."[56, pp. 2–5, 6] Funding is often compartmentalized and inflexible, with no clear point of accountability. According to the IOM, public health financing needs more rigorous and uniform budgeting systems. Additionally, these budgeting systems also need to be more clearly tied to measures of program activities and outcomes. Without these features, it is difficult for public health agencies to directly show how their activities have led to positive outcomes. The credibility of public health is correspondingly diminished in the eyes of budget policymakers, so public health loses out when funding choices are made.

Getting Quality into the Public Health System

All of these reform areas tie into the growing imperative for quality improvement in public health. Not surprisingly, with deficiencies in coordination, financial management, and outcomes research, public health has lagged behind other healthcare areas in terms of applying quality concepts and techniques in service delivery. There are currently growing efforts, centered in the U.S. Department of Health and Human Services, to implement a "Consensus Statement on Quality in the Public Health System."[57] This consensus states that quality improvement depends on ensuring that the U.S. public health system is population-centered, equitable, proactive, health-promoting, risk reducing, vigilant, transparent, efficient, and effective.[58] Inevitably, significant additional research will be needed to develop the concepts and methods appropriate for public health.

Of course, political leadership and determination will be needed to achieve any of these possible reforms, which brings us back to the beginning of this chapter. There are clearly forces working in favor of a greater nationwide emphasis on public health. As a growing body of research has shown, public health activities improve environmental and community health, and these aspects of health are as essential for good health outcomes as individually directed health service provision.[59] Public health "works"; however, it does so less dramatically than other forms of health care, and its beneficiaries are not specifically targeted. All members of society benefit from public health, but few of them appreciate it, or even think much about it. Public health does not have the public visibility and respect of health care provided by physicians and hospitals, for example. This reduced visibility and respect translates into fewer resources and fewer political "wins."

Unfortunately, there is no easy or quick way to solve this problem. Public health organizations and professionals must compete in the policy marketplace for resources and authority (the "who gets, what, when, how" of politics). The stronger the substance of public health, the more effective it will be in this competition. That means maintaining currently successful activities, but also enhancing them through quality improvement efforts. It also means having public health organizations with better budgeting systems and outcomes research units, so that they can more clearly see *how* they work well, and how their funding relates to successful outcomes.

All of this is necessary but not sufficient. Policymaking is not just about substance, but also about political skill—the ability to publicize and advocate a cause by connecting with both policymakers and members of the public on rational and emotional levels. Public health therefore needs political leaders in addition to talented epidemiologists, laboratory workers, inspectors, physicians, and nurses. Those already in public health need to develop better political talents in order to develop winning coalitions in the policy marketplace. Those entering public health need to know that their profession is not just about health and science. It is also about peoples' wants, needs, and fears. To deal with these while advancing the field and the community's health, the 21st-century public health professional will need to be an effective politician as well.

Discussion Questions

1. Can you find examples of "the tragedy of the commons" in your own community? Describe and explain these. What should public and community health professionals do to respond to these "tragedies"?

2. The chapter notes that the constitutional structure of U.S. government limits the ability to conduct system-level health policymaking. Do you feel that the United States should amend its Constitution to reduce or remove those limiting features (especially federalism and separation of power)? Why or why not?

3. Look at your own community to find an example of the policy marketplace in action with respect to the individuals and groups involved in health policymaking. Who are the suppliers and demanders? Which individuals and groups seem to be most successful in the case, and why?

4. This chapter describes the case of autism and vaccines, noting that there is a conflict between the imperatives of science and individual and family choice. Can you think of another example of public health where this conflict exists? Describe and analyze this example.

5. Consider the issues surrounding the provision of health care to undocumented immigrants in the United States. To what extent are those issues similar to the ones discussed in the example provided in this chapter of global public health and infectious disease? Explain.

References

1. Public Health Functions Steering Committee. Public health in America. Available at: http://www .health.gov/phfunctions/public.htm. Accessed May 7, 2012.
2. Samuelson PA. The pure theory of public expenditure. *Rev Econ Stat.* 1954;36(4):387–9.
3. Hardin G. The tragedy of the commons. *Science.* 1968;162(3859):1243–8.
4. Lasswell H. *Politics: Who Gets What, When, How.* New York: World Publishing Company; 1951.
5. Feldstein PJ. *The Politics of Health Legislation: An Economic Perspective.* Chicago: Health Administration Press; 2006.
6. Olson M. *The Logic of Collective Action.* Cambridge, MA: Harvard University Press; 1965.
7. Longest BB. *Health Policymaking in the United States.* Chicago: Health Administration Press; 2006.
8. Forman C. Grassroots victim organizations: Mobilizing for personal and public health. In: Cigler AJ, Loomis BA, eds. *Interest Group Politics*, 4th ed. Washington, DC: Congressional Quarterly Press; 1995.
9. Denenberg R. The community: Mobilizing and accessing resources and services. In: Cohen FL, Durham JD, eds. *Women, Children and HIV/AIDS.* New York: Springer Publishing Company; 1993.
10. Koyanagi C, Bevalacqua JJ. Managed care in public mental health systems. In: Hackey RB, Rochefort DA, eds. *The New Politics of State Health Policy.* Lawrence, KS: University Press of Kansas; 2000:186–206.
11. Weissert CS, Weissert WG. *Governing Health.* 3rd ed. Baltimore, MD: Johns Hopkins University Press; 2006.
12. Easton D. *A Systems Analysis of Political Life.* Chicago: University of Chicago Press, 1979.
13. Crenson MA. *The Unpolitics of Air Pollution.* Baltimore, MD: Johns Hopkins University Press; 1971.
14. Yankelovich D. The debate that wasn't: the public and the Clinton plan. *Health Aff.* 1995;14(1):7–23.
15. Skocpol T. The rise and the resounding demise of the Clinton plan. *Health Aff.* 1995;14(1):66–85.
16. Edelman M. *The Symbolic Uses of Politics.* Urbana, IL: University of Illinois Press; 1964.
17. Brown LD. Getting there: the political context for implementing health care reform. In: Brecher C, ed. *Implementation Issues and National Health Care Reform.* Washington, DC: Josiah Macy, Jr. Foundation; 1992:13–46.

18. Thompson FJ. The evolving challenge of health policy implementation. In: Litman TJ, Robins LS, eds. *Health Politics and Policy*. 3rd ed. New York: Delmar Publishers; 1997:155–75.

19. Pressman JL, Wildavsky A. *Implementation*. Berkeley, CA: University of California Press; 1973.

20. Sparer MS, Brown LD. States and the health care crisis: limits and lessons of laboratory federalism. In: Rich RF, White WD, eds. *Health Policy, Federalism and the American States*. Washington, DC: Urban Institute Press, 1996:181–202.

21. Wenk E. *Margins for Survival: Overcoming Political Limits in Steering Technology*. New York: Pergamon Press; 1979.

22. Aaron HJ, Schwartz WB. *Can We Say No?* Washington, DC: Brookings Institution Press; 2005.

23. Moon M. *Medicare Now and in the Future*. 2nd ed. Washington, DC: Urban Institute Press; 1996.

24. Oberlander J. *The Political Life of Medicare*. Chicago: University of Chicago Press; 2003.

25. Madison J. No. 10. In Hamilton A, Madison J, Jay J. *The Federalist Papers*. New York: The New American Library of World Literature: 1961.

26. Courtois S. Conclusion: why? In: Courtois S, Werth N, Panné JL, et al. *The Black Book of Communism: Crimes, Terror, Reprssion*. Cambridge, MA: Harvard University Press; 1999:727–57.

27. Liptak A. Supreme Court is asked to rule on health care. *New York Times*, September 28, 2011. Available at: http://www.nytimes.com/2011/09/29/us/justice-dept-asks-supreme-court-for-health-care-ruling.html. Accessed February 16, 2013.

28. *Frontline*, PBS-TV. Obama's deal. Broadcast April 13, 2010. Available at: http://www.pbs.org/wgbh/pages/frontline/obamasdeal/. Accessed May 5, 2012.

29. Centers for Disease Control and Prevention. Vaccines and preventable diseases. Available at: http://www.cdc.gov/vaccines/vpd-vac/default.htm. Accessed May 1, 2012.

30. Wakefield A, Murch SH, Anthony A, et al. Ileal-lymphoid-nodular hyperplasia, non-specific colitis, and pervasive developmental disorder in children. *Lancet*.1998;351(9103):637–41.

31. Gerber JS, Offit PA. Vaccines and autism: a tale of shifting hypotheses. *Clin Infect Dis*. 2009;48(4): 456–61.

32. McNeil DG. 3 rulings find no link to vaccines and autism. *New York Times*, March 12, 2010: Available at: http://www.nytimes.com. Accessed on May 5, 2012.

33. Generation Rescue. A message from Jenny McCarthy, Generation Rescue President. Available at: http://www.generationrescue.org/home/about/jenny-mccarthy/. Accessed March 16, 2012.

34. Booz & Co. Pharma business model is broken, say industry execs. *Quality Digest*, March 30, 2012. Available at: http://www.qualitydigest.com/inside/health-care-news/survey-pharmaceutical-executives-view-business%20model%20broken.html. Accessed April 25, 2012.

35. Jaffe ME. Regulation, litigation, and innovation in the pharmaceutical industry: an equation for safety. In: Hunziker JR, Jones TO, eds. *Product Liability and Innovation*. Washington, DC: National Academies Press; 1994:120–8.

36. The Independence Institute. The drug development and approval process. Available at: http://www.fdareview.org/approval_process.shtml. Accessed March 5, 2012.

37. U.S. Court of Federal Claims. Vaccine Program/Office of Special Masters. Available at: http://www.uscfc.uscourts.gov/vaccine-programoffice-special-masters. Accessed April 6, 2012.

38. CNN Health. Vaccine court finds no link to autism. March 12, 2010. Available at: http://articles.cnn.com/2010-03-12/health/vaccine.court.ruling.autism_1_vaccine-autism-federal-claims?_s=PM:HEALTH. Accessed March 12, 2012.

39. Barnes R. Supreme Court rules vaccine makers protected from lawsuits. *Washington Post*, February 22, 2011. Available at: http://www.washingtonpost.com/wp-dyn/content/article/2011/02/22/AR2011022206008.html. Accessed March 7, 2012.

40. Brower J, Chalk P. *The Global Threat of New and Reemerging Infectious Diseases*. Santa Monica, CA: RAND Science and Technology; 2003.

41. Bradsher K. SARS ebbs in East Asia, but financial recovery is slow. *New York Times*, May 31, 2003. Available at: http://www.nytimes.com/2003/05/31/business/worldbusiness/31ASIA.html?pagewanted=all. Accessed April 22, 2012.

42. Shilts R. *And the Band Played On*. New York: St. Martin's Press; 1987.

43. World Health Organization. The WHO agenda. Available at: http://www.who.int/about/agenda/en/index.html. Accessed March 3, 2012.

44. Bradshaw S. Vatican: condoms don't stop AIDS. *The Guardian*, October 9, 2003. Available at: http://www.guardian.co.uk/world/2003/oct/09/aids. Accessed March 5, 2012.

45. Centers for Disease Control and Prevention. Vision, mission, core values and pledge. Available at: http://www.cdc.gov/about/organization/mission.htm. Accessed April 10, 2012.

46. Young A. U.S. Congress eyes CDC's lingering morale problems. *Lancet*. 2007;370:207–8.

47. Banks W. Mold, mildew, and the military role in disaster response. *Jurist*. October 17, 2005. Available at: http://www.jurist.org/forumy/2005/10/mold-mildew-and-military-role-in.php. Accessed February 16, 2013.

48. Gilson L, Sen PD, Mohammed S, et al. The potential of health sector non-governmental organizations: policy options. *Health Policy Plan*. 1994 9:14–24.

49. U.S. Department of Health and Human Services. Global Health Initiative. Available at: http://www.globalhealth.gov/global-programs-and-initiatives/global-health-initiative/. Accessed April 25, 2012.

50. Institute of Medicine. Attitudes toward U.S. foreign assistance: perception and reality. In: *America's Vital Interest in Global Health: Protecting Our People, Enhancing Our Economy, and Advancing Our International Interests*. Washington, DC: National Academies Press; 1997:19–23.

51. Institute of Medicine. *The Future of the Public's Health in the 21st Century*. Washington, DC: National Academies Press; 2003.

52. Friedman TL. *The World Is Flat*. New York: Farrar, Straus and Giroux; 2005.

53. Turnock BJ, Atchison C. Governmental public health in the United States: the implications of federalism. *Health Aff*. 2002;21:68–78.

54. Public Health Preparedness in the 21st Century, testimony by Nicole Lurie, RAND Corporation, before the Health, Education, Labor and Pensions Committee Subcommittee on Bioterrorism and Public Health Preparedness, U.S. Senate, March 28, 2006. Testimony No. CT-257.

55. U.S. Department of Health and Human Services, Office of Minority Health, Robert Wood Johnson Foundation. *Public Health Systems Research Expert Panel Summary and Recommendations*. Washington, DC: 2008.

56. Institute of Medicine. *For the Public's Health: Investing in a Healthier Future*. Washington, DC: The National Academies Press; 2012.

57. U.S. Department of Health and Human Services. Consensus statement on quality in the public health system. Available at: http://www.hhs.gov/ash/initiatives/quality/quality/phqf-consensus-statement.html. Accessed February 16, 2013.

58. Honore PA, Wright D, Berwick D, et al. Creating a framework for getting quality into the public health system. *Health Aff*. 2011;30:737–45.

59. U.S. Department of Health and Human Services. Determinants of health. Available at: http://www.healthypeople.gov/2020/about/DOHAbout.aspx. Accessed March 11, 2012.

Public Health Finance

Peggy A. Honoré and Louis Gapenski

LEARNING OBJECTIVES

- To describe how public health programs are financed
- To compare the allocation of health resources to medical care and public health
- To explain the role of federalism in funding public health
- To discuss variations in public health funding
- To identify which public health financial management skills are most important

---

Chapter Overview

Public health practice consists of organized efforts to improve the health of communities. The field of finance plays a major part in this process. Generally, the role of finance is to plan for, acquire, and use resources to maximize the efficiency and value of the organization.[1] More specifically, **public health finance** is defined as a field of study that examines the acquisition, utilization, and management of resources for the delivery of public health functions and the impact of these resources on population health and the public health system.[2] Its primary focus is on the resources needed for the delivery of essential public health services and how those resources are acquired and managed.

Although many significant achievements can be credited to the public health system, public health services, like most public services, are provided within a financially constrained environment. According to a Trust for America's Health analysis, the U.S. public health system has been chronically underfunded for decades. At the federal level, funding has remained relatively flat and at an insufficient level for years. At the state and local levels, public health budgets have been reduced drastically in recent years as evidenced by the fact that local health departments have lost a total of 34,400 jobs due to budget cuts. Such funding deficiencies have prevented federal, state, and local public health departments from adequately performing many core functions.[3] With bleak federal, state, and local government revenue projections, it is unlikely that the chronic underfunding will be reversed in the near future.

As the scarcity of financial resources increases, the role of public health finance increases in importance. Each dollar that is available must be spent wisely and productively to produce the greatest benefit at the least cost. In addition, public health organizations must be proactive in protecting existing funding as well as recognizing and accessing potential new funding sources from the public and private sectors. Public health managers at all levels and from all disciplines, including senior leadership, unit administrators, finance specialists, and program managers, must be engaged in financial activities, so a knowledge of public health finance is critical to system productivity and sustainability.

Sources of Public Health Funds

It is impossible to provide services of any kind without funding. For example, at the federal, state, and local levels, public health organizations need money for facilities, personnel, equipment, supplies, and many other purposes.

Public health programs are financed through a combination of federal, state, and local governmental appropriations and, especially at the local level, from local taxes, fees, and other reimbursements from sources such as Medicaid and Medicare received directly for services provided. In its current configuration, public health is a public good and, as such, relies heavily on government sources for funding. In this financing structure, each level of government has different, but important responsibilities for protecting the public's health.

Financing public health functions at different levels of government is grounded in the basic theory of **fiscal federalism**. Historically, the fiscal federalism framework assigns responsibility for specific functions to national, state, and local levels of government and puts in place proper financing mechanisms to fulfill those functions.[4] Fiscal federalism lies within the field of public finance and the financing instruments such as federal grants that are used to transfer funds to state and local levels for the delivery of public health services are covered in detail later in this chapter. The transfer of funds for purposes specified at the federal level provides some perspective on the influence that the federal government can exert over establishing public health program priorities at the lower levels. As an example, the federal government provides an incentive for states to establish policies like setting the legal drinking age at 21 as a condition for receiving federal funding.

While public health plays a critical role in population health interventions, far more of the health resources of the United States are allocated to the provision of medical care as opposed to the promotion of health. Nationally, only a small percentage of the total funds spent on health care are allocated to public health. For example, of the roughly $2.6 trillion total health expenditures in 2010, only 3.2% was spent on governmental public health activities.[5] Put another way, Americans spent $8,402 per person on medical care but only $267 per person in public health spending.

Federal spending accounts for about 30% of total public health expenditures while state and local spending cover the remaining 70%. Unfortunately, data on public health funding are not completely reliable because of the large number of funding sources, differences in accounting practices, and even problems in separating public health from other healthcare activities.

Understanding the financing of public health services is critical to understanding the public health system. In essence, the "follow the money" rule helps public health managers understand the role that different entities play in providing public health services to the U.S. population. The purpose of this section is to introduce the financing structure of the public health system.[6]

Federal Funding Mechanisms

Federal funds are distributed through its system of agencies. It is each agency's responsibility to manage the distribution of funds utilized for public health services, including ensuring that the funds are used for the purposes stated in the enabling legislation and in a prudent manner. The funds are provided to beneficiaries, or recipients, such as states, local health departments, and other health services providers, through hundreds of individual programs, such as the Maternal and Child Health Program. Each program, which is assigned a unique name to distinguish it from other programs, is created for a specific purpose. For administrative purposes, programs are assigned to offices or operating divisions within a federal agency and may include administrative personnel who work directly or indirectly with the program.

Program funds are distributed to recipients through federal grants (awards), which use funds that are allocated from general revenues. Recipients must first apply for the award directly to the federal agency that administers the program. The agency then determines the amount of assistance to be awarded and notifies the recipient of the award. In order for an award to be considered official, a grant agreement (contract) between the agency and the recipient, which delineates the purpose of the award as well as restrictions and limitations, is signed by both parties.

Federal awards typically specify a time period, called the period of availability, during which the recipient may use the funds. Most grants have a term of 1 year (although some may have a longer lifespan), and the recipient must use the grant funds within that timeframe. The expiration of funds is a consequence of the federal budget process, which dictates that any funds not used within the specified time limit revert to other uses. As a condition of receiving federal grants, recipients must agree to comply with the applicable laws and regulations to avoid potential penalties or legal charges.

Types of Federal Grants

The federal government has several different types of grants, each with its own unique way of awarding and/or operating:

- *Categorical grants.* These are the main source of federal aid to state and local governments for public health services.
  - *Project basis.* Such grants are awarded competitively. Project grants are the most common form of grants in terms of numbers (not dollar value), and most grants are found in scientific research, technology development, education, social services, and the arts.

Examples of project grants for health services include the Community Health Centers, Head Start, and health disparities in minorities programs.

- *Formula basis.* These grants are awarded on the basis of a precise formula often specified in the legislation that creates the program. Formula grants are typically funded on the basis of measurable factors, such as overall population, proportion of population below the poverty level, or infant mortality rate. The specified formula informs potential recipients, typically states, precisely how they can calculate the quantity of aid to which they are entitled, as long as the recipient qualifies for such assistance under the stipulations of the program. Usually, the elements in the formula are chosen to reflect characteristics related to the purpose of the aid. Examples of formula grant programs include the Ryan White HIV/AIDS Program and the Substance Abuse and Mental Health Services.

- *Block grants.* 1966 marks the initial year that block grants were introduced as a federal funding mechanism. With the creation of nine new or revised block grants, the Omnibus Budget Reconciliation Act of 1981 renewed the focus on this type of funding. Block grants typically are large amounts of funding awarded to state or local governments with only general provisions for the way the grant is to be spent. This is in contrast to other types of grants, which contain very specific provisions regarding how the funds are to be used. Block grants allow state and local governments to use different approaches to solving problems as well as allow the funds to be used to address needs determined by the recipient to be most worthwhile.

- *Mandatory (earmark) grants.* These are explicitly specified in appropriations by the U.S. Congress. They are not competitively awarded and are subject to the vagaries of the political process.

Federal Pass-Through Grants

The federal government permits certain recipients to act as **pass-through entities**, which allows the initial recipient to provide the funds to another recipient. The pass-through entity is still considered the recipient of the grant, but the assistance provided in the grant may be "passed on" to another recipient, who is called a subrecipient. This process is used when the federal granting agency does not have the organizational capability to provide assistance directly to the final recipient and hence requires administrative support from an intermediate entity.

For example, the Women, Infants, and Children (WIC) program is a federally funded nutrition program that provides nutrition assessments, diet counseling, and food coupons to low-income women. The funds are granted to states (and similar governmental jurisdictions), but then are further allocated through subgrants to counties and municipalities, typically ending up in local health departments. The original recipients, the states, are the pass-through entities and the counties and cities are the subrecipients, all of which share the responsibility of supporting the original purpose of the program. Subrecipients may in turn pass some or all of the funds to another subrecipient if it supports the purpose of the program. Therefore, a recipient may be considered a pass-through entity and a subrecipient at the same time.

Pass-through entities and subrecipients are equally responsible for the management of all federal funds received. The federal government monitors the federal aid provided to any recipient and requires all pass-through entities to monitor the aid they pass on. Noncompliance of a federal regulation on the part of a subrecipient may be attributed to the pass-through entity because it remains responsible for the management of the funds that it passes on.

Federal Funding Amounts

As mentioned earlier, the primary federal agencies involved with funding state and local public health efforts are the Health Resources and Services Administration (HRSA) and the Centers for Disease Control and Prevention (CDC).

HRSA distributes approximately 90% of its total funding in grants to states and territories, public and private healthcare providers, and health professions training programs. The bulk of HRSA funds are in its two largest programs, the community and migrant health centers and the Ryan White HIV/AIDS Program, which are awarded on a competitive basis and/or based on disease burden. In 2011, HRSA distributed about $7.5 billion to a variety of public health entities, which amounts to $23.75 per person (per capita). However, the amount of funding spent for key health programs varied from state to state, with a per capita low of $12.77 in Nevada to a high of $82.95 in Alaska. The amount of funding also varied regionally, with the Midwest averaging a per capita low of $20.20 and the Northeast averaging the high of $27.31. The West and South fell in the middle at $25.24 and $22.09 respectively.[3]

Approximately 75% of the CDC's budget is distributed to states, localities, and other public and private partners to support services and programs. Some of the CDC's funding is based on the number of people in a state or on a need-based formula. Other funds are based on competitive grants. States can apply to the CDC for grants for a specific program area, but typically there are insufficient monies available to fund all requests. In 2011, the CDC distributed about $6.3 billion to various public health entities, which translates to a per capita amount of less than $20.28. However, as with HRSA funding, CDC funding was highly variable, ranging from a per capita low of $14.20 in Ohio to a high of $51.98 in Alaska. The funding also fluctuated regionally, with the Midwest averaging a per capita low of $17.65 and the West averaging a high of $21.94. The Northeast and South fell into the middle at $20.70 and $19.91 respectively.[3]

The combined annual federal funding from the CDC and HRSA to state and local public health entities in 2011 was approximately $13.8 billion, or about $45 per person. Although there is some rationality to the differences in per capita amounts distributed to individual states, it is likely that the funding variation does not totally represent disparities in public health needs.

Currently, most of the federal funding from the CDC to states is distributed for specific programs (categories). While each category provides important funding for serious public health concerns, the funding is not allocated based on priority goals for reducing disease and injury rates, such as those outlined in the *Healthy People 2020* initiative, or to programs that have demonstrated effectiveness in reducing disease.[7] Furthermore, although many federal programs do help alleviate a number of health problems, the funding typically is not well coordinated among federal agencies or with state and local funding programs.

Funding at the State and Local Levels

States and localities have the following public health responsibilities:[7]

- Fulfill core public health functions such as diagnosing and investigating health threats, informing and educating the public, mobilizing community partnerships, protecting against natural and manmade disasters, and enforcing state health laws.
- Provide relevant information on the community's health and the availability of essential public health services. This information should be integrated with reporting from local hospitals and healthcare providers to show how well public concerns and health threats are being addressed. Furthermore, this information should be publicly available and utilized by public health departments to work collaboratively with hospitals, physicians, and others that have a role in public health to set health goals.
- Work collaboratively with the multiple stakeholders who influence public health at the community level to design appropriate programs and interventions that address key health problems and improve the health of the region.
- Deal with complex, poorly understood problems by acting as "policy laboratories" to take advantage of the fact that states and localities are closer to the people and to the problems causing ill health than is the federal government.

There are three types of organizational structures for state public health departments: stand alone, umbrella, and mixed function. Stand-alone public health agencies are independent from other agencies in the state and have a dedicated public health mission. State public health agencies that fall under larger agencies like a state department of health services are called umbrella agencies. Lastly, mixed-function state agencies function independently but perform other functions in addition to public health such as Medicaid and health insurance regulation. Although organizational differences have a significant impact on the administration of the state public health function, organizational structure does not appear to affect the amount of state funding devoted to public health activities.

There are approximately 2,600 local health departments (LHDs) in the United States serving a diverse assortment of populations ranging from less than 1,000 residents in some rural jurisdictions to about 9 million people, the number served by the New York City Department of Health. LHDs are structured differently, depending on state, and may be centralized (controlled at the state level) or decentralized (controlled at the local level). Therefore, the level of responsibility and services provided by LHDs varies among states, and consequently so does the way that funding levels are established and allocated.

State-Level Funding

States and local communities have chosen a variety of ways to fund public health activities and services, hence the amount of funding is highly variable. To illustrate, although the median per capita revenue at the local level in 2010 was $44, funding ranged from less than $10 to more than $100 and the annual budgets of LHDs ranged from less than $10,000 to more than $1 billion. Roughly 25% of LHDs had annual funding of less than $500,000, while 17% had funding of more than $5 million.[8]

Table 9.1   State Health Department Funding Sources

Source	National Average
Federal	45%
State general funds	23%
Other state funds	16%
Fees and fines	7%
Other sources	5%
Medicare and Medicaid	4%

Source: Data from Association of State and Territorial Health Officials (ASTHO). Profile of state public health. Vol. 2 (2011), Arlington, VA: ASTHO. Available at: http://www.astho.org/uploadedFiles/_Publications/Files/Survey_Research /ASTHO_State_Profiles_Single[1]%20lo%20res.pdf. Accessed February 17, 2013.

Table 9.1 lists the 2009 national average funding sources of state health departments. The largest funding source was the federal government with 45%, followed closely by state sources that totaled 39%.[9] Note that approximately 60% of the federal funding and more than half of the total amount of state-level funding were used to support local health departments and community-based organizations. In general, the amount of funding and distribution of those funds at the state level is controlled by the legislature and governor as part of the state budgetary process.

Local-Level Funding

Table 9.2 lists the 2010 national average revenues (funding) of LHDs by source.[8] Note that local and state appropriations provided 48% of the funding, while federal appropriations provided 23% of the funding, for total governmental appropriations funding of 71%. That means that on average, 29%, or almost one-third, of the funding of LHDs came from sources other than appropriations. These sources included Medicaid reimbursements (13%), service fees (7%), and Medicare reimbursements (3%). Other nonappropriation sources consist primarily of private foundation grants.

Table 9.2   Local Health Department Revenue Sources

Source	National Average
Local	27%
State direct	21%
Federal pass-through	17%
Medicaid	13%
Fees	7%
Federal direct	6%
Other	6%
Medicare	3%

Source: Data from National Association of County and City Health Officials (NACCHO). 2010 national profile of local health departments, Washington, DC: NACCHO. Available at: http://www.naccho.org/topics/infrastructure/profile /resources/2010report/upload/2010_Profile_main_report-web.pdf. Accessed February 17, 2013.

The data in Table 9.2 highlight two important points. First, a significant proportion of public health funding at the local level is generated from services provided to the community and foundation grants, which typically can be influenced by local managerial actions more than the amount of government appropriations. Second, national average data are just that: averages. Thus, revenue percentages at the local health department level are highly variable. For example, some LHDs do not provide clinical services to individual clients, and hence their revenues do not include clinical service fees.

It is important to note that public health does not finance local services to a great degree with dedicated property taxes.[10] While other public entities such as school districts and police and fire departments historically finance services with dedicated property taxes, only 12 states in the nation have authorized their local governments to levy a dedicated tax for public health purposes. Local governments do use property tax revenues held in their general funds to fund local public health services, but the lack of a tax levy specifically dedicated for public health exposes those agencies to annual appropriation fluctuations that jeopardize the continuation of services.

Geographic Variations in Public Health Funding

State and local public health departments are on the front line of the nation's "prevention delivery" system and hence are responsible for keeping Americans healthy and safe and preventing disease and injury. But in order for this system to work efficiently, all Americans must have more-or-less equal access to disease-prevention programs, disaster-response plans, food-safety inspections, and other services provided by local public health departments.

Although the median per capita funding of public health services at the local level in 2010 was $44, funding ranged from under $10 to over $100. This variation, and its implications, was highlighted in a 2009 report by the Robert Wood Johnson Foundation.[11] The report, which summarized the results of an academic study, confirmed that public health funding varies widely across communities, suggesting that people have greater or lesser access to critical public health services depending on where they live.[12] Also, communities with high proportions of racial and ethnic minority populations were much more likely to have experienced reductions in public health spending over the past decade than were their counterparts. It is believed that this funding variation is due to the fact that public health funding decisions typically are determined by a complex interaction of economic, political, bureaucratic, and population health–related factors that place some communities at a disadvantage in securing resources.

In addition, communities that spend more on public health services were the same communities that have been shown to have lower levels of medical care spending, which suggests that the availability of public health resources in a community reduces the need for medical care in that community by limiting disease and injury.

Variations also exist in financing public health through the use of dedicated property taxation at the local level. While dedicated property taxation for public service purposes is aggressively used for functions such as public education, fire, and police services, local governments in only 12 states have authority to levy and collect a property tax dedicated for public health services.

Geographic variation in medical care spending has long been a source of policy concern because it implies large inefficiencies and inequities in resource availability. As policymakers struggle with how to reform the healthcare delivery system and how to pay for it, prevention must be front and center. Many of the costly chronic diseases that Americans are suffering from can be prevented. If certain communities spend more on prevention, do they need to spend less on medical care to treat patients? If communities are spending more on medical care, does this mean they are not spending enough to keep people from getting sick in the first place? These are the tough questions policymakers face as they work to make decisions about how to improve the health system and the health of all Americans.

As the nation's health system reforms and evolves, it is critical that policymakers examine both the delivery and prevention sides of the system. The current close examination of the health system presents an opportunity to make an historic and strategic investment in community-based prevention programs that will help Americans live healthier lifestyles and keep them out of doctors' offices and hospitals.

However, to accomplish this worthy goal, every dollar allocated to public health must be spent wisely. By measuring spending levels in specific programs, such as tobacco control, obesity prevention, and communicable disease control, policymakers and public health officials will be able to identify exactly how funding is being used and the value of each type of investment. A uniform tracking system also will enable policymakers to correct wasteful and inequitable variations in public health spending.

Uses of Public Health Funds

Building on an understanding of how public health organizations are funded, the next logical step is to examine how those funds are spent.

Spending at the Federal Level

Because much of the public health spending at the federal level involves the transfer of funds to local and state levels, this discussion focuses on how state and local agencies use their funding. However, to get some feel for how one federal agency spends its funds, consider the CDC. **Table 9.3** shows the uses of the CDC's 2010 funding, with emphasis on the top five uses.[13] Because there are 25 listed uses in the 2010 budget, only the top five are presented; they comprise 76% of the agency's roughly $11 billion budget.

Table 9.3   Uses of CDC Funding

Funding Use	Percentage of Total Budget
Vaccines for children	35%
Bioterrorism preparedness	15%
HIV/AIDS, hepatitis, STD, and TB prevention	10%
Chronic disease prevention	9%
Immunization and respiratory diseases	7%
All other activities	24%

Source: Data from U.S. Department of Health and Human Services, Centers for Disease Control and Prevention (CDC). Justification of estimates for appropriation committees, Washington, DC: CDC. Available at: http://www.cdc.gov/fmo /topic/Budget%20Information/appropriations_budget_form_pdf/FY2011_CDC_CJ_Final.pdf. Accessed February 17, 2013.

The data in Table 9.3 show that more than one-third of CDC spending is for children's vaccines, while another quarter is spent on bioterrorism prevention and selected disease prevention. Remember, though, that only about 25% of CDC's budget is spent in house; the remaining 75% is distributed to state and local public health entities. Although there is no doubt that federal spending on public health services accomplishes a great deal in keeping the population healthy, critics of such government spending claim that much of the money is spent without hard evidence that the benefits match the costs.

Spending at the State Level

Although spending on public health activities at the federal level is crucial to the population's health, most of the delivery of public health services occurs at the state and local levels. To begin the discussion of public health spending at the state level, consider **Table 9.4**, which lists how states, on average, allocated their 2009 revenue dollars.[14]

To better understand these data, the categories are defined as follows:

- **Improving consumer health**—includes all clinical programs such as those for Alzheimer's disease, adult day care, medically handicapped children, AIDS treatment, renal disease, breast and cervical cancer treatment, TB treatment, emergency health services, and assistance to LHDs
- **WIC**—includes all expenditures related to the Women, Infants, and Children program, including nutrition education and voucher dollars
- **Infectious disease**—includes TB prevention, family planning education programs, and AIDS and STD prevention and control; also includes immunization programs (including the cost of vaccine and administration) and infectious disease control

Table 9.4   State Public Health Expenditures by Category

Category	Percentage of Total Budget
Improving consumer health	24%
Women, infants, and children (WIC)	24%
Infectious disease	13%
Chronic disease	8%
Quality of health services	6%
All hazards preparedness and response	5%
Environmental protection	5%
Administration	5%
Injury prevention	2%
Health laboratory	2%
Health data	1%
Vital statistics	1%
Other	4%

Source: Data from Committee on Public Health Strategies to Improve Health, Institute of Medicine. *For the public's health: investing in a healthier future*, Washington, DC: Institute of Medicine; 2012. Available at: http://books.nap.edu/catalog.php?record_id=13268#toc. Accessed February 17, 2013.

- **Chronic disease**—includes chronic disease prevention such as heart disease and cancer programs as well as substance abuse prevention programs including tobacco programs; also includes programs such as disease investigation, screening, outreach, and health education

- **Quality of health services**—includes quality-regulation programs such as health facility licensure and certification, regulation of emergency medical systems, health-related boards or commissions, and licensing boards; also includes the development of health access planning and financing activities

- **All hazards preparedness and response**—includes disaster preparedness programs (including bioterrorism), and the costs associated with disaster response such as shelters and emergency healthcare facilities

- **Environmental protection**—includes lead poisoning and air quality programs, solid and hazardous waste management, and water quality and pollution control; also includes food service and lodging inspections

- **Administration**—includes all costs related to public health department management such as human resources, information technology, supplies, finance, and facilities; also includes expenses related to health reform and policy development not otherwise embedded in program areas

- **Injury prevention**—includes programs such as consumer product safety, fire injury prevention, defensive driving, child abuse prevention, occupational health, and boating and recreational safety

- **Health laboratory**—includes costs related to state health laboratories such as those for personnel, administration, facilities, and supplies

- **Health data**—includes the costs of data collection, data analysis (including vital statistics analysis), report production, monitoring of disease and registries, monitoring of child health accidents and injuries, and death reporting

- **Vital statistics**—includes all costs related to vital statistics administration, including records maintenance, reproduction, generation of statistical reports, and customer service at the state level

- **Other**—includes forensic examination and infrastructure funds provided to local public health agencies

It is important to recognize that most of the state-level expenditures are not spent at the state level, but rather are sent to local health departments and community-based organizations. To illustrate, in 2008 and 2009 state health departments sent a total of $5.3 billion to fund local health departments and $2.5 billion in grants to communities for nonprofit health organizations. These funds were distributed as follows: 60% to local health departments, 21% to regional/district health department offices, and 19% to nonprofit health organizations.[14]

Spending at the Local Level

Because most of the public health services are provided at the local level, it is important to understand how local health departments spend their funds. **Table 9.5** lists the 10 activities

Table 9.5 Ten Most Frequent Activities and Services Provided Directly by LHDs

Activity or Service	Percentage of LHDs
Adult immunization	92%
Communicable/infectious disease surveillance	92%
Child immunization	92%
Tuberculosis screening	85%
Food service inspection	78%
Environmental health surveillance	77%
Food safety education	76%
Tuberculosis treatment	75%
Schools/daycare center inspection	74%
Population-based nutrition services	71%

Source: Data from U.S. Department of Health and Human Services, Centers for Disease Control and Prevention (CDC). Justification of estimates for appropriation committees, Washington, DC: CDC. Available at: http://www.cdc.gov/fmo /topic/Budget%20Information/appropriations_budget_form_pdf/FY2011_CDC_CJ_Final.pdf. Accessed February 17, 2013.

and services most frequently provided directly by LHDs, and **Table 9.6** lists those activities and services most frequently provided through LHD contracts with other organizations.[13]

These tables indicate that most activities and services are provided directly by LHDs. Furthermore, the most common activities are immunization programs and communicable/infectious disease surveillance. Of the activities and services that are contracted to other organizations, the most common are laboratory services and communicable/infectious disease screening and treatment.

Recommendations for Change

In spite of the many successes of the public health system, there is no doubt that funding inadequacies, coupled with an overall lack of coordination and focus of services offered, have kept

Table 9.6 Ten Most Frequent Activities and Services Provided by LHDs Through Contracts with Other Organizations

Activity Service	Percentage of LHDs
Laboratory services	21%
HIV/AIDS treatment	12%
Cancer screening	11%
HIV/AIDS screening	11%
STD screening	9%
Tobacco prevention	9%
Oral health	9%
Tuberculosis treatment	9%
STD treatment	9%
Child immunization	9%

Source: Data from U.S. Department of Health and Human Services, Centers for Disease Control and Prevention (CDC). Justification of estimates for appropriation committees, Washington, DC: CDC. Available at: http://www.cdc.gov/fmo /topic/Budget%20Information/appropriations_budget_form_pdf/FY2011_CDC_CJ_Final.pdf. Accessed February 17, 2013.

the system from reaching its full potential. A recent Institute of Medicine (IOM) report assessed the financial challenges facing the public health infrastructure and provided recommendations for stable and sustainable funding as well as its optimal use by public health agencies.[14]

The report contained several recommendations regarding reforming public health and its financing, including the following:

- Public health agencies at all levels of government should endorse the need for a minimum package of public health services.
- To enable the delivery of the minimum package of public health services, Congress should double the current appropriation for public health and make periodic adjustments to reflect changes in the cost of the minimum package.
- Public health departments should focus their activities on population health and work with other public and private providers to provide clinical care. (This recommendation assumes that healthcare reform will provide health insurance for almost all citizens.)
- State and local health departments should have greater flexibility in the use of federal grant funds to achieve state and local population health goals.

If these recommendations are followed, the potential exists for a significant change in both the level of public health system financing and how those funds are spent.

Public Health Financial Management

In the introduction to this chapter public health finance was defined as the field of study that examines the acquisition, utilization, and management of resources for the delivery of public health functions and the impact of these resources on population health and the public health system. As the scarcity of financial resources increases, the role of finance in the management of public health services increases in importance. Each dollar that is available must be spent wisely and productively to produce the greatest public benefit at the least cost.

This section provides an overview of the financial activities conducted by public health managers to help ensure that financial resources are being well utilized. It begins with a discussion of essential public health finance competencies, then provides some insights into selected areas of public health financial management, including accounting for costs, budgeting, financial reporting, and grant management. Of course, this section merely scratches the surface of public health financial management; the purpose here is to provide some of the specific finance competencies that are required of public health managers and the activities needed to achieve those competencies.

Public Health Finance Competencies

It is now widely recognized that public health managers must have some finance skills, but which are most important? This question is best answered by examining public health finance competencies. Contemporary examinations of essential finance competencies for public health managers trace their lineage back to a 1993 report released by the Public Health Faculty/Agency Forum.[15]

While the finance recommendations of this panel were stated only in general terms, they did serve to lay the foundation for a greater understanding of the field of public health finance.

Following the initial impetus, researchers and practitioners from across the United States collaborated on several studies that drew on secondary analysis of existing public health finance competencies as well as the collection of original data through surveys, focus groups, and expert panels. The goals of these studies were to consolidate the results of previous efforts and to develop a better understanding of the public health finance competencies that are relevant to public health managers. These efforts culminated in the 2009 publication of consensus public health finance competencies.[16]

The study identified 39 essential competencies. Although the competencies focus on public health finance, they were developed using an organizational systems (holistic) perspective that integrates finance with strategy, operations, human resources, information systems, law, ethics, and cultural competence.

Another feature of the study is that competencies were identified for both public health financial specialists and general managers. The intent was to identify those competencies that are unique to either financial or nonfinancial managers. Interestingly, the set of competencies required of both financial and nonfinancial managers are the same, which implies that generalist managers must have some understanding of the same finance principles and concepts as do specialists.

The study also focused on the amount of knowledge required for each competency. To accomplish this, the competencies were broken down into three knowledge levels: basic, which implies familiarity with the concept; knowledgeable, which requires a working knowledge of the subject; and proficient, which implies expert knowledge of the concept. Not surprisingly, most of the competencies require expert knowledge for financial managers but only basic knowledge for nonfinancial managers.

Table 9.7 lists 10 of the identified public health finance competencies along with the knowledge level suggested for nonfinancial managers. These are the basic finance competencies suggested for generalist public health managers.

Note that 8 of the 10 competencies listed require only basic knowledge by nonfinancial managers. However, the "knowledge and ability to manage monetary (cash) resources" competency requires working knowledge. Furthermore, two competencies require expert knowledge: "assesses the financial status of the organization and develops any necessary corrective measures" and "sets the strategic financial direction of the organization."

The key point here is that public health finance knowledge is too important to leave to the financial specialists. Any manager in a public health setting, whether a program manager, a local health department director, or a senior executive at state or national levels, must have at least a basic proficiency in public health finance.

It is also important that the appropriate educational, training, and professional development opportunities be available for public health students and professionals. Reviews of finance-related coursework for this audience revealed insufficient content specific to public health. Additionally, while professional associations for healthcare finance and management were established as early as 1926, there is no professional home for this area of public health.

Table 9.7   Selected Public Health Finance Competencies and Knowledge Level

- Demonstrates knowledge of general accounting principles and other appropriate standards (B)
- Gathers, interprets, and reports financial data and communicates data and information according to standards (B)
- Assesses the financial status of the organization and develops any necessary corrective measures (P)
- Develops budgets and financial data according to prescribed submission formats and specifications (B)
- Uses cost, managerial accounting, and economic evaluation approaches and applies these skills to the practice of public health (B)
- Integrates knowledge of the grant-making process with financial management practices (B)
- Applies knowledge of basic financial and business processes (e.g., procurement, accounts payable, accounts receivable) (B)
- Applies management, evaluation methods, and performance measurement to monitor program performance and track achievement of program objectives (B)
- Demonstrates the knowledge and ability to manage monetary resources (K)
- Sets the strategic financial direction of the organization (P)

Note: (B) = basic knowledge (familiarity); (K) = working knowledge; (P) = expert knowledge

Financial Activities

Public health managers have many financial responsibilities. The more important ones include planning for the future, establishing policies that control the operations of the organization, and overseeing day-to-day financial activities. One of the key steps in the planning process is to estimate the future demand for programs and services and see to it that the organization has the facilities, staff, and supplies necessary to meet the forecasted demand. This task is accomplished primarily with budgets that use forecasted future volume to estimate the resources needed to meet expected community needs.

All of these financial activities require great deal of information. Furthermore, this information has to be presented in a format that facilitates analysis, interpretation, and decision making. Without timely and relevant financial information, public health managers would be making decisions in the dark. Of course, accurate information does not ensure good financial decision making, but without it the chances of making good decisions are almost nil.

The National Association of County and City Health Officials (NACCHO) recently launched the Public Health Uniform National Data System (PHUND$) to improve the availability of valid and reliable public health financial data.[17] Designed as a web-based portal for the collection of financial data, PHUND$ provides users with values on financial and operational ratios and trends and also with comparative analysis to peer agencies. In addition to aiding agency decision making for predicting and avoiding declines, the analytical capacities of PHUND$ have also been shown to facilitate agency turnarounds from a deficit to a surplus position.[18]

Grants Management

Because a significant amount of public health funding comes in the form of grants, grant management is an important part of the overall financial management process. This section covers some basic principles of good grant management.

Suppose your organization just received a grant—that's the good news. The bad news is that now the grant must be managed. Regardless of whether you're a seasoned professional at the state level or a new LHD program manager, the job of grant manager at receiving organizations involves a difficult balancing act: ensuring that program staff have the latitude to accomplish the grant's purpose without violating any of the funding agency's requirements.

To begin the process, a good grant manager will study the terms and conditions of the award and compare them to the approved grant application. Occasionally, the grantor will make a mistake or include inappropriate terms and conditions in the final grant agreement. If corrections or clarifications are needed, it is important to raise the issue as promptly as possible.

The next step is to hold a project initiation briefing with the project manager and all staff responsible for carrying out the grant activities. This briefing should ensure that everyone involved with the grant understands the essential terms and conditions of the grant as well as their individual responsibilities. At a minimum, the project manager and staff must have a workable plan of action for carrying out each approved activity.

In addition to the program activities, the grant agreement will contain a set of compliance requirements. To ensure that all compliance responsibilities are met, it is prudent to develop a checklist of all the compliance actions required, and then document the actions taken to meet each requirement. Often this can be accomplished by placing the compliance documentation in a dedicated file that can be provided to the grantor if necessary.

Another essential component of good grant management is the establishment and maintenance of a sound financial control system. Good financial control has three major components: 1) an accounting system that meets generally accepted accounting principles for public and nonprofit organizations; 2) a system of controls that ensures proper cost allocation and that complies with cost-management requirements imposed by the grantor; and 3) a reporting system that fairly and accurately documents the expensing of grant funds. The process of allocating, charging, and documenting costs is vitally important to good grant management. Grant managers, project administrators, and organizational financial managers must have a thorough understanding of how costs are defined, composed, allocated, and charged to one or more authorized grants.

In many grants, the largest expense item is personnel. Federal grant assurance requirements dictate that organizations maintain a system of personnel administration that is merit based and nondiscriminatory. In essence, when federal grant funds are used for personnel, the organization must hire on merit and avoid practices that violate state and federal laws concerning discrimination, equal opportunity, and nepotism. Grant-funded personnel must be treated the same as other organizational employees, although they may be considered as conditional employees whose employment is subject to the availability of grant funding.

Regular audits are a sound business practice for any organization. State or local law usually mandates annual audits for municipalities and state-supported institutions, and many foundations are reluctant to award grants to organizations that do not conduct periodic audits. As applied to grant funding, an audit examines whether the financial transactions are properly recorded and documented according to generally accepted accounting principles.

While most grantees have well run grant programs, a few do not. Unfortunately, even within excellent programs there can be individuals who bend the rules or commit outright fraud or larceny. Organizational and personal conflicts of interest are matters that can affect every type of grant-funded program. All organizations must have written policies that prohibit employees from personal gain associated with grant funding. Employees who work on funded programs should be required to disclose any personal or organizational relationship that might compromise the integrity of the program. To help protect the organization from both personal and property liability, grantees should carry liability insurance that includes grant assets and personnel. Furthermore, key managers and employees who handle grant receipts and payments should be bonded.

Finally, grant managers must monitor program performance in its entirety as well as the progress and completion of grant-funded activities. To accomplish this task, managers must create performance metrics that measure program progress and activity completion. This process might indicate that program success will require a reallocation of funds among program activities. Most grantors will permit organizations to make minor budget reallocations, but major budget changes require approval by the grantor.

This section has presented the financial management competencies required of public health managers along with some tools to manage financial resources as efficiently as possible. It is our hope that this overview of public health has stimulated your interest to learn more and, perhaps, to pursue a career as a public health finance specialist.

Future Outlook

Building a vision to set a future course of action for financing and management of resources in public health could benefit from a critical analysis of the past. The current predicament of underfunding, perceived lack of accountability, and absence of financial management educational and professional development opportunities are interrelated. As a general observation, professionals trained in finance-related disciplines have never been heavily recruited and integrated into the leadership of public health. Consequently, these professionals, for the most part, are not attracted to careers in public health. Evidence of this can also be seen in the marginal and, in most cases, absence of invitations to finance professionals to participate in national committees convened to examine public health finance and other topics.[19] It is highly plausible that without the infusion of knowledge from these disciplines on how to build economic models for financial strength, public health has succumbed to a position of overreliance on unsustainable financing structures.

An overreliance on traditional public health funding methods, such as those presented in this chapter, is not a sustainable strategy. Projected economic conditions do not favor increases in federal government grant funding and flat revenue collections have a direct impact on state and local allocations to public health budgets. These conditions represent a new normal that requires a shift in how public health leadership should plan for sustainability. It is possible that public health may be better positioned by transitioning from overreliance on government budget allocations to building product lines that generate diversified revenues.

Models for population health consistently show the marginal influence of medical care on improving health status when compared to other determinants. When exploring future directions, public health could use this reality to identify new avenues for revenue generation and diversification. The financial inefficiencies of 85% of national health consumption expenditures on personal health care[5] that impact only 20% of population health improvements[19] could be used to support the creation of public health innovations that influence improvements in health.

Data collection and analysis are well established public health activities that are perfectly aligned with contemporary investment interest in information diffusion and technology. Public health innovations that turn this established niche into revenue-generating business models are plausible opportunities. Growing calls to strengthen the integration between public health and medical care to produce health improvements provides a potential existing market for such services.

For these innovations to be successful, public health must also ensure that managers with appropriate financial management skills are folded into all levels of the profession. This will happen when demands are placed on academic institutions to offer appropriate levels of education and training and when value is placed on this segment of the public health workforce.

Public health must evolve into a 21st-century enterprise that is capable of long-term sustainability. Being categorized for the most part as a public good does not erase expectations of long-term sustainability supported with nongovernmental revenue sources. Reliance on financing models that originated in the 19th century will not translate into 21st-century sustainability.

Discussion Questions

1. What is the definition of public health finance?
2. Describe fiscal federalism.
3. Discuss the role of federal agencies in the distribution of federal funding.
4. Describe how public health services are funded at the state and local levels.
5. Describe the variability of public health funding at the state and local levels.
6. List some of the most common activities of local public health agencies.
7. What is the role of financial management in public health agencies?
8. Describe the selection of public health financial management competencies for nonfinancial managers as provided in the chapter.
9. What are some critical steps in the grant-management process?

References

1. Gapenski LC. *Healthcare Finance: An Introduction to Accounting and Financial Management*. Chicago: Health Administration Press; 2012.
2. Honoré PA, Amy BW. Public Health finance: fundamental theories, concepts, and definitions [editorial]. *J Public Health Manag Pract*. 2007;13(2):89–92.
3. Trust for America's Health. Investing in America's health: a state-by-state look at public health funding and key health facts. Available at: http://healthyamericans.org/assets/files/Investing.pdf. Accessed February 17, 2013.
4. Oates WE. An essay on fiscal federalism. *J Economic Literature*. 1999;XXXVII:1120–49.
5. Centers for Medicare and Medicaid Services. Table 1: National health expenditures aggregate, per capita amounts, percent distribution, and average annual percentage change: selected calendar years

1960–2010. Available at: http://www.cms.gov/Research-Statistics-Data-and-Systems/Statistics-Trends-and-Reports/NationalHealthExpendData/NationalHealthAccountsHistorical.html. Accessed February 17, 2013.

6. For historical data on public health funding, see Kinner K, Pellegrini C. Expenditures for public health: assessing historical and prospective trends. *Am J Public Health*. 2009;99(10):1780–91; Haldeman JC. Financial local health services. *Am J Public Health*. 1955;45(8):1780–91.

7. U.S. Department of Health and Human Services, Office of Disease Prevention and Health Promotion. *Healthy People 2020: Topics and Objectives*. Available at: http://www.healthypeople.gov/2020/default.aspx. Accessed February 17, 2013.

8. National Association of County and City Health Officials. 2010 National Profile of Local Health Departments. Available at: http://www.naccho.org/topics/infrastructure/profile/resources/2010report/upload/2010_Profile_main_report-web.pdf. Accessed February 17, 2013.

9. Association of State and Territorial Health Officials. Profile of State Public Health, Vol. 2. Available at: http://www.astho.org/uploadedFiles/_Publications/Files/Survey_Research/ASTHO_State_Profiles_Single[1]%20lo%20res.pdf. Accessed February 17, 2013.

10. Honoré PA, Fos PJ, Wang X, et al. The effects on population health status of using dedicated property taxes to fund local public health agencies. *BMC Public Health*. 2011;11:471.

11. Robert Wood Johnson Foundation. *Geographic Variations in Public Health Spending: Correlates and Consequences*. Available at: http://www.rwjf.org/content/dam/web-assets/2009/10/geographic-variations-in-public-health-spending. Accessed February 17, 2013.

12. Mays GP, Smith SA. Geographic variations in public health spending: correlates and consequences. *Health Services Research*. 2009;44(5):1796–817.

13. U.S. Department of Health and Human Services, Centers for Disease Control and Prevention. Justification of estimates for appropriation committees. Available at: http://www.cdc.gov/fmo/topic/Budget%20Information/appropriations_budget_form_pdf/FY2011_CDC_CJ_Final.pdf. Accessed February 17, 2013.

14. Committee on Public Health Strategies to Improve Health, Institute of Medicine. *For the public's health: investing in a healthier future*. Available at: http://books.nap.edu/catalog.php?record_id=13268#toc. Accessed February 17, 2013.

15. Sorenson AA, Bialek RG. *The Public Health Faculty/Agency Forum: Linking Graduate Education and Practice—Final Report*, Gainesville, FL: University of Florida Press; 1991.

16. Honoré PA, Costich JF. Public health financial management competencies. *J Public Health Manag Pract*. 2009;15(4):311–8.

17. National Association of County and City Health Officials. Public Health Uniform National Data System. Available at: http://phuds.naccho.org/1320/login. Accessed February 17, 2013.

18. Honoré PA, Stefanak M, Dessens S. Anatomy of a public health agency turnaround. *J Public Health Manag Pract*. 2012;18(4):364–71.

19. County Health Rankings. Available at: http://www.countyhealthrankings.org/. Accessed April 1, 2013.

The Public Health Workforce

Gerald M. Barron, Linda Duchak, and Margaret A. Potter

LEARNING OBJECTIVES

- To outline the characteristics of the public health workforce
- To describe workforce enumeration by comparing its strengths and weaknesses
- To explain the framework of the Core Competencies for Public Health Professionals
- To list the major historical and health system factors that influence the demand for public health workers
- To list the present demographic, political, and economic conditions that are influencing the employment of public health workers

---

Chapter Overview

The public health system's most essential resource is its workforce. The U.S. public health workforce consists of individuals from a wide variety of professions, technical disciplines, and educational backgrounds. This diversity both challenges and motivates efforts to define and assess the composition of the workforce. By understanding workforce skills, training needs, and practice settings, public health decision makers can design programs and policies that make optimal use of this resource.

This chapter defines and describes the current public health workforce, considers what influences the demand for and the supply of public health workers, reports on current estimates of the workforce size and distribution, and examines strategies for educating and training those who provide essential public health services to the nation's communities.

Who Are Public Health Workers?

A management focus on population health requires a broadly inclusive definition of the **public health workforce**. Its composition includes those working in governmental public health agencies as well as official voluntary or not-for-profit public health agencies, community-based private organizations, healthcare organizations, and businesses. Hence, an inclusive definition can be stated as:

> The public health workforce is composed of individuals whose primary work focus is delivery of one or more of the essential services of public health, whether or not those individuals are on the payroll of an official, voluntary, or not-for-profit public health agency.[1]

For any practical application, this inclusive and encompassing approach to defining the public health workforce requires some limitation. There are many individuals whose work contributes only incidentally to the population's health. These might include the intensive care nurse who appropriately reinforces the reduction of tobacco use by limiting smoking by a patient's visiting family members or the highway patrol officer who reduces injuries by enforcing speed limits on interstate highways. Although the contributions of these persons to public health is important, it is nevertheless secondary to the main responsibilities of their employment; rarely are public health goals considered in the plans for their day-to-day work.

Competencies

Competency sets describe: 1) an acceptable level of performance, 2) the skill needed to perform the work, and 3) the actual conditions under which the work is executed. As a foundation for professional definition, competency sets can be used to develop educational curricula, establish standards for professional certification, write job descriptions, and evaluate performance. When used properly, competencies can contribute to the delivery of the essential services in any program area or community.[2]

Any one competency set may apply broadly to many or all public health workers or be specific to a small subset. Well-established competency sets exist for preventive and occupational medicine, dental public health, health education, law, and several other specialized areas.

The Core Competencies for Public Health Professionals, originally published and validated by the Council on Linkages Between Academia and Public Health in 2001 and revised in 2010, are a set of skills desirable for the broad practice of public health.[3] Domain—or major category of knowledge or skill—and three levels of responsibility group the competencies. The domains are analytic and assessment skills, policy development and program planning skills, communication skills, cultural competency skills, community dimensions of practice skills, public health science skills, financial planning and management skills, and leadership and systems thinking skills. These competencies describe what professionals in the field as a group should be able to do, rather than the abilities or attributes of separate professions or occupations. **Figure 10.1** shows the percentage of local health departments using competency sets by purpose of the competencies; it is based upon the findings of a 2008 National Association of County and City Health Officials (NACCHO) survey of local health departments.

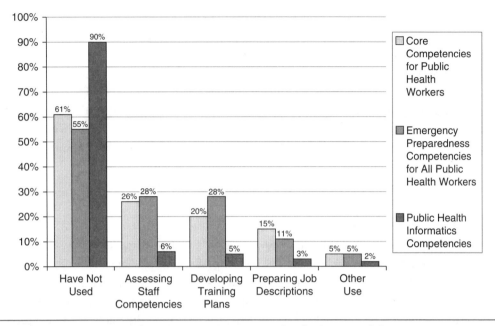

Figure 10.1 Percentage of LHDs Using Competency Sets by Purpose of Competencies
Source: NACCHO, "The Local Health Department Workforce: Findings from the 2008 National Profile of Local Health Departments." Available at: http://www.nacho.org/topics/infrastructure/ profile/upload/NACCHO_WorkforceReport_FINAL.pdf.

Educational Background

No single degree or professional credential defines all public health workers or all public health professionals. Rather, the public health workforce includes individuals from almost every discipline and profession associated with health services as well as from numerous professions outside of the health arena. Each of these brings to public health a special combination of knowledge, skills, abilities, and, perhaps most importantly, worldview. This diversity is essential to the vitality and success of public health efforts.

The **master of public health (MPH)** degree is most closely associated with expertise in public health practice. However, only a small fraction of those in the workforce have attained the MPH degree, in part because the capacity of the nation's schools and programs in public health is insufficient.[4] Most public health careers begin with some other educational course such as basic, applied, social or behavioral science; nursing; education; or social work. The MPH degree includes a basic introduction to epidemiology, biostatistics, environmental health, behavioral science, and management. Graduates can also specialize in one of these fields, or in a program area such as maternal and child health (MCH), international health, or public health laboratory science. A large proportion of those seeking the MPH have had some work experience in a public health organization and expect to return to a position of greater responsibility. Others follow the MPH with study for the **doctor of public health (DrPH)** or the doctor of philosophy (PhD) degree in a field of science related to public health—training that provides an opportunity for deeper specialization and development of research skills. The DrPH is a practice degree, supporting a higher level of leadership or innovation in service organizations; its role in relation to occupational categories is not specific. The field currently has a limited number of such graduates. Most schools describe the role of the PhD as preparing students for academic careers.

The single largest group of professionals in public health practice is nursing, and most nurses do not have an MPH degree. To be considered a public health nurse, graduation from a bachelor's degree program is considered essential. Nursing schools also offer graduate degrees in public health nursing and community health nursing. Other disciplines such as environmental engineering, social work, and nutrition offer graduate degrees that are highly relevant to public health. Many of those seeking graduate degrees may have begun work in public health with less training, and they use formal education as a strategy for career advancement.

Professional Certification

There is, at present, no governmental or private organization that licenses public health as a separate and distinct profession. Some public health professions (medicine, nursing, dentistry) require licensure to practice in every state. Other professionals, such as sanitarians, are licensed in some states, certified or registered in others, or left to voluntary standards in still others. The National Commission for Health Education Credentialing may certify public health educators at an entry or advanced level, though in most areas, state law does not require this.

The interest in certification and credentialing in public health gained momentum with a 2003 Institute of Medicine report, which called for voluntary certification of new master of public health graduates.[5] In 2005, the Association of Schools of Public Health (ASPH) and the American Public Health Association (APHA) moved forward in establishing a National Board of Public Health Examiners whose purpose is to ensure the competence of public health graduates through a voluntary credentialing examination that is based on the ASPH competencies and demonstrates mastery of the core principles of public health.[6] The inaugural **Certified in Public Health (CPH)** examination was offered across the world in 2008. The academic public health community is embracing the CPH exam, with some schools and programs requiring completion of the CPH exam for graduation and many providing full or partial financial support for eligible students, alumni, faculty, and staff to become credentialed. To date, more than 2,300 graduates and students from Council on Education for Public Health–accredited schools and programs have passed the exam. Because the United States does not currently require any license to practice public health, the voluntary individual-level credentialing strategy is helping to brand and elevate the field of public health. In early-adopter agencies, the CPH bestows preference for recruitment, hiring, promotion, and support for professional development.

Occupational Classifications and Employment Status

Occupational classifications and job titles define public health workers by what work performance is required of them. Any number of such classification systems exists among governments and private-sector employers.

The national system of listing and categorizing the employed workforce is the Standard Occupational Classification (SOC) System of the U.S. Department of Labor, Bureau of Labor

Statistics (BLS).[7] The SOC system classifies workers into occupational categories for the purpose of collecting, calculating, and disseminating uniform national data to employers, educators, and others interested in documenting or tracking employment numbers and trends. The SOC system creates a comprehensive occupational framework within four levels of aggregation: 23 major groups, 97 minor groups, 461 broad occupations, and more than 824 detailed occupations. As listed in **Exhibit 10.1**, at least 55 SOC titles designate some aspect of public health work, as used in a workforce enumeration study.[8]

Not all workers counted among the occupations listed in Exhibit 10.1 in the BLS's periodic surveys would meet even the inclusive definition of the public health workforce, provided earlier. For example, an individual counted as an epidemiologist might work in a healthcare setting, such as a hospital, studying outcomes of surgical procedures and as such would not necessarily be delivering an essential public health service. Whether all individuals included in the listed public health occupations should be counted as members of the public health workforce depends on the purpose: Employers assessing workforce supply and demand for population health agencies and organizations would need a count more narrowly focused on those work settings than the currently configured SOC data can provide.

Employment status can affect the representation of public health workers in national labor statistics based on SOC. The inclusive definition provided at the beginning of this chapter recognizes that contract workers and volunteers comprise important groups who contribute to the delivery of essential public health services. Public health efforts are often the result of a mix of volunteers, paid individuals, professionals, and laypersons. This is in no way a detriment and, in fact, is one of public health's major strengths. Particularly as public health efforts become more focused on the socioeconomic and behavioral determinants of health, this blending becomes more important to the success of public health programs. Nevertheless, the BLS's methodology for surveying employers includes full- and part-time wage and salary workers, omitting contractors and volunteers.

Finally, public and private employers use job titles designed for or adapted to their respective needs. Each state government and many local governments use civil service job titles and descriptions that emphasize educational, technical, scientific, and/or military criteria to recruit and employ workers across many types of agencies; therefore, these titles may lack any specification of population health qualifications or responsibilities. Thus, for example, a "statistical specialist" in a state civil service system might be employed in a state agency that monitors insurance rates or one that monitors health trends. Similarly, private community-based organizations, healthcare firms, and other businesses may maintain job titles that require public health competencies or that define population health responsibilities; but, if such titles differ from SOC codes, the incumbent individuals could be omitted from national labor statistics.

Worksites

The public health workforce is found in both population-based and institutional services. The wide distribution of these workers throughout the public and the private sectors rests on contemporary realities of the U.S. public health system. Governmental resources will always be limited relative to needs, making essential the ongoing role of private-sector workers. Further,

Exhibit 10.1   Classification Scheme for Public Health Occupations as Developed by Columbia University Center for Health Policy and U.S. Bureau of Health Professions

Administrative

Health Administrator

Professional

Administrative/Business Professional

Attorney/Hearing Officer

Biostatistician

Clinical, Counseling, and School Psychologist

Environmental Engineer

Environmental Scientist and Specialist

Epidemiologist

Health Economist

Health Planner/Researcher/Analyst

Infection Control/Disease Investigator

Licensure/Inspection/Regulatory Specialist

Marriage and Family Therapist

Medical and Public Health Social Worker

Mental Health/Substance Abuse Social Worker

Mental Health Counselor

Occupational Safety and Health Specialist

PH Dental Worker

PH Educator

PH Laboratory Professional

PH Nurse

PH Nutritionist

PH Optometrist

PH Pharmacist

PH Physical Therapist

PH Physician

PH Program Specialist

PH Student

PH Veterinarian/Animal Control Specialist

Psychiatric Nurse

Psychiatrist

Psychologist

Public Relations/Media Specialist

Substance Abuse and Behavioral Disorders Counselor

Other Public Health Professional

Technical

Computer Specialist

Environmental Engineering Technician

Environmental Science and Protection Technician

Health Information Systems/Data Analyst

Occupational Health and Safety Technician

PH Laboratory Specialist

Other PH Technician

Investigations Specialist

Other Protective Service Worker

Community Outreach/Field Worker

Other Paraprofessional

Clerical/Support

Administrative Business Staff

Administrative Support Staff

Skilled Craft Worker

Food Service/Housekeeping

Patient Services

Other Service/Maintenance

Volunteers

Volunteer Health Administrator

Volunteer PH Educator

Volunteer Paraprofessional

PH = public health
Source: Bureau of Health Professions, National Center for Health Workforce Information and Analysis. The public health workforce, enumeration 2000. Washington, DC: U.S. Department of Health and Human Services, Health Resource and Services Administration; 2000.

population health depends on expert performance in six functional areas: infectious disease control, environmental safety, injury prevention, behavioral health risk avoidance, disaster response and recovery, and assurance of healthcare services. Each of these areas has its own resource bases, stakeholders, and scientific, sociopolitical, and professional institutions.

Public Agencies

The core of public health workers lies in the federal agencies of public health service and in the designated agency of every U.S. state and many local jurisdictions having responsibility for public health functions. Other public-sector agencies at the federal, state, and local levels share responsibility for the various functional areas affecting population health, and thus they too employ a portion of the public health workforce. For example, public health–related programs exist in departments of environment, agriculture, labor, education, natural resources, social welfare, transportation, and policy—in other words, nearly every department of federal and state governments. However, due to budget cuts, positions in public and nonprofit agencies are being reduced. The Association of State and Territorial Health Officials (ASTHO) did a 2012 State Budget Cuts Impact Survey and NACCHO did a public health workforce survey in 2012, which are informative to the issue of the governmental public health workforce.[9,10] The major federal worksite for public health personnel is the U.S. Department of Health and Human Services (HHS).

The job titles, qualifications, and duties of public employees are defined by civil service personnel systems at the federal, state, and local levels. These personnel systems reflect a variety of public policy interests, including fair employment practices, equal employment opportunity, military service, and job security—above and beyond educational background and job-related competencies. This and the typically slow pace of change in governmental systems make it difficult to update job specifications on a regular basis, with particular attention to the evolving needs of public health practice. For this reason, *Healthy People 2020* Objective PHI-1.1 calls for public health agencies to incorporate core competencies for public health professionals into job descriptions and performance evaluations.[11]

Private Organizations and Businesses

Public health workers are also employed in numerous settings outside the government, including for-profit and nonprofit enterprises. In the personal health services, many individuals work to promote community health, gather and report health statistics, track nosocomial infections, and plan health-promotion and health-education programs. In many hospitals and community health clinics, they also implement and evaluate community-based programs.

In for-profit industries throughout the economy, many corporations have come to recognize the impact of health on productivity and profitability and therefore have undertaken public health initiatives such as health promotion and education. Although often focused on employee populations, some such businesses have extended these initiatives to entire communities. Workers in labor unions often monitor health impacts or threats to health and inform their members about health issues.

Some for-profit industries in the health field employ public health professionals as essential to their core business. They work in pharmaceutical companies developing and testing vaccines and drugs, in health insurance and health maintenance organizations monitoring the health status of enrolled populations, developing programs and policies aimed at sustaining good health, and evaluating the quality and effectiveness of programs of disease prevention and health promotion.

Private nonprofit associations, such as the American Cancer Society, the American Diabetes Association, and the American Heart Association, have sizable workforces that monitor the target disease in the population, provide education, and evaluate treatment options. These associations often collaborate with governmental health agencies. Communities receive public health services from a vast array of **community-based organizations (CBOs)**. In some rural and underserved areas, the presence of these organizations may match or exceed that of official governmental public health agencies.[12] Some CBOs have regular full-time staff, others rely on volunteers, and many combine professional and volunteer staffs. Often, CBOs are affiliated with local charity, religious, or political institutions. Some CBOs address a specific health or other social problem; others are more concerned with the general health and wellbeing of the community. The elementary, secondary, or college school setting, with a concentrated population of children or young adults, presents challenges and opportunities to public health. At the high school level, the direct provision of personal health care has been developed with school-based health and dental clinics. In some jurisdictions the local health agency provides nurses for some or all K–12 school settings. In many others, including colleges and universities, these nurses and other health professionals are employed by the school and should be considered a part of the public health workforce.

Occupational Description

In this section, the characteristics of some of the most important public health occupations are summarized.

Epidemiologists

Epidemiology is the study of the distribution and determinants of health-related states or events in specified populations and the application of this study to the control of health problems. By this definition, nearly all people who work in public health may be **epidemiologists** in some sense, but those considered to be experts in public health's core science generally have a graduate degree in epidemiology and focus their work on the surveillance of health problems and the effectiveness of interventions. Epidemiology can be the primary specialty for a graduate or postgraduate degree, generally a master of science (MS), MPH, or PhD. It can also be a graduate specialization added to initial preparation in medicine, nursing, or another health field. Although epidemiologists previously were concerned exclusively with infectious and vector-borne diseases, some now specialize in other areas such as occupational and environmental hazards, violence and injury, and chronic diseases.

Epidemiologists have typically worked in public-sector agencies and academia but are increasingly being employed by managed care organizations and in hospitals, medical centers, and hospital systems in programs to control nosocomial infections. Some are employed in the private sector in consulting firms and other corporations. These positions may be in conducting research, consulting, or providing oversight on scientific investigations.

Biostatisticians

The work of epidemiologists frequently overlaps with that of **biostatisticians**. Although also an undergraduate area of concentration, biostatistics education also occurs at the MS, MPH, and

PhD levels in schools of public health. In such graduate programs, biostatisticians focus primarily on statistical theory, techniques, and methods to identify and analyze health problems, to evaluate the effectiveness of health services, and to analyze data for planning and policy development. Many are employed in the research divisions of pharmaceutical companies and academic medical centers as well as in specialized federal public health agencies.

Educators and Behavioral Scientists

The public health workforce also needs to include an adequate number of individuals with skills in education and behavioral sciences. The more that is known about human behavior, the more important becomes the application of behavioral tools for disease prevention and intervention. For example, efforts to control sexually transmitted diseases (STDs) frequently address human sexual behavior and decision making. In efforts to prevent chronic disease, behavioral science drives program planning for promoting increased exercise, changing individual eating patterns, and reducing stress. All of the public- and private-sector organizations engaging in health promotion, health education, and risk communication for general or special populations employ social and behavioral scientists and professionals.

Environmental Health Specialists

Environmental health specialists ensure a safe and healthy environment through the control and management of air and water quality, food safety, toxic substances, solid wastes, and workplace hazards. Job titles for individuals working in environmental health are extremely varied, but include scientist, engineer, geologist, hydrologist, toxicologist, risk assessor, industrial hygienist, and sanitarian.

The lead national agency that employs environmental health specialists is the Environmental Protection Agency. However, environmental specialists are found in almost all federal offices. Within state governments, environmental workers are frequently employed in departments of environmental quality, environmental health, or environmental protection. Locally, environmental specialists work in local health departments and in the environmental agencies of some large cities.

Environmental health workers are also employed by private consulting and engineering firms whose clients need help in assessing environmental risks and complying with environmental regulations. All organizations associated with the preparation of food products—from mills and bakeries to meatpacking houses and restaurants—use a variety of sanitarians and environmental health specialists.

Nurses

Public health nursing in the United States originated with the work of Lillian Wald at the Henry Street Settlement House in New York City, established in 1895. Wald and her colleagues targeted a wide range of disease-prevention and health-promotion efforts at vulnerable immigrant populations.[13] Since then, **public health nurses** have remained distinct from other nursing specialties by their focus on populations rather than individuals and on disease prevention rather than acute or chronic care. Although public health agencies often employ nurses with a diploma or associate degree, a public health nurse generally has a bachelor's degree. In larger agencies, nurses with public health education and experience work in community-based programs or hold leadership positions. Other nurses are limited to clinical or support positions. Public health nursing covers most aspects of public health but are most visible in infectious disease–control programs such as directly observed therapy for tuberculosis, maternal and child health programs, and immunizations. Newer programs in which nurses have been active include lead poisoning identification and abatement, tobacco control, injury prevention, and mental health services.

Physicians

Physicians practicing in public health come from almost every specialty of medicine, but mainly the primary care specialties including pediatrics, obstetrics, internal medicine/infectious disease, emergency medicine, and pathology. Physicians have traditionally held leadership positions in public health agencies at all levels of government as well as in public health academia. Public health programs require physicians' knowledge of human health and disease as well as their advanced education and leadership skills. Often physicians learn about public health on the job in community- and population-based programs.

Some, however, are certified specialists in population health. Postgraduate medical education in the form of structured preventive medicine residencies is provided for three specialties: general preventive medicine/public health, aerospace medicine, and occupational medicine.

Nutritionists

Given the influence of dietary habits on health outcomes, it is no surprise that **nutritionists** are part of the public health workforce. Nutritionists plan and supervise the preparation and service of institutional meals, assist in the prevention and treatment of illnesses by advising on healthy eating habits, and evaluate dietary trends in the population. The advent of the U.S. Department of Agriculture's (USDA) Special Supplemental Food Program for Women, Infants, and Children (commonly known as WIC) demonstrates the value of nutritional interventions as one of the nation's most successful public health programs.

Cultural competence plays a unique role in public health nutrition. Although cultural competence is an asset and requirement of any public health program, the need for culturally competent nutritionists is perhaps greater than for any other public health specialty. The continued flow of immigrants from around the globe means that most communities must regularly update food-related activities and information to accommodate the habits and preferences of those from other cultures.

Health Service Administrators

Managing public health programs is a unique challenge; funding streams are usually complex, and the programs are not easily analyzed using the tools appropriate for the private sector. With every resident of the service community as a client, analysis of cost–benefit and investment payoffs does not fit a sales or customer model. Many of those served by public health may not know that they have been served or may not be happy about the experience (e.g., a restaurant forced to close temporarily because of a food-handling problem).

Because public health recruits managers not only from public health training programs but also from business settings and public administration training programs, public health leaders need to ensure that the new recruits are adequately oriented to a public health perspective. That said, it is also important for public health managers to listen to and learn from those trained in settings such as industrial administration, business management, human resource management, information technology, and other business management specialties. To cross-fertilize managerial perspectives and expertise, public health organizations can exchange staff with other national, state, and local agencies and institute a variety of training strategies.

Dental Health Workers

Many public health agencies employ dentists and dental hygienists in preventive and restorative roles. In addition to supporting the fluoridation of public water supplies, public health agencies promote children's dental health through education, the application of sealants, and the application of topical fluoride in areas without fluoridated drinking water. Those agencies with clinical services may also provide dental examinations and restorative dentistry as a part of ensuring care for those individuals without other sources of care.

Generalists and Specialists

Many public health workers are generalists, trained and experienced in a variety of perspectives and capable of functioning across a broad array of day-to-day public health services. The lone public health nurse in a small local agency may, for example, provide immunizations, give advice on elder health, conduct prenatal education, administer directly observed TB therapy, counsel those at risk of HIV infection, and interpret vital records reports and infectious disease summaries. Generalists must recognize when to call for consultation by a specialist and require support by a system of regular updates and refreshers on public health topics.

Most programs benefit from specialized staffs that are able to devote their knowledge and skills full time to single areas of public health concern, especially when dealing with larger populations. Such areas can be defined as a single kind of threat to health (e.g., vector control), a single disease area (e.g., STDs), a single health resource (e.g., outreach and access to care), or a single public health skill (e.g., epidemiology, microbiology, or health education). Finding the right number of specialists, providing them with the resources necessary to fulfill their potential, and linking them appropriately with each other and with generalists is one of the enduring challenges for public health leaders and managers. With the growth of new knowledge concerning health and the determinants of health, it is likely that the need for specialists will continue to grow and that their numbers will increase throughout the public health workforce.

How Many and What Kind of Workers Are Needed?

History reveals the variety of factors that influence the fluctuating need for public health workers of various professions. Important factors at any given time may include prevailing health threats to the population, the availability of complementary healthcare resources, and the social and political allocation of responsibilities between governmental public health and private healthcare providers. Ideally, there would be a performance-based standard for establishing optimal numbers and qualifications of public health workers, but that is still an effort in progress.

Historical Perspective

An historical perspective reveals that major population trends in morbidity and mortality have influenced the perception of need for public health workers having particular backgrounds and skills. At the founding of the nation's public health services, Lemuel Shattuck's 1850 Report of the Massachusetts Sanitary Commission called for physicians who would keep records of vital statistics and patient contacts as well as for nurses and sanitary scientists.[14] In the early decades of the 1900s, infectious diseases were the predominant cause of mortality. In 1922, the Committee on Municipal Health Department Practice prescribed the workforce needed to staff a city health department serving a population of 100,000: a health officer, physicians to lead divisions of epidemiology and communicable diseases, nurses for clinical and preventive functions (one nurse to each 2,000–2,500 persons), and sanitary and nuisance inspectors (one for approximately 25,000 people).[15] The bacteriologic revolution and increased acknowledgment of the depth of knowledge needed to effectively protect the public's health brought further breadth and specialization to the public health workforce. By 1945, the list of recommended personnel included health educators and differentiated statistical clerks from other clerks, health officers from other administrative medical personnel, and engineers from sanitarians.[16]

Since the latter half of the 1900s, public health priorities have shifted from predominately infectious diseases to include behavior-related conditions such as cancers and cardiovascular disorders, thus increasing the need for health educators and behavioral scientists. With research advancing the understanding of environmental health factors—such as lead paint in houses, air quality, and waterborne pollutants—the need for workers with engineering and technical backgrounds has increased as well.

In the mid-1990s, an expert panel in Washington state estimated the number and job titles of personnel needed to carry out the 10 essential services of public health[17] as 21.25 full-time equivalent employees for every 50,000 persons in an agency's jurisdiction.[18] The panel recognized that the selected population size was fairly arbitrary and that many other factors could legitimately influence the estimated need for personnel.

Present and Future Perspectives

The needed numbers, distributions, and skill sets of the public health workforce depend on the availability, affordability, and quality of healthcare resources. To ensure that individuals are linked to needed care is an essential service of public health. If and when insurance for healthcare services becomes widely accessible and affordable, public health agencies may no longer need to provide direct clinical services. To the extent that various functions and services of public health are staffed by workers in nongovernmental entities, the "public" portion of the public health workforce may have fewer numbers, different skill sets, and/or different distribution patterns. Not all of the 10 essential services are inherently governmental. Recently, local health departments have reported partnerships and collaborations in which healthcare providers are taking on responsibility to assure that clinical service and other public health services are available to underserved populations.[19] Present budget constraints facing local governments explain the growing frequency of such reports: Clinical services are expensive and may be provided more efficiently in the private and nonprofit sectors. Nevertheless, cost savings for governmental public health must be balanced by the need to maintain public accountability and oversight—tasks for public health leaders and evaluators.

How Many and What Kind of Workers Are There Now?

From 1923 to 1946, the U.S. Public Health Service bulletins regularly included reports that summarized the public health workforce.[20,21] From 1946 until the mid-1960s, the U.S. Public Health Service continued to gather and report data on local health units and their employees using a standardized report of public health personnel. Local jurisdictions wishing to receive state or federal monies were required to provide workforce data, and under a variety of titles, survey results were reported nearly every year. Recognizing their importance to the public health system, government officials conducted a separate census of public health nurses nearly every year between 1940 and 1960.[22] But in the late 1960s, legislative changes brought an end to the public health workforce surveys, and no consistent, longitudinal assessments of the public health workforce were conducted for the remainder of the 20th century. Between the 1970s and the 1990s, a series of reports to Congress on the status of health personnel in the United States continued to develop estimates based on old data. One such report stated that the nation had approximately 500,000 public health workers—250,000 public health workers in the primary public health workforce and another 250,000 ancillary workers.[23]

At the state level, the public health workforce is estimated at approximately 130,000 full-time equivalent (FTE) positions.[24] The highly variable staffing patterns across state health departments reflect the diversity of services and functions for which each department is legally responsible and the health priorities it seeks to address. This is not unlike the situation for local health departments. Compared with local districts, however, states, because of their fiscal, regulatory, and policy-setting responsibilities, have a larger proportion of their employees in managerial and oversight positions and fewer providing direct services. Surveys of the public workforce have been motivated by specific legislative or policy initiatives.

Workforce Enumeration

A national **workforce enumeration** system is important for the assessment, advocacy, and accountability of the public health workforce. Reliable, quantifiable data that accurately depict the number and characteristics of those providing the essential public health services and the impact of variations in workforce characteristics on community health are necessary for developing constructive, relevant workforce policy. According to Moore, the lack of clear definitions and good data make it difficult to fully assess the sufficiency of the supply of qualified public health workers in relation to the demand for them, and the adequacy of their skills and competencies in relation to their roles and responsibilities.[25] The most credible recent national study to enumerate the public health workforce was commissioned and carried out in the late 1990s. The findings of that study, titled "The Public Health Workforce: Enumeration 2000,"[8] were based on existing state and local reports, and on nationally available federal employment information. It yielded the often-quoted figure of 448,244 workers or one for every 635 persons in the United States. Nearly 3 million volunteers augment the efforts of these employed workers. The distribution of workers across levels of government illustrates the concentration of professionals with research and analytic skills at the national and state levels and of professionals with direct service skills at the local level.

"Enumeration 2000" might be challenged for lacking original data or failing to meet the inclusive definition of a public health worker. But its shortcomings are attributable to systematic deficits of definition and data sources as well as inconsistency in counting the public health workforce over many decades. Recognizing these issues, the Health Resources and Services Administration, the Centers for Disease Control and Prevention, and the Public Health Foundation jointly convened a study in 2011 to assess the usability of currently existing public health workforce data sources and develop strategies for conducting a national enumeration of governmental public health workers. They report that much remains to be done before researchers can accurately estimate public health workforce composition and supply. Issues include uncoordinated, fragmented studies that use multiple survey methodologies; lack of clear, concise, mutually exclusive public health profession classification schemes and categories; an absence of consistent public health professional credentialing requirements; and a professional workforce educated in such specific disciplines as medicine, nursing, dentistry, or administration but lacking formal public health training.[26]

Future Trends in Workforce Demand and Supply

It is uncertain whether the demand for public health workers will grow. Recent surveys indicate that state agencies are cutting employment rolls, with already high position vacancy rates and a large proportion of retirement-eligible workers.[27] The possible future shift away from government agencies providing clinical services could reduce the need for public employment of physicians, nurses, other medical practitioners, and health technicians. The federal investment in preparedness for public health emergencies that increased FTEs in state and local health departments since the early 2000s[28] may not continue in the foreseeable future. Additionally, many workers are progressing toward retirement, and there is high turnover in key leadership positions.[29] Whether these positions will be filled—and by what occupational categories—remains to be seen.

The 2003 IOM report, *Who Will Keep the Public Healthy?*[4] recognized eight fields of expertise newly growing in importance for public health practice: informatics, genomics, communication, cultural competence, community-based participatory research, global health, public health policy and law, and public health ethics. Although not all of these fields are likely to require large numbers of additional workers, they do predict areas of expertise that public health agencies are likely to need in the foreseeable future.

What Strategies Can Enhance Workforce Capacity?

Despite government's primary responsibility for core public health functions, the private sector may have an advantage in the competition to hire skilled workers and therefore to deliver highly technical or specialized services. The broader policy interests of civil service hiring systems, the lower compensation levels, and the lower perceived prestige or status of public-sector employment may disadvantage public health agencies. One approach to countering these disadvantages is the credentialing of public health workers. Other approaches are targeted at increasing educational programs at graduate and undergraduate levels for entry into public health work, maintaining and enhancing the skills of currently employed workers, and providing career development opportunities.

Graduate Education

The continuing interest in public health has led to the growth in schools of public health and graduate programs offering the MPH degree. In 2006, there were 36 accredited schools, and 64 accredited graduate programs. In 2012, there were 49 accredited schools and 85 accredited graduate programs in the United States—some of which were preparing to seek school-level accreditation. Faculty for these schools and programs are often scholars with limited experience in the practice of public health. This may be problematic, as noted in *Who Will Keep the Public Healthy?*,[4] as schools need both research-oriented and practice-focused faculty members. Changes needed for the immediate future include the development of faculty with practice expertise, increased student involvement in public health agencies for fieldwork, and active efforts to provide continuing education to the already-employed workforce.

Undergraduate Public Health Education

The 2003 Institute of Medicine report on the public health workforce strongly recommended that at least some public health courses be offered to undergraduate students as a way to increase the public health literacy of the population and to attract students to graduate study in public health.[30] Such workers could provide much needed entry-level field staff for public health programs and services, particularly at the local level; certainly, baccalaureate nursing programs have been and will likely continue to educate entry-level public health workers. An ASPH survey of its member's in 2010 reported that 15 of the 38 schools of public health that responded to the survey offered an undergraduate major in public health, and 11 schools offered a minor in public health.[31] The Association of American Colleges and Universities performed a survey in 2008. Of 837 institutions surveyed, 137 (16%) offered a major, minor, or concentration in public health.[32]

Training for Employed Public Health Workers

Public health workers arrive on the job with diverse educations and experience. Much of this educational preparation is specific to a single professional practice area and may or may not include specific public health content. Thus, many workers need not only on-the-job and technical/vocational training for a specific task, but also general orientation to public health. Even with an appropriate public health background, staff development and continued learning opportunities are a necessity.

Worksite-Based Training Programs

Beginning in the late 1990s, the U.S. Health Resources and Services Administration (HRSA) and the Centers for Disease Control and Prevention (CDC) introduced workforce development programs designed to enhance access by working professionals. In 1996, the CDC awarded competitive 3-year grants to schools of public health to develop distance-accessible MPH programs for the agency's field assignees as well as other interested students. The success of those programs enabled employed workers—even those from out of state—to earn the advanced degree while maintaining their regular employment. In 1999, HRSA piloted another workforce development approach: to develop a competency-based training curriculum suitable for distance media and providing a series of short courses. In the next 2 years, HRSA awarded six grants to launch the Public Health Training Center (PHTC) network. In 2010, the Patient Protection and Affordable Care Act increased funding for HRSA's network to $16.8 million so that there are now 38 training centers covering almost every state. The PHTCs are partnerships between accredited schools of public health, related academic institutions, and public health agencies and organizations. The network improves the nation's public health system by strengthening the technical, scientific, managerial, and leadership competence of current and future public health professionals through the assessment of learning needs, provision of accessible training, and delivery of organizational development services to meet other strategic planning, education, and resource needs.

Online Training Resources

Mode of delivery is a major consideration in training employed public health workers. Although many are in urban areas with extensive resources and short distances to educational centers, many others work in small and isolated agencies that require extensive travel to training sites. Distance learning technologies, often available without fees or copyright restrictions, help to relax the constraints imposed by decreasing travel funds and limited staff to assume the responsibilities of those who attend training events.

The original example of web-based learning resources is the Supercourse, a repository of lectures on global health and prevention designed to improve the teaching of prevention. It currently has a network of more than 56,000 scientists in 174 countries who are sharing for free a library of 5,300 lectures in 31 languages.

The Public Health Foundation has supported online access to training resources since early 2001. The federal investment in state-level preparedness training and education drove many states to explore the use of learning management systems (LMS), developed in the 1990s for corporate training. About half the states developed or adopted their own LMS, and the other half combined resources to subscribe to the Public Health Foundation's learning management system, TRAIN. Nonsubscribers lack access to TRAIN's management and tracking capabilities, but can nevertheless access its course inventories.

In 2011, the Institute of Medicine, the public health community, and others called for improvements to better prepare the public health workforce. In answer to this call, the CDC began to expand e-learning through the CDC Learning Connection and CDC TRAIN as priorities within its mission to support state, tribal, local, and territorial public health workforce development.

Career Development

The 2010s promise to bring dramatic change to the field and to bring greater opportunities for creative leadership. *The Future of the Public's Health in the 21st Century* reviews the nation's public health capabilities and notes that public health leaders must have mastery of the skills to mobilize, coordinate, and direct broad collaborative actions within a complex public health system.[30]

Succession planning and individual career development are understood in the private sector as essential to a business success plan. *Who Will Keep the Public Healthy?* strongly suggested that all agencies and all individual public health professionals accept responsibility for such efforts.[4] The national and regional public health leadership institutes have provided an important impetus to this effort. Rather than teaching specific techniques for managing individual programs, these creative programs have emphasized the leadership skills needed to move the public health enterprise forward and have made the commitment to lifelong personal growth an explicit expectation of scholars.

Future Outlook

As described in this chapter, there are many uncertainties about the needs of the U.S. population for public health services and the extent to which workers in governmental agencies will meet those needs. Regardless of how those issues may resolve, there are several considerations of importance for workforce professionalism, performance, and policy: professional credentialing, systems research, and quality management.

Credentialing

The National Board of Public Health Examiners (NBPHE) now oversees the credentialing of public health professionals. It supports a national set of standards for competency and awards the Certified in Public Health credential to those who pass its examination. State and local governments have not yet begun to require the certification for positions in civil service, but doing so in the future could raise the qualification standard for public health employment.

Credentialing also formalizes the process of continuing education for the public health profession. A person who earns the Certified in Public Health credential must maintain it by accumulating credits through ongoing training and retaking the examination at periodic intervals.

The potential importance of credentialing is limited at present because only a small proportion of public health workers meet the NBPHE's prerequisite: a graduate degree from an accredited school of public health. Recently, the NBPHE has indicated its openness to relaxing that requirement. Doing so will extend the incentives of credentialing and continuing education to a greater number of public health workers.

Public Health Systems Research

In 2003, the Institute of Medicine's Committee on Assuring the Health of the Public for the 21st Century found insufficient evidence for recommending precisely the number and types of public health workers needed by states and localities.

At about the same time, a CDC-sponsored public health workforce initiative recommended an agenda for public health workforce research with five top-priority elements:[33]

1. Predictive relationship—Determine the relationship between performance indicators for workforce systems and health outcomes controlled for community context.
2. Competency development—Identify effective methods for building individual competency.
3. Workforce performance—Determine the best indicators for measuring workforce performance.
4. Workforce monitoring—Establish a system to track and monitor data about the public health workforce.
5. Labor market forces—Describe the components of the system for employment in public health . . . and its influences on recruitment and retention.

Since 2003, public health systems research has begun to address these priorities. The resulting insights can guide decision making for challenges about the number of types of workers needed to fulfill the responsibilities of governmental public health.

Quality Management

The voluntary public health agency accreditation activities, which are being administered by the Public Health Accreditation Board (PHAB), will have a profound effect on the public health workforce. The goal of accreditation is to improve the performance and capacity of public health agencies to perform the 10 essential public health services. Several of the domains and their standards in the accreditation requirements involve workforce competencies, which are relatively new to public health agencies. Domain 9, which has two standards, requires that agencies use a performance management system to monitor achievement of organizational objectives and the development and implementation of quality improvement processes which are integrated into the organizational practices, programs, processes, and interventions. The governmental public health agency workforce has not been well trained in these areas, and this will require a new skill set.

Discussion Questions

1. What is the definition of the public health workforce? Give some examples of the type of agencies in which they work.

2. Give examples of the professions that encompass the public health workforce and discuss the primary essential services they carry out.

3. Given present trends, where are employment opportunities for public health professionals most likely to arise in the coming years?

4. What knowledge and skills are likely to be needed by public health workers in the future that are different from those of the past?

5. The number and type of the public health workers needed depends on such factors as the health priorities of the population, the availability of healthcare services, and the social and political allocation of responsibility between government and the private sector. Discuss how these factors change over time and, as a result, impact the public health workforce.

References

1. Public Health Functions Project. *The Public Health Workforce: An Agenda for the 21st Century.* Washington, DC: U.S. Department of Health and Human Services; 1997.

2. Gebbie KM. *Competency-to-Curriculum Toolkit: Developing Curricula for Public Health Workers.* Rev ed. New York: Center for Health Policy, Columbia University School of Nursing, Association of Teachers of Preventive Medicine; 2008.

3. Public Health Foundation. Core competencies for public health professionals, 2010. Available at: http://phf.org/resourcestools/Pages/Core_Public_Health_Competencies.aspx. Accessed February 18, 2013.

4. Moore F. *Analysis of the Public Health Workforce, Final Report.* Washington, DC: Health Resources and Services Administration; 1985.

5. Institute of Medicine. *Who Will Keep the Public Healthy? Educating Public Health Professionals for the 21st Century.* Washington, DC: National Academies Press; 2003.

6. Calhoun J, Ramian K, Weist EM, et al. Development of a core competency model for the master of public health degree. *Am J Public Health.* 2008;98:1598–607.

7. U.S. Department of Labor, Bureau of Labor Statistics. Standard Occupational Classification. Available at: http://www.bls.gov/soc/home.htm. Accessed September 24, 2005.

8. Center for Health Policy, Columbia University School of Nursing. The public health workforce: enumeration 2000. Available at: http://bhpr.hrsa.gov/healthworkforce/reports/phwfenumeration2000.pdf. Accessed February 18, 2013.

9. Association of State and Territorial Health Officials, *Budget Cuts Continue to Affect the Health of Americans*, December 2012. Available at: http://www.astho.org/Advocacy/2013-Advocacy-Materials/2013-Hill-Day-Budget-Cuts-Brief/. Accessed February 28, 2013.

10. National Association of City and County Health Officials, *Local Health Department Job Losses and Program Cuts: Findings from January 2012 Survey.* Available at: http://www.naccho.org/advocacy/upload/Overview-Report-Mar-2012-Final.pdf. Accessed February 28, 2013.

11. *Healthy People 2020.* Objective PHI-1.1. Available at: http://www.healthypeople.gov/2020/topics objectives2020/objectiveslist.aspx?topicId=35. Accessed February 28, 2013.

12. University of Pittsburgh, Center for Rural Health Practice. Bridging the health divide. The rural public health research agenda, April 2004. Available at: http://www.upb.pitt.edu/uploadedFiles/About/Sponsored_Programs/Center_for_Rural_Health_Practice/Bridging%20the%20Health%20Divide.pdf. Accessed February 18, 2013.

13. Mason DJ, Leavitt JK. *Policy and Politics in Nursing and Health Care.* 3rd ed. Philadelphia: W.B. Saunders; 1998.

14. Shattuck L. *Report of the Sanitary Commission of Massachusetts, 1850.* Cambridge, MA: Harvard University Press; 1948.

15. Winslow CEA, Harris HL. An ideal health department for a city of 100,000 population. *Am J Public Health.* 1922;12(11):891–907.

16. Emerson H, Luginbuhl M. *Local Health Units for the Nation*. New York: The Commonwealth Fund; 1945.

17. Public Health Functions Steering Committee. Public health in America. Available at: http://www .health.gov/phfunctions/public.htm. Accessed February 18, 2013.

18. Libbey PM. Correspondence of February 13, 2002, and enclosed unpublished 1994 Washington State Public Health Improvement Plan Capacity Standards, Resource Estimate, and Technical Advisory Committee's Narrative Description of Its Assumptions, Cost Estimate Calculations, and the Cost Estimate of the Minimum Staffing Pattern (cited with permission).

19. Richardson JM, Pierce JR, Jr., Lackan N. Attempts by one local health department to provide only essential public health services: a 10-year retrospective case study. *J Public Health Manag Pract*. 2012;18(2):126–31.

20. Mountin JW, Hankla EK, Druzina GB. Ten Years of Federal Grants in Aid for Public Health: 1936–1946 (U.S. Public Health Bulletin No. 300). Washington, DC: Superintendent of Documents; 1949.

21. Treasury Department, U.S. Public Health Service. *Report of the Committee on Municipal Health Department Practice*. Washington, DC: U.S. Government Printing Office; 1923.

22. U.S. Department of Health and Human Services, Public Health Service. *Nurses in Public Health*. Washington, DC: U.S. Government Printing Office; 1960.

23. U.S. Department of Health and Human Services, Public Health Service, Health Resources Administration. *Public Health Personnel in the United States, 1980*. Washington, DC: U.S. Government Printing Office; 1992.

24. Public Health Foundation, State Health Agency Staffs. *1991 Final Report of a Contract with DHHS-PHS-HRSA*. Washington, DC: Public Health Foundation; 1992.

25. Moore, J. Studying an ill-defined workforce: public health workforce research. *J Public Health Manag Pract*. 2009;15(6 Suppl), S48–53.

26. University of Michigan/Center for Excellence in Public Health Workforce Studies, University of Kentucky/Center for Excellence in Public Health Workforce Research and Policy. *Strategies for Enumerating the U.S. Government Public Health Workforce*. Washington, DC: Public Health Foundation; 2012.

27. Association of State and Territorial Health Officials. Public health workforce. Key findings on state health agency workforce from the 2010 profile of state public health. Available at: http://www.astho .org/Research/Data-and-Analysis/2010-Profile-Survey-Slide-Decks/2010-Profile-Survey-Slide-Decks/. Accessed February 18, 2013.

28. Association of State and Territorial Health Officials. *Profile of State Public Health, Volume 1, page 37*. Available at: http://www.astho.org/Research/Major-Publications/Profile-of-State-Public-Health-Vol-1/. Accessed June 5, 2006.

29. Association of State and Territorial Health Officials. ASTHO Profile of State Public Health. Available at: http://www.astho.org/Research/Profile-of-State-Public-Health/. Accessed February 18, 2013.

30. Institute of Medicine. *The Future of the Public's Health in the 21st Century*. Washington, DC: National Academies Press; 2003.

31. Association of Schools of Public Health, Undergraduate Survey 2010. Available at: http://www .asph.org/UserFiles/Undergraduate%20Survey%20Data%202010.clean_ForTaskForceWebsite.pdf. Accessed February 28, 2013.

32. Association of American Colleges and Universities. *Catalog Scan of Undergraduate Public Health Programs, 2008*. Available at: http://www.aacu.org/public_health/catalog_scan.cfm. Accessed February 28, 2013.

33. Cioffi JP, Lichtveld MY, Tilson H. A research agenda for public health workforce development. *J Public Health Manag Pract*. 2004;10(3):186–92.

Human Resource Management for Public Health

Janet E. Porter

LEARNING OBJECTIVES

- To learn elements of an effective human resources function in public health
- To identify best practices in human resources that are practical and implementable by public health organizations
- To understand the market forces and trends in management of public health professionals

---

Chapter Overview

The purpose of **human resources management** in public health is to select and develop an engaged workforce capable of meeting organizational and community goals. Traditional personnel management consists of an array of functions including job analysis, recruitment and selection, orientation and onboarding, compensation and benefits, employee and labor relations, coaching, training, and performance appraisal. Workforce planning, management and leadership development, diversity, cultural competency, mentoring, and culture enrichment are increasingly important.

If human resources management is effective, staff are motivated and engaged and the organization is more effective. Research has consistently demonstrated that an engaged workforce is a key determinant of organizational success. The degree of engagement of staff of any organization determines its failure or success, its strengths or weaknesses, its accomplishments, and its disappointments. Since the late 1970s, the Gallup organization has interviewed over a million employees to assess their commitment—commonly known as engagement—to the organization. They determined that the strength of a workplace can be measured by simply asking the following 12 questions:[1]

1. Do I know what is expected of me at work?
2. Do I have the materials and equipment I need to do my work right?
3. At work, do I have the opportunity to do what I do best every day?
4. In the last 7 days, have I received recognition or praise for doing good work?
5. Does my supervisor, or someone at work, seem to care about me as a person?
6. Is there someone at work who encourages my development?
7. At work, do my opinions seem to count?
8. Does the mission/purpose of my company make me feel my job is important?
9. Are my coworkers committed to doing quality work?
10. Do I have a best friend at work?
11. In the last 6 months, has someone at work talked to me about my progress?
12. This last year, have I had opportunities at work to learn and grow?

Historically, organizations have measured staff satisfaction. But the satisfaction of the staff is not the same as employee engagement—or connectedness to the mission of the firm. This chapter addresses how public health organizations can put systems in place so that staff respond positively to these core questions, which are linked to improved organizational outcomes.

Public health administrators can tend to place emphasis on the management of community programs, financial resources and information resources, but often the most important determinant of institutional success is how well human resources are managed. Personnel management includes all of the functions and activities that allow an organization to manage its workforce. For example, a key function of human resources personnel is the development of organizational procedures and procedures that assure consistent hiring, promoting, feedback, staffing, and compensation practices (see **Box 11.1**).

Although core personnel management activities are usually organized in a designated human resources office, all managers and all supervisors engage in personnel management every day. These midlevel managers rely on a centralized human resources office to provide consistent information, guidance, and support with routine practices and thorny personnel issues.

Organizations strive to hire and staff a human resources or personnel office with staff educated and experienced in human resources. Such human resources staff members bring an understanding of the theory and the practice of personnel management, and they also understand current employment law and the practices and policies of any parent organization, such as the county or state government. However, most human resources personnel do not start out thinking this will be their career; they come to human resources from all kinds of backgrounds. Oftentimes in public health, managers who have proven themselves effective in other departments are called upon to consider human resources as a career. Regardless, the complexity and importance of human resources means that investments must be made in continuing education for human resources personnel to assure they are promoting contemporary practices. Staff in human resources must

---

Box 11.1   Public Health Human Resources Challenge

Current trends indicate that the U.S. public health workforce is aging, with many workers retiring or near retirement. For example, the average age of the public health nurse, an integral part of the public health workforce, is 49.5 years.[2] In addition, up to 43% of the state public health department will retire or be eligible for retirement by 2006.[3]

To counteract this growing crisis, public health leaders have begun discussing potential strategies to do the following:[4]

- Strengthen the skills and competence of the existing workforce to fill the experience void left as workers retire.
- Effectively prepare and recruit students and professionals from other disciplines to enter and remain in the practice of public health to ensure adequate numbers of workers in the right places with the right skills to protect and improve the health of the American public.
- Examine the working environment of public health agencies in order to formulate changes that could bolster retention and recruitment.
- Coordinate recruitment and retention efforts to reduce duplication and maximize efficiency and effectiveness.

---

have an understanding of employment law, personnel recruitment and selection, counseling, mediation, position classification, compensation, and information management.

Typically, the human resources director and office are positioned in a central part of the organization, such as directly reporting to the public health director or to a director of administration. For an organization to accomplish its mission and objectives, the practices and policies of human resources must support the organization's direction (**Figure 11.1**). In addition, the human resources office must work closely with the accounting, budgeting, planning, and payroll functions of the organization for effective routine operations and for development of new programs.

Human resource activities can be viewed as a cycle that includes workforce planning; job analysis; recruitment and selection; onboarding; training and development; coaching and

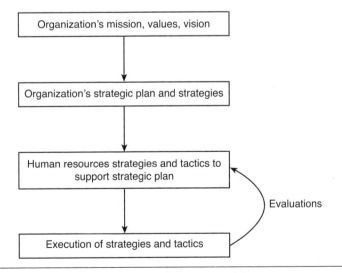

Figure 11.1   Relationship of HR Strategies to Organizational Strategies

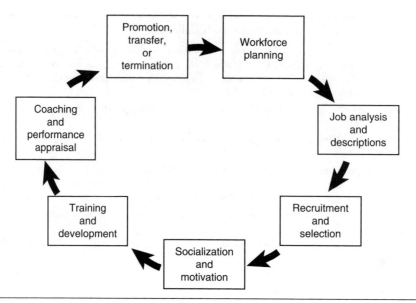

Figure 11.2 Cycle of Human Resource Activities

performance appraisal; and promotion, transfer, or termination (**Figure 11.2**). This chapter is organized to provide useful information that will guide managers through these processes.

Workforce Planning

Human resource experts should be integrally involved in developing an organization's strategic plan, strategies, and tactics. After all, without skilled staff, the plans cannot be executed. For most public health organizations, 80% of the budget is personnel expense. The strategic planning process should be iterative with various scenarios developed, workforce and other expenses calculated, and estimates as to impact on the community and budget determined.

When public health departments develop plans for a new initiative, more and more they are schooled in the development of public health business plans. Those business plans typically hinge on the recruitment of the requisite personnel. For example, if a health department wants to open a pediatric dental clinic, the major barrier to accomplishing that objective is the recruitment of a suitable pediatric dentist. Thus, human resources must be integrated into the planning at all levels.

As Figure 11.1 illustrates, after the organization's strategic plan is developed, human resources must identify strategies and tactics to support the strategic plan. Human resources' progress on those strategies should be reviewed at least quarterly so that adjustments in the plans or schedule can be made. The human resources plan is essentially a **workforce plan** that identifies the number and types of qualified personnel necessary along with the expected salary and benefits necessary to fully staff those positions. Furthermore, additional personnel require space for desks, computers, phones, and other supplies, so planning for additional personnel needs to consider far more than just the additional personnel expense.

Job Analysis and Job Description

The primary building block for any human resources department is **job analysis**. It is important that the organizational needs of the organization are thoughtfully considered before any recruitment or selection takes place. Managers are oftentimes anxious to get started and have some idea of the type of person they want to hire and how many people are needed. But the time devoted to the steps of job analysis and **job description** will pay off with better decision making about who is hired, how they are oriented and trained, the resources they are provided with, and their placement in the organizational structure. Perhaps most important is that thoughtful job analysis will improve the accuracy of the way the job is described to prospective candidates, which will impact the quality and quantity of the candidate pool.

Job analysis refers to separating the whole into its parts in order to examine and interpret each part.[5] To conduct a job analysis, human resource departments must collect data from a variety of sources, determined by the following:[6]

- Job content—Identifies and describes activities such as tasks and duties
- Job requirements—Outlines the knowledge, skills, and attributes (KSAs) a candidate should possess
- Job context—Identifies the purpose of the position, responsibilities of the employee, working conditions, and supervision arrangements

Using this information, a job description can be created. The job description should begin by listing the job title, department, grade or classification, and supervisor title. The next section of the job description includes a job summary, which is a brief paragraph outlining the specific duties performed in the job. A well-written job summary can be utilized in subsequent recruitment materials. The final portion of the job description is a job task section that identifies all of the tasks required for the job. It can be helpful to organize these tasks into categories that represent important areas of the work performed. This provides a clear overview of the work expectations. The job analysis and job description can be useful tools in the performance appraisal process discussed later in this chapter.[6]

Recruitment

The ease in recruiting public health workers is heavily dependent on issues such as salary and benefits, the supply of workers with the needed skills, the strength of the private sector, the responsiveness of the personnel system to changes in the marketplace, the reputation of the organization, the morale of the current workforce, and the skill of those charged with recruiting. It is often said that public health agencies do not feel like they have much choice in whom they hire due to their low pay scales. But this section explains what public health agencies can do to assure they have the largest pool—and best candidates possible—to fulfill their plans. The good news is that research consistently shows that pay is not a prime motivator in staff remaining in their jobs: Satisfaction with their work, flexibility, and connection to the mission, for example, are much stronger determinants of tenure than salary.

The most difficult person to recruit is usually the organization's senior administrator. A local or state health official is ideally a doctoral level professional, with either a doctor of medicine (MD) or a doctor of philosophy (PhD) degree in another health profession. Experience in public health practice and public sector administration is often helpful to administrators in these positions. Significant public health experience may offset the need for extensive academic training. The ability to offer tenure in office, such as a contract for a specified period of appointment, promotes continuity and increases the supply of qualified applicants willing to serve in these high-level positions.[7]

A large proportion of the public health workforce falls into five professional groups: physicians, nurses, environmental professionals, administrators, and health educators. These professions are in high demand in the private sector and the public sector, making **recruitment** and retention important to the success of the public health organization.

Many of the limitations imposed by merit systems and comparable civil service systems are not always under the control of the public health organization, but some are. For example, the supply of workers with the skills needed may be limited, so the challenge lies in how to increase the supply. One way is to develop relationships with academic institutions and their faculty to help channel referrals to the organization. Offering internships or other summer employment can expose young students to a career in public health. Another technique is to recruit internally and create opportunities for existing staff to increase their skill level within the organization. A third example is to pay for employees to enhance their professional and technical skills through external education and training, perhaps even paying the tuition for graduate programs.

Managers should never assume that personnel systems are unchangeable. They are only unchangeable if the managers never seek flexibility or improvements. An important role for senior administrators and other high-level managers is to develop relationships with decision makers that allow input into the process of developing rules, procedures, and laws that govern the personnel systems of the organization. For example, following difficult recruitment efforts by one state health agency for a high-level regulatory manager, the agency suggested that out-of-state moving expenses be included in the state's fiscal rules. At the next hearing for changes in fiscal rules, that change was made for the state. This effort was appreciated by all of the state agencies. Managers of other agencies simply had not thought to ask.

Another creative solution includes the incorporation of private-sector techniques for recruitment. In the past, these techniques might have been viewed as foreign to the public sector, but in fact they allow greater success in recruiting difficult-to-find talent. They include signing bonuses, pay matching to allow a counteroffer when an employee or potential employee is being recruited by others, referral awards to existing staff for helping recruit hard-to-fill positions, and temporary pay differentials to compensate for such responsibilities as acting duties or special projects. These types of incentives in the public sector are fairly recent phenomena and are driven by talent shortages that can occur in such areas as nursing and computer specialists. Asking employees to assist with recruitment is especially useful because staff will often have a developed network of contacts in their field and enjoy being part of the promotion of the agency.

Recruitment may be targeted or broadly reaching. Traditional recruitment techniques have included newspaper ads, professional organizations' job lines or newsletters, and the posting of announcements through bulletin boards. But these have become less common with the rise of Internet-based recruiting, which is typically much less expensive and faster. A growing percentage of employees in public health report that they learned of the opportunity on the Internet—either on the public health agency's website or on other geographically or professionally focused websites. Job fairs may be helpful for certain types of recruitment, and using internships to identify talented individuals who are still in training is an excellent technique that allows both the intern and the organization to see if there is a good fit. Recruiting broadly or even targeting specific minority groups is critical to diversifying the workforce.

Minimal information to include in any job announcement includes a brief and accurate job summary, minimal qualifications, salary range, how to apply for the position and receive additional information, and a closing date for applications. It is also helpful to open the announcement with a positive description of the agency that creates the image of an exciting place to work.

Diversity in the Workplace

Customers to public health organizations include people of myriad languages and cultures. In addition to issues of ethnicity, religion, race, sexual orientation, and culture, a well-balanced organization includes a broad range of age levels and people with disabilities. The recruitment, testing, and selection of staff need to be designed to reduce any potential adverse effects on protected classes. Adverse effects are defined as using a "selection process for a particular job or group of jobs that results in the selection of members of any racial, ethnic, or sex group at a lower rate than members of other groups."[8, pp. 28–30] Agencies and organizations that work proactively to encourage diversity incorporate fair selection practices, targeted recruitment, and employee training in diversity. They also use an employee–manager committee to encourage diversity in the workforce and appoint a staff member to function as an equal opportunity counselor. Furthermore, there are several laws governing equal opportunity and affirmative action, including Title VII of the Civil Rights Acts of 1964 and 1990, Executive Order 11246 (amended by Executive Order 11375), the Equal Pay Act of 1963, the Age Discrimination in Employment Act of 1967, the Americans with Disabilities Act, and state and local laws.[9]

Selection of Applicants

The most important decisions that any manager makes are those of selecting and promoting employees. Unfortunately, the personnel selection process is too often hurried, incomplete, and inappropriate, resulting in huge costs in productivity and morale, as well as potential legal actions. The selection process in any organization is usually governed by specific rules and laws. The intent in the public agency is to maintain a system that is based on merit or the meeting of minimal qualifications. Most agencies will use a combination of reviewing resumes, testing for knowledge or skills, role playing, and checking references prior to interviewing the final candidates. The human resources office will usually wish to partner with the program manager or senior administrator to determine the best techniques to match the candidates with the job requirements (see **Box 11.2**).

Box 11.2   Hiring the Best

It is theorized that most hiring mistakes can be prevented by looking beyond the resumes and references and concentrating instead on identifying a candidate's work habits.[11] "Eighty-five percent of all job failures have to do with a lack of appropriate work habits, not technical skills," said Still. "Technical skills are very easy to identify. On the other hand, how the person does the job and what kind of habits they bring in is in many cases more important to identify than technical skills."[11] A candidate's ability to perform well in your organization can best be assessed by exploring that person's past work behaviors and habits. It is not enough to ask candidates what they did during their previous employment, but rather, how they did it.[12]

Asking behavior-based questions places the interviewer in the role of an analyst. One example of a behavior-based question is asking the candidate to describe an incident in which he or she had a disagreement with a coworker. Human relations experts suggest that this method allows candidates to reveal aspects of their personalities obscured by other interviewing techniques. Based on their answers, the interviewer gets a history of the candidate's ability to work with others, a key indicator of future success.[11]

The basic principles of psychology—primacy and recency—apply to communication with prospective employees. Primacy means that people form a lasting first impression based upon the first contact, or the first few minutes of an encounter. One public health organization conducted "stay interviews" with long-term employees to determine what factors contributed to longevity. What was surprising to the human resources staff conducting the interviews was that virtually every employee started by talking about their first day at work—regardless of whether they had been there 15, 20, 25, or even 30 years—or their first contact with the organization through human resources. Thus, the employees whom prospective candidates meet first—receptionists, secretaries, human resources staff—have tremendous impact on candidates' impressions of the professionalism of the organization. A manager must spend time making sure that the job description is professionally presented, that the address for mailing resumes or applications is correct, and that the person answering questions is knowledgeable and welcoming to candidates. Conversely, staff will form a lasting impression from their last week or day on the job. Because former staff can be potential recruiters for the organization, assuring that staff depart with recognition for their efforts is important.

Interviewing candidates for employment is key to wise selection. The interview process is most effective if the hiring manager has clarity about the job expectations and has established a systematic process during the interviews for garnering information from the candidates. The interview process is usually limited to the final few (usually three) candidates who have been selected through the initial screening process. A manager may select the final three candidates or involve a formal or informal search committee to assist with the review and selection of candidates. It is usually advisable to invite peers to interview candidates. This can help to clarify for the candidates what the job really is and peers can provide insight into candidates' fit with the position. Perhaps a team of stakeholders and others with whom the applicant must work and interact can provide input to the appointing authority. The appointing authority is defined as the individual who has the authority to make the actual offer of employment. The appointing authority should be the direct supervisor of the new hire. This may be a department head, a program manager, or perhaps the senior administrator or health officer.

A good interview is conducted in a comfortable setting and includes introductions to all the parties involved, along with an explanation of why they have been asked to participate. Questions have been prepared ahead of time and are consistently asked of all the candidates. Questions should be experientially based ("Tell us about your experience.") and open ended. The behavioral interview asks candidates to describe situations in which they have exhibited the behavior required in the position. Laws prohibit the asking of questions related to race, religion, sexual preference, or ethnic origin. All staff in the public health agency should be trained in interviewing techniques to assure that they ask relevant questions and avoid illegal questions.

The Mountain States Employers Council has identified the following 10 common errors made when interviewing candidates:[10]

1. Failing to establish rapport with the applicant—There are two excellent reasons to put the applicant at ease. First, he or she will respond better to the interview and provide a clearer representation of talents and experience. Second, while the interviewee is marketing him- or herself to the organization, the interviewer is also marketing the agency as a good place to work. Having the applicant think positively about the interviewer and the organization is important for successful recruiting. Some ways to ease into the interview are to offer the applicant a cup of coffee, or to show the candidate the office, laboratory, or site where the candidate would be working.

2. Asking direct instead of open-ended questions—Applicants will offer more information if they are asked questions that cannot be answered with yes, no, or a brief statement. For example, "Have you ever investigated a disease outbreak?" is less useful than, "Tell me what experience you have had with disease investigations."

3. Asking questions that are too general—Questions that are too general provide too little useful or specific information to assist in the selection process. Requiring an answer that lends itself to specific timeframes, experience, skills, events, and so forth will yield more useful information. For example, "Tell me about your nursing career," may reveal less than, "Please discuss your last position as a visiting nurse for a local health department."

4. Asking multiple questions within the same question—If lengthy and complex questions are asked, the applicant is likely to answer only a portion of the question or answer the question as he or she interpreted its meaning.

5. Failing to ask reflective questions—If an answer is not clear or seems incomplete, the interviewer should ask for additional information. For example, if asked why he or she left a previous position, a brief answer of, "There were layoffs due to reduced funding," might not provide sufficient information to evaluate the reasons why the individual left. By adding another question such as, "Tell me more about the agency's decision to terminate your position," additional information may be obtained regarding the termination.

6. Asking leading questions—Too much information included in the question can lead the applicant in the direction that will yield the most acceptable answer. However, that answer may not be indicative of how the applicant really feels about the topic. For example, the question, "Our agency is very interested in keeping abreast of the latest technology. How

do you feel about learning new software when we upgrade our computers?", can bias the applicant toward a positive response.

7. Not allowing enough time for the applicant to respond to questions—The interviewer should avoid rushing the applicant. Providing sufficient time to give a complete answer is important.

8. Asking questions that identify or single out a candidate's protected group status—Only questions that are related to the job should be asked. Questions that tend to identify or discuss a person's race, religion, sex, age, disability, or national origin should not be mentioned.

9. Spending too much time talking—The purpose of the interview is to hear from the applicant, not the interviewer. A good rule of thumb is that the applicant should be talking approximately 80% of the time.

10. Failing to demonstrate active listening—The interviewer should provide both verbal and nonverbal messages that show whether he or she is listening, attentive, and interested in the answers.

Reference Questions

A key part of the selection process includes the verification of previous employment and the discussion that occurs with previous employers or other references. Applicants might typically provide three or more references, with two of them from previous direct supervisors. Applicants should be asked for written authorization to contact previous employers and references. Many agencies or companies have a policy to release only the dates of employment and the titles of the positions held.

Questions asked of references should include how the individuals know the applicants and how they might have worked together, as well as questions that will indicate the work ethics and skills of the applicant. One way to elicit useful information is to describe the qualities and skills sought and then ask if the applicant has those qualities and skills. Objective questions are useful, such as, "Did the applicant use Excel spreadsheets in his work in your office?" Work attendance history may be useful to indicate work practices. It is sometimes useful to ask the individuals whether they would hire the applicant themselves, and, if so, why. Just as in an interview, any questions that appear to indicate an attempt to determine religion, race, age, sexual orientation, or national origin should be avoided.

It is important in checking references to have someone who is skilled in eliciting information. For example, a chief nursing officer was hiring a key person and checked the candidate's references herself, with mixed results, so a professional reference-checking firm was hired. While the chief nursing officer had been told that the candidate "worked well independently," the professional firm got the message that the candidate was not a team player and did not work well with others. The chief nursing officer did not have the skills needed to dig into answers to correctly interpret the message. The offer to the candidate needed to be withdrawn based upon the more thorough reference checking.

Socialization and Motivation

Socialization

After the newly recruited employee becomes a member of the organization, preparation is needed so that the former applicant learns and becomes committed to the organization's goals, objectives, and operations.[13] **Organizational commitment** involves three factors: 1) belief in the goals and values of the organization, 2) willingness to exert considerable effort on behalf of the organization, and 3) desire to continue to work with the organization. This concept is not limited to organizational loyalty, rather it reflects a desire by the individual to further the success of the organization. Better work performance is correlated with the employee's commitment to the organization.[14] There is also a positive relationship between organizational tenure and job commitment.[15] High levels of organizational commitment are associated with low levels of employee turnover (see **Box 11.3**).[16]

What enhances employee commitment to organizations, including public health organizations? The attachment the employee brings to the organization on the first day of work correlates with the employee's propensity to develop a stable attachment and long stay with the organization.[10,13,14] The implications for astute recruitment and employee orientation are evident.

Public health agencies need to spend time thinking about the orientation of all new hires. Often organizations see that as a time to review policies and procedures when, in fact, it should be a time to orient new hires to the organization's culture and values. If a core value is customer service, have a customer come to talk; if a core value is teamwork, have a team come and talk about how they work together. The most important thing at the end of the first day is not that the new staff member understands policies and procedures, but that they go home feeling that they are a fit with the organization and they are energized to make a difference. Nothing that happens during their tenure will influence their impression more than their first encounters with the organization through the hiring process and their first day at work.

Box 11.3   Teamwork

Because public health is an amalgam of disparate disciplines—environmental health, nursing, nutrition, epidemiology—glued together by a common mission of improving community health, effective teamwork is necessary.[20] Every member of the team has to appreciate that each person's role is equally important. For example, in a workshop to challenge staff to think about creating their vision for the future, a receptionist stood up and presented drawings illustrating her view of the team. One of her three drawings was of machinery with interlocking cogs and wheels—all different sizes but obviously interdependent. She simply stated,

> We all need to operate like a well oiled machine. Like all machines, some parts are bigger than others, but all are equally important for even if the smallest cog breaks, the machine stops. And, the oil that lubricates our working parts is the love we have for each other and for the communities we serve.

With her hand-drawn pictures she eloquently described that everyone was equally important to the overall functioning of the team no matter how seemingly insignificant their tasks.[20] Fostering the sense of team and respect for all positions is a cornerstone for effective human resource management in public health.

Motivation

Human resources are especially important to public health organizations, because staff are undoubtedly the most important asset in achieving improvements in population health. A chief priority of senior and middle managers within the organization is to excel at the motivational challenge to increase employee participation and production at work. Managerial approaches to **motivation** are examined in this chapter, including employee development, mentoring, job training, quality management, and recruitment. Additionally, human resource systems and processes frequently encountered by public health managers are examined, including merit systems, job classification systems, labor relations processes, and contract development processes.

Patterns of managerial motivation are shown in **Table 11.1**. According to the Porter and Lawler model, employee effort is determined by two factors: 1) the value placed on certain outcomes by the individual, and 2) the extent to which the person believes that his or her effort will lead to attainment of these rewards.[17,18] Other theories of successful managerial motivation also emphasize the role of individual expectancy with respect to the assigned job. If people are assigned to tasks for which they lack capability, their expectancy for accomplishment and resulting performance will be low. Human resources managers sensitive to the importance of these self-efficacy beliefs in job performance typically rely on the following four methods to strengthen employee confidence:[18]

1. Performance successes strengthen a person's perception of his or her capability. Building experience through stages of success can help to overcome limitations in training, supervision, and mentoring.
2. Modeling ideal performance using other employees can convey to observers effective strategies for responding effectively to different work situations.
3. Social persuasion, including realistic encouragement, can increase individuals' beliefs that they possess the necessary capabilities to do the job.
4. Reducing job stress levels using stages of successes, performance models, and social persuasion can improve performance over time.

The foundation of the human resources model is positive reinforcement of employee performance, rather than use of punishment for undesirable behaviors, and concentration on building strengths. Positive reinforcement is a widely recommended strategy that is supported in both the scientific and professional literatures on human performance. Positive reinforcement enhances an individual's commitment to the organization and can be achieved by fulfilling the individual's core professional needs for job security, social support, and achievement.

Guidelines for positive reinforcement include the following:[19]

- Do not reward every worker in the same way; differentiate rewards based on performance.
- Do something. Nonaction by managers also influences employee behavior, but there may be negative consequences to nonaction on performance.
- Tell the individual worker what he or she can do to receive positive reinforcement.
- Tell the worker what he or she is doing wrong.

Table 11.1   General Patterns of Managerial Approaches to Motivation

Traditional Model	Human Relations Model	Human Resources Model
Assumptions		
1. Work is inherently distasteful to most people. 2. What people do is less important than what they earn for doing it. 3. Few want or can handle work that requires creativity, self-direction, or self-control.	1. People want to feel useful and important. 2. People desire to belong and to be recognized as individuals. 3. These needs are more important than money in motivating people to work.	1. Work is not inherently distasteful. 2. People want to contribute to meaningful goals that they have helped establish. 3. Most people can exercise far more creative, responsible self-direction and self-control than their present jobs demand.
Policies		
1. The manager's basic task is to closely supervise and control subordinates. 2. He or she must break tasks down into simple, repetitive, easily learned operations. 3. He or she must establish detailed work routines and procedures, and enforce them firmly but fairly.	1. The manager's basic task is to make each worker feel useful and important. 2. He or she should keep subordinates informed and listen to their objections to his or her plans. 3. The manager should allow subordinates to exercise some self-direction and self-control on routine matters.	1. The manager's basic task is to make use of "untapped" human resources. 2. He or she must create an environment in which all members may contribute to the limits of their ability. 3. He or she must encourage full participation on important matters, continually broadening subordinates' self-direction and self-control.
Expectations		
1. People can tolerate work if the pay is decent and the boss is fair. 2. If tasks are simple enough and people are closely controlled, they will produce up to standard.	1. Sharing information with subordinates and involving them in routine decisions will satisfy their basic needs to belong and to feel important. 2. Satisfying these needs will improve morale and reduce resistance to formal authority—subordinates will "willingly cooperate."	1. Expanding subordinate influence, self-direction, and self-control will lead to direct improvements in operating efficiency. 2. Work satisfaction may improve as a "byproduct" of subordinates making full use of their resources.

Source: Adapted from Miles RE, Porter LW, Craft JA. Leadership attitudes among public health officials. *Am J Public Health.* 1966;56(12):1990–2005.

- Do not correct the worker in front of others.
- Make the consequences equal to the behavior; reward good workers and counsel employees with unsatisfactory performance.

It is important to think about how the team functions effectively and to reinforce positive team behavior over time. Team motivation is a function of leadership, individual drive, clear goals, resources to do the job, and rewards for positive behavior.

Training and Development

Professional development of employees pays off in two key ways. First, such development leads to greater job satisfaction by the employees, improved morale, reduced turnover, and enhanced performance. Second, the organization benefits from a staff with a breadth of skills, knowledge, and attitudes. Creativity and ownership in the success of the organization come from enhancement of the quality of the workforce. Employee development includes training and education, mentoring programs, and employee involvement in organizational improvement and decisions. Public health organizations are often at a competitive disadvantage in the pay and working conditions that they are able to offer employees relative to other employers. However, the intrinsic satisfaction that can come from making a difference in the community is a highly motivating characteristic of public health work. Employees who feel valued and see tangible investments in their growth will often develop a commitment to the organization that is as powerful a motivator or more powerful than compensation.

Every organization needs a training budget that is recognized as being just as important as other expenses, such as utilities and equipment maintenance. A common error in organizations is to assume that the training budget is discretionary and thus subject to reduction during difficult budgetary times. Each employee needs a personal development plan that includes specific skills and personal growth components. This plan should be negotiated during each annual work planning session and updated to reflect changing roles in the organization and new technologies. For example, clinical responsibilities within an organization may be declining as these responsibilities are assumed by private-sector managed care plans, but the need for community health assessment may be growing. This shift in organizational and community needs should be reflected in the skills that management makes available to staff through training opportunities.

Training initiatives must also reflect the evolving competencies required of public health professionals, such as designing and interpreting health status indicators or surveillance data for specific risk factors and disease outcomes and crafting and monitoring service contracts to achieve specific results consistent with the rules and laws of the local jurisdiction. Almost every job in public health now requires information technology and information analysis skills. Likewise, effective communication skills—both written and verbal—are required in almost every position in order to connect with the community. Another reason staff diversity is so critical is that cultural competency—understanding the cultures of the community the agency serves—is essential to effective communication with constituents.

Professional competencies may be quite different from the tasks that were expected of staff in the recent past, when more clinical services were directly provided by public health organizations. As the role of public health organizations changes, staff must be transitioned to new responsibilities. New technologies create a constant need for new skills as information tools and scientific options evolve. A developmental plan for each employee needs to recognize these changes.

Coaching and Performance Appraisal

Employees are most likely to be successful if an organization recognizes the following:

- Performance improves most when clear goals are mutually established.
- Coaching is at the core of every interaction every day.
- Coaching comes from supervisors, peers, and direct reports.
- The key element of organizational learning is individual learning, and individual learning comes from many sources, one of which is coaching.

Coaching occurs regularly between individuals working together in organizations to improve performance. However, at least annually, organizations require a formal performance appraisal—a review of the employee's performance relative to goals.

Although most managers will eagerly agree that personnel management is a key responsibility, many do not relish the tasks and roles required for effective performance management. Formal **performance appraisals** are an important part of supervisory responsibilities in most organizations. Appraisals are for the benefit of the organization, and ideally, for the benefit of employees. They are used to inform organizational decisions that determine salary, promotions, transfers, layoffs, demotions, and terminations. They also provide the mechanism and opportunity for employees to receive useful coaching and suggested changes in behavior, attitudes, knowledge, and skills. However, if left to their own devices, many managers and supervisors would never administer a performance appraisal. Therefore, the organization usually creates prescribed procedures with common forms and other tools. However, the formal appraisal process should not provide information to the employee about their performance that is new; with regular coaching the employee should have received feedback all year long about their performance and should be attuned to strengths and areas for improvement.

Successful performance appraisal systems take time to implement, and yet most supervisors spend only 4 to 8 hours a year per employee in performance management, including preparation, paperwork, and discussion.[21] It is therefore not surprising that most employees do not see a link between their performance and their pay.

Many options are available to an organization regarding the instrument used for appraisals. These can include a numeric rating scale or a nonnumeric rating. For example, the instrument may be developed with a maximum number of points set at 100. Other instruments may focus on categories of performance such as exceeds objectives, fully meets objectives, partially meets objectives, and unsatisfactory. Some agencies use unsatisfactory, fully competent, and peak performer, which align with numeric ranges. Some instruments focus on behavior; others focus on traits and skills. The factors evaluated, such as communications, leadership, or problem solving, may be weighted so that some are recognized as more crucial than others. The instrument itself is less important than how it is administered and how plans are developed against which the employee is evaluated.

An organization is more likely to have successful **performance management** if: 1) supervisors and employees are trained regarding the appraisal process and how to develop meaningful objectives and work plans, 2) supervisors are trained to be coaches and mentors, and 3) performance management is seen as a meaningful mechanism for development. Performance management starts with the job, not the form, and both parties have a responsibility regarding its success. The phases of performance management include the following:[10, p. 21]

- Performance planning, in which objectives, standards, competencies, and a development plan are mutually determined
- Performance execution, which involves the actual work being accomplished
- Performance assessment, which includes both parties independently assessing how the plan was achieved
- Collection of data from other parties, such as subordinates, peers, or customers
- Performance review, where the results are discussed
- The renewal of the agreement or contract for the following performance period

Typically, a performance appraisal should include four parts:

- The employee's self-assessment of his or her performance ("How do you think things are going?")
- The supervisor's feedback on the employee ("Let me provide you with feedback on how you are doing relative to your goals.")
- The employee's feedback on working more effectively with the supervisor ("What can I do to make you more successful in your position?")
- The development of a plan for performance improvement ("So this is your development plan for next year.")

The stage for the entire performance appraisal is set by the employees talking about how they are feeling about their performance. The conversation is entirely different for employees who are feeling overwhelmed and as if their performance is low compared to the employees who think they are top performers. Thus, the supervisor needs to first gauge the connection between the employee's perspective and the supervisor's assessment of performance.

The employee needs commitment to the objectives and goals, solicitation of feedback from others, communication that is open and regular with the supervisor, the collection of performance information or data, and preparation for the review. The supervisor is responsible for creating an environment that encourages open communication and motivation, observing and documenting performance, updating and revising objectives and standards, explaining the relationship between the overall goals of the organization and the employee's objectives, creating developmental paths, and reinforcing effective behavior. The employee's work plan should reinforce and integrate with a unit or program work plan. Objectives at both the program and the employee level should be specific, measurable, achievable, results oriented, and timely. Organizations facilitate the connection between organizational goals and individual goals by:

- Having a participative process of organizational goal setting
- Prominently displaying organizational goals in conference rooms and common work spaces

- Using forms that ask employees to identify what organizational goals each of their individual goals supports
- Setting staff meeting agendas around organizational goals and asking staff to report on their accomplishments relative to the goals
- Recognizing and rewarding milestones in organizational goals

One public health manager annually had the staff make up a "We Would Be Proud" list of desired accomplishments for the next year. Whenever one of those goals was accomplished, a staff meeting was held and key staff who got to cross that goal off their list were recognized.

Some of the most common errors in performance management include the following:[21]

- Contrast effect—The employee is compared with another employee or employees.
- First impression error—An initial observation rules the supervisor's thinking even though it is no longer applicable.
- Halo or horns effect—One aspect of the employee's performance is generalized to the entire performance.
- Like me effect—The supervisor rates employees who are similar to him or her higher than others.
- Skews to the center, negative, and positive—The supervisor has a tendency to rate employees in the middle, or at the high or low end of the scale.
- Attribution bias—The supervisor has a tendency to attribute failing to factors that are under the control of the employee and successes to outside causes.
- Recent effect—The supervisor remembers the most recent event(s) instead of the full performance period.
- Stereotyping—The supervisor ignores the individual and generalizes across groups or work units.

Some organizations directly link pay to performance, while others do not. In governmental agencies, salary increases are often based more on seniority than on performance. In unionized organizations, union rules and contracts may dictate salary levels to a greater extent than the supervisor does. The success of performance management does not require a link to pay, although that link may make employees and supervisors more aware of the importance of appraisals and planning activities. The need to include as much objectivity as possible in appraisals increases with the link to pay. If there is no obvious linkage, supervisors may have a tendency toward "grade inflation" or leniency in ratings. Supervisors generally find it more comfortable to discuss positive ratings and results than to focus on areas where objectives are not being met. This tendency leads to a sense of unfairness in the workforce and discounts the opportunities that performance planning and appraisal provide.

A successful performance appraisal occurs when a supervisor and employee reach a better understanding of the employee's performance level and develop a plan to further improve performance.

Transfer, Promotion, and Termination

Evaluations can be helpful in determining the strengths and areas in need of improvement for employees. The evaluation process can also yield information that assists the human resources staff with decisions related to the most useful placement of employees. One of the most important functions of a human resources department is identifying the best position fit for employees. Effective transfer and promotion strategies are an essential component of this process. Transferring and promoting existing employees allows individuals to grow within the organization. The opportunity to progress within the organization is a major factor in retaining productive employees.[22]

Human resources personnel must also recognize situations in which the best move for the employee is out of the organization. Though this is the most difficult component of human resources, it is necessary and crucial for success of the organization. Failure to address problem employees can limit organizational effectiveness (see **Box 11.4**).

Human resource departments have traditionally focused on schedules, benefits, pay structure, and grievance procedures. Yet, a great opportunity exists for human resources to impact the effectiveness of the organization by working with managers to match employees with the position or work that needs to be done. And, perhaps more importantly, to address those employees who are not suited to the position or the organization.[1]

Box 11.4   Dealing with Difficult Employees

While in training at the University of North Carolina at Chapel Hill, Public Health Leadership Institute scholars from across the United States had 1,158 peers, superiors, subordinates, and clients complete the Center for Creative Leadership's (CCL) Benchmarks assessment to evaluate their skills in meeting job challenges, leading people, and respecting self and others. The results over the three cohorts were remarkably consistent. For all three, the number one leadership deficit was in "confronting problem employees."[23] You might say this is not a leadership skill but a basic personnel management skill.

Leaders in public health will say they are rated poorly at confronting problem employees because they work within civil service systems, with unions and government bureaucracies that limit their flexibility. However, the 88,731 private-sector respondents who have evaluated their leaders with the CCL's Benchmarks instrument, also identified "failure to confront problem employees" as the number one deficit for more than 10,000 leaders who work in Fortune 500 companies, associations, nonprofits, the military, and the government.[23] Clearly, public health is not unique in not having the skills—or the incentives or support systems—to address problem employees.

Supervisors should be clear about their expectations and the staff member's performance relative to that expectation; then a plan to close the gap should be developed. A commitment should be made to meet regularly to determine whether the gap is being closed. Ideally, this coaching model works. But when coaching fails it is the responsibility of the supervisor to take action. Taking action may mean finding another job in the organization where the employee's skills are a better fit. But sometimes the employee needs to be terminated. The inexperienced supervisor lacks confidence that they have been clear about their expectations and feedback and avoids addressing the performance gap. The keys to an effective termination are to be direct and clear about the performance gap, the exit arrangements and any severance.

Personnel Policies

Policies that implement basic rules of the organization and provide management intent are important to successful personnel management. At a minimum, an organization should have specific agency or organizational policies on such topics as affirmative action, violence in the workplace, the use of drugs and alcohol by employees, outside employment, use of the various types of leave, work hours, disability accommodations, employee grievances, and sexual harassment. Many of these policies are determined by the need to clarify how the agency or organization will respond to legal questions and challenges. With specific policies in place, an organization is better equipped to deal with employee behavior issues and lawsuits. It is important that each employee has a copy of the current policies. These should be provided at a new employee orientation and followed with periodic issuance of policies to all staff members. Policies should be signed by the top-level manager to illustrate that they are organization-wide policies and decisions. Policies should cite relevant law and other directives such as state or local rules.

Future Outlook

With the passage of the Accountable Care Act, the incentives and focus for healthcare systems is no longer on treatment of illness but rather on the management of health of populations. The transformation of the nation's healthcare system will take place over several years as the rules take effect of the most significant healthcare legislation since Medicare and Medicaid. Healthcare organizations are turning to their public health colleagues to collaborate with them on effective ways to improve the dental, physical and mental health of the community. The demand for experts in environmental health, health communication, health administration, biostatistics, epidemiology has never been greater. This is an opportune time for public health professionals to have broad community impact.

Discussion Questions

1. What is the major purpose of human resources management?
2. What are the key components of workforce planning?
3. What are the major challenges for public health human resources management?
4. Describe the recruitment process.
5. Discuss the common motivation strategies and illustrate how to use them to motivate employees.
6. What is performance appraisal? How might it be conducted?
7. Why is it important to address problem employees in a workplace?
8. What can organizations do to retain high-performing employees?

References

1. Buckingham M, Coffman C. *First, Break all the Rules.* New York: Simon & Schuster; 1999:27–28.
2. Association of State and Territorial Health Officials, Council of State Governments, National Association of State Personnel Executives. *State Public Health Worker Shortage.* Washington, DC: Association of State and Territorial Health Officials; 2004.
3. Council of State Governments, National Association of State Personnel Executives. *The Trends Alert: State Employee Workforce Shortage.* Lexington, KY: Council of State Governments; 2002.
4. Council on Linkages Between Academia and Public Health Practice. *Evidence-Based Forum on Effective Recruitment and Retention Efforts.* Washington, DC: Council on Linkages; 2004.
5. Hornsby JS, Kuratko DF. *Frontline HR: A Handbook for the Emerging Manager.* Mason, OH: Texere; 2005:43–60.
6. Hornsby JS, Kuratko DF. Human resource management: critical issues for the 90s. *J Small Business Manage.* 1990;28:9–18.
7. Thielen L, et al. *A Guide for the Recruitment, Selection and Retention of a State Health Officer.* Washington, DC: Association of State and Territorial Health Officials; 1993.
8. Shafritz JM, et al. *Personnel Management in Government: Politics and Process.* New York: Marcel Dekker; 1986:28–30.
9. McConnell CR. *The Effective Health Care Supervisor.* 4th ed. Gaithersburg, MD: Aspen Publishers; 1997:461–71.
10. Mountain States Employers Council. *Top Ten Errors Made by Interviewers.* Denver, CO: Mountain States Employers Council; 1999.
11. Still DJ. *High Impact Hiring: How to Interview and Select Outstanding Employees.* Dana Point, CA: Management Development Systems; 2001:27–53.
12. Siering M. Interview techniques can separate prime candidates from 'wannabes.' *Denver Business Journal.* November 14, 1997.
13. Neale MA, Northcraft GB. Factors influencing organizational commitment. In: Steers RM, Porter LW, eds. *Motivation and Work Behavior.* 5th ed. New York: McGraw-Hill; 1991:290–7.
14. Steers RM. Antecedents and outcomes of organizational commitments. *Admin Sci Q.* 1977;22:46–56.
15. Koch JL, Steers RM. Job attachment, satisfaction and turnover among public employees. *J Vocational Behav.* 1978;12:199–228.
16. Angle H, Perry J. An empirical assessment of organizational effectiveness. *Admin Sci Q.* 1981;26:1–14.
17. Miles RE, Porter LW, Craft JA. Leadership attitudes among public health officials. *Am J Public Health.* 1966;56(12):1990–2005.
18. Pinder CC. Valence-instrumentality-expectancy theory. In: Steers RM, Porter LW, eds. *Motivation and Work Behavior.* 5th ed. New York: McGraw-Hill; 1991:144–64.
19. Hammer WC. Reinforcement theory and contingency management in organizational settings. In: Steers RM, Porter LW, eds. *Motivation and Work Behavior.* 5th ed. New York: McGraw-Hill; 1991:61–87.
20. Porter J, Baker EL. The management moment: management is a team sport. *J Public Health Manage Practice.* 2004;10:564–6.
21. Grote D. *The Complete Guide to Performance Appraisal.* New York: Amacon; 1996.
22. Fried BJ. Recruitment, selection, and retention. In: Fried BJ, Fottler MD, Johnson JA, eds. *Human Resources in Health Care: Managing for Success.* 5th ed. Washington, DC: AUPHA; 2005:163–204.
23. Porter J, Baker EL. The management moment: the coach in you. *J Public Health Manage Pract.* 2004;10:472–4.

Leadership for Public Health

Claudia S. P. Fernandez and David P. Steffen

LEARNING OBJECTIVES

- To better understand leadership in public health organizations
- To gain an understanding of various theories of leadership
- To develop skills useful in public health leadership positions
- To appreciate the unique environment in which public health works
- To learn about the roles and responsibilities of public health leaders

---

Chapter Overview

Developing leaders across the spectrum of public health has been a priority area since the 1980s in the United States.[1-7] Yet, there have been some differences in implementation that have led to divergent paths of leadership skills development. To some, developing leaders means developing individual professionals with cutting edge technical "hard skills" critical to a discipline—for example, medical, statistical, science, research, or intervention skills. These skills are of key importance in furthering the discipline-specific base of knowledge and practice in a field. Truly these programs promote leadership through supporting the role of the individual contributor and by pushing the boundaries of a discipline farther.

The other path, perhaps less taken, is to focus on the type of skills that are not discipline-specific, but rather are strategic in nature, cross-disciplinary, and are applied particularly in inter-professional contexts. These are the "soft skills" related to working with and through others: skills that have applications and relevance across every particular public health discipline, including areas such as maternal and child health, environmental health, health behavior, health policy, clinical care, and academics. These skills have similar relevance in non-public health fields like technology, finance, and government. This type of leadership development does not focus on the individual contributor, but rather on the type of leadership skills that promote the necessary infrastructure that allows the enterprise to be successful by doing "whatever it takes"[8] to identify and achieve the mission and vision. The very nature of these leadership skills is boundary spanning, as they are not tied to any particular discipline of practice. Developing these skills in individuals helps them to become boundary-spanning leaders. These types of skills help leaders interface with those from outside, and inside, their area of technical expertise to communicate and advocate persuasively with them. As such, these skills help individuals become boundary-spanning ambassadors for the field of public health as well.

In both paths, the students of leadership hone skills that allow them to serve others better. It is the "others" who differ—that end audience for which the leader is being prepared to impact. For a technical discipline leader, the end target is the patient or community member who serves to benefit from the expertise of the individual, or other providers who learn from the advancing technology or theory in a field. For the boundary-spanning leader, the target audience is typically the organization itself. In the private, for-profit sector, the "organization" is the brick-and-mortar entity that produces a good of some commercial value, commonly referred to as "a widget." In the public or nonprofit sector—where the vocabulary and the goals are different from for-profits—correspondences can still be made:[9,10] the organization can be the brick-and-mortar institution, or, ideally, it can be the alliance of community groups or the policies that impact a wide swath of the population in order to improve the community health. These are the targets on which the leader focuses her or his skills. These relate to the infrastructure-building and population-based services that make up the foundation of the Maternal and Child Health Pyramid of Health Services.[11]

Even the greatly celebrated scientist, Albert Einstein, echoed the crucial role played by skills outside the technical realm:

> The development of general ability for independent thinking and judgment should always be placed foremost, not the acquisition of special knowledge. If a person masters the fundamentals of his subject and has learned to think and work independently, he will surely find his way and besides will better be able to adapt himself to progress and changes than the person whose training principally consists in the acquiring of detailed knowledge.[12, p. 62]

This chapter addresses the concept of boundary-spanning leadership training—from the theoretical underpinnings to the execution of curricula. This chapter examines leadership development in public health the United States, the history of leadership thought over time, the essential skills and competencies for public health leadership, and salient issues in developing leaders, including crucial topics, assessment tools, and mentoring. This chapter presents some of the core considerations for developing leaders across the spectrum of public health, reviewing several leadership theories and applications in public health, with a focus on the essential skills and tools for leadership development of contemporary public health leaders.

A Brief History of Leadership Development in Public Health, 1988–2014

The critical need for leadership training has long been noted[1,13–15] and public health as a field has gone to great lengths to promote this boundary-spanning style of leadership development in addition to promoting technical expertise. After the call in 1988 for leadership development to amend a public health system that was "in disarray,"[16] the director at the Centers for Disease Control and Prevention (CDC), Dr. William Roper, called for implementing leadership training across the spectrum of governmental public health.[17] Subsequently, the CDC funded an elite, individual model of public health leadership development, the National Public Health Leadership Institute (PHLI) in 1991.[18]

Public health and its leadership were greatly shaken by the September 11, 2001, terrorist attacks and the subsequent anthrax threats. These events put public health leadership in the public's eye and necessitated a heightened emphasis on preparedness, risk communication, and reassuring logistical and emotional readiness.[19] A specialized form of collaborative leadership, "meta-leadership," was promoted among preparedness professionals emphasizing precrisis partnerships and "connectedness."[20] In 2002, the Institute of Medicine (IOM) released follow-up reports to its earlier one in 1988[16]—*Who Will Keep the Public Healthy?*[21] and *The Future of the Public's Health in the 21st Century*[22]—concluding that public health leadership had improved but still faced significant challenges: "We must be led by those who have mastery of the skills to mobilize, coordinate and direct broad collaborative actions in the complex public health system . . . these skills need constant refinement and honing." The report called for lifelong learning based on the transdisciplinary, socioecological model of health. It noted, "The focus on preparing individuals for leadership roles and senior practice positions requires redesign of curricula and teaching approaches to incorporate enhanced participation in the educational process by those in senior practice positions with comparable experiences." This report also broadened the concept of who, in addition to traditional governmental public health, was to be counted as major players in the public health system: media, health care, communities, academia, and business.

The CDC's commitment to leadership training reflected the IOM report's conception of a broader public health system beginning in PHLI year 10. For the first time, participants as preestablished teams from communities utilized action-learning team projects with coaching to learn collaborative work, as well as individual leadership development.[23] Similarly fueled by these key studies of the state of public health, states and territories eventually developed more than 20 state or regional leadership programs covering all but a handful of states,[24] which were funded by the CDC until 2011. In that year, CDC shifted PHLI leadership funding commitments to an even greater emphasis on leadership in community in the National Leadership Academy for the Public's Health, with participants being four-member community teams, much of the training taking place in their localities, and the desired results measured by community health outcomes.

Since the first IOM report, many categorical leadership institutes were also begun at a national level, among them programs serving environmental professionals, state health officials, and those in oral health, nursing, and health education. Similarly, the Maternal and Child Health (MCH) Bureau training program in the Division of Research, Training and Education responded to the need for ongoing leadership development for mid- to senior-level leaders—funding training that is specific to MCH public health leaders, grounded in a central core of leadership values, and with the goal of creating measurable impact.[4,25,26]

Formal leadership training is valued in order to avoid two common scenarios: 1) individuals being promoted, based upon their technical expertise, into positions requiring additional skills that they had yet to develop; and 2) individuals suddenly becoming leaders from being thrust into positions of authority where the potentially blinding spotlight of leadership expectation immediately hits them despite their having little or no training in leadership, per se. It was recognized that even those who might not seek positions of leadership could find that the spotlight was thrust upon them by chance or circumstance as public health issues emerged. Formal leadership training also helps to accomplish a third scenario: the United States has the highest expenditures on health care in the world yet has consistently had fundamental indices of health in the middle of the pack.[27] If resources are to be devoted to public health and communities are to be rallied to develop community health assessments and improvement plans, then leadership training that inspires and prepares trainees to collaborate with others external to the world of public health is imperative. That is, true public health leaders must be boundary-spanning leaders if they are to have a significant impact.

A Brief History of Leadership Theory: The "Born With It" Factor Debate

The interest in and debate about leadership has raged for thousands of years, with research in the past 100 years creating theories about predicting and teaching leadership. More than 2,000 years ago, Aristotle taught that some are marked from birth for subjugation and others for command. This became known as the "Great Man" (or more contemporarily, "Great Woman") theory for millennia, with the idea that only "great people are worthy."[28] Today, scholars surmise that it is easy to identify great leadership in hindsight when history has recorded the end of the story. Predicting the future, however, remains challenging, and thus a great deal of leadership research has been undertaken to examine this elusive, yet much sought after quality.

In the perpetual nature versus nurture argument, trait theories clearly fall into the nature camp,[29] seeking that essential "it" factor of leadership. Early theories of leadership postulated that certain personal characteristics, such as mental, physical, or cultural attributes, separated great leaders from followers or unsuccessful leaders.[29,30] Hence the "Great Person" theory of leadership was embraced for many years. While contemporary traits of leadership portray a laudable list of qualities, research has failed to reveal any individual traits that predict leadership effectiveness or success or even to separate leaders from followers.[29,31–33] Thus, possession of a specific trait does not guarantee leadership success; rather, it is the behaviors employed by individuals that have the greater impact on their leadership performance.[28,29,34–37] Indeed, it would seem that these traits are important at every level throughout an organization—as is the behavioral skill to implement them with eloquence and ease.

The 1950s and 1960s brought research that suggested the role of *behaviors* rather than traits is the underpinning of great leadership, with the benefit that nearly anyone could *learn* the behaviors of leadership.[28,29,36,38,39] Researchers looked at behavioral dimensions being *task/production* oriented versus being *people* oriented,[40–42] arguing that leadership is about the transactions between workers and leaders. From this era we have inherited the "carrots and sticks" theories of leading by offering rewards and punishments. While this approach has limited effectiveness, it laid the groundwork for the next evolutionary stage of leadership theory, as researchers examined the complexity of the roles leaders play. For the first time research acknowledged that leaders must adjust their behaviors, situationally, based on differing target audiences. This is when the idea emerged that in some ways we are all leaders, followers, doers, and thinkers.[41–44] This discovery, in turn, led the way for the introduction of emotional intelligence into the leadership literature, which became popular just before the turn of the century[30,45,46] and remains a core of contemporary leadership thought, research, and leadership development in practice.[47–49]

The theory of emotional intelligence developed concurrently with the transformational and servant leadership models. Transformational theories acknowledge the power and influence of individuals who have the gift for more than just leading their organizations—but rather transforming their organizations through envisioning, energizing, and enabling. Researcher George Burns voiced the idea of **transformational leadership** in the late 1970s,[50] with theorists Bennis and Nanus[51] providing lists of steps for individuals to follow in their pursuit of becoming transformational leaders of their organizations.

Many of these steps later became core principles of the total quality management, continuous quality improvement, and systems thinking era of leadership thought.[52,53] Transformational leadership quickly became a popular, although not uncriticized,[54,55] leadership theme with contemporary authors. While transformational leadership was the buzzword of the 1990s, its reliance upon case studies of individuals coupled with the lack of empirical studies, rigorous research, and definitions failed to adequately support its efficacy and contributed to its fading from the foundations of contemporary thought.

The next key set of theories to emerge falls into the category of **principled leadership**. These are leadership models based on ethics and principles that embrace higher and less self-centered values. Many people in public health, for example, feel closely aligned with Robert Greenleaf's model of servant leadership. While he wrote of this as early as 1970, it took more than 30 years for it to become widely influential.[56] Sadly, it was not until the many shocking revelations of corruption and deceit in corporate America, such as the economy-rocking scandals of Enron and Arthur Andersen in 2001, that principled leadership began to truly take hold in and thus open the minds of leaders to the potential benefits of skills like emotional intelligence.

Principled leadership topics got another unfortunate backhanded endorsement in 2008–2009 when the AIG scandals and the mortgage-backed securities debacle initiated a global economic meltdown. The casting of millions into joblessness and poverty, many of them children, furthered the cry from the populace and the U.S. Administration alike for ethics- and values-based leadership from all sectors of the U.S. economy.[57,58] This opened the door for principle-centered leadership to take center stage in the ongoing dialogue of what makes a great leader.

Table 12.1   Universal Attributes in Leadership from the GLOBE Study

Universally Positive Leader Attributes		Universally Negative Leader Attributes
Trustworthy	Dynamic	Loner
Just	Motive arouser	Asocial
Honest	Confidence builder	Noncooperative
Foresight	Motivational	Irritable
Plans ahead	Dependable	Nonexplicit
Encouraging	Intelligent	Egocentric
Positive	Decisive	Ruthless
Effective bargainer	Administrative skills	Dictatorial
Win-win problem solver	Communicative	
Team builder	Excellence oriented	

Source: Data from House RJ, Hanges PJ, Javidian M, et al., eds. *Culture, Leadership, and Organizations: The GLOBE study of 62 societies.* Thousand Oaks, CA: Sage; 2004.

Indeed, the ideas of principle-centered leadership provided the foundation for the opening of the 2012 meeting of the World Economic Forum in Davos, Switzerland.

Given the increasingly international nature of business and travel today, this brief history of leadership theory would not be complete without examining the concept of universally heralded or decried leadership attributes. The GLOBE study sheds valuable light here with the most extensive report on global leadership to date, which involved more than 160 investigators in 62 countries or regions.[59] The GLOBE study revealed clear differences in expectations and preferences of leadership across cultures, however, some expectations of leaders are universal. The GLOBE study identified 22 leadership attributes universally liked and 8 disliked (see **Table 12.1**). Note that many of the universally negative attributes are related to poor emotional intelligence and to poor communication or interactions between leaders and followers, which is addressed later in this chapter.

The Leadership–Management Relationship

While this is a chapter on leadership, it is important to note that management roles are also vital, and in reality many public health leaders must execute both of those functions on a daily basis. Few are the positions that have only leader-related duties. Thus, it is more useful to think of the *functions* of leadership and management rather than the *individuals* who wear those labels in an organization. Alone, each is necessary but insufficient for organizational success; rather, they are equally important, interdependent, and complementary functions of every organization. **Table 12.2** lists common descriptors of managers and leadership. Excellent management is needed to better focus upon and execute proven processes and strategies in order to close the documented "Knowing–Doing Gap" that wastes billions of dollars annually.[60,61] Similarly, during times of increased complexity, uncertainty, risk taking, and growth, management is vitally important.[62] **Leadership** is about the future and discontinuous or disruptive change that must take place to ensure the organization's survival in the chaos ahead. Leadership assures

Table 12.2   Common Descriptors Ascribed to Managers and Leaders

The Traditional View of Managers	The Traditional View of Leadership
Mission and purpose oriented	Vision and goal oriented
Focused is internal, on status quo and rules	Focus is external, on strategic change and unbridled possibilities and opportunities
Knows many different subjects they have mastered	Most important skill set is knowing how to learn how to learn anything
Initially approaches all issues as technical problems	Distinguishes between adaptive and technical issues with initial comfort with ambiguity
Leads by authority and direction	Leads with vision and charisma
Works within their span of control	A boundary spanner
Develops individuals for line and supervisory positions within organization	Develops others who can play a boundary-spanning role in the community
Does things right	Does the right things
Fosters and manages incremental change, continuous quality improvement (CQI)	Leads disruptive, significant change processes
Supports the ideals and symbols of the organization	Epitomizes the ideals of and symbolizes the organization to internal and external constituencies
Works through contracts and other formal, narrowly demarcated exchange agreements	Works through interest and curiosity, fostering open and longer term exchange relationships
Is an excellent linear thinker and accomplisher	Is an excellent systems thinker and strategic planner
Is most focused on maintaining order and consistency	Values creativity, inspiration, and collaborative change
Reinforces the values and guiding principles of organization	Establishes and embodies organizational values culture
Efficiently follows protocols and formal guidance	Exercises judgment, discernment, and contextual wisdom in order to make sound decisions
Negotiates with others via a positional approach	Negotiates through a "win-win" appreciation of separate and shared interests
Is an active "doer"	Is a reflective learner who applies insights to actions

that the organization has an appropriate vision of the future informed by boundary spanning and external connections, and it tests this vision's viability through calculated risk taking via "mini-experiments."

Management's focus is on the present, assuring that operations that support the vision and mission are run efficiently and effectively. Incremental, continuous quality improvement is the province of the management role. For example, in a health department setting, leadership would set a stretch goal for the agency of achieving the highest possible quality improvement recognition by going through the most rigorous accreditation process or competing for the Malcolm Baldrige National Quality Award. Management would then operationalize and oversee the step-by-step progress toward that goal, managing people and resources along the way. Leadership scans the external environment to make sure that the best evidence-based practices are brought back to its agency, then management implements those new practices precisely.

Management is responsible for following current best practice, while leadership finds the next practice.

Marcus Buckingham and Curt Coffman synthesized a large Gallup poll of more than 80,000 managers and 1 million of their reports and concluded,

> The most important difference between the great manager and the great leader is one of focus. Great leaders look outward . . . at the competition, out at the future, out at alternative routes forward. They focus on broad patterns and connections, cracks . . . . They must be visionaries, strategic thinkers, activators; they don't have much to do with the challenge of turning one individual's talents into performance.[63]

Great managers on the other hand,

> look inward . . . inside the company into each individual, and the differences in style, goals, needs, and motivations of each person. The differences are small and subtle but great managers need to pay attention to them . . . . They guide them toward the right way to release each person's unique talents into performance.[63]

Leadership as a Life Course

Developing into an effective leader is a lifelong process. Many authors talk about leadership pathways or journeys and levels of leadership through which one must advance. Leaders should ideally master a competency area at the level that is appropriate to their experiential level, then, after additional professional and personal experience, add a more advanced level they'd like to address in that same skill area, but in a new, richer, and deeper way. A metaphor for this progressively increasing skill attainment over time is the most common symbol found in Southwestern Native American hieroglyphs, the ever-ascending spiral.

The development of individual leadership can be likened to the life-course model, which posits that there are stages of life with associated critical developmental tasks that must be achieved at particular points in life or one falls behind.[64] Everyone has a projected leadership development trajectory and potential that can be fulfilled if they receive appropriate "assessment, challenge and support"[65] at the appropriate points in time. Like a runner trying to develop a faster time, they must be given "stretch" assignments that push them past their comfortable speed for longer periods of time than they think they can handle in order to grow faster. This can only be done at certain times for an appropriate duration of time or the athlete can become burned out, like a greyhound pacesetter dog. If this life-course window of opportunity is taken advantage of, then growth, confidence, and readiness for another such generative experience are gained. Bennis calls these challenging experiences "crucible" times in which large leaps of leadership lessons can be learned.[66] Reflective practices that consolidate the experience and its meaning and place it in one's overall development plan are key to taking advantage of the challenging experience.[67] The ultimate goal is for leaders to "learn how to learn" leadership and build their adaptive capacity, which puts them in position to respond creatively and appropriately to almost any new leadership challenge they might face.[68]

One of the most common mistakes public health leaders and managers make is confusing a technical problem with an adaptive problem. According to Heifetz and Linsky, technical problems are defined and have clear solutions; an expert in the field can easily solve these problems if they carefully follow the established protocols, procedures, and instructions. Adaptive challenges, on the other hand, have:

> no simple, painless solutions—problems that require us to learn new ways .... Uncompetitive industry, drug abuse, poverty, poor public education, environmental hazards .... Making progress on these problems demands not just someone who provides answers on high, but changes in our attitudes, behavior, and values .... To meet challenges such as these, we need a different idea of leadership and a new social contract that promotes our adaptive capacity, rather than inappropriate expectations of authority.[69,70, p. 754]

Most of the problems identified in public health's socioecological model of health are these complex and "wicked" types of issues that require an adaptive approach. This is common in other fields as well, as the Center for Creative Leadership estimates that 43% of problems are technical challenges solvable with current techniques, 37% are adaptive challenges, 10% are critical challenges needing a crisis response, and the remainder are a mix.[71] Health care and healthcare reform provide us with a clear example of this confusion of technical issues for adaptive issues. The typical office visit to a clinician is designed to take 7–10 minutes. Because of the short timeframe, clinicians push to identify the patient's chief complaint. Once this diagnosis is reached, then a technical solution can be imposed as each diagnosis triggers a preestablished cascade of treatments and medicines to fit each diagnostic code. This often works with stable, chronic disease patients; however, for diabetes and alcoholism and most other health issues, more adaptive changes need to be made.

Similarly, many technically sufficient plans have been put forward for healthcare reform including the Affordable Health Care for America Act. However, there has not been consensus on the values, purpose, and responsibility for health care. Is health care a right, a privilege, something you earn by living healthily and participating in your community/society, or a commodity you buy on the market just like any other good? Until leaders meet the adaptive challenge and have the dialogue that can lead to changes in people's attitudes, values, and behaviors, there will be no broadly supported system.

In **adaptive leadership**, leadership is a relational, social process through which the leader first addresses stakeholders, communities, and those responsible for issues to carefully define their thoughts and feelings about an issue. These groups must go through the process of distinguishing what is important from what is truly expendable, taking responsibility themselves, and reaching an acceptable approach to significant issues. Leadership modulates the stress involved in the process so that it can help the issue ripen or simmer and assures that the work is accomplished despite the discomfort and loss people are sure to feel. Through this process cognitive shifts can take place which, at a minimum, allow a bridging connection to grow between two or more different views on the subject, and ideally an agreement to take action a third way. It takes persistence, time, and willingness to understand others opinions and feelings, and it takes great caring, commitment, and courage.[72]

Other leadership development experts ascribe to this staged approach to development. In their 2010 article, "Outcome-Based Workforce Development and Education in Public Health," Koo and Miner described their modification of the Dreyfus five-level model of learning levels from novice to expert into a seven-level model that adds the two higher levels—"advanced expert" and "luminary."[73] Internal organizational strategic leadership and mentoring those within their organization begins at the fifth level of "expert." Trans-agency strategic alliances and extensive mentorship is a leadership practice at the sixth level of "advanced expert." During the final stage of "luminary," the leader is involved in establishing benchmarks for the country or globally and is also a mentor of mentors. At each of these successively elevated levels, the leadership competencies of mentoring and giving and accepting direction are learned and practiced at successively higher levels until the highest level of the spiral is reached.[73]

The Future of Developing Public Health Leaders: Essential Skills and Competencies for Public Health Leadership

The same dynamic of different levels of learning and practice competencies is found in the three-level set established in 2009 by the Council on Linkages Between Academia and Public Health.[74] Eight unique domains of competencies are used; each has a nonmanager, program manager or supervisor (master of public health [MPH] degree with 5 years of work experience or 10 years' experience), and senior manager or agency leader category. The most relevant domains to public health leadership and management are systems thinking and leadership skills and financial planning and management skills, although others, such as communication and cross-cultural skills, are also critical at times. The systems thinking and leadership skills domain covers systems thinking, visioning, promotion of learning, mentoring, CQI, concurrence with modern public health and societal systems, and change management. These competencies are crosswalked with the 10 Essential Public Health Services.[75]

A final set of public health leadership competencies for practitioners was developed by the National Public Health Leadership Development Network (NLN) in 2005 under the auspices of the University of St. Louis Heartland Center for Community and Public Health Leadership.[76] These competencies were originally named the "Public Health Leadership Competency Framework," but were updated in 2009 to include emergency preparedness;[77] therefore, this set of competencies is now called "The Public Health and Crisis Leadership Competency Framework." These competencies were widely used by state and regional public health leadership institutes during their creation and development and include five broad categories: core transformational, political, transorganizational, team-building, and crisis leadership competencies. The first four domains have a total of 115 subcompetencies while the last domain, crisis leadership, has 106 on its own. There is no distinction among the competencies for experience level in public health or any other factors. The strength of this system is the very strong focus on leadership in all of the competencies, which points out the relative limitations of the other models for leadership in public health.

The Association of Schools of Public Health (ASPH) competencies are designed specifically for MPH graduates.[78] The April 2006 version consists of five public health core discipline competency domains and seven cross-cutting domains. A total of 118 competencies are in the model. ASPH offers an optional exam for certification as a public health professional. A strength of the ASPH model is its excellent section on professionalism, which outlines the ethos of public health very well. There are also leadership and systems thinking sections among the cross-cutting competencies. Because these competencies are designed specifically for MPH graduates, there is no distinction made for levels of expertise or any other factors.

What leadership competencies are currently the most important? The answer would seem to be those that allow public health leaders to address the most pressing challenges, opportunities, and issues of the day. In addition, this information must be combined with a gap analysis between the current capacities the individual leader possesses and those she will need for the future. Customized or personalized competency development on an individual basis is most important for higher level public health leaders.[79] At this level, public health leaders are able to learn how to learn almost any skill they need through a combination of information gathering, reflection, meaning making, coaching and/or mentoring, and repeated practice. Leaders take responsibility for their learning and assemble a "personal board of directors" of people to assess, challenge, and support them in their leadership journey.[80]

In this new modern era, change is constant and learning is essential to keep ahead of the "tsunami" of change. Reg Revans, one of the founders of action learning, famously said, "Learning must be greater than the rate of change" or obsolescence, decay, and death will occur for an organization.[81] This concept is evidenced by a significant proportion of the Fortune 500 falling out of the list by thinking they had "arrived" and that what got them there would keep them there. In the private sector, Level 5 leadership is associated with company success. In this model of leadership, the leader possesses a paradoxical combination of humility and persistent focus on high standards and quality execution in order to reach its lofty goals.[10] In the social sector, leadership is, at its best, a social process in which leadership can be exercised at any level and involves providing direction, gaining alignment, and receiving commitment from followers.[82] When leaders and managers are mutually respected, interdependent partners, public health can better achieve its vision, which is the desired end of leadership.

Special Areas of Concern for Public Health Leaders: Emotional Intelligence and Cultural Competence

Emotional Intelligence

Public health leaders cry, "we must assure those conditions in which people can be healthy," in order to achieve *healthy people in healthy communities*—a mission and vision that uniquely situates them between science and the complexities of people, politics, and economic realities. For public health leaders, intelligence and leadership do not equate. More is required— significantly more. Public health as a field is cast against a background of unending, complex needs coupled with limited resources in a multicultural context that is impacted by events in the political arena. Intellect is an asset, but it is only one of many factors of success for public health leaders. Perhaps there is no field in which emotional intelligence is more critical than in public health. While intellectual ability is a necessity, research has found that across fields only 6% of career success can be attributed to intelligence quotient (IQ), while between 27% and 45% can be attributed to what is colloquially referred to as "EQ," for emotional quotient.[83] As a differentiated construct, the term **emotional intelligence (EI)** is comprised of the personal-emotional-social components of general intelligence.[45,84–86] EQ tends to be used more often when referring to measurement of EI, such as with a variety of psychological assessment instruments (see Table 12.4 later in this chapter).[47,48,84–89]

While the great recession of the new millennium thrust the challenges of budgetary constraints and shrinking staff resources more heavily to the fore than in the decades preceding, it only increased the interpersonal challenges that arise requiring soft skills—the misunderstandings of either word or intent, the inability of some to grasp the impact of their actions on others, the disillusionment and low morale of overly stressed employees, and the hurdles created by organizational culture issues. Across health fields, it is these challenges that leaders find the most time and resource consuming.[48,90–93]

Emotional intelligence is a must because leaders set the EI culture of their organizations.[94] This culture directly impacts staff morale,[91] turnover,[92,95] relationships with colleagues,[91,93,96–99] and ultimately patient relationships as well.[99–101] Organizational culture guru Edgar Schein notes that the primary duty of a leader is to create the culture of the organization.[94] Clearly EI is a foundational skill that is a prerequisite for good leadership in public health situations.[102–104]

Personal competence is the foundation of emotional intelligence, and is comprised of self-awareness and self-management. Social competence is the "other half" of EI, and grows out of a solid foundation in Personal Competence. It is comprised of social awareness and relationship management.[28,45,46,48,105] These types of skills are essential when understanding, engaging, and motivating a team come into play, and when transforming conflict into constructive dialogue is a necessity. Smoothly managing complexity in all its forms is one of the benefits of highly developed emotional intelligence. Unlike IQ, which is thought to remain fairly stable over the course of a life, EQ is thought to improve with development.[28, 45,46,105]

Emotional intelligence broadly translates into skills in self-perception, self-expression, stress management, decision making, social awareness, interpersonal relationships, and relationship management.[83–85,89,106] These are commonly seen as one's ability to conduct constructive interpersonal interactions, communicate, and maintain professionalism even under stress.[96–98] They also relate to being able to understand the emotions of others and to help them constructively harness them in professional settings.[107] In looking back at Table 12.1, you might notice that the GLOBE study's list of universally esteemed leadership attributes bear some similarities to those identified by EI research as foundational to leading in an emotionally intelligent fashion. Training public health leaders to develop these skills generally involves a combination of assessment tools to provide valid and reliable objective feedback (both self-assessment and 360-degree assessments are available) coupled with interpersonal skills–based training in managing difficult conversations.[108,109] At times, physical skills training—such as in mind–body techniques that promote calmness, objectivity, and the ability to listen "with the intensity usually reserved for speaking"—can also provide some foundational skills in this area. It is vital that any leadership development program or individual development activities in which public health leaders engage are founded on a core of emotional intelligence skills, principles, and practices.

Cultural Competence and the Public Health Leader

Increasingly, public health professionals must operate as boundary-spanning ambassadors, reaching out to those from other groups and sectors to help them understand the importance and interconnectedness of public health. In order to serve in this role effectively, public health leaders must be culturally competent—in multiple ways. The field of public health has gone to great lengths to promote **cultural competence** in terms of improving the health of people from a variety of racial backgrounds, ethnicities, and religions and to eliminate health disparities. These are highly important foci of work, but public health leaders must also think of how to communicate with those from a variety of economic and educational backgrounds in addition those from cultures rooted in other global communities.

This global aspect of public health leadership becomes important as international travel and relocation become more commonplace and communication becomes a more pervasive factor influencing political movements, economic opportunity, and health choices. In effect, public health leaders operate in a world that is growing ever smaller. Thus, even leaders in smaller communities might face the same challenges as their counterparts in large cities or on the other side of the globe—from bedbugs to the global spread of H1N1 influenza, from SARS and HIV to the international marketing of tobacco and higher fat foods, all of which have made solving public health issues a global enterprise. Public health leaders must convene and direct virtual teams as they become more frequently used—many being global and multicultural in nature. These issues in public health are now commonplace and present complex leadership challenges to the health leader in communities large and small, who must be cross-culturally intelligent in making decisions, motivating workers, and leading.

Culture is crucial for a public health leader to address, because it exerts a significant influence on health-seeking behaviors, attitudes, diet, choice of healthcare resource (e.g., modern, traditional, self-treatment, no treatment), and so on. But it also exerts an influence on work performance behaviors, which directly impact the efforts of the enterprise to influence community health status. In addition, there is a culture of the workplace that public health leaders are responsible for, and this culture, too, impacts the organizations' ability to achieve its mission. **Organizational culture** impacts employee engagement, which in turn impacts worker commitment and productivity.[57,58,110] In order to impact community health, public health leaders must focus on cultures, communication, and health behaviors. But in leading an enterprise or managing an office, a leader must think about organizational culture. Indeed, with culture operating at global, national, state, local, organizational, team, and family levels, the job of the public health leader becomes quite complex.

There is synergy here with Heifetz's theory of adaptive leadership.[69,70,111] What a public health leader needs to understand is that changing an organizational culture, just like the culture of any community, is a slow process. Community members fear many aspects of change:

In organizations people resist change because of fear of loss of competency, because of their ingrained habitual ways of doing things, and out of a feeling of disloyalty to those who created the current culture. Leading a successful organizational culture change requires clear and often repeated statements of the vision, helping team members understand their role in the organization, training them in the appropriate and expected behaviors, holding them accountable for performance using these new behaviors, and rewarding success.[55]

Thinking from a global perspective, the culture of organizations within a region is greatly affected by the context in which it operates and from which it draws its workers—the local and national culture. The focus on cultural competence in public health outreach programs can help a leader think about how to impact the organizational culture of the workplace. Gardenswartz and Rowe[112] present a model of how this personal sense of culture comes to interface with the organizational sense of culture: where the public health leaders' worlds of cultural competence collide, as it were. Their four-layer model of diversity starts with a core layer of personality factors, which relate to individual style and characteristics. Indeed, every leadership development program should have a strong foundation in understanding human personality, motivation, and communication styles. These can be taught particularly well when grounded in psychological assessment tools that are debriefed not only for personal understanding, but debriefed to improve understanding of others, to improve communication strategies, and to strengthen personal flexibility.

Gardenswartz and Rowe's[112] next layer out presents internal dimensions, which are aspects of the individual that are relatively unchangeable (e.g., age, gender, race, sexual orientation, ethnicity, physical abilities). The third layer presents external dimensions, over which an individual has some choice or influence (e.g., work experience, marital status, education, religion, income). The final and most outer layers are the organizational dimensions, which are defined by work-based factors such as field and work content, union status, management status, work location, seniority, and so on. In leading the enterprise, a public health leader must work at this outer layer and yet take all the inner layers that influence and flavor that outer layer into account.

Each of these four levels represents areas of focus for cultural competence skills, since the public health workforce can be valued or devalued, respected or disrespected, engaged or alienated at any of these levels. Moodian asserts that all of these dimensions represent areas that offer similarities and common ground as well as differences which, when managed well, "have the potential to bring new perspectives, ideas and viewpoints needed by the organization. However, if mismanaged, they can sow the seeds of conflict and misunderstanding that sabotage teamwork and productivity and hinder effectiveness."[113, p. 36]

According to the National Center for Cultural Competence,[114] there are five essential elements that contribute to an individual's, institution's, or agency's ability to become more culturally competent (see **Table 12.3**). Based in gaining awareness and knowledge, a public health leader would subsequently need to take appropriate actions to improve the cultural competency and cultural elasticity of the organization. Public health leaders can focus on these five elements in policy making, administration, and practice as well as in the attitudes, structures, policies, and services of the organization.

Table 12.3   The Five Essential Elements of Cultural Competence

1. Valuing diversity
2. Having the capacity for cultural self-assessment
3. Being conscious of the dynamics inherent when cultures interact
4. Having institutionalized culture knowledge
5. Having developed adaptations to service delivery reflecting an understanding of cultural diversity

Source: National Center for Cultural Competence, Cultural and Linguistic Competence: Rationale, Conceptual Frameworks, and Values. Available at: http://www.nccccurricula.info/framework/B3.html. Accessed March 1, 2013.

The previously mentioned GLOBE project clearly identified differences in preferences of leadership style for potential international leaders and provides clear direction in terms of improving communication skills for effective cross-cultural leadership.

Cultural competence is an essential skill for public health leaders—on many levels. Of all the leadership skills, it is likely the most complex and relies most heavily upon mastery of many other challenging leadership skills. Earley, Ang, and Tan[107] refer to the term "CQ," for cultural intelligence, which forms the critical third intelligence needed by effective leaders in addition to IQ and EQ.

Measuring Leadership Growth and Development

One question most good leaders ask is, "How am I doing as a leader?" In order to address this question, it is important to understand how leadership is measured. Due to the influence of situational factors, the progressive and repetitive nature of learning, and the time it takes to move from a theory one espouses to a theory one puts into use, it can be difficult to assess how far one's leadership ability has come. Several psychological assessment instruments can help with leadership development and self-insight. The primary focus of these tools is to help the leader understand him- or herself better, to promote self-reflection, and to apply knowledge about him- or herself and others into leadership practice. The goals of development using such instruments are: to help the individual appreciate the contributions of others; to understand effective communication styles with a variety of people; to gain insight into creating and sustaining an organizational culture that allows for normal differences in perspectives, types, and temperaments; to motivate and empower him- or herself and others; and to understand how his or her own behavior can be interpreted or "read" by others in organizations.

It is estimated that at any given time about 2,300 leadership assessment instruments are available, yet only 3–5% of these have scientific validity or reliability testing to support them.[86] While instruments that do not have scientific rigor might help start an interesting conversation about leadership, there is a distressing tendency for individuals to self-label after receiving instrument feedback, thus such nonscientifically grounded instruments should be used with extreme caution. **Table 12.4** lists a sample of scientifically sound leadership instruments and

Table 12.4   Leadership Assessment Instruments and Applications

Instrument	Instrument Focus	Areas of Application
360 Instruments		
A variety of instruments exist that examine skill sets by industry, level of seniority, etc. *Example*: A public health–specific 360 is available from Discovery Learning (available from https://www.discoverylearning.com/c-7-360-leadership-assessments.aspx) *Example*: MBTI 360 and VOICES The VOICES instrument is fully customizable (available from http://leadership-systems.com/assessments.aspx) *Example*: LPI (available from http://www.pfeiffer.com/WileyCDA/Section/id-811878.html) *Example*: EQ-i 2.0 (available from http://ei.mhs.com/)	Provide feedback on a specific set of organizationally desirable behaviors from boss, superiors, peers, direct reports	Provide a "snapshot" of leadership performance along many domains
360 Instruments		
Example: The Kaplan Leadership Versatility Index 360 assesses the capacity to strike balances across the opposite types of leadership (available from http://www.kaplandevries.com/whatwedo/3/C26/21/)	Provide feedback on specific domains of skill from boss/superiors and peers	Balance in skills and assessment of over-leveraging of skills in areas of natural tension (e.g., forceful and enabling leadership)
Personality Inventories		
Example: Myers-Briggs Type Indicator (MBTI) (available from Consulting Psychologists Press at https://www.cpp.com/products/mbti/index.aspx or via https://www.skillsone.com/contents/mbti/mbti.aspx)	Personality type preferences for interacting with others, gathering information, evaluating information, and lifestyle choices	Organizational culture, understanding others, communication, building effective teams
Behavior Inventories		
Example: Fundamental Interpersonal Relationships Orientation-Behavior (FIRO-B) (available from Consulting Psychologists Press at https://www.cpp.com/products/firo-b/index.aspx or via https://www.skillsone.com/Contents/firo-b/firo-b.aspx)	How behaviors are read by others in organizations	Communication, leading others, motivating others
Example: California Psychological Inventory 260 (CPI 260) (available from Consulting Psychologists Press at https://www.cpp.com/products/cpi/index.aspx or via https://www.skillsone.com/contents/cpi260/cpi260.aspx)	Benchmarks 26 behavior sets against "ordinary people"	Leading others, gaining insight into how one's behaviors are similar to or different from others
Example: CPI 260 Coaching Report for Leaders (available from Consulting Psychologists Press at https://www.cpp.com/en/cpiproducts.aspx?pc=66 or via https://www.skillsone.com/contents/cpi260/cpi260.aspx)	Benchmarks 20 behavior sets against those of senior leaders and managers	Leading others, gaining insight into how one's behaviors are similar to or different from other successful leaders

Table 12.4   Leadership Assessment Instruments and Applications (continued)

Instrument	Instrument Focus	Areas of Application
Example: Dominance, Influence, Steadiness, Compliance (DiSC) (available from http://www.discprofile.com/)	Examines behaviors and emotions relevant to interacting and working with others	Communication, gaining commitment, building effective teams, resolving/preventing conflict, gaining credibility or influence
Example: Leadership Practices Inventory (LPI) Available as self-assessment and also with other-observer assessments (available from http://www.pfeiffer.com/WileyCDA/Section/id-811878.html)	Gathers self-assessment data on five behaviors: modeling the way, inspiring a shared vision, challenging the process, enabling others to act, encouraging the heart	Understanding how one engages (or how others sees one engage) in leadership practices that impact the organizational climate
Change Inventories *Example*: Change Style Indicator (available from http://www.discoverylearning.com/p-1-change-style-indicator.aspx)	Approach to change: originator, pragmatist, or conserver	Dealing with change, understanding how others approach change, communication around change, adapting to situational change, selling change to stakeholders
Emotional Intelligence *Examples*: Bar-On EQi, EQ-i 2.0, and the Mayer-Salovey-Caruso Emotional Intelligence Test (MSCEIT) *Example*: EQ-i 2.0 (all available from http://ei.mhs.com/)	Ability to solve emotional problems and perform tasks either by subjective assessment of perceived emotional skills or by ability-based skill measures	Dealing with people skills, soft skills, and areas that require "noncognitive" intelligence; communicating with others, creating organizational culture, motivating others
Creativity/Innovation Tools *Example*: FourSight (available from http://www.FourSightOnline.com)	Help individuals and teams better understand how they approach solving problems through creative thinking (through clarifying, generating ideas, developing solutions, or implementing plans)	Creativity, innovation, team building, communication
Conflict Tools *Example*: Thomas-Kilman Conflict Mode Instrument (available from https://www.skillsone.com/contents/tki/tki.aspx)	Methods of dealing with conflict, including competing, collaborating, compromising, avoiding, and accommodating	Dealing with conflict, anger, and relating to others

the topic areas for which they may be useful. This is not a comprehensive list of the 140 or so quality instruments available, but it does survey some of those most respected and broadly used. Certification programs are available for many of these assessment tools, most requiring a 4-year degree as a prerequisite for entering the training program.

It is vital to note that **leadership assessment instruments** are designed to inform the learner about his or her style, behaviors, perspective, biases, and beliefs in relation to the larger, outside world. These instruments should be administered and debriefed (counseled) by a professional with the appropriate background, usually certification in the instrument. Instruments are not intended to be used for decisions about hiring (selection), workload assignment, or downsizing, as they are generally not skill-based inventories. Since many of these are self-report instruments, it is essential that the individuals completing them understand that they are: 1) confidential between the coach/counselor and themselves; 2) for their personal use, insight, and leadership development; 3) are not intelligence tests; and 4) are not skill-based assessments and thus have no right or wrong answers. Leadership instruments help individuals objectively view and understand the impact of their behavior on others, both positively and negatively. Thus, they help individuals to make informed choices about how they interact with others.

These psychological assessment instruments are not designed to be implemented in a test–retest fashion, as if to imply that a different score would be more desirable. Statistical test–retest validation studies actually examine the stability of the instrument. Furthermore, the importance of context cannot be overemphasized. Context is one of the primary tasks of the coach to explore during the debriefing process. When objectives such as a "higher score" are a part of the assessment, the quality and truthfulness of the answers must be called into question. For example, if a job candidate who completes the Myers-Briggs Type Indicator (MBTI) believes that someone with an extraverted personality is desired for the position, she might answer falsely in order to appear as a stronger candidate for the position, rather than for what is her true preference. Continuing with this example, applying leadership assessment tools to hiring decisions also inaccurately implies that someone who prefers an introverted style could not execute the job equally well as someone with an extraverted personality preference. There is no relationship between scores on an instrument like the MBTI, FIRO-B, CSI, TKI, or FourSight and skills at implementing tasks commonly associated with the preferences. These tests do not measure skills—they measure preference. There are other skills-based inventories which do measure intelligence, mathematical ability, and logical deductive reasoning, for example. While these may be used in hiring decisions,[115] they are not used in leadership development and are not addressed here. Similarly, most of the assessment tools discussed in Table 12.4 are not intended for use in selection or promotion systems. In most cases to use them as such is not legally defensible.

The cornerstone instrument for many programs is a 360 feedback instrument. These tools provide a snapshot of current leadership performance as assessed in the individual's current work environment by his or her direct reports, peers, and superiors (some versions of these instruments are "180s" and do not include feedback from direct reports). It is quite insightful for leaders to have 360 feedback as they consider the information from other leadership instruments which may be used. While psychological assessment instruments have some limitations, participants generally find them invaluable as part of their leadership development, particularly when between three and seven instruments are used over a period of time (i.e., 1 year) and the participant is able to work confidentially with a coach to examine the threads or themes in the feedback given. It is often helpful to administer/debrief no more than three instruments in one leadership session (for example during a week-long leadership retreat) and to allow for many months of ongoing consideration and reflection as part of a leadership development program. For all instruments, the coach and the leader should discuss how the insights and items assessed play out in the leader's day-to-day leadership experience.

While it might seem tempting to readminister a 360 assessment to measure leadership growth, research has shown quite disappointing results due to response shift bias.[116] Education on any topic typically results in one having a far greater appreciation of their previous ignorance on a topic, and leadership is no different. The same holds true for external observers: Repeatedly asking a stakeholder to rate performance results in lower ratings over time, primarily because of their increased attention on the attribute—regardless of the actual changes in performance on the candidate's part. Furthermore, these assessments are time consuming for organizations, which can also impact the quality of the feedback when used sequentially. When outcomes are used to reward, penalize, or judge, it is doubtful the leader will be able to complete the instruments with the openness and honesty required for them to serve a useful purpose. Finally, it is inappropriate to use leadership assessment instruments other than how they were designed, since the statistical and validity measures that support them do not apply outside of the design parameters.

Mentoring: A Vital Aspect of Leadership Development

Many successful leaders cite having a mentor as crucial to their leadership development and career progression. A mentoring relationship is usually one in which the mentor instructs, shares his or her perspective and experience, and gives advice to the mentee. By providing another perspective, mentors can elucidate issues that their mentees do not grasp and clarify organizational culture—in short, they identify and open doors that mentees do not even know exist. These relationships are often characterized by a deep level of respect and personal regard. The mentor has an investment in developing the career of the mentee, and thus strives to make opportunities happen for the mentee, by providing introductions and giving "off the record" advice on complex situations. This relationship is considered private and the items discussed are to be held in confidence. Mentoring is completely different from coaching in that it would be inappropriate for a mentor to advise on interpretation of leadership assessment tools, for example.

One of the challenges to mentoring is that few people have had training in how to be a good mentor. The time commitment can be unclear, as can be the goals and objectives. When asked to serve as a mentor, individuals should carefully consider whether they want to mentor the requestor and whether they have the time to devote to this relationship. Often mentors meet with mentees once a month or sometimes once a quarter. Meeting less frequently, at least initially, probably renders the relationship meaningless. These meetings are often face-to-face but phone- or email-based relationships can also be productive. All mentors should have a clear idea of what the mentee hopes to gain from this relationship and what their expectations are. Since this is a highly rewarding and personal relationship that often involves sharing ideas, perspectives, and experiences with another, more junior, person, it is understandable that when asked one would want to choose a mentee carefully, and choose someone who is both respected and trusted. It is appropriate for potential mentors to decline the invitation if they feel the personal chemistry is not right or if the trust is insufficient. Mentors should not be the "sole source" for leadership development for their mentees. The mentor can encourage mentees to read books and articles, engage in leadership development experiences, or undertake stretch assignments. The role of a mentor is to give advice and perspective. Mentors often make connections and opportunities happen for their mentees, as they nurture their careers. Mentoring can be successful between two individuals when one formally reports to the other in an organization, between individuals from separate departments or different organizations, or between individuals from different locations—perhaps across the country.

Mentees have more clearly defined responsibilities in this relationship. It is up to the mentee to manage and nurture this connection, setting initial expectations when the request is made. Mentees should ask for the frequency of meeting schedule, type of meetings, and have questions or topics prepared when they meet with their mentors. If they are engaged in a formal leadership development program, such as a leadership institute, they should inform their mentor of those experiences. Always, mentees should be sensitive to the mentor's time, and similarly they should always thank the mentor, usually formally for their time and wisdom. Absolutely, confidences should be respected between mentors and mentees.

Future Outlook

For many years, the subject of leadership and management has been discussed and debated and that dialogue will undoubtedly continue for years to come. Many questions will be asked during these discussions, but the most important one is how the individual, the organization, and the community answer the call to leadership. Leaders can choose to renege and play it safe, or select the option of taking a risk and living dangerously by entering the heated, reforming crucible of leadership development. If they become students of leadership, they will not be preoccupied with whether they were "born a leader." They will be continually working to learn more about themselves and others, studying the essential skills of leadership and management, experiencing how to lead—even without authority, utilizing adaptive leadership, increasing their emotional intelligence, assessing their leadership growth, inviting feedback and reflecting upon it, maintaining resilience in the face of criticism, and growing.

Most importantly, while leaders will know that leadership cannot be taught, they will be certain that leadership can be learned and that learning can be facilitated by reflection, conscious goal setting, emphasizing soft skills, practice, assessment, challenge, and support. They will be asking the questions, "How can I learn more?" and "What does this mean?", as they first develop their own individual leadership skills. Then they will begin to facilitate community social leadership, thereby increasing human capital and social capital—leading to improved health status.

Great leaders will know to push the field forward by advancing technical skills, but will not assume that those necessary tools will be sufficient to meet their needs—or anyone else's. They will constantly work to hone the skills that foster their abilities to serve as boundary-spanning leaders, and reach out in order to build bridges to connect others from disciplines, organizations, and communities different from their own. The field of public health is full of diversity and requires great leadership to create the coalitions that will help solve the pressing public health issues facing the world today. Great public health leaders will walk a divergent path from many others in that they will seek to blend the benefits of many abilities as they work to serve the greater good.

Discussion Questions

1. What is leadership? Does it differ from management? If so, how?
2. Identify and discuss two leadership theories. Which makes the most sense to you? Why?
3. What are the unique challenges leaders in public health face?
4. Describe the knowledge, skills, and abilities that might be employed by public health leaders.
5. Identify two public health leaders, from history or the present, and describe them. What were their accomplishments?
6. Interview a public health leader or ask them to come speak to your class. Find out what it is like to "walk in their shoes" on a daily basis.

References

1. Halverson PK, Mays GP, Kaluzny AD, et al. Developing leaders in public health: the role of executive training programs. *J Health Adm Educ.* 1997;15(2):82–100.
2. Maternal and Child Health, Public Health Leadership Institute. What is MCH-PHLI? Available at: http://www.mchphli.org. Accessed March 1, 2013.
3. Maternal and Child Health Bureau. Maternal and Child Health Bureau strategic plan: FY 2003–2007. Available at: http://mchb.hrsa.gov/about/strategicplanfy200307.pdf. Accessed March 1, 2013.
4. Health Resources and Services Administration. Maternal and Child Health Training Program. Available at: http://mchb.hrsa.gov/training/. Accessed March 1, 2013.
5. Health Resources and Services Administration. MCH Training Program: Strategic plan. Available at: http://mchb.hrsa.gov/training/strategic_plan.asp. Accessed March 1, 2013.
6. MCH Training Program. National MCH Training Plan 2012–2020 Working Draft (6/14/12). Available at: http://www.aucd.org/docs/lend/2012_0614_mch_str_plan_draft4.pdf. Accessed March 1, 2013.
7. Dodds J, Vann W, Lee J, et al. The UNC-CH MCH Leadership Training Consortium: building the capacity to develop interdisciplinary MCH leaders. *Matern Child Health J.* 2012;14(4):642–8.
8. Center for Creative Leadership. *Addressing the leadership gap in healthcare. What's needed when it comes to leader talent? A white paper.* Available at: http://www.ccl.org/leadership/pdf/research/addressing leadershipGapHealthcare.pdf. Accessed March 1, 2013.
9. Collins, J. *Good to Great: Why Some Companies Make the Leap...and Others Don't.* New York: HarperBusiness; 2001.
10. Collins J. *Good to Great and the Social Sectors: A Monograph to Accompany Good to Great.* New York: HarperBusiness; 2005.

11. Health Resources and Services Administration. MCH Programs Overview. Available at: http://mchb .hrsa.gov/programs/. Accessed March 1, 2013.

12. Einstein A. *Ideas and Opinions*. New York: Crown Publishers; 1954:62.

13. Drath WH. Approaching the future of leadership development. In: McCauley CD, Moxley RS, Van Velsor E, eds. *The Center for Creative Leadership Handbook of Leadership Development*. San Francisco: Jossey-Bass; 1998:262–88.

14. Liange AP, Renard PG, Robinson C, et al. Survey of leadership skills needed for state and territorial health officers, United States, 1988. *Public Health Rep*. 1993;108(1):116–20.

15. O'Neil EH, Pew Health Professions Commission. *Recreating health professional practice for a new century. The fourth report for the Pew Health Professions Commission*. San Francisco: Pew Health Professions Commission; 1998.

16. Institute of Medicine. *The Future of Public Health*. Washington, DC: National Academies Press; 1988.

17. Roper WL, Baker EL, Dyal WW, et al. Strengthening the public health system. *Public Health Rep*. 1992;107(6):609–15.

18. National Public Health Leadership Institute. About PHLI. Available at: http://www.phli.org/about/ index.htm. Accessed March 1, 2013.

19. Baker E. Public health leadership after September 11th. *Leadership in Public Health*. 2004;6(4):9–12.

20. Marcus L, Ashkenazi I, Dorn B, et al. Meta-leadership: expanding the scope and scale of public health. *Leadership in Public Health*. 2008;8(1–2):31–7.

21. Institute of Medicine. *Who Will Keep the Public Healthy? Educating Public Health Professionals for the 21st Century*. Washington, DC: National Academies Press; 2002.

22. Institute of Medicine. *The Future of the Public's Health in the 21st Century*, Washington, DC: National Academies Press; 2002.

23. Umble K, Steffen D, Porter J, et al. The national public health leadership institute: evaluation of a team-based approach to developing collaborative public health leaders. *Am J Public Health*. 2005;95:641–4.

24. Trevino F, Mains D, Gonzalez A, et al. Comparison of public health leadership institutes in the United States: a descriptive study. *Leadership in Public Health*. 2004;6:(4):37–50.

25. Mouradian W, Huebner C. Further directions in leadership training of MCH professionals: cross-cutting MCH leadership competencies. *Matern Child Health J*. 2007;11:211–8.

26. MCH Leadership Competencies. MCH Leadership Competencies. Available at: http://leadership .mchtraining.net/. Accessed March 1, 2013.

27. Institute of Medicine. Roundtable on Value & Science-Driven Health Care. Available at: http://www .iom.edu/Activities/Quality/VSRT.aspx. Accessed March 1, 2013.

28. Zaleznik A. Managers and leaders: are they different? *Harvard Bus Rev*. 2004;82(1):74–81.

29. Pointer DD, Sanchez JP. Leadership: a framework for thinking and acting. In: Shortell SMK, Arnold D, eds. *Health Care Management: Organization Design and Behavior*. 4th ed. Albany, NY: Delmar, Thompson Learning; 2000:106–29.

30. Goleman D. Leadership that gets results. *Harvard Bus Rev*. 2000;March-April:78–90.

31. Bennis W. The challenges of leadership in the modern world. *Am Psychol*. 2007;62(1):2–5.

32. Bowditch JL, Buono AF. *A Primer on Organizational Behavior*. 4th ed. New York: John Wiley & Sons; 1997.

33. Lord RG. An information processing approach to social perceptions, leadership and behavioral measurement in organizations. In: Cummings LL, Staw BM, eds. *Research in Organizational Behavior*. Greenwich, CT: JAI Press; 1985.

34. Kouzes JM, Posner BZ. *The Leadership Challenge: How to Get Extraordinary Things Done in Organizations*. San Francisco: Jossey-Bass; 1988.

35. Kouzes JM, Posner BZ. *The Team Leadership Practices Inventory (TEAM LP): Measuring Leadership of Teams, Participant's Workbook*. San Francisco: Jossey-Bass Pfeiffer; 1995.

36. Van Vleet DD, Yukl GA. A century of leadership research. In: Rosenbach WE, Taylor RL, eds. *Contemporary Issues in Leadership*. Boulder, CO: Westview Press; 1989:65–90.

37. Kouzes JM, Posner BZ. *The Leadership Challenge: How to Make Extraordinary Things Happen in Organizations*. San Francisco: Jossey-Bass Pfeiffer; 2012.

38. Tichy NM, Cohen E. *The Leadership Engine: How Winning Companies Build Leaders at Every Level*. New York: HarperBusiness; 1997.

39. Tichy NM, Devanna MA. The transformational leader. *Train Dev J*. 1986;July(a):27–32.

40. Hersey P, Blanchard KH, Johnson DE. *Management of Organizational Behavior: Utilizing Human Resources*. 7th ed. Upper Saddle River, NJ: Prentice-Hall; 1996.

41. Hersey P, Blanchard KH. *Management of Organizational Behavior: Utilizing Human Resources*. Englewood Cliffs, NJ: Prentice-Hall; 1977.

42. Hersey P, Blanchard KH. *The Management of Organizational Behavior*. 2nd ed. Englewood Cliffs, NJ: Prentice-Hall; 1984.

43. Argyris C. Teaching smart people how to learn. *Harvard Bus Rev*. 1991;May–June:99–102.

44. Blanchard K. *Situational Leadership: The Article*. Escondido, CA: The Ken Blanchard Companies; 1994.

45. Goleman D. *Emotional Intelligence: Why It Can Matter More Than IQ*. New York: Bantam Dell; 1996.

46. Goleman D, Boyatzis R, McKee A. Primal leadership: the hidden driver of great performance. *Harvard Bus Rev*. 2001;December:42–51.

47. Fernandez CSP. Emotional intelligence in the workplace. *J Public Health Manag Pract*. 2007;13(1): 80 –2.

48. Fernandez CSP, Peterson HB, Holmström SW, et al. Developing emotional intelligence for health care leaders. In: Di Fabio A, ed. *Emotional Intelligence—New Perspectives and Applications*. New York: InTech; 2012:239–60.

49. Freshman B, Rubino L. Emotional intelligence: a core competency for health care administrators. *Health Care Manag*. 2002;20:1–9.

50. Burns JM. *Leadership*. New York: Harper & Row; 1978.

51. Bennis WG, Nanus B. *Leaders: The Strategies for Taking Charge*. New York: Harper & Row; 1985.

52. Senge PM. *The Fifth Discipline*. New York: Doubleday; 1990.

53. Senge PM, Ross R, Smith B, et al. *The Fifth Discipline Fieldbook—Strategies and Tools for Building a Learning Organization*. New York: Doubleday; 1994.

54. Kotter JP. What leaders really do. *Harvard Bus Rev*. 1990:43–50.

55. Kotter JP. Leading change: why transformation efforts fail. *Harvard Bus Rev*. 1995;March–April:59–67.

56. Greenleaf Center for Servant Leadership. What is Servant Leadership? Available at: https://www.greenleaf.org/what-is-servant-leadership/. Accessed March 1, 2013.

57. EEngagement. Towers Perrin: Employee Engagement/Global Workforce Study. Available at: http://employeeengagement.com/2011/09/towers-perrin-employee-engagement/. Accessed March 1, 2013.

58. BlessingWhite. *Employee Engagement Report: Beyond the Numbers: A Practical Approach for Individuals, Managers and Executives*. Available at: http://www.blessingwhite.com/eee__report.asp. Accessed March 1, 2013.

59. House RJ, Hanges PJ, Javidian M, et al. eds. *Culture, Leadership, and Organizations: The GLOBE Study of 62 Societies*. Thousand Oaks, CA: Sage; 2004.

60. Bossidy L, Charan R, Burck C. *Execution: the discipline of getting things done*. New York: Crown Publishing; 2002.

61. Pfeffer, J, Sutton RI. *The Knowing-Doing Gap: How Smart Companies Turn Knowledge into Action*. Cambridge, MA: Harvard Business School; 2000.

62. Yukl G, Lepsinger R. Why integrating the leading and managing roles is essential for organizational effectiveness. *Org Dynamics*. 2003;34(4):361–75.

63. Buckingham M, Coffman C. *First Break All the Rules: What the World's Greatest Managers Do Differently*. New York: Simon and Schuster; 1999.

64. Lu MC, Halfon N. Racial and ethnic disparities in birth outcomes: a life-course perspective. *Matern Child Health J*. 2003;7(1):13–30.

65. McAuley CD, Martineau JW. *Reaching Your Development Goals*. Greensboro, NC: The Center for Creative Leadership; 1998.

66. Bennis, W. The challenges of leadership in the modern world. *Am Psychol*. 2007;62(1):2–5.

67. Booth C, Segon M. A leadership and management practice development model. *Int Rev Bus Res Papers*. 2009;5(2):19–41.

68. McGonagill G, Reinelt C. Leadership development in the social sector: a framework for supporting strategic investments. *Foundation rev.* 2011;2(4):57–72.

69. Heifetz R. *Leadership Without Easy Answers.* Cambridge, MA: Harvard University Press; 1994.

70. Heifetz R, Linsky M, Grashow A. *The Practice of Adaptive Leadership: Tools and Tactics for Changing Your Organization and the World.* Cambridge, MA: Harvard Business Press; 2009.

71. Martin A. *The Changing Nature of Leadership: A CCL White Paper.* Greensboro, NC: The Center for Creative Leadership; 2007.

72. Ospina S, Foldy E. Building bridges from the margins: the work of leadership in social change organizations. *The Lead Quarterly.* 2010;21:292–7.

73. Koo D, Miner K. Outcome-based workforce development and education in public health. *Annu Rev Public Health.* 2010;31:253–69.

74. Public Health Foundation. Council on Linkages Between Academia and Public Health Practice. Available at: http://www.phf.org/programs/council/Pages/default.aspx/index.htm. Accessed March 1, 2013.

75. Centers for Disease Control and Prevention, National Public Health Performance Standards Program. 10 Essential Public Health Services. Available at: http://www.cdc.gov/nphpsp/essentialservices.html. Accessed March 1, 2013.

76. National Public Health Leadership Development Network. Public Health Leadership Competency Framework. Available at: http://www.heartlandcenters.slu.edu/nln/about/framework.pdf. Accessed March 1, 2013.

77. Association of Schools of Public Health. Public Health and Crisis Leadership Competency Framework. Available at: http://www.asph.org/userfiles/Competencies-Resources/22_CL-CompsFrame.doc. Accessed March 1, 2013.

78. Association of Schools of Public Health. MPH Core Competency Model. Available at: http://www.asph.org/document.cfm?page=851. Accessed March 1, 2013.

79. Antonakis J, Day DV, Schyns B. Leadership and individual differences: at the cusp of a renaissance. *Lead Quarterly.* 2012;23(4):643–50.

80. Thomas R, Jules C, Light DA. Making leadership development stick. *Org Dynamics.* 2012;41:72–7.

81. International Management Centres & Revans University. Career Success Through Action Learning at Work. Available at: http://www.i-m-c.org/resources/download/imc_corporate_brochure.pdf. Accessed March 1, 2013.

82. Meehan D. A New Leadership Mindset for Scaling Social Change. Available at: http://www.leadership foranewera.org/page/A+New+Leadership+Mindset. Accessed March 1, 2013.

83. Stein SJ, Book HE. *The EQ Edge: Emotional Intelligence and Your Success.* 2nd ed. Toronto, Canada: Multi-Health Systems; 2006.

84. Bar-On R. *EQ-I Technical Manual.* Toronto, Canada: Multi-Health Systems; 1997.

85. Bar-On R. *EQ-I Technical Manual.* Toronto, Canada: Multi-Health Systems; 2002.

86. Pearman R. *Emotional Intelligence For Self-Management and Enhanced Performance v 5.2 (Bar-On Emotional Quotient Training Manual).* Winston-Salem, NC: Qualifying.Org; 2003.

87. Ackley, D. *EQ Leader Program Manual.* Toronto, Canada: Multi-Health Systems; 2006.

88. Mayer JD, Salovey P, Caruso DR. *Mayer-Salovey Emotional Intelligence Tests (MSCEIT) User's Manual.* Toronto, Canada: Multi-Health Systems; 2002.

89. Stein SJ. *The Complete EQ-I 2.0 Model (technical manual).* Toronto, Canada: Multi-Health Systems; 2011.

90. Pfifferling JH. Physicians' "disruptive" behavior: consequences for medical quality and safety. *Am J Medical Quality.* 2008;23:165.

91. Freshman B, Rubino L. Emotional intelligence: a core competency for health care administrators. *Health Care Manag.* 2002;20:1–9.

92. Gifford BD, Zammuto RF, Goodman EA. The relationship between the hospital unit culture and nurses' quality of work life. *J Health Care Manag.* 2002;47:13–25.

93. Cummings GC, MacGregor T, Davey M, et al. Leadership styles and outcome patterns for the nursing workforce and work environment: a systematic review. *Int J Nurs Studies.* 2010;47:363–85.

94. Schein EH. *Organizational Culture and Leadership.* San Francisco: Jossey-Bass; 2010.

95. Hill KS. Practitioner Application (organizational culture of nursing units). *J Health Care Manag.* 2002;47:25–6.

96. Porath CL, Pearson CM. The cost of bad behavior. *Org Dynamics.* 2009;39(1):64–71.

97. O'Toole J, Bennis W. What's needed next: a culture of candor. *Harvard Bus Rev.* 2009;June:54–61.

98. Awad SS, Hayley B, Fagan SP, et al. The impact of a novel resident leadership training curriculum. *American J Surg.* 2004;188:481.

99. Mrkonjic L, Grondin SC. Introduction to concepts in leadership for the surgeon. *Thoracic Surg Clin.* 2011;21:323–31.

100. Levinson W, D'Aunno T, Gorawara-Bhat R, et al. (2002). Patient-physician communication as organizational innovation in the managed care setting. *Am J Managed Care.* 2002;8:622–30.

101. Wagner PJ, Moseley GC, Grant MM, et al. Physician's emotional intelligence and patient satisfaction. *Fam Med.* 2002;34(10):759–4.

102. Schwartz RW, Pogge C. Physician leadership: essential skills in a changing environment. *Am J Surg.* 2000;180:187–92.

103. Levinson W, D'Aunno T, Gorawara-Bhat R, et al. (2002). Patient-physician communication as organizational innovation in the managed care setting. *Am J Managed Care.* 2002; 8:622–30.

104. Lattore P, Lumb PD. Professionalism and interpersonal communications: ACGME competencies and core leadership development qualities. Why are they so important and how should they be taught to anesthesiology residents and fellows? *Sem Anesth Periop Med Pain.* 2005;24:134–7.

105. Goleman D, Boyatzis R. Social intelligence and the biology of leadership. *Harvard Bus Rev.* 2008;September:74–81.

106. Bar-On R. The Bar-On model of emotional-social intelligence (ESI). *Psicothema.* 2006;18:13–25.

107. Earley C, Ang S, Tan JS. *Developing Cultural Intelligence at Work.* Stanford, CA: Stanford University Press; 2006.

108. Fernandez CSP. Managing the difficult conversation. In: Baker EL, Menkens AJ, Porter JE. eds., *Managing the Public Health Enterprise.* Sudbury, MA: Jones & Bartlett Learning; 2010:145–50.

109. Patterson K, Grenny J, McMillan R, et al. *Crucial Conversations Tools for Talking When Stakes Are High.* 2nd ed. McGraw-Hill; 2009.

110. Fernandez CSP. Employee engagement. In: Baker EL, Menkens AJ, Porter JE, eds. *Managing the Public Health Enterprise.* Sudbury, MA: Jones & Bartlett Learning; 2010:31–5.

111. Linsky M, Heifetz R. *Leadership on the Line: Staying Alive Through the Danger of Leading.* Cambridge, MA: Harvard Business Press; 2002.

112. Gardenswartz L, Cherbosque J, Rowe A. Emotional intelligence and diversity: a model for differences in the workplace. *J Psychological Iss Org Culture.* 2010;1:1:74–84.

113. Moodian M, ed. *Contemporary Leadership and Intercultural Competence.* Thousand Oaks, CA: Sage; 2009.

114. National Center for Cultural Competence, Cultural and Linguistic Competence: Rationale, Conceptual Frameworks, and Values. Available at: http://www.nccccurricula.info/framework/B3.html. Accessed March 1, 2013.

115. Winsborough D. CEOs aren't like us. Available at: http://www.hoganassessments.com/sites/default/files/CEOs_Arent_Like_Us_R3.pdf. Accessed March 1, 2013.

116. Rohs FJ. Response-shift bias: a problem in evaluating leadership development with self-report pre-test post-test measures. *J Agricult Educ.* 1999;20:4.

Public Health Information Systems and Management

Bernard J. Kerr, Jr., Jean Popiak-Goodwin, and Andrew T. Westrum[*]

LEARNING OBJECTIVES

- To describe the contemporary concepts and applications of health information systems (HISs) and health information management (HIM) in public health
- To define the core concepts of information systems architecture
- To list at least three common databases available for public health
- To summarize the publics' concerns regarding the privacy of personal health information
- To explain and defend the value of data warehousing in public health

---

Chapter Overview

Public health organizations require well-designed information systems in order to make optimal use of the mounting supply of health-related data. Organizations rely on these systems to inform managerial decision making and improve operations in areas such as epidemiologic surveillance, health outcomes assessment, program and clinic administration, program evaluation

---

[*]The authors wish to acknowledge the work of Stephen Parente, James Studnicki, Donald J. Berndt, and John W. Fisher, the authors of the previous versions of this chapter.

and performance measurement, public health planning, and policy analysis. Key design considerations in developing information systems include service-based and population-based application objectives, units of analysis, data sources, data linkage methods, technology selection and integration strategies, and information privacy protections. A growing collection of models and resources now exists for developing effective information systems for public health organizations.

Information systems are an essential public health tool, providing real-time data to guide public health decisions. The escalating importance of **health information systems (HISs)** has three fundamental drivers: 1) the expanding breadth of data available from multiple public and private sources, 2) advances in information technology (IT), and 3) the growing recognition of the power of information management (IM) in public health decision making. Data from public and private health service providers and insurers contain an electronic history of healthcare utilization and costs. Government surveys provide an unprecedented level of detailed information on health status, functional status, medical care use and expenditures, nutrition, sociodemographics, and health behaviors. Analyzing public and private data can then inform decision makers, and the findings can be used to develop strategies and tactics to address public health challenges and opportunities.

HISs support a wide variety of public health system objectives, including the following:

- Epidemiologic disease and risk factor surveillance
- Medical and public health outcomes assessment
- Facility and clinic administration (billing, inventory, clinical records, utilization review)
- Cost-effectiveness and productivity analysis
- Utilization analysis and demand forecasting
- Program planning and evaluation
- Quality assurance and performance measurement
- Policy development, analysis, and revision
- Clinical and managerial research
- Health education and health information dissemination

IT and IM have now advanced to the point that the Medicare program's 2011 claims history— approximately 1.2 billion observations—can be stored, manipulated, and analyzed on a high-end personal computer (PC) workstation. Advances in IT and IM are dramatically influencing public health organizations and their historical roles in collecting and disseminating data and leveraging information as organizational assets. Vital statistics and disease registries—critical functions of public health departments at the local and national levels—are being transformed by IM and an emphasis on evidence-based decision making. Yet, HIS resources remain difficult to develop and manage in addressing current public health challenges. Data sets are located in a disparate array of separate computing platforms with little interconnectivity. For HISs to be effective, the full spectrum of public health personnel must have full access to available data sources, the skills to extract information and formulate decision-support knowledge, and the insights to capitalize on the benefits derived from these systems.

This chapter examines concepts, resources, and examples of HISs for public health organizations. Issues and implications for public health management are explored in the following six areas:

1. Contemporary concepts and applications of HISs in public health
2. Information systems architectures
3. Sources of data for information systems
4. Common databases available for public health
5. HIS applications in public health administration
6. Privacy and security issues

Contemporary Concepts and Applications

What is public health information? A more telling question may be, "What is not public health information?", because the scope of data required to examine and interpret the multiple and overlapping health, social, and environmental factors that affect a population can be enormous. Traditionally, public health or epidemiologic data have consisted of vital statistics, disease registries, and other surveillance-based resources. However, these resources are often limited in scope due in part to the lack of standardization in core data elements.[1] Uniformity among data sets enables trend analysis and forecasting and more precise development of initiatives and performance metrics targeting groups with special needs. Managing limited resources efficiently and effectively at the population level requires comprehensive data resources to predict and measure cost against outcomes relative to policies and interventions.

An examination of public health applications of HISs is facilitated by an understanding of the two most common applications of these systems in practice. First, information systems are used to store and make available service data that reflect activities performed by public health organizations and other health-related entities. Second, information systems store and make available population-based data that are important for surveillance, program evaluation, policy making, and priority setting in public health. These two common applications are not separate; they are synergistic and interact extensively.

For example, routinely collected service data by local public health agencies often include the results of blood lead screening of children under 5 years of age, immunization status, and encounter data recording the results of client visits for tuberculosis (TB) and sexually transmitted diseases (STDs). Other routinely collected service data include records of individual client encounters in the federal Special Supplemental Nutrition Program for Women, Infants, and Children (WIC) and other early intervention programs. These service data are important for the effective management of individual care by public health and ambulatory care providers. Importantly, these data reflect individual transactions and can be used to monitor program performance and to describe a group of users at a particular facility. However, the data cannot be generalized to an entire community or population.

An important practical distinction exists between the service-based application of HISs and the population-based application, which offers information about defined communities and population groups of interest. To support this latter application, information systems must integrate data from major population-wide sources such as vital statistics registries and disease surveillance systems. In some cases, service data may also contribute to population-based information.

For example, the National Notifiable Diseases Surveillance System (NNDSS), formed more than a century ago, serves as a major source of population-wide data. This system captures information on disease incidence for more than 65 diseases for which accurate and timely information is essential to effective prevention and control. The Centers for Disease Control and Prevention (CDC) receives disease reports from the 50 states, two cities (New York City and the District of Columbia), and five territories.[2] The NNDSS database is exceedingly useful to public health agencies because of its ability to enable trend analysis and comparisons of disease incidence between and among communities.

Population-based information systems may also be constructed from service-level data. Immunization registries have been implemented by many state and local public health agencies and provide an excellent example of this use. These registries record immunization status and vaccinations provided to all children residing within a defined geographic area, making this information available not only to the initial provider, but also to other providers, health plans, and schools. Many of these registries incorporate birth certificate data for children born in the community, adding a population denominator. This is an example of an information system that provides service-level information that is helpful to individual providers and their patients, while also providing population-level information that is helpful to public health organizations for surveillance, program evaluation, and policy making. As more records are entered into immunization registries, validity and reliability of the information increases. Forty-nine of 50 states have registries. More than 19,800 records were found for children and adolescents displaced after Hurricane Katrina, saving more than $4.6 million in revaccination expenses.[3]

State-of-the art computing technology has enabled public health organizations to collect health data rapidly and extract meaningful information about community health status.[4] The major challenge is to integrate data sources and develop networks that make this information available to public health organizations at all levels of government as well as to appropriate entities in the private sector. New service-oriented computing architectures are intended to build these types of networked information systems. The current impetus to having a surveillance capability supported by a national network of public health HISs is fueled by concerns about bioterrorism and emerging infectious diseases, resulting in sizeable investments by the CDC for constructing linked information systems.

Major practical goals for the future development of HISs for public health organizations include the following:

- Integrating the multiple data sources available for public health purposes
- Networking information systems to make interaction and information flow between different entities largely seamless
- Using healthcare information systems to produce public health information regarding preventive services, preventable diseases, and quality of care
- Employing geographic information system (GIS) technology to better inform public health planning and investment[5,6]

Integration

Government public health agencies have historically designed computer-based information systems for single programs. For years, the same data were entered and maintained in disparate, often incompatible systems that supported different public health programs.[7] This duplicative and fragmented information infrastructure hindered the ability of public health managers to know what data existed and how to access them. For example, most local public health agencies maintain multiple programs for children, including lead toxicity prevention, immunization, WIC, and early intervention services. Meanwhile, the local departments of social services enroll families in Medicaid. Despite the fact that Medicaid and public health programs serve client populations that overlap substantially in most communities, the databases used to manage these programs are commonly separate. Information systems integration can offer opportunities for improved service delivery and enhanced population-based decision making and management while avoiding costly redundancies.

The ongoing surveillance and community assessment activities that represent core public health functions require HISs to accumulate and integrate data for continuous use via widely available data warehousing technologies. Data warehousing should become a core technology in the public health arena, providing data cubes that can be "sliced and diced," in turn providing meaningful, actionable information. Vital statistics, hospital discharge data, and disease registries can be integrated with demographic and economic data to populate public health data warehouses.

Public health agencies are also beginning to innovate by using unconventional data sources such as market research databases. For example, electronic information compiled from grocery and drug store sales can be used as part of an HIS to identify the purchase of cigarettes concomitantly with products associated with pregnancy or infants, such as diapers. This information by ZIP Code can help target or evaluate public health intervention programs, such as efforts to prevent tobacco use in the perinatal period.

Networks

Another major function of HISs in public health is to create linked networks of information that can strengthen public health operations by: 1) facilitating communication among public health practitioners, 2) enhancing the accessibility of information, and 3) allowing swift and secure exchange of public health data.[8] As a prominent example, the CDC initiated the Public Health Information Network (PHIN) in 2004 (http://www.cdc.gov/phin/). The CDC has been the major supporter of efforts to create networks that link public health information from localities and states with that of federal agencies. Information networks of this type are increasingly indispensable for disease surveillance activities, particularly in cases of local disease outbreaks that have the potential to spread regionally and nationally. In this way, HISs can help to create and sustain effective interorganizational relationships among public health organizations.

An example of health information systems at work is the CDC's Epi-X: The Epidemic Information Exchange (http://www.cdc.gov/epix/), a web-based communication system connecting CDC officials, state and local health departments, poison control centers, and other public health professionals. Designated experts in health care are able to rapidly report food-borne outbreaks involving multiple jurisdictions, investigate travelers with potentially contagious diseases, and share preliminary health surveillance information over a secure data network. From 2000–2012, more than 6,700 reports were posted to this system.[9]

Utilization of Healthcare Delivery Systems

Public health organizations can also benefit from timely access to healthcare services information from providers of personal healthcare services.[8] For example, immunization registries must acquire information on immunization status from multiple community providers who deliver vaccinations. In a growing number of communities, public health organizations are able to obtain relevant and timely information from the systems that are maintained by healthcare delivery organizations. Large delivery systems can offer information on the delivery and utilization of preventive services (including missed opportunities for prevention), the incidence of preventable diagnoses and comorbidities, and the quality of medical facilities and providers (such as medical errors and mortality rates).

These types of resources drive the contemporary development of HISs among public health organizations, and they reflect a basic change of thought regarding the delivery of medical and public health services subsequent to the 1993 federal health reform initiative. This initiative accentuated the need for informed decision making by consumers, providers, employers, and governments. For example, the Clinton administration reform plan relied solely on analyses of the 1987 National Medical Expenditure Survey (NMES) to draw conclusions about the future demand for and cost of health care in the United States. Between the time the NMES was fielded and 1993, the dominance of fee-for-service care gave way to managed care as the primary health-financing mechanism for the private and public insurance markets. As a result, the 1987 NMES could not reliably estimate the impact of the administration's healthcare reform proposal without significant and possibly questionable assumptions. The data limitations increased the administration's interest in an annual survey that could provide better estimates of a rapidly changing market.

In 1996, the Agency for Health Care Policy and Research fielded the Medical Expenditure Panel Survey (MEPS), providing a national annual survey instrument to track changes in healthcare use and cost as well as health status and insurance coverage. A similar demand for information came from employers, who wanted health plans to provide standardized information on the value of their products. The result was a cooperative effort between employers and health insurers though the National Committee for Quality Assurance to develop a common set of health plan performance measures known formally as the Healthcare Effectiveness Data and Information Set (HEDIS). Some of the HEDIS measures were prevention oriented and thus illustrated the principle of obtaining public health information from a healthcare information system.[8] Health plans can compare their performance against other health plans for 76 measures across 8 domains of care. More than 90% of health plans use HEDIS data.[10]

Building new databases for multiple purposes such as MEPS and HEDIS required a clear identification of HIS objectives and knowledge of the strengths and weaknesses of established data structures. This knowledge is essential in determining which structures can be recycled in building a new database, such as using existing health insurer records for HEDIS, and which structures need to be newly constructed, such as designing medical record abstraction protocols for obtaining disease and outcomes data for HEDIS. With appropriate design, medical encounter (service) data can be used for several population-based purposes, including community health assessment, surveillance, and evaluation.

Information Systems Architectures

A common misperception in developing HISs for public health applications is the expectation that such systems are analogous to their counterparts in IT-intensive industries such as banking or manufacturing. Health and health care are a combination of many uncertain inputs. These inputs range from the unique biologic and behavioral characteristics of the individual patient or population under study, to health insurance characteristics and the accessibility of health resources, to the practice styles of physicians and other health professionals, to thousands of possible diagnoses, comorbidities, risk factors, and interventions. In combination, these inputs generate millions of possible outcomes for a given health-related episode. Consequently, the HISs used to support public health applications and decision making may need to be more complex and costly than the systems supporting applications in other industries and professions.

In building an HIS, the field of health informatics constitutes a multidisciplinary core of expertise, including specialists in, but not limited to, the following fields: computer science, electrical engineering, medicine, nursing, allied health management, finance, accounting, economics, sociology, survey design, geography, epidemiology, and statistics. These disciplines work in combination to produce HISs to serve the public health system objectives described earlier. In designing and managing HISs, public health administrators require the ability to: 1) distinguish among data, information, and actionable decision support; 2) define units of analysis for the level of data aggregation; (3) understand the health IT architecture of system(s) to be used; and (4) leverage the IM capability of the system(s).

Collaboration is taking place to improve the exchange of information between the public and private sectors. The Nationwide Health Information Network (NwHIN) is a civilian health network that brokers health data, locates health records, and records patient data.[11] The Public Health Information Network (PHIN) is used for monitoring data, capturing intervention and prevention data, and sending out communication and health alerts. For instance, PHIN captures animal disease data and vector-control information while NwHIN captures clinical data for these diseases. To facilitate interoperability, the two systems are developing national standards for messaging, vocabulary, directories, and security.

Data Versus Information Versus Knowledge Versus Wisdom

There have been endless discussions on the differences between data, information, knowledge, and wisdom. In public health, data are obtained from a variety of sources ranging from patient history from clinical visits to health insurance claims to bacteriology laboratory reports. Data are raw facts and statistics that are collected as part of the normal functioning of a business, clinical encounter, or research experiment. Information is data that has been processed in a structured, intelligent way to obtain results that are directly useful to managers and analysts. This is often the case once data have been organized in a database management system. Knowledge is obtained by using information to explain the context of a problem or situation. Finally, wisdom is knowledge tempered by experience.

Service-Oriented Computing

Healthcare planners and administrators are likely to interact with large-scale information systems as end users and as participants on implementation teams charged with the responsibility of deploying new technologies. Even direct providers of care can use an increasingly integrated set of information systems to capture patient-level data in electronic medical records, as well as more general knowledge for clinical decision support systems. This section explores the architectural considerations of large-scale information systems as computing power continues to dramatically improve with each technological iteration and the growth of networking, which is providing increasingly reliable interconnections.

Service-oriented computing (SOC) is not new, but maturing standards support the approach and make implementing complex service-based systems practical. Service-oriented computing standards, such as Extensible Markup Language (XML), Simple Object Access Protocol (SOAP), and Web Service Description Language (WDSL), govern the structure, transmission, and description of services. Registry standards such as the Universal Description, Discovery, and Integration (UDDI) protocol provide a method for publishing, retrieving, and analyzing services as components of complex systems. These standards allow developers to implement high-quality, tightly focused computing services that can be published and serve as components of large information systems.[12]

Among the most important goals of well-designed information system architectures are scalability to meet growing demands, flexibility to meet changing demands, and reliability or fault tolerance so systems are continually available to meet all demands. Achieving organizational agility demands the flexibility to quickly and decisively change business processes and supporting information systems by adding or modifying components. This is particularly challenging given the number of independent or quasi-independent providers that coordinate to deliver health services. A key advantage of service-oriented computing is the loose coupling between components. No detailed knowledge of the internal operation of a service is required and all coordination is managed through standardized protocols. Using this approach, services can be reused, rearranged, and new services can be added as systems are adapted in the pursuit of new opportunities and challenges.

Computer Networking

Computer networking and communication technologies provide the glue that binds the different components or services that form complex, distributed information systems. Typically, networking tasks are separated by the general nature of the connection and the underlying technologies used to handle the communications. The major technology classes are wide area networking (WAN), local area networking (LAN), and storage area networking (SAN).

Wide area networking is the term applied to the task of interconnecting large numbers of geographically dispersed computers. This is typically accomplished in piecemeal fashion by interconnecting smaller networks to create more global connectivity—the Internet being the quintessential example. Internetworking relies on standard protocols or rules of engagement that allow data to be routed through cooperating networks. Although there have been many competing proposals, the current standard that governs the Internet is the Transmission Control Protocol/Internet Protocol (TCP/IP). The Internet Protocol provides for routing or message delivery through cooperating networks, with the most basic service being best effort delivery of a message (with no guarantees). The Transmission Control Protocol provides a reliable end-to-end delivery service that costs a bit more (computationally speaking). These WAN protocols provide the foundation for the emerging service-oriented computing approaches discussed earlier.

An LAN spans an office, the floor of building, or similarly restricted geographic area. There can be many computers in this small area that are typically interconnected by shared media. Ethernet is the dominant technology in this arena because of its very low costs, wide availability, and continually improving speeds. In a clinical environment, local area networks are likely to interconnect departmental devices, including handheld wireless devices that are becoming increasingly common and value added.

SAN technologies provide an infrastructure for the lower levels of tiered architectures. Database systems, file transfers, document handling, and image storage and retrieval all require the transmission of large amounts of data. Storage area networks provide a high-performance alternative for such demanding tasks. SAN technologies allow storage to be centralized and flexibly reallocated through network addressing.

Cloud Computing

Cloud computing may be the next logical step in the evolution of public health information systems. The National Institute of Standards and Technology defines cloud computing as "a model for enabling ubiquitous, convenient, on-demand network access to a shared pool of configurable computing resources that can be rapidly provisioned and released with minimal management effort."[13] Cloud computing is the delivery of computing as a service, not as a product. In other words, cloud computing involves the migration of software programs away from desktop computers or servers maintained locally to remotely located hosts linked by a network or the Internet.[14] Cloud computing allows public health organizations to deliver technology infrastructure services, such as processing power and data storage, beyond the organization's physical perimeter. Facebook and LinkedIn are social networking examples of cloud computing services.

The three most common cloud architecture models are the public cloud, private cloud, and the community cloud.[13] A public cloud consists of a service provider making resources, such as storage and applications, available to the general public over the Internet. A private cloud (also called internal cloud or corporate cloud) refers to a proprietary computing architecture that provides hosted services to a determined number of users behind a firewall. The community cloud

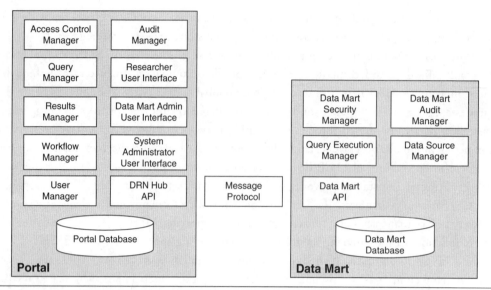

Figure 13.1   Distributed Research Network System Architecture
Source: Reproduced from Agency for Healthcare Research and Quality, Enhanced Functionality for the Distributed Research Network Pilot, Distributed research network system architecture. Retrieved February 28, 2013 from http://effectivehealthcare.ahrq.gov/index.cfm/search-for-guides-reviews-and-reports/?productid=1027&pageaction=displayproduct.

infrastructure is typically shared by several organizations. Community clouds may be managed by an organizations or a third party and physically located anywhere.

Several service models are used in cloud computing. The three most common ones are: Software as a Service (SaaS), Infrastructure as a Service (IaaS), and Platform as a Service (PaaS). SaaS is a software distribution model characterized by applications that are hosted by a service provider and made available to customers over a network, typically the Internet. IaaS is a provision model in which an organization outsources the equipment used to support operations, including hardware, servers, networking components, and storage. In this service model, the service provider owns the equipment and is responsible for housing, operating, and maintaining it. The option that is most relevant to public health is PaaS.[15] The PaaS model is used for delivering core services and interchangeable applications over the Internet without installation or downloads (**Figure 13.1**). The operating system and related networking features are clones of each other, which reduces the level of expertise required for interoperability (**Figure 13.2**).

One example of the use of cloud computing in public health is the National Electronic Disease Surveillance System (NEDSS) Base System application service provider version.[16] This CDC-supported program offered states a web-based SaaS model for accessing the NEDSS Base System software using a private cloud model. The states were required to subscribe to the service and share the infrastructure and support costs with the CDC. In return, each state was able to leverage this centralized service.

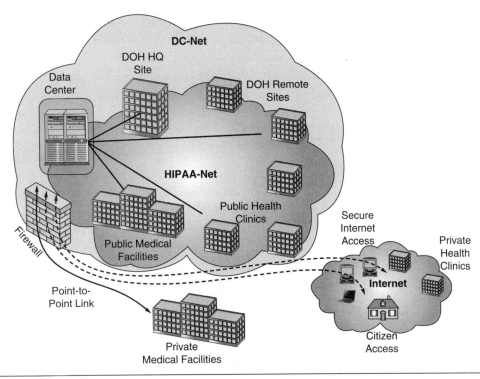

Figure 13.2 Platform as a Service Public Health Cloud With Three Public Health Departments, Each with Its Own Copy of the Platform with Different Applications Based on the Same Core Services
Source: Reproduced from The District of Columbia, Health Solutions. Retrieved February 28, 2013 from http://www.dcnet.dc.gov/DC/DCNET/Solutions/Health+Solutions.

Sources of Data for Information Systems

The heart of any public health information system is the data that it contains. Understanding the fundamental characteristics of databases is essential for effectively structuring and employing database technologies. Public health information databases share many characteristics with business enterprise data warehouses. That is, the systems are generally "subject oriented, integrated, nonvolatile, time variant collection[s] of data in support of management's decisions."[17]

Dimensional model data warehouses are constructed of two main components—fact tables and dimension tables. Facts are most often numeric, continuously valued, and additive measures of interest. For instance, a hospital discharge record includes such fields as length of stay and charge data that can be summed or averaged across various population groupings. Most commonly, however, the discharge counts are aggregated to compute event rates for specified demographic population segments.

Dimensions, on the other hand, are textual and discrete, providing a rich query environment for investigating associations between the dimensions and outcomes. Common hospital discharge dimensions include race, age, gender, physician, diagnosis, procedure code, payer, and so on. In order to facilitate analysis, many of these dimensions are refined to create hierarchies for aggregation. For instance, instead of comparing the hospitalizations for every age by individual years, records are "rolled up" or aggregated by age bands, which are simply predefined age groupings. Similarly, a geographic hierarchy (ZIP Code, community, county, state, region, or nation) identifies multiple levels of aggregation for comparing hospitalization rates.

Data Characteristics

Grain

Data granularity refers to the level of aggregation, or distance from individual events of the fact tables. The finest grain of data is the individual transactions themselves, such as birth or death certificates or individual hospital discharge records. As data are aggregated or summarized, there is a commensurate loss of information. For instance, death records are commonly rolled up geographically, temporally (quarterly or annual rates), by gender, race, and causes (combining various International Disease Classification [ICD]-9 or -10 codes). Virtually all reports are aggregated data. Although these aggregates are useful for comparing rates, they cannot be later disaggregated without access to the underlying transaction records. In general, the finer the grain of the fact tables, the greater the flexibility in aggregating and analyzing the data.

Determining the granularity in a data warehouse is one of the critical design decisions, providing a lower bound on subsequent analyses. Therefore, database designers typically err on the side of more rather than less detail. Data warehouses provide a flexible query environment by allowing users to "roll up" or summarize data, enabling a decision maker to choose a unit of analysis. The unit of analysis determines a level at which data are aggregated and analyzed in order to generate information. The most common units of analysis in public health are person/patient, vendor/supplier, region/population, and program.

Scope

Scope is a measure of breadth of coverage across any of the dimensions. For instance, geographic grain describes the unit of coverage, such as census tract–level data and geographic scope, providing the coverage of all tracts in a county or state. Temporal grain reflects the finest unit of time, and temporal scope reflects the total units available (e.g., monthly or annual data covering the last 5 years).

Source Type

Public health data can be gathered from a variety of source types, with a broad spectrum of reliability. Vital statistics and hospital discharges (and their derived aggregations) are generally among the most accurate, as their sources are individual events recorded by objective individuals and subject to post-collection cleansing efforts by official agencies. Moreover, the formatting and coding systems are often standardized across the states to facilitate ease of reporting to the CDC, which compiles state data into national reports. Similarly, state registries most commonly collect information through questionnaires completed in real time by third parties at the point of service and are generally validated for accuracy and completeness before entering the database.

In contrast, data sets such as the Behavioral Risk Factor Surveillance System (BRFSS) are collected using survey instruments that are completed by individuals with varying levels of commitment to completeness and accuracy. Moreover, surveys are, by their very nature, partial samplings of the total populace and results must be projected to include the whole population. This necessarily introduces sampling error and the potential for selection bias (respondents may selectively opt out of embarrassing questions).

Finally, some data, such as demographic changes between census years or estimates of per capita income, are simply estimated based on observations of proxy events, such as school registrations, vehicle registration changes, and voter rolls. Different agencies use different methods for arriving at their estimates with necessarily different results. It is important that the estimate sources used not be mixed in the database.

Regardless of the source of the data, however, it should be checked for completeness and consistency before being added to the data repository. A clear policy for handling missing or inconsistent data elements must be thought out and enforced, unit definitions understood and reconciled, and records containing erroneous data flagged or removed.

Metadata

Central to the maintainability of the data repository is keeping a clear record of its contents. This record is called **metadata**, or data about the data. Elements such as sources of the data and the agencies responsible for its collection, definitions of each of the fields, the date the data set was last updated, and the number of records each update contains can be invaluable for performing data quality checks and providing needed context for end users. Making such metadata available to end users should be an integral part of any information system, but it is particularly important for health information systems, where timeliness and context are critical for proper interpretation.

Common Data Problems

Not all data are created equal, and the prudent investigator chooses sources carefully. Fuzzy data element definitions, inconsistent collection and screening processes, changing variable definitions or scales, and intentional hiding of data values are a few of the threats to data quality that must be considered and addressed before bringing new data sources into the data warehouse.

Race is a particularly problematic dimension because it is generally self-reported and poorly understood. Many individuals responding to surveys or questionnaires confuse race with ethnicity or nationality and may classify themselves as multiracial or "other" if their nationality is not listed as a racial option. This confusion was magnified by the significant expansion of racial and ethnic categories offered in the 2000 census. From the single selection from the relatively simple four racial categories offered in the 1990 census, respondents in 2000 could select from an expanded list of more than 30 options. Moreover, since this same smorgasbord of racial options is generally not duplicated in most event data–collection instruments (e.g., hospital discharge records or vital statistics forms), reconciling event data with demographics requires careful conformation of racial definitions. That is, the demographic value categories must be conformed to the definitions used in the event records. The CDC has created a bridging methodology for reconciling the different race categorization schemes. In an effort to better collect the changing demographics of the U.S. population, the 2010 census revised the questions related to race and ethnicity, delineating Hispanic origin; however, capturing demographic data becomes more challenging as racial, national, and ethnic groups assert their distinctiveness.

A related, more general, data concern is the tendency of data-collection agencies to change the definition of data elements or the circumstances of collection. For example, ZIP Code boundaries change frequently, with approximately 5–10% of the codes changing each year. Besides the obvious problem of aligning the numerator (event) values with the denominator (population estimates) for rate calculations, the creation and deletion of ZIP Codes each year presents challenges when trying to trend data over time.

More serious are changes to definitions of the data. ICD-9/-10 changes most often involve additions or deletions of codes, rather than changes in definitions themselves; however, aggregations based on these codes often do change. Communicable disease reports, for instance, may simply report hepatitis C incidence one year, and then split the data out to report acute, chronic, and congenital incidences the next year. Unless the change is detected and the new subcategories are aggregated, the data values will be in error.

A subtler problem with public-use data sets may arise from privacy concerns. Many government agencies responsible for collecting and distributing event-level data will mask one or more of the fields that may be used to identify individuals. Masking simply replaces the actual value of the masked field(s) with one or more placeholder values for some predetermined percentage of the records. The most commonly masked fields are ZIP Codes, age, gender, and race.

Common Databases Available for Public Health

A solid understanding of health IT and data structure is required for the optimal design of public HISs. Fortunately for public health managers, there are rich data resources available at federal and state levels. This section provides an overview of the most common databases available to health managers and researchers in developing HISs. Most of the databases described here are federal or state specific in their focus. Although a federal focus may be too broad for local and regional health policy issues, federal surveys can still provide two significant benefits. First, national databases provide field-tested survey instruments or data-abstraction tools that can be applied to a more focused information system. Second, federal surveys can provide a comparison database for information systems that also use state and local data sources in order to gauge the effectiveness of local initiatives.

It is worth noting the distinction between health statistics databases and health reports. Websites that serve as data sources, such as the U.S. Centers for Medicare and Medicaid Services (http://www.cms.gov) and some state departments of health, allow users to execute relatively broad queries that return fine-grain data across the full scope of one or more dimensions. Report sites, on the other hand, provide either preformatted reports, often in fixed formats such as PDF files, or point queries that return aggregated data for a limited scope. The U.S. Centers for Medicare and Medicaid Services site, for instance, allows end users to generate comprehensive queries covering a large number of available indicator statistics. The data are available as downloadable files that can be directly imported into database programs for end-user manipulation.

At the other end of the spectrum is the Florida Youth Substance Abuse Survey that presents aggregated county data in individual PDF files, without the benefit of race, gender, or grade-level breakdowns (http://www.dcf.state.fl.us/programs/samh/publications/fysas/). This requires manual conversion of the data tables into spreadsheet format but still precludes any end-user reaggregation of the data or creating different dimensional views.

Most sites fall between these two extremes. For example, the Florida Community Health Assessment Resource Tool Set (CHARTS) allows users to return statewide incidence counts and rates for hundreds of diseases and injuries, grouped by county, ZIP Code, gender, race, or age bands and formatted in spreadsheets for easy importation into a database (http://www.floridacharts.com/charts/QASpecial.aspx). A comprehensive view of the health status of communities across the state can be generated very quickly using this system.

Government Survey Data

The federal government collects a broad array of data that may be used by public HISs. The U.S. Department of Health and Human Services (HHS) has the largest health data–collection responsibility. However, other federal government departments such as Defense, Labor, and Commerce also collect critical health data.

The phrase "national probability sample" describes a survey instrument that has been deliberately designed to reflect the U.S. national population's sociodemographic variation in age, gender, race, income, and education. If a state-level analysis were attempted, the survey could produce misleading estimates if survey respondents were over- or underweighted to reflect their proportional representation within the nation.

Another important concept is the panel survey. In this design, a panel or cohort of survey participants is followed during several rounds of the questionnaire. For example, some surveys such as the MEPS and the Medicare Current Beneficiary Survey (MCBS) follow participants for at least 2 years to track health status and cost. Panel surveys are valuable to assess long-term impacts in health care, such as a lack of health insurance or follow up for a massive heart attack.

Most federal surveys are collected on an annual basis and are generally available as public use files 1 to 2 years following the completion of the data-collection period. These data are available for a small fee to cover the cost of producing the databases. A list of nearly all of the government surveys used for health is available via the National Center for Health Statistics webpage (http://www.cdc.gov/nchs).

Several examples of government-sponsored survey data are provided in the following paragraphs.

Current Population Survey (CPS)

This survey is completed monthly by the U.S. Census Bureau for the Department of Labor and updated annually. It contains basic information on healthcare use and can be queried online at http://www.census.gov/cps/data/cpstablecreator.html. It is often available before any other federal survey with health data. The sample consists of approximately 52,000 housing units and the persons in them. The survey's primary goals are to provide estimates of employment, unemployment, and other socioeconomic characteristics of the general labor force, of the population as a whole, and of various subgroups of the population.

National Health Interview Survey (NHIS)

This survey, collected by the National Center for Health Statistics (NCHS) within the HHS, is a national probability sample of the health status of the population (http://www.cdc.gov/nchs/nhis.htm). A two-part questionnaire is used with a sample size of approximately 49,000 households yielding 127,000 persons. The NHIS has had continuous data collection since 1957 for national estimates through household interviews by U.S. Census Bureau interviewers. The NHIS provides the sampling frame for other NCHS surveys and is linked to the National Death Index (http://www.cdc.gov/nchs/ndi.htm). A core survey of demographic and general health information and a supplement focusing on different populations are deployed.

Administrative/Claims Data

Administrative (claims) data are defined as the data elements that are generated as part of a healthcare organization's operations. For example, health insurers generate claims data to record the services that are reimbursed by the insurer. There are three significant advantages to using administrative data. First, the data cover a large breadth of services ranging from inpatient services to prescription drug use and immunizations. Second, administrative data are an inexpensive source of data when contrasted with other forms of health service data such as medical records. The third advantage is the timeliness of availability when compared with government surveys and other data sources. The most commonly used administrative databases are: state hospital discharge records, state Medicaid claims data, and the Medicare National Claims History.

HIS Applications in Public Health Administration

There are several operating public HISs of note. These initiatives range in scope from federal to local sponsorship. Some provide a general database for a full range of public health issues, while others are designed for specific disease tracking or program evaluation.

The CDC's INPHO

The Information Network for Public Health Officials (INPHO) system was developed as a framework for public health information and practice based on a state-of-the-art telecommunications network.[8] The INPHO is part of a strategy to strengthen public health infrastructure. The three concepts of the INPHO are linkage, information access, and data exchange. First, the CDC works with state and local area health agencies to build local and wide area networks. Second, the CDC has expanded "virtual networks" through the use of CDC Wide-ranging Online Data for Epidemiologic Research (WONDER). This is a software system that provides access to data in the CDC's public health databases. Third, the CDC has encouraged each state to connect to the Internet to gain access to information.

Georgia (discussed in more detail later in the chapter) pioneered the program in early 1993. By 1997, 14 more states made the INPHO vision integral to their public health information strategies: California, Florida, Illinois, Indiana, Kansas, Michigan, Missouri, New Jersey, New York, North Carolina, Oregon, Rhode Island, Washington, and West Virginia. A second round of INPHO projects was funded through a cooperative agreement program, with awards made in the spring of 1998. The program promotes the integration of information systems, with special emphasis on immunization registries. The cooperative agreements were funded as either implementation projects (Florida, Georgia, Missouri, and New York) or demonstration projects (Iowa, Maryland, Montana, Nevada, and Texas). More information on the initiative is available at http://www.cdc.gov/learning.

CDC WONDER

CDC WONDER was designed by the CDC to put critical information into the hands of public health managers quickly and easily. Originally a PC-based system, it is now available from any computer with an Internet connection, solving the problem of dedicating workstations to a specific database. As such, it is one of the few truly national public health data resources available with real-time access to anyone in the world. With CDC WONDER, one can do the following:

1. Search for and retrieve *Morbidity and Mortality Weekly Report* articles and prevention guidelines published by the CDC.
2. Query dozens of numeric data sets on the CDC's mainframe and other computers via fill-in-the blank request screens. Public use data sets about mortality, cancer incidence, hospital discharges, AIDS, behavioral risk factors, diabetes, and many other topics are available for query, and the requested data can be readily summarized and analyzed.
3. Locate the name and email addresses of the CDC staff and registered CDC WONDER users.
4. Post notices, general announcements, data files, or software programs of interest to public health professionals in an electronic forum for use by CDC staff and other CDC WONDER users.

For more information on CDC WONDER, refer to http://wonder.cdc.gov.

State Public HISs

States have multiple public HISs mirroring the complicated array of categorical programs with different funding sources. Commonly maintained information systems include computerized immunization registries, lead toxicity tracking, early intervention databases for children with a disability, congenital disease registries, in addition to vital statistics data, Medicaid utilization, and disease reports. The need for integrated information systems and the support of the INPHO project has spurred models in a number of states. The next sections describe efforts in Missouri and Georgia.

Missouri

The Missouri Department of Health had a problem with 67 information systems that ran on different platforms and could not communicate with one another.[7] To solve this problem, the

Missouri Health Strategic Architectures and Information System (MOHSAIC) was developed. An integrated client service record was an important component of this initiative. From the client's perspective, it was irrelevant if the services were labeled WIC, prenatal care, diabetes, Maternal and Child Health Services block grant, or local funding. Considerable effort and staff resources were committed to develop this system. Also, integrated systems magnify concerns about confidentiality. Benefits include increased capability for community health assessment, coordination of services, outreach, and linkages to primary care delivered by larger networks.[7]

Georgia

Georgia was the first site of the CDC INPHO initiative. Georgia was able to develop quickly as a demonstration site through a unique consortium of state agencies with academic health partners and IT partners. For example, members of the consortium included the Medical College of Georgia, the Georgia Center for Advanced Telecommunications Technology, and the Emory University School of Public Health. The program also had initial funding from the Robert Wood Johnson Foundation.[4] The infrastructure includes 81 clinics and 59 county health departments.

The Georgia INPHO system includes local and wide area computer networks, office automation and email, a public health calendar, an executive HIS, and electronic notification of public health emergencies. Before the project began, the state public health office operated 13 small, unlinked local area networks. With the INPHO project, hardware and software were consolidated into one integrated network system.

Privacy and Security Issues

The public's concern for the privacy of personal health information has become a major policy issue. Unfortunately, this concern is not easily addressed. At the heart of this issue is the paradox that health data must be identifiable if they are to be valuable for public health interventions. Complicating the issue is that even an encrypted personal identifier still yields a personal identifier. HISs must remain responsive to these evolving data privacy and confidentiality issues.

Public health data are provided to public health managers and researchers as an act of trust. If one individual or organization violates that trust, the public's confidence may erode immediately. Harris poll results show consistently that health data confidentiality and security issues are an important public concern.[18]

Two federal government regulations have advanced the privacy and security debate: the Health Insurance Portability and Accountability Act (HIPAA) and the Health Information Technology for Economic and Clinical Health Act (HITECH Act). Enacted in 1996 by the Clinton administration, HIPAA consists of two sections: Title 1: Health Care Access, Portability, and Renewability; and Title 2: Preventing Health Care Fraud and Abuse, Administrative Simplification, Medical Liability Reform. Title 1 involves the regulation of the availability of group health plans and certain health policies. Title 2 created programs to control fraud and abuse within the healthcare system and established civil and criminal penalties and numerous administrative simplification rules, including extensive privacy and security rules for protected health information.

The HIPAA **Privacy Rule** prohibits the disclosure of individually identifiable health information, otherwise known as **protected health information (PHI)**, without the consent of the patient (or guardian), except for three purposes: payment, medical treatment, or healthcare operations (e.g., care coordination, case management, quality assessment).[19] PHI consists of individually identifiable health data that are transmitted or maintained in electronic media and related to the physical or mental health of an individual, the healthcare services provided to an individual, or the payment for those services provided to the individual. For covered entities using or disclosing PHI, the Privacy Rule establishes a range of health information privacy requirements and standards, including procedures for notification of individuals, internal policies and procedures, employee training, and technical and physical data security safeguards.

Public health practice and research uses protected health information to perform many of its required functions, including public health surveillance, outbreak investigation, program operations, and terrorism preparedness. Public health authorities have a long history of protecting the confidentiality of individually identifiable health information and were given significant latitude in the Privacy Rule, which expressly permits PHI to be shared for specified public health purposes. Covered entities may disclose PHI to a public health agency legally authorized to collect information for the purpose of preventing or controlling disease, injury, or disability, without separate authorization. It should be noted, however, that in addition to using PHI from covered entities, a public health agency may itself be a covered entity, providing services and producing electronic transactions.[20]

HIPAA created a timetable for the adoption of national medical privacy legislation by the year 2000. The combination of HIPAA and privacy laws also created the first national policy to prosecute those persons who breach the medical privacy of an individual. The penalties can range from fines to prison.

While the Privacy Rule pertains to all paper and electronic PHI, the HIPAA Security Rule specifically addresses electronic protected health information (EPHI). The Security Rule requires appropriate technical, physical, and administrative safeguards to ensure the integrity and security of EPHI. It also imposes organizational requirements for documenting processes analogous to the Privacy Rule. The Security Rule took effect in April 2003.

Security Rule technical safeguards involve controlling access and enabling covered entities to protect communications containing EPHI being transmitted over open networks from being accessed by any third parties. Covered entities are required to authenticate any other entities they communicate with through password systems, token systems, telephone callbacks, and two- or three-way handshakes. Information systems storing EPHI must utilize intrusion-protection systems. Data encryption must be used for transmissions over open networks. All HIPAA policies and procedures must also be documented and provided to the government to ensure compliance.

Physical safeguards consist of controlling physical access to protect data from unauthorized access. Required access controls include facility security plans, visitor sign-in records, and escorts. Access controls must also address the introduction of hardware and software from an organization's network by properly authorized individuals. Disposal of network equipment must also be addressed to ensure that EPHI is not compromised.

Administrative safeguards consist of policies and procedures for organizational compliance. Covered entities are required to adopt a written set of security procedures and designate a security officer for implementing and enforcing all policies and procedures. These policies identify specific individuals or types of employees who are given access to EPHI. The procedures must address employee access authorization and termination. A contingency plan for backing up data and defined disaster recovery procedures is also required for responding to emergency situations.

The HITECH Act also addresses the privacy and security concerns associated with EPHI. Enacted as part of the American Recovery and Reinvestment Act of 2009, the HITECH Act extends all HIPAA Privacy Rule and Security Rule requirements to include business associates of covered entities. This legislation also included new notification requirements for the breach of any unsecured EPHI for all covered entities and their business associates. Additionally, the HITECH Act implemented new rules for the accounting of any disclosures of EPHI by any covered entities using an electronic health record.

Future Outlook

The broad range of public HIS applications developed over the past decade demonstrates how managers are seeking to improve the scope and quality of their data systems. HIS experts consistently state that the future lies in building an infrastructure that is both easy to use and able to demonstrate value for its investment.[18,21] To build such an infrastructure requires data standards and translators for different standards to help bridge the transition from the current system.[22]

Opportunities for developing HISs are becoming less technical and more political. Public concerns about the privacy of health-related information in this new environment are motivating new policies for information use that, it is hoped, will build the public's trust in emerging health information applications while preserving the ability of public health organizations to use health data for essential surveillance, research, and management activities. Both HIPAA and the HITECH Act have mandated privacy and security standards to be applied to the development of HISs. The operations of all covered entities and business associates dealing with PHI and EPHI must now be in continuous compliance with these government regulations. As a result, the innovation required for further HIS development also requires the lock-step participation of the federal government to ensure that all privacy and security concerns are addressed.

The transition of the medical profession from an arcane paper-based data collection world toward e-commerce for business-to-business applications is gaining greater attention. The HITECH Act is, in part, intended to enhance the reimbursement of healthcare providers for the meaningful use of electronic healthcare records systems.[19] Clinical providers will receive incentive payments to exchange specified types of data, such as immunizations, with the public health system. Clearly, the health industry is moving toward linking health services data with public health data for greater overall health awareness. However, to facilitate this type of exchange of information, the information architectures of public health information systems will need to adapt to accept the types of data proposed for exchange. This shift will require a meaningful and sustained commitment on the part of industry and substantial funding from the government.

One of the most promising developments is the use of the Internet as the platform to collect data, turn data into information, and monitor the health of the population. Public health administrators should consider following other non-health industries in the growing trend toward cloud computing. This approach offers the advantages of scalability of performance, customizability for individual users, disaster resilience, and reductions in organizational infrastructure costs. Other potential areas for HIS research include technology-driven advances in evidence-based medicine, personalized medicine, and social media.[23]

Conclusion

The value of health information systems to public health administration is inarguable. Public health organizations heavily rely on these systems to inform managerial decision making and improve their operations for public health planning, policy analysis, health outcomes assessment, epidemiologic surveillance, program evaluation, and performance measurement. Future developments in this field will continue to be less technical and more political in nature. Privacy and security issues will serve as prominent driving forces for the next generation of health information systems. Public health organizations will need to continue to push forward with developing state-of-the-art information systems to meet the future health information management needs of the populations they serve.

Discussion Questions

1. What is service-oriented computing and how does it apply to health information systems?
2. What are the core concepts of information systems architecture?
3. What are the three major network types used in public health?
4. What are the key elements of the HIPAA Security Rule?
5. How might cloud computing principles be applied to public health information systems?

References

1. Abernethy NF, DeRimer K, Small PM. Methods to identify standard data elements in clinical and public health forms. *AMIA Annu Symp Proc.* 2011;2011:19–27.
2. Koo D, Wetterhall SF. History and current status of the National Notifiable Diseases Surveillance System. *J Public Health Manage Pract.* 1996;2(4):4–10.
3. Boom JA, Dragsbaek AC, Nelson CS. The success of an immunization information system in the wake of Hurricane Katrina. *Pediatrics.* 2007;119(6):1213–7.
4. Chapman KA, Moulton AD. The Georgia Information Network for Public Health Officials (INPHO): a demonstration of the CDC INPHO concept. *J Public Health Manage Pract.* 1995;1(2):39–43.
5. Dubowitz T, Williams M, Steiner ED, et al. Using geographic information systems to match local health needs with public health services and programs. *Am J Public Health.* 2011;101(9):1664–5.
6. Nykiforuk CI, Flaman LM. Geographic information systems (GIS) for Health Promotion and Public Health: a review. *Health Promot Pract.* 2011;12(1):63–73.
7. Land GH, Stokes C, Hoffman N, et al. Developing an integrated public health information system for Missouri. *J Public Health Manage Pract.* 1995;1(1):48–56.

8. Corrigan JM, Nielsen DM. Toward the development of uniform reporting standards for managed care organizations: the Health Plan Employer Data and Information Set. *J Joint Commission Qual Improv.* 1993;19(12):566–75.

9. Centers for Disease Control and Prevention, Epi-X. What's being shared on *Epi*-X? Available at: http://www.cdc.gov/epix/#3. Accessed February 28, 2013.

10. National Committee for Quality Assurance. HEDIS & performance measurement. Available at: http://www.ncqa.org/HEDISQualityMeasurement.aspx. Accessed February 28, 2013.

11. HealthIT.gov. Nationwide Health Information Network. Available at: http://www.healthit.gov/policy-researchers-implementers/nationwide-health-information-network-nwhin. Accessed February 28, 2013.

12. Huhns M, Singh M. Service-oriented computing: key concepts and principles. *IEEE Internet Comput.* 2005;9(1):75–81.

13. Mell P, Grance T. *The NIST Definition of Cloud Computing. National Institute of Standards and Technology.* Gaithersburg, MD: Department of Commerce; 2011.

14. Rosenthal A, Mork P, Li MH, et al. Cloud computing: a new business paradigm for biomedical information sharing. *J Biomed Inform.* 2010;43(2):342–53.

15. Lenert L, Sundwall DN. Public health surveillance and meaningful use regulations: a crisis of opportunity. *Am J Public Health.* 2012;102(3):e1–7.

16. CSC. Disease surveillance system exchanges public health data to protect U.S. citizens. Available at: http://www.csc.com/public_sector/success_stories/9236-nedss_exchanges_public_health_data. Accessed February 28, 2013.

17. Inmon W. *Building the Data Warehouse.* 3rd ed. New York: John Wiley and Sons; 2002.

18. Milio N. Beyond informatics: an electronic community infrastructure for public health. *J Public Health Manage Pract.* 1999;1(4):84–94.

19. Burde, H. The HIGHTECH ACT—an overview. *Virtual Mentor.* 2011;13(3):172–5.

20. Centers for Disease Control and Prevention, Epidemiology Program Office. HIPPA Privacy Rule and public health. *MMWR.* 2003;52:1–12.

21. Baker EL Jr, Ross D. Information and surveillance systems and community health: building the public health information infrastructure. *J Public Health Manage Pract.* 1996;2(4):58–60.

22. Lumpkin J, Atkinson D, Biery R, et al. The development of integrated public health information systems: a statement by the Joint Council of Governmental Public Health Agencies. *J Public Health Manage Pract.* 1995;1(4):55–9.

23. Fichman R, Kohli R, Krishnan R. The role of information systems in healthcare: current research and future trends. *Information Systems Research.* 2011;22(3):419–28.

Geographic Information Systems for Public Health

Alan L. Melnick and Brendon Haggerty

Chapter Overview

From its inception, public health has relied on information as a core component of practice. Public health practitioners have used epidemiology, one of the core sciences underlying public health, to analyze information on the distribution of health and disease within populations. While accurate geographically based data have always been necessary to improve the health status of communities, relatively recent changes in technology and information management have created quite a revolution in public health practice. Much more data from varied sources are available, and technological tools to analyze the data have become easier to obtain. This chapter describes one of the most exciting technological developments available to public health practitioners, **geographic information system (GIS)** technology. Geographic information systems integrate several functions, including the incorporation, storage, and retrieval of data with a spatial or geographic component. For example, analysis and display of the data on maps provide public health practitioners with a tool to assist in understanding disease and disease risks related to environmental exposures for diverse populations. Like other new technologies, GIS technology presents threats as well as opportunities. On one hand, GIS technology has the capacity to bring community health assessment to the neighborhood level by making data much more meaningful to neighborhood residents, non-public health professionals, and policy makers, while giving public health officials an opportunity to engage their constituents in meaningful conversations and projects around community health improvement. On the other hand, the technology could provide a setup for abuse through violations of confidentiality and misinterpretation of results. Consequently, public health officials, including administrators, should not leave the use of this technology solely to technicians. This chapter is written for public health students and public health officials, including administrators, who will need a basic understanding of the technology. The chapter provides a brief history of GIS; the components of GIS, including hardware, software, and data; a basic description of the map-making process; and its uses in epidemiology, including environmental epidemiology, community health assessment, community health improvement, and a relatively new application—health impact assessments. In addition, the chapter includes a discussion of the potential pitfalls in using GIS, including challenges related to data quality, workforce capacity, community definitions, confidentiality, and misinterpretation of results. Finally, the chapter describes the future of GIS, including the role that public health officials can play in using and sharing this wonderful technology with their communities.

History of GIS in Public Health

As early as 1854, John Snow, the father of modern epidemiology, plotted the geographic distribution of cholera deaths in London, demonstrating the association between the deaths and contaminated water supplies.[1] In doing so, he linked forever the new science of epidemiology with the use of geographic information to reveal relationships between environment and disease.[2]

Of the three core epidemiologic variables—time, place, and person—place has always been the most difficult and time consuming to analyze and depict.[2] In the past, when public health practitioners focused mainly on communicable disease control, pushpins or dots drawn on maps usually proved effective in helping to analyze and control disease outbreaks. The modern public health practitioner, however, is responsible for analyzing and responding to complex health issues in a rapidly changing, diverse environment. The social, environmental, and behavioral determinants of health have a strong geographic component. To work effectively with communities in improving health status, modern public health practitioners and their community partners will need easy, immediate access to accurate, geographically based data.[3] New developments in GIS technology are making this possible.

Limitations of Pre-GIS Analysis

For several reasons, local health consumers and health planners have rarely used health data collected routinely by local and state governments. First, the data are not timely. For example, up to 2 years can elapse before states report vital statistics data. Second, many different agencies at the local, state, and federal level collect and maintain health-related data in different formats in different locations, making the data less accessible for consumers, health planners, and local health departments. Third, data analyzed and reported at the county level and above are not useful for assessing the health of diverse communities within large or even medium sized counties. Such macro-level data fail to capture the unique essential characteristics of the individual communities, leaving little opportunity for local public health professionals to seek dialogue and strengthen relationships with populations within their counties. By providing easy access to a variety of data that are analyzable at the community level, modern GIS promise to address these problems, enabling public health practitioners to engage diverse communities in a partnership to improve community health.[4]

Emergence of Modern GIS

Several factors contributed to the development and increasing use of GIS in many sectors. Computers became smaller, faster, more accessible, and less expensive. Software became easier to use. Landscape and census data became available in digital format, allowing the linkage of health-related data sets to a geographic map.[5] In addition, online applications have allowed for rapid innovation and wide distribution of spatial data, changing the way that we use and interact with maps.[6]

Features of GIS

Definition

GIS are automated computer packages that are defined more by their functions than by what they are.[5] GIS integrate several functions, including the capture and incorporation of data sets, the storage of data, the retrieval of data, the statistical manipulation of data, data analysis, data modeling, and the display of the data on maps.[5,7] The incorporated data must have a spatial or geographic component. Because much of the data collected today have some geographic reference, such as a street address, GIS have the potential to revolutionize public health practice. With GIS, public health practitioners can map health-related issues, such as mortality and birth rates, at the neighborhood or street level.[8] In addition, GIS are tools for understanding and displaying disease or disease risks related to environmental exposures for diverse populations.[2] For example, studies have used GIS to demonstrate the relationship between childhood lead poisoning cases by census block with older housing stock.[9] The public health uses of GIS are described later in this chapter.

Data Acquisition and Storage: Creating Spatial Databases

To perform geographic analyses, GIS require a foundation of spatial, or geographic, data. The creation of the U.S. Bureau of the Census Topologically Integrated Geographic Encoding and Referencing (TIGER)/Line files as a foundation database contributed to the development of modern GIS.[10] Updated, easily obtainable versions of the TIGER/Line files include detailed street and address range information, along with political and administrative boundaries such as counties, ZIP Codes, census tracts, and census block groups.[11] TIGER/Line files are available to order at the U.S. Census Bureau TIGER home page (http://www.census.gov/geo/maps-data/data/tiger.html). Updated geographic data files are also available from commercial vendors, but may be expensive.[8] Many state and local governments maintain spatial data, which they often make available online.

The next step in a GIS analysis is to obtain the attribute data and link them to points in space through a geographic database.[11] To do this, GIS use a projection system that adapts a mathematical model of the Earth's curved surface to the two-dimensional extent of a map.[12] Attribute data relate to any public health issue of interest, and can include health, social, and environmental data. Examples of attribute data include the U.S. Census Bureau's extensive demographic, economic, and social data sets; state and local vital statistics (perinatal and mortality data); and law enforcement data (reported arrests). To link to the geographic foundation, the attribute data must include a geographic reference, such as an address field. For example, to analyze birth rates by geography, each record in the birth database must include a field with the mother's street address. GIS can analyze any attribute database, such as arrest data, that includes a field with a location.

Geocoding is the process by which GIS software matches each record in an attribute database with the geographic files. The GIS software converts each address in the attribute file to a point on a map. The software then compares each address with the corresponding information in the foundation spatial database. A match occurs when the two agree.[11]

Map Making and Data Analysis

Once stored and geocoded, the data are ready for analysis and display. The power of GIS technology stems from its ability to allow users to analyze and display health-related data in new and effective ways.[5] The simplest form of display would be analogous to a pushpin depiction with events, such as reported cholera cases, displayed as dots on a map. In one study, local public health planners created a map showing the home locations of children who had high blood lead levels (**Figure 14.1**).[11] Areas with larger numbers of children with reported high lead levels show up as clusters of triangular-shaped black dots. Like other epidemiologic studies, this map raised an additional question. Was clustering a reflection of high blood lead prevalence or a reflection of greater screening efforts? A second map, in which circular clear dots displayed all children

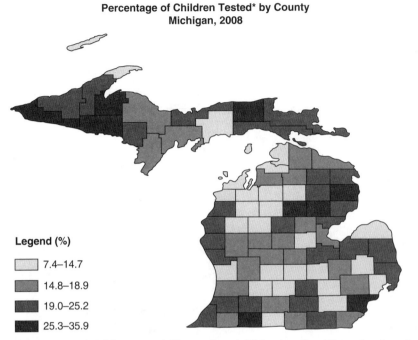

**Percentage of Children Tested* by County
Michigan, 2008**

Legend (%)

- [ ] 7.4–14.7
- [ ] 14.8–18.9
- [ ] 19.0–25.2
- [ ] 25.3–35.9

*Percentage of children tested: The number of children less than 72 months of age tested for blood lead divided by the total number of children less than 72 months of age based on 2000 U.S. Census data, multiplied by 100.

Figure 14.1   Children with Elevated Blood Lead Level
Source: Centers for Disease Control and Prevention. Michigan data, statistics and surveillance. Available at: http://www.cdc.gov/nceh/lead/data/state/midata.htm#2008tested. Accessed February 28, 2013.

screened, answered the question, revealing the varying patterns of children with high and low blood lead levels (**Figure 14.2**).[11]

Of course, GIS can perform much more complex tasks than a simple mapping of events.[5] There are many tools and analysis methods available in GIS software. Overlays and buffers are among the most common. The overlay capability allows the user to display more than one attribute on a map at a time. For example, the Centers for Disease Control and Prevention (CDC) has identified older housing as the most significant risk factor for lead exposure in young children. Local public health planners might be interested, then, in identifying the location of older housing in targeting lead exposure prevention efforts. If the data were available, a map could overlay the triangular black dots of reported childhood lead cases with the location of houses built before 1960. In this case, dots of different colors and shapes could represent older housing. Alternatively, the user could overlay the reported lead cases with a map showing the percentage of homes built before 1960 by census tract or census block group.[11] Each census block group could be colored or shaded based on its range of percentage of housing built before 1960. This

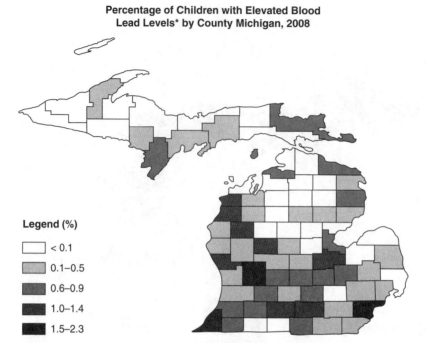

Figure 14.2   Children Screened for Blood Lead Poisoning
Source: Centers for Disease Control and Prevention. Michigan data, statistics and surveillance. Available at: http://www.cdc.gov/nceh/lead/data/state/midata.htm#2008tested. Accessed February 28, 2013.

type of map, in which a given area, or polygon, is shaded with different colors to depict variations of features such as the percentage of older housing stock, is called a **choropleth map**. Public health planners in Duval County, Florida used overlays to create such a map. Census block groups were shaded based on the percentage of older housing, with reported childhood lead poisoning cases displayed as black dots (**Figure 14.3**).[13] This map was quite useful in focusing blood lead screening efforts.

With buffering, another powerful feature of GIS analysis, users can create polygons based on the distance from a target object.[8] Buffers are particularly useful in identifying people at risk of exposure to environmental hazards. A GIS study of childhood lead risk could define a 25-meter zone around main roads to identify areas with potentially high levels of lead-contaminated soil from past use of leaded gasoline (**Figure 14.4**).[14] The same study could then identify and locate children living within these areas who would benefit from lead screening. Another study used buffering to evaluate potential health risks and health risk perceptions of minority populations living within 0.2 miles of businesses that store hazardous chemicals (**Figure 14.5**).[15] A different study examined the availability of supermarkets within a 1-mile buffer of survey respondents' homes, finding an association between nearby supermarket density and diet.[16]

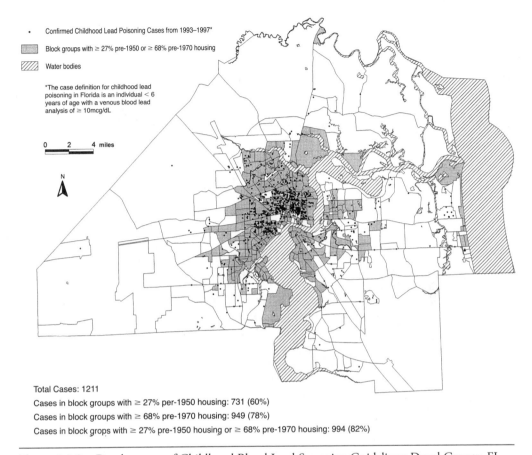

- • Confirmed Childhood Lead Poisoning Cases from 1993–1997*

Block groups with ≥ 27% pre-1950 or ≥ 68% pre-1970 housing

Water bodies

*The case definition for childhood lead poisoning in Florida is an individual < 6 years of age with a venous blood lead analysis of ≥ 10mcg/dL

0   2   4   miles

N

Total Cases: 1211
Cases in block groups with ≥ 27% per-1950 housing: 731 (60%)
Cases in block groups with ≥ 68% pre-1970 housing: 949 (78%)
Cases in block grops with ≥ 27% pre-1950 housing or ≥ 68% pre-1970 housing: 994 (82%)

Figure 14.3   Development of Childhood Blood Lead Screening Guidelines: Duval County, FL
Source: Bureau of Environmental Epidemiology, Duval County, Florida.

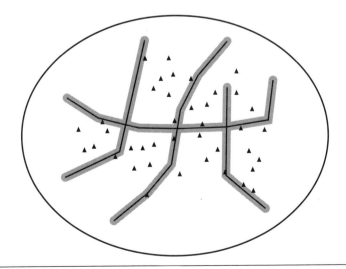

Figure 14.4   25-meter Zones Around Main Roads
Source: Reprinted from Vine MF, Degnan D, Hanchette C. Geographic information systems: their use in environmental epidemiological research. *Environ Health Perspect.* 1997;105(6):598–605.

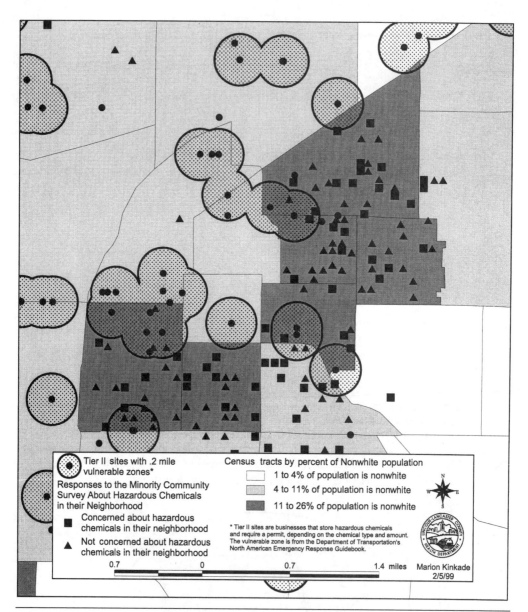

Figure 14.5   Responses to the Survey of Environmental Health Hazard Risks in the Minority Community, in Relation to the Primary Minority Census Tracts and the Evacuation Zones for Tier II Sites in Lincoln, NE, February 1999
Source: Lincoln-Lancaster County Health Department, Lincoln, Nebraska.

Public Health GIS Applications

Given that many determinants of health have strong geographic components, GIS technology has many public health applications. These applications range from epidemiology—including research—to community health assessment and community health planning.

Epidemiology

Perhaps the most direct use of GIS technology is as a tool for understanding and displaying disease or disease risks related to environmental exposures.[2] GIS technology can assist in environmental epidemiologic investigations in several ways:[17]

- By defining the population potentially exposed: For example, cohort studies have used GIS to identify populations with risk of exposure to magnetic fields from high-powered electrical lines,[14] populations potentially exposed to hazardous waste near landfill sites,[18,19] and pregnant women exposed to industrial toxic release emissions.[20]
- By identifying the source and potential routes of exposure: For example, GIS studies have depicted nitrate or trichloroethylene levels in drinking water,[21,22] dioxin in air around industrial plants in Denmark,[23] childhood lead poisoning cases by housing age,[9,13] and proximity to traffic, highways, and/or point source air pollution emitters in case control studies of asthma[24,25] and autism.[26]
- By estimating environmental levels of contaminants: For example, a GIS study of iodine-131 releases from the Hanford Nuclear Reservation estimated the amount of I-131 that might have been present in milk,[27] a Swedish lung cancer study used GIS to estimate air pollutant concentrations,[28,29] and a Durham County, North Carolina study used GIS and industrial source dispersion monitoring to characterize the spatial distribution and ambient concentration of glycol ethers.[30] In addition, a Spanish study exploring the association between air pollution exposure during pregnancy and low birth weight used land use regression (LUR) modeling to estimate exposures to nitrogen dioxide, benzene, toluene, ethylbenzene, p-xylene, and o-xylene.[31]

Since the 1980s, several studies have identified an unequal distribution of environmental hazards across racial, ethic, and socioeconomic groups.[32] An accompanying increase in health disparities based on social class and ethnicity has led to concerns that these disparities have environmental causes. Although many factors, such as differential healthcare access, genetic variations, health behaviors, occupation, and discrimination contribute to health disparities, differential environmental hazard exposures probably contribute significantly. GIS technology has been helpful in understanding and addressing these disparities by identifying the extent to which low-income and minority populations are disproportionately exposed to environmental hazards.[32] For example, the U.S. Environmental Protection Agency (EPA) has been developing the Community-Focused Exposure and Risk Screening Tool (C-FERST). Local governments and community-based organizations will be able to use this GIS-based tool to identify populations at risk for environmental exposures and to obtain information necessary for developing interventions and policies necessary for eliminating the hazards.[33]

By integrating GIS with statistical methods, epidemiologists can use GIS for modeling, a spatial analysis process that can identify disease risk factors. A study of Lyme disease in Baltimore, Maryland obtained data for 53 environmental variables at the residences of Lyme disease patients. Combining GIS with a logistic regression analysis, researchers rapidly identified Lyme disease risk factors over a large area.[34] A case-control study of breast cancer on Cape Cod used a three-dimensional model of groundwater developed by the U.S. Geological Survey (USGS) to estimate exposures to environmental contaminants in drinking water.[35]

Many diseases cluster geographically whether or not they are related to environmental exposure.[2] One of the most useful features of GIS is their ability to identify and analyze space–time clusters or "hotspots" of disease.[5] An early GIS application called the Geographical Analysis Machine (GAM) was used to evaluate whether spatial clusters of childhood leukemia were located near nuclear facilities in Britain.[5,36] More recently, investigators have used GIS to identify spatial clusters of cancer in Illinois,[37] spatial clusters of neural tube birth defects in Shanxi Province, China,[38] cancer mortality in Appalachian populations exposed to coal mining activities,[39] and breast and lung cancer clusters near two rivers in Michigan.[40] Although these ecologic studies do not prove an association between environmental factors and disease, they raise questions useful for follow-up case control and cohort studies.[37]

Community Health Assessment and Planning

For public health practitioners, the most exciting aspect of GIS technology may be its potential to revolutionize the process of community health improvement by improving access to health-related data. Every community or neighborhood has assets and capacities in addition to needs.[41] GIS will enable communities to assess many of these factors, strengths, and weaknesses related to community wellbeing and allow them to evaluate actions they take to improve their health status.[4] This potential is a consequence of several features inherent in GIS.

The relational and overlay features of GIS encourage the rapid incorporation of multiple attribute data sets, including data sets not traditionally viewed as related to public health. Attribute data are available from many sources, both government and commercial.[42] Census data, available from the U.S. Census Bureau, include demographic and socioeconomic data at various levels of geographic resolution. Demographic data, useful as denominator data in calculating rates, contain information on age, gender, race, and ethnicity. Socioeconomic data include educational level, poverty level, employment, and age of housing.[42]

Depending on the state and locality, many data sets are easily obtainable, such as vital statistics data (perinatal and mortality), healthcare expenditures, access to primary care data, hospital discharge data, and behavioral risk factor data.[42] **Table 14.1** lists a few examples of commonly available data sets. Data sets yield varying levels of resolution depending on the data type and summary level. For example, state-level data will not allow comparisons at geographies smaller than states, but census block groups provide a fine-grained comparison. The most flexible type of data is point data, which ascribe attributes to points in space. This allows for summary and analysis at any geographic level.

One vision for community health assessment suggests other data such as high school dropout rates, commuting time, and domestic abuse.[4] Depending on the locality or state, registries not included in Table 14.1 may be available. For example, one study used an out-of-hospital cardiac arrest registry available through the Rochester, New York Emergency Medical Services program to identify clusters of out-of-hospital cardiac arrests.[43] Communities can add data on neighborhood assets, such as local businesses, libraries, social clubs, and religious and cultural organizations.[41,44]

Table 14.1 Types and Potential Sources of Attribute Data

Category (examples)	Source (varies by state)	Level of Analysis (varies by state and locality)
Demographic data (e.g., age, sex, race, and ethnic distribution)	U.S. Bureau of Census	Census block group, county, state
Perinatal indicators by age and population subgroups (e.g., births, repeat births, prenatal care, low birth weight)	State vital statistics	Census block group (if address included on birth certificate), county, state
Pregnancies; abortions	State vital statistics	County (abortion data do not contain street address), state
Mortality (by age and population subgroups) including years of potential life lost	State vital statistics	Census block group if address included on death certificate; otherwise county, state
Hospitalization (causes by age and population subgroup)	Depends on state—may be Medicaid agency	Varies (census block group, ZIP Code, county, state—depending on how residence is reported)
Ambulatory encounter data (by diagnosis age and population subgroup) for Medicaid population	State Medicaid agency	Census block group, county, state
Reportable disease (communicable disease, including sexually transmitted disease, lead poisoning, pesticide exposure)	Local health department, state epidemiologist	Census block group, county, state
Immunization of 2-year olds	Depends on state – may be state health department	Varies
Cancer incidence (by age and population subgroup)	State cancer registry	Census block group, county, state
Behavioral risk factors	Centers for Disease Control and Prevention (CDC)	ZIP Code, state
Youth risk behaviors (Youth Risk Behavior Survey)	CDC, state health department	School (elementary through grade 6, middle school through grade 8, high school through grade 10, school district, state
Synar Reports (reports of tobacco outlet inspections)	Depends on state—agency responsible for alcohol and drug treatment planning	Census block group, county, state
Arrests by residence (causes by age and population subgroup)	County law enforcement (e.g., sheriff's office), state justice department	Census block group, county, state

Sources: Data from Melnick A, Seigal N, Hildner J, et al. Clackamas County Department of Human Services community health mapping engine (CHiME) geographic information systems project. *J Public Health Manag Pract.* 1999;5(2):65; Lee CV, Irving JL. Sources of spatial data for community health planning. *J Public Health Manag Pract.* 1999;5(4):9–13, Table 1.3.

The feature of unlimited scale of analysis is particularly helpful when performing community health assessments and program evaluations in densely populated counties. Large counties often contain many diverse and sizable communities whose borders do not necessarily coincide with county boundaries. As a result, summaries based on these boundaries may not accurately capture community characteristics. For example, a large county may have low teen birth rates compared to the state, whereas several communities within the county may have markedly elevated rates. In this instance, county-level data are not useful in targeting teen pregnancy prevention efforts. Using GIS, public health practitioners and their community partners can analyze and display the data at the local, sub-county, community level. They can compare their teen birth rate measures statistically with state data, national data, and benchmarks. They can also display available resources for teen pregnancy prevention by overlaying physical features such as health and social work facilities, roads, public transit routes, and travel time.[4,45] Over time, they can use the analytic features of GIS to evaluate the outcomes of pregnancy prevention or other public health efforts within their communities.[4]

The flexibility to define community geographically is invaluable in community health planning. GIS software can aggregate data into a variety of geographic definitions, such as high school attendance areas or legislative districts. Likewise, GIS software can aggregate attribute data, such as vital statistics data, into the same areas for analysis. For example, a GIS prototype application analyzed teen birth rates, teen male arrest rates, and adequacy of prenatal care by high school attendance area, and compared these rates with overall county rates, state rates, and benchmarks.[4] Overlays allow users to look at two variables simultaneously so they can visualize spatial patterns and relationships. For example, GIS could depict teen birth rates with Youth Risk Behavior Surveillance System (YRBSS)[46] results for high school attendance areas. Alternatively, those persons interested in improving prenatal care could evaluate the percentage of first trimester care and income level by legislative district.

Another example of a GIS application in public health is its use in Health Impact Assessments (HIAs). Health departments and their local partners are increasing their use of HIAs to evaluate the health impacts of policy decisions related to the built environment.[47] For example, an HIA could estimate the reduction in the risk of injury from traffic crashes associated with a new street design. GIS can aid public health professionals in assessing impacts by identifying areas in which expected impacts coincide with the location of vulnerable populations. In a 2012 HIA conducted in Minnesota, analysts overlaid demographic data, such as racial and ethnic composition, with a map of areas impacted by a new light rail line. This assessment informed the rezoning decisions that accompanied the light rail line, highlighting the consequences of displacing low-income households.[48] The Atlanta Beltline HIA, a similar example, examined the impacts of a land use and parks plan on vulnerable populations by mapping differences in health outcomes across the project area.[49]

GIS programs can be Internet compatible, making them easily accessible. Most communities have access to Internet-capable libraries, where they could create customized maps to meet their needs.[4] GIS Internet packages can be designed for users without formal epidemiologic skills, and tutorials can be added. For example, tutorials can provide explanations of concepts such as incidence rates, prevalence, confidence intervals, and the need for age adjustment when evaluating mortality rates.[4,50]

Perhaps the greatest strength of GIS technology is that its product is a picture.[2] Epidemiologists often portray analyses in formats that are only comprehensible by other epidemiologists. Program managers, policy makers, and others who must act on results need these results in a way they can digest and therefore believe. GIS take complex data and translate them into easily understandable information. This feature promises to enhance collaboration between all partners involved in community health improvement.

Lessons Learned and Challenges

Like any other new technology, GIS comes with limitations and a potential for problems. Limitations include limited availability of data, inconsistent data quality, lack of a trained workforce, and costs. Potential problems include community definitions, confidentiality, and misinterpretation of results.

Data Availability and Quality

As with any analysis, useful GIS output is dependent on useful input. Many commonly used databases, such as mortality data or hospital discharge data, frequently lack an address. Public health professionals will have to encourage their data-sharing partners to include address fields to make their data useful for community health planning. In addition, public health professionals who decide to contract with commercial vendors for geocoding must be careful to select vendors based on match rates, accuracy, and reliability.[51] Encouraging data producers to geocode the data before release will further facilitate incorporation of the data set into effective GIS applications.

Many important data sets are not available, and when they are, users must be careful to evaluate their quality.[2,14] Quantitative information regarding the measured factor, such as environmental hazard exposure, must be present and accurate. Numerator address data may be missing, wrong, or (particularly in rural areas) impossible to match.[2,14] Inaccuracies may exist in denominator data and in the geographic data file, especially if they are outdated. The match rate between geospatial and attribute databases is directly dependent on their quality. Misspellings, empty address fields, and geographic files that are not up to date with the latest road maps lead to low match rates. For example, new housing developments often create new roads that may not be present in an old file. Low match rates, in turn, lead to selection bias in subsequent analyses. Public health professionals need to ensure that GIS users carefully assess and account for these limitations in their analyses. Depending on the quality of the data, unmatched records often need to be evaluated one at a time, a potentially cumbersome process. To solve these problems, agencies, professionals, and commercial vendors using GIS will need to incorporate and adhere to standards for currency, quality, and completeness of data. Government and commercial suppliers will have to provide metadata—data about the data—allowing users to evaluate data quality in relation to these standards.[8,15]

Trained Workforce and Costs

Many local public health departments will have to invest in hardware, software, and trained staff to apply GIS successfully. In a small study conducted by the National Association of County and

City Health Officials (NACCHO) several years ago, the cost to complete relatively small projects was $10,000–$15,000, beyond the reach of many small, rural health departments.[15] Staff time is required to acquire data sets, geocode the data, check the quality of the data, perform the analyses, and answer questions concerning the data. Increasing the availability of geocoded data would help cut this time.[8] For example, if state health departments released geocoded vital statistics data, they would encourage the use of GIS. At the local level, public health departments can reduce costs and improve collaboration by sharing data sets, trained staff, software, and hardware with other community partners. The proprietary nature of some data sources can pose a barrier or cost to public health departments. For example, marketing data and intercensal estimates are often proprietary and must be purchased.

Defining Community

When using GIS for community health improvement, public health officials and their partners will need to be careful and flexible in how they define communities. How to portray a community will be constrained by the quality of the data and the perceptions of those within the depicted community. Although GIS projects can define communities in many geographic ways—ZIP Codes, census tracts, census block groups, high school attendance areas, legislative districts, cities, and counties—in any given situation, all are not equally appropriate.[2] The same data, presented with different geographic boundaries, can result in different interpretations. For example, maps portraying the proportion of homes built before 1950, a risk factor for childhood lead exposure, provide different information when using different geographic levels (see **Figure 14.6**).[52]

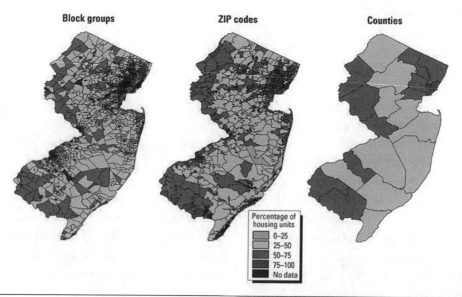

Figure 14.6   Percentages of Homes Built Before 1950 in New Jersey Based on U.S. Census Data Reported at the Block Group Level of Resolution. The Three Major Maps Depict the Same Data at Three Different Scales: U.S. Census Block Group, ZIP Code, and Counties.
Source: Reprinted from Elliot P, Wartenberg D. Spatial epidemiology: current approaches and future challenges. *Environ Health Perspect.* 2004;112(9):998–1006.

Due to the influence of urban areas, compared to the block group and ZIP Code scale maps, the county scale map of pre-1950 overlooks many rural areas with older housing.[52] On a case-by-case basis, public health officials can share their community maps with community partners to obtain comments. Then, using GIS, they can easily redraw the community boundaries, selecting the most appropriate mapping strategy.[2]

Confidentiality

Confidentiality issues pose a significant limitation for public health officials intending to share health-related data with community partners or to place data on the Internet. Data containing personal addresses can be as identifying as data with names. Without appropriate, clear laws, guidelines, and standards regarding confidentiality and data release, health agencies and consumers may be unwilling to provide needed information.[10] Those persons responsible for maintaining the data files should ensure appropriate precautions in order to prevent unauthorized access. Great care and thought must precede the depiction of address data linked to confidential information.

One possible solution is to remove identifiers such as name or address, presenting aggregated data only. State and federal agencies have traditionally reported data aggregated at the county, state, and federal levels. Public health officials can do the same for geocoded community-level data by aggregating it into any selected community definition. For example, public health officials could share GIS software with hospitals unwilling to release discharge data. Local hospitals could then use the wizard to geocode the personal health data and aggregate it by legislative district boundaries. Then, they could remove the personal identifiers such as name and address and release the aggregated data to the public health officials for incorporation into the web-based GIS. In this way, public users would only view data that was aggregated at the legislative district level.

When small numbers (numerator or denominator) are involved, the possibility exists that aggregated data could still be ascribed to individuals. This is particularly true when GIS users stratify their community health analyses by multiple demographic variables, such as gender and ethnicity. To avoid this, public health officials must develop safeguards, built into the software, that restrict the analysis, reporting, and depiction of very small numbers.[4] For example, standards could prohibit the release of a health statistic, such as teen birth rate, if the population denominator (teenage females) were less than 50. If the denominator were a cohort defined by an event, such as all births, a standard could prohibit release of percentage of outcomes (e.g., first trimester care) for a community with fewer than 10 events (births). Alternatively, GIS applications can allow users to analyze data aggregated over 2 or more years when rates for a single year are unstable due to small numbers.

Even if GIS studies do not identify individuals, group disclosure, especially in studies of environmental exposure, can lead to financial risk for individuals in an exposed community, including decreased property values[52] and increased insurance cost.[53] GIS technology is just one more reason to develop a nationally uniform framework of information sharing that protects privacy while permitting public health practice.[2]

Misinterpretation of Results

Ironically, the strength of GIS technology may be its biggest shortfall. The elegance of GIS is that they integrate many complex data sets into an easily understandable picture—a map. Because of this, GIS technology is becoming available to a diversity of users, many with little understanding of public health and epidemiologic principles. Many determinants of health, such as age, ethnicity, socioeconomic status, and education, cluster geographically. Consequently, most GIS analyses will find an association between geography and health outcomes. Usually, however, these outcomes will cluster geographically because of underlying population characteristics, not because of the geography itself. Users without epidemiologic training may be tempted to misinterpret why geographic clustering is occurring, often as proof of a pet theory.[2]

The conflicting analyses of the 1854 London cholera epidemic provide a perfect example. For John Snow, geographic analysis of cholera death clustering implicated the Broad Street pump. However, using the same data, the England General Board of Health was convinced that nocturnal vapors from the Thames River were responsible.

As a communication and analysis tool, increased access to spatial data holds tremendous potential for translating research findings to policy actions. For example, a map showing differences in access to parks is a fast and effective planning tool for elected officials. However, as GIS technology becomes more widely available, inexperienced users, including those in policy-making positions, may be tempted to make individual-level inferences from ecologic data and make false assumptions concerning the nature of associations between exposure and health.[2,14] The job of public health officials is to ensure that any interpretation of geographically referenced health data looks beyond maps to a wider range of analytic tools. For example, a superficial analysis of the geographic variation in childhood asthma hospitalization rates could have led to the conclusion that different populations have different burdens of illness. Closer study revealed that geographic variation in hospital bed supply and hospital proximity, not asthma itself, were independent predictors of admission.[54]

Public health officials can help prevent these mistakes by building safeguards into Internet-based GIS applications. For example, pop-up help screens could contain messages discussing the concept of ecologic fallacy and the need for caution about drawing conclusions when cause-and-effect relationships have not been established previously.[4,50] In addition, built-in links to appropriate county health officials would allow inexperienced users to obtain consultation.

Getting Started with GIS

Before a local health department invests in a GIS application, it should determine whether it really needs the application or if other, cheaper alternatives might suffice.[55] For example, a small jurisdiction with limited resources and small numbers of residents may not benefit from a detailed geographic analysis. In many cases, other local government or private agencies may have already developed a GIS application and would welcome partnership with the local health department.

Future Outlook: GIS and the Role of Public Health Officials

As GIS technology evolves and becomes more widely available, the role of public health officials will undoubtedly evolve with it. Many more data sets—containing information on a broad range of social, demographic, and health-related data—will become available on the web. The same information now available only to public health officials will become available to the public.[56]

Rather than posing a threat, the new technology poses incredible opportunities for public health officials and their communities. GIS technology is eminently compatible with the core public functions of assessment, policy development, and assurance.[57] Public health managers will have many important roles to play, such as building data systems, mobilizing community partnerships, serving as resources, inserting (and teaching) science, and ultimately facilitating community health improvement.

Building Data Systems and Mobilizing Community Partnerships

GIS will encourage public health officials and communities to form partnerships to assess community health status. Through dialogue with their public health partners, communities will decide what data are relevant for community health improvement. Public health officials will then help obtain the data sets and incorporate them into an effective assessment system. They will essentially create a "one-stop" shopping data system, eliminating the need for users to search for data from multiple sources.

An example of one such application is the food retail database developed in Clark County, Washington. Public health assessment staff joined with local food safety inspectors to categorize food retail establishments as grocery stores, supermarkets, convenience stores, full-service restaurants, and fast food restaurants (see **Figure 14.7**). This data set allowed the agency to assess differences in access to food across the jurisdiction, and offers potential for linking to other data, such as BRFSS[58] survey responses.

Diffusing the Technology, Serving as Resources, and Inserting the Science

Public health officials who want dialogue and strengthened relationships with local communities and who want to develop policy through collaboration will have to make health information readily available. The information will have to be of high quality and adequately referenced. Health officials at all levels—local, state, and federal—will have to work with their public and private partners to develop guidelines for metadata. These guidelines should include standards for geocoding and data quality. In addition, health officials at all levels will have a responsibility, with their public and private partners, to develop guidelines on data sharing and confidentiality. Adequate guidelines should lead to the development of new and improved data sets, such as morbidity data, that will be relevant to every community.

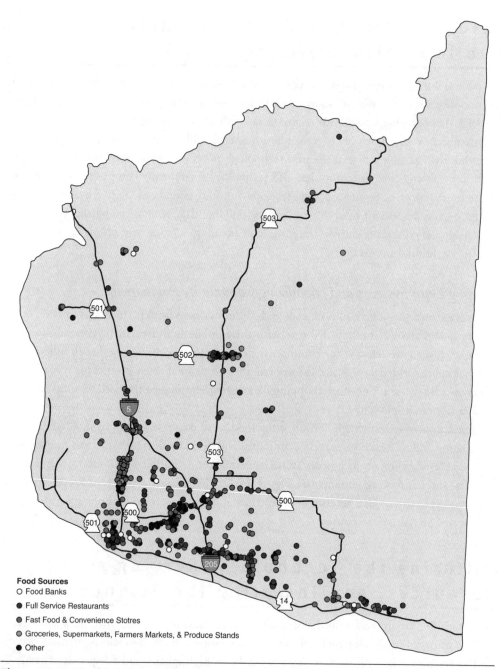

Food Sources
○ Food Banks
● Full Service Restaurants
● Fast Food & Convenience Stotres
◉ Groceries, Supermarkets, Farmers Markets, & Produce Stands
● Other

Figure 14.7 Food Retail Locations, 2011
Source: Clark County Public Health.

Once data become readily available, public health officials will have an additional responsibility to work with their partners in teaching them basic concepts in epidemiology and ensuring that they use the data appropriately. Fortunately, GIS are compatible with existing community planning tools, such as Mobilizing for Action through Planning and Partnership (MAPP)[59] and the Protocol for Assessing Community Excellence in Environmental Health (PACE EH), are compatible with GIS.[60]

In many communities, a major issue has been how to assess community health given the chaotic location of health-related data. Consequently, many states and communities have amassed data on interactive Internet sites that permit community partners to assess health and health-related issues, including the social determinants of health, at the county, and in some cases, neighborhood level. Each of these websites has strengths and weaknesses, as indicated in **Table 14.2**. These activities accelerated in 2010 with the development of the U.S. Department of Health and

Table 14.2   Interactive Internet Sites for Community Health Issues

Jurisdiction	Description
South Carolina Department of Health and Environment, Division of Biostatistics and Health GIS http://scangis.dhec.sc.gov	User can select from births, deaths, cancer, teen pregnancy, childhood lead poisoning, fetal deaths, hospital discharge, infant mortality, health disparities initiative, etc. using multiple combinations of variables. Output is a table with options for a variety of charts. The output appears as a pop-up window, taking some time to generate. Users can create choropleth maps by ZIP Code, county, or Department of Health and Environmental Control (DHEC) region. The user specifies quartiles or quintiles. The legend title includes rate denominator, interstates, and county boundaries—user may add senate or house districts. Map prints with legend and title, but does not save as image.
Florida Department of Health Community Health Assessment Resource Tool Set (CHARTS) http://www.floridacharts.com/charts/default.aspx	Users create maps of vital statistics data and census data. The user interface is a bit clunky, and users can map only one variable at a time. The application provides good labeling and user tools. Vital statistics are available in 5-year aggregations. Users can choose an entire state or county; map shows variables down to tract level. Identify tool shows census profile for a selected county. Map can be saved as html including title, legend, and disclaimers and printed up to 34 × 44".
Georgia Online Analytical Statistical Information System (OASIS) http://oasis.state.ga.us/oasis/	Users can create maps of vital statistics, hospital discharge, emergency room visit, STD, motor vehicle crash, population, and other data. Depending on the data set, analysis available by year or aggregates of several years; also some data available only at district or county level can be performed by year or aggregated over several years. Some data not available after 2007. Users can also create maps of automobile crashes at the county level by severity and environmental conditions (2008 and earlier).
Baltimore Neighborhood Indicators Alliance http://www.bniajfi.org/	Data are available for 55 Community Statistical Areas (CSAs). "Clusters of Baltimore neighborhoods have been created along census tract boundaries to form 55 CSAs. This clustering was necessary for the creation of statistical areas since most of the 270+ neighborhoods in Baltimore City do not have boundaries that fall along census tracts." User can choose choropleths of indicators (one at a time) for census data, crime data, housing, sanitation, etc. Health-related data are available at the community level in table format only.

(continues)

Table 14.2   Interactive Internet Sites for Community Health Issues (continued)

Jurisdiction	Description
Network for a Healthy California—GIS Map Viewer http://www.cnngis.org/	Provides online viewing of mapped health data, including nutrition and school programs, WIC grocery stores, and demographics.
Sonoma County Network of Care http://sonoma.networkofcare.org/ph/index.aspx	Data for a variety of "dashboard" indicators are available at the county level, with a limited number of measures available at ZIP Code levels. Indicators include health data and data related to social determinants of health, such as employment and housing. Users can compare Sonoma indicators with other counties and the state. Mapping and analysis at other geographic levels are not available
California Environmental Health Tracking Program http://www.ehib.org/page.jsp?page_key=65	Contains online geocoding service allowing registered users to geocode attribute data to points and political boundaries, including census block groups; has tools for mapping pesticide use at township and section levels; has tool for mapping drinking water system boundaries; another tool allows users to evaluate traffic volume by various buffers around point locations. Several forms of health outcome data are available but most available only at county or ZIP Code level. Some maternal and child health data are available at census tract.

Human Services (HHS) Community Health Initiative and passage of the Patient Protection and Affordable Care Act (ACA). The goal of the HHS initiative, "Putting Data and Innovation to Work to Help Communities and Consumers Improve Health," was to provide free public access to health-related data in several formats, including an online data warehouse.[61] In addition, the initiative encouraged local communities and states to add locally generated data, and it encouraged the development of applications for data analysis and display. The ACA requires nonprofit hospitals to conduct a community health needs assessment every 3 years as a condition for maintaining their nonprofit status.[62] Subsequently, private vendors began developing Internet-based assessment applications, including applications involving GIS technology, for use by hospitals, public health governmental agencies, and community partners, such as the Network of Care community health websites. One example, the Sonoma County Network of Care website (see Table 14.2) features a data warehouse containing a variety of health-related data and data related to the social determinants of health, including education, employment, housing, transportation and environmental conditions. Most of these communities are just beginning to add health data at the sub-county level, mostly by ZIP Code, and many will be looking to their local governmental public health partners for support in analysis and interpretation.

Facilitating Community Health Improvement

Like other analytic tools, the greatest promise of GIS technology lies in raising additional questions rather than in coming up with answers. The map will begin or advance, but not end, the process of community health improvement. In this way, the development of GIS and other new technologies may change the fundamental roles of public health officials. The public health professional of the 21st century will work closely with his or her community partners to ask questions about community health at the neighborhood level. Together, they will use the new technology to develop neighborhood-based programs that rely on community strengths and meet community needs. Public health officials will serve as resources and facilitators in gathering data, ensuring data quality, and inviting their partners to the community health improvement table. As the technology and information become more available, public health officials will lead the way in promoting assessment, policy development, and assurance as community responsibilities rather than government responsibilities.

Discussion Questions

1. Besides the software itself, what are the basic components of a public health GIS application, and how are they obtainable?
2. What are the potential benefits of the use of GIS technology?
3. For what health issues would you consider using GIS?
4. How could you use GIS in evaluating health equity?
5. Describe the steps you would take to create a map of a specific health issue. In doing so, how might you use the tools commonly available?
6. What are the pitfalls involved in the use of this technology?
7. Describe a situation where you would not use GIS technology and discuss why.
8. How would you use GIS in conducting health impact assessments?
9. What do you consider the future uses of GIS, and what is the role of public health officials in ensuring the appropriate use of the technology?

References

1. Snow J. *On the Mode of Communication of Cholera.* 2nd ed. New York: Commonwealth Fund; 1936.
2. Melnick AL, Fleming DW. Modern geographic information systems—promise and pitfalls. *J Public Health Manag Pract.* 1999;5(2):viii–x.
3. Roper WL, Mays GP. GIS in public health policy: a new frontier for improving community health. *J Public Health Manag Pract.* 1999;5(2):vi–vii.
4. Melnick A, Seigal N, Hildner J, et al. Clackamas County Department of Human Services Community Health Mapping Engine (CHiME) Geographic Information Systems Project. *J Public Health Manag Pract.* 1999;5(2):64–9
5. Clarke KC, McLafferty SL, Tempalski BJ. On epidemiology and geographic information systems: a review and discussion of future directions. *Emerg Infect Dis.* 1996;2(2):85–92.
6. Haklay M, Singleton A, Parker C. Web mapping 2.0: the neogeography of the geoweb. *Geography Compass.* 2008;2(6):2011–39.
7. Tim US. The application of GIS in environmental health sciences: opportunities and limitations. *Environ Res.* 1995;71:75–88.
8. Rogers MY. Getting started with geographic information systems (GIS): a local health department perspective, *J Public Health Manag Pract.* 1999;5(4):22–33.
9. Wilkinson S, Gobalet JG, Majoros M, et al. Lead hot zones and childhood lead poisoning cases, Santa Clara County, California, *J Public Health Manag Pract.* 1995 5(2):11–2.

10. Croner CM, Sperling J, Broome FR. Geographic information systems (GIS): new perspectives in understanding human health and environmental relationships. *Stat Med.* 1996;15:1961–77.

11. McLafferty S, Cromley E. Your first mapping project on your own: from A to Z. *J Public Health Manag Pract.* 1999;5(2):76–82.

12. Melnick AL. *Introduction to Geographic Information Systems in Public Health.* Sudbury, MA: Jones and Bartlett Publishers; 2002.

13. Duclos C, Johnson T, Thompson T. Development of childhood blood lead screening guidelines, Duval County, Florida, 1998. *J Public Health Manag Pract.* 1999;5(2):9–10.

14. Vine MF, Degnan D, Hanchette C. Geographic information systems: their use in environmental epidemiologic research. *Environ Health Perspect.* 1997;105(6):598–605.

15. Bouton PH, Fraser M. Local health departments and GIS: the perspective of the national association of county and city health officials. *J Public Health Manag Pract.* 1999;5(4):33–41.

16. Moore LV, Diez Roux AV, Nettleton JA, et al. Associations of the local food environment with diet quality—a comparison of assessments based on surveys and geographic information systems: the multi-ethnic study of atherosclerosis. *Am J Epidemiol.* 2008;167:917–24.

17. Nuckols JR, Ward MH, Jarup L. Using geographic information systems for exposure assessment in environmental epidemiology studies. *Environ Health Perspect.* 2004;112(9):1007–15.

18. Dolk H, Vrijheid M, Armstrong B, et al. Risk of congenital anomalies near hazardous-waste landfill sites in Europe: the EUROHAZCON study. *Lancet.* 1998;352(9126):423–7.

19. Fielder HMP, PoonKing CM, Palmer SR, et al. Assessment of impact on health of residents living near the Nant-Gwyddon landfill site: retrospective analysis. *BMJ.* 2000;320:19–22.

20. Braud T, Nouer S, Lamar K. Residential proximity to toxic release sites and the implications for low birth weight and premature delivery. *J Environ Health.* 2011;73:8–13.

21. Ralston M. Elevated nitrate levels in relation to bedrock depth, Linn County, Iowa, 1991–1996. *J Public Health Manag Pract.* 1999;5(2):39–40.

22. Reif JS, Burch JB, Nuckols JR, et al. Neurobehavioral effects of exposure to trichloroethylene through a municipal water supply. *Environ Res.* 2003;93(3):248–58.

23. Poulstrup A, Hansen HL. Use of GIS and exposure modeling as tools in a study of cancer incidence in a population exposed to airborne dioxin. *Environ Health Perspect.* 2004;112(9):1032–6.

24. Oyana TJ, Rogerson P, Lwebuga-Mukasa JS. Geographic clustering of adult asthma hospitalization and residential exposure to pollution at a United States-Canada border crossing. *Am J Public Health.* 2004;94(7):1250–7.

25. Cook AG, DeVos AJ, Pereira G, et al. Use of a total traffic county metric to investigate the impact of roadways on asthma severity: a case-control study. *Environ Health.* 2011;10:52.

26. Volk HE, Hertz-Picciotto I, Delwiche L, et al. Residential proximity to freeways and autism in the CHARGE Study. *Environ Health Perspect.* 2011;119(6):863–77.

27. Henriques WD, Spengler RF. Locations around the Hanford Nuclear Facility where average milk consumption by children in 1945 would have resulted in an estimated median iodine-131 dose to the thyroid of 10 rad or higher, Washington. *J Public Health Manag Pract.,* 1999;5(2):35–6.

28. Bellander T, Berglind N, Gustavsson P, et al. Using geographic information systems to assess individual historical exposure to air pollution from traffic and house heating in Stockholm. *Environ Health Perspect.* 2001;109(6):633–9.

29. Nyberg F, Gustavsson P, Jarup L, et al. Urban air pollution and lung cancer in Stockholm. *Epidemiol.* 2000;11(5):487–95.

30. Dolinoy DC, Miranda ML. GIS modeling of air toxics releases from TRI-reporting and non-TRI-reporting facilities: impacts for environmental justice. *Environ Health Perspect.* 2004;112(17):1717–24.

31. Aguilera I, Guxens M, Garcia-Esteban R, et al. Association between GIS-Based exposure to urban air pollution during pregnancy and birth weight in the INMA Sabadell Cohort. *Environ Health Perspect.* 2009;117(8):1322–7.

32. Sheppard E, Leitner H, McMaster RB, Tian H. GIS-based measures of environmental equity: exploring their sensitivity and significance. *J Expo Anal Environ Epidemiol.* 1999;9:18–28.

33. Zartarian BG, Schultz BD, Barzyk TM, et al. The Environmental Protection Agency's Community-Focused Exposure and Risk Screening Tool (C-FERST) and its potential use for environmental justice efforts. *Am J Public Health*. 2011;101(Suppl 1):S286–94.

34. Glass GE, Schwartz BS, Morgan JM 3rd, et al. Environmental risk factors for Lyme disease identified with geographic information systems. *Am J Public Health*. 1995;85(7):944–8.

35. Gallagher LG, Webster TF, Aschengrau A, et al. Using residential history and groundwater modeling to examine drinking water exposure and breast cancer. *Environ Health Perspect*. 2010;118(6):749–55.

36. Openshaw S, Wymer C, Craft A. A mark 1 geographical analysis machine for the automated analysis of point data sets. *Int J Geographic Information Systems*. 1987;1(4):335–8.

37. Wang F. Spatial clusters of cancers in Illinois 1986–2000. *J Med Systems*. 2004;28(3):237–56.

38. Wu J, Wang J, Meng B, et al. Exploratory spatial data analysis for the identification of risk factors to birth defects. *BMC Public Health*. 2004;18(4):23.

39. Hendryx M, Fedorko E, Anesetti-Rothermel A. A geographical information system-based analysis of cancer mortality and population exposure to coal mining activities in West Virginia, United States of America. *Geospat Health*. 2010;4(2):243–56.

40. Guajardo O, Oyana TJ. A critical assessment of geographic clusters of breast and lung cancer incidences among residents living near the Tittabawassee and Saginaw Rivers, Michigan, USA. *J Environ Public Health*. 2009;2009:1–16.

41. McKnight JL, Kretzman JP. *Mapping Community Capacity. The Asset-Based Community Development Institute. Institute for Policy Research* (Rev. 1996). Evanston, IL: Northwestern University; 1990.

42. Lee CV, Irving JL. Sources of spatial data for community health planning. *J Public Health Manag Pract*. 1999;5(4):7–22.

43. Lerner EB, Fairbanks RJ, Shah MN. Identification of out-of-hospital cardiac arrest clusters using a geographic information system. *Acad Emerg Med*. 2005;12(1):81–4.

44. Mason M, Cheung I, Walker L. Substance use, social networks, and the geography of urban adolescents. *Substance Use Misuse*. 2004;39(10–12):1751–77.

45. Gordon A, Womersley J. The use of mapping in public health and planning health services. *J Public Health Med*. 1997;19(2):139–47.

46. Centers for Disease Control and Prevention. Youth Risk Behavior Surveillance System (YRBSS). Available at: http://www.cdc.gov/HealthyYouth/yrbs/index.htm. Accessed February 28, 2013.

47. National Research Council of the National Academies, Committee on Health Impact Assessment. *Improving Health in the United State: The Role of Health Impact Assessment*. Washington, DC: National Academies Press; 2011.

48. Malekafzali S, Bergstrom D. Healthy corridor for all: a community health impact assessment of transit-oriented development policy in Saint Paul, Minnesota. Available at: http://www.healthimpactproject.org/news/project/body/Healthy-Corridor-Technical-Report_FINAL.pdf. Accessed February 28, 2013.

49. Ross CL, Leone de Nie K, Dannenberg AL, et al. Health Impact Assessment of the Atlanta Beltline. *Am J Prev Med*. 2012;42(3):203–13.

50. Morgenstern H. Ecologic studies. In: Rothman KJ, Greenland S, eds. *Modern Epidemiology*. 2nd ed. Philadelphia: Lippincott-Raven Publishers; 1998:459–80.

51. Whitsel EA, Rose KM, Wood JL, et al. Accuracy and repeatability of commercial geocoding. *Am J Epidemiol*. 2004;160(10):1023–9.

52. Elliot P, Wartenburg D. Spatial epidemiology: current approaches and future challenges. *Environ Health Perspect*. 2004;112(9):998–1006.

53. Cox LH. Protecting confidentiality in small population health and environmental statistics. *Stat Med*. 1996;15:1895–905.

54. Goodman DC, Wennberg JE. Maps and health: the challenges of interpretation. *J Public Health Manag Pract*. 1999;5(4):xiii–xvii.

55. Thrall SE. Geographic information system (GIS) hardware and software. *J Public Health Manag Pract*. 1999;5(2):82–90.

56. Thrall GI. The future of GIS in public health management and practice. *J Public Health Manag Pract*. 1999;5(4):75–82.

57. Institute of Medicine. *The Future of Public Health*. Washington, DC: National Academies Press; 1988.

58. Centers for Disease Control and Prevention. Behavioral Risk Factor Surveillance System (BRFSS). Available at: http://www.cdc.gov/brfss/. Accessed March 1, 2013.

59. National Association of County and City Health Officials. Mobilizing Action through Planning and Partnership (MAPP). Available at: http://www.naccho.org/topics/infrastructure/MAPP.cfm. Accessed February 28, 2013.

60. National Association of County and City Health Officials. *PACE EH Demonstration Site Project: Communities in Action, January 2005*. Available at: http://www.naccho.org/topics/environmental/documents/PACE_EH_proof.pdf. Accessed November 20, 2005.

61. U.S. Department of Health and Human Services. *Putting data and innovation to work to help communities and consumers improve health*. Available at: http://www.hhs.gov/news/press/2010pres/06/20100602a.html. Accessed February 28, 2013.

62. Internal Revenue Services. *New requirements for 501(c)(3) hospitals under the Affordable Care Act*. Available at: http://www.irs.gov/Charities-&-Non-Profits/Charitable-Organizations/New-Requirements-for-501%28c%29%283%29-Hospitals-Under-the-Affordable-Care-Act. Accessed February 28, 2013.

Public Health Surveillance

Benjamin Silk and Ruth Berkelman

LEARNING OBJECTIVES

- To understand the purposes of public health surveillance
- To gain an appreciation for the importance of surveillance in public health
- To become familiar with the framework of surveillance and some of its technology
- To better understand the knowledge and skills needed for effective surveillance
- To gain awareness of the range of stakeholders, especially for the community being studied

Chapter Overview

Surveillance is a primary mechanism through which public health organizations acquire information concerning population health. Surveillance approaches vary widely in both structure and function. Consequently, the optimal system design is contingent on an organization's specific information needs and resources as well as the characteristics of the populations and health issues under study. In developing and maintaining surveillance systems, public health administrators must use current epidemiologic knowledge in tandem with effective managerial strategies.

Public health **surveillance** is a primary mechanism through which health agencies generate and process information for use in management, policy, and practice. Effective public health management requires an iterative cycle of formulating objectives, designing and implementing interventions, measuring the impact of programs, and using that information to revise program interventions and objectives. Described as the "continuous and systematic collection, analysis, interpretation and dissemination of descriptive information for monitoring health problems,"[1, p. 435] surveillance provides essential input for this cycle. Public health surveillance data allow organizations to measure the prevalence of risk factors and healthy behaviors, monitor the effects of interventions, and assess trends in disease and other health outcomes.[2] Conclusions drawn from this information process are used for decision making and action at multiple levels of the public health and healthcare systems.

This chapter provides an overview of surveillance systems and strategies that are relevant to the public health administrator. The first section describes the various functions that surveillance systems serve in public health and the common forms of surveillance. This is followed by an overview of key design and operation considerations, including administrative and managerial activities to maintain surveillance programs. Readers seeking a more detailed discussion of public health surveillance are directed to other texts written for epidemiologists and others responsible for surveillance operations.[3–8]

Function and Form of Public Health Surveillance Systems

Functions: What Purpose Does Surveillance Serve?

Although surveillance originally signified monitoring contacts of persons with communicable diseases for onset of symptoms,[9] public health surveillance applications expanded dramatically in the second half of the 20th century.[10] Surveillance systems now monitor infectious and chronic disease, injury and disability, occupational health and safety, environmental exposures, maternal and child health, health awareness and behavior, and the use of healthcare services.

Surveillance activities support public health management at many levels, beginning with the establishment of health objectives. Health officers rely on surveillance data to select targets for public health action, including populations at higher risk for morbidity and mortality and associated risk factors (e.g., tobacco use, physical inactivity, microbial infection, and exposure to toxic agents). Further, public health officers use surveillance to monitor the effects of changes in healthcare practice and policy.[11] For example, documented underutilization of preventive health services, such as immunization or early disease detection through screening, may point to the need for public health intervention to increase the use of these services. Once officials establish priorities for public health interventions, they continue to rely on surveillance data to design and direct specific programs. Surveillance provides information about the characteristics of people most affected by health conditions and the communities to which they belong. Programs can be formulated to reach targeted populations and address health priorities. With interventions operationalized, surveillance data can also be used to measure program impact. By analyzing trends in specific outcomes, policy makers evaluate whether their program is achieving its desired effect. Surveillance data can then support programmatic decision making about whether interventions should be continued, modified, expanded, or terminated.

Surveillance systems often identify emerging public health problems and epidemics, triggering more intensive surveillance, public health investigation, and disease-control interventions. A 1999 outbreak of salmonellosis in the United States serves as an example.[12] (*Salmonella* infection can cause diarrhea, abdominal cramping, fever, and dehydration.) Health officials in

Washington state were notified of 85 cases of salmonellosis that occurred between June 10 and July 9, 1999. An investigation revealed that 67 cases had consumed a particular brand of unpasteurized orange juice. Meanwhile, in Oregon 57 cases of salmonellosis were identified by health officials; all had occurred in the latter half of June. Thirty-nine cases drank the same brand of orange juice. After collaborative investigations by the two states and discussions with the U.S. Food and Drug Administration (FDA), the manufacturer voluntarily issued a recall of the juice. Further investigations identified *Salmonella* in samples of the juice, dispensers in restaurants, and the juice factory. Smaller outbreaks among individuals who drank the juice during the same period were reported in 13 other states.

Surveillance systems can monitor large cohorts over time, producing databases that contain longitudinal information on disease occurrence and revealing issues that warrant an in-depth investigation through formal epidemiologic research. The U.S. Renal Data System (USRDS), which tracks outcomes related to end-stage renal disease (ESRD) in the United States, exemplifies the broad scope of surveillance (http://www.usrds.org). The goals of the USRDS include monitoring trends in the frequency of ESRD-related morbidity and mortality and providing a foundation for research through the provision of national datasets.[11] To achieve these goals, the system integrates data from the Centers for Medicare and Medicaid Services (CMS), the United Network for Organ Sharing (UNOS), the Centers for Disease Control and Prevention (CDC), the ESRD networks, and special USRDS studies.[13] Data on demographics, clinical measures, biochemical laboratory testing results, dialysis and transplantation, and all other medical services reported as Medicaid claims are used to generate a comprehensive Annual Data Report, also known as the Atlas of End-Stage Renal Disease in the United States.[14] The report demonstrates that inclusion of data on incident (new) and prevalent (existing) diseases and conditions may be important for monitoring chronic disease trends (**Figure 15.1**). The number of incident

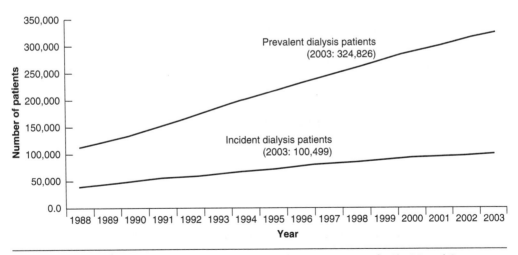

Figure 15.1   Trends in Incident and Prevalent Dialysis Patient Counts for the United States, 1988–2003
Source: Adapted from the U.S. Renal Data System (USRDS). 2005. ADR/Atlas. Available at: http://usrds.org/atlas.htm.

dialysis patients increased gradually from 1988 to 2003 in the United States. Because the number of prevalent patients is a function of the incidence and duration of the condition, prevalence increased markedly in the same period.

Surveillance System Forms

Surveillance systems take on a variety of forms depending on the health-related events being monitored, the availability of resources, and each system's intended purposes. Several references have characterized sources of health-related information that are either obtained from surveillance systems or used for public health surveillance.[2,15] Major types of surveillance approaches and their strengths and weaknesses are described in the following sections.

Notifiable Disease Reporting

Public health agencies monitor diseases, conditions, and events of importance by designating them as notifiable, thereby requiring persons with knowledge of their occurrence to report. Most **notifiable diseases** are communicable, though other occurrences, including animal bites, birth defects, cancer diagnoses, elevated blood lead levels, poisonings, and illness clusters, are often reportable.[16] Typically, clinicians, infection control professionals, and laboratories report patients whose clinical descriptions and laboratory diagnoses meet case definitions for the diseases under surveillance.[17] In the United States, states have the legal authority to mandate reporting of notifiable diseases.[18] Although each state's list of notifiable diseases varies in accordance with local public health priorities, the majority of states and territories require reporting of most nationally notifiable diseases. In collaboration with the CDC, the list of nationally notifiable diseases is revised yearly by the Council of State and Territorial Epidemiologists (CSTE), whose members include the state epidemiologists responsible for collection and use of notifiable diseases data within their jurisdictions.

Infectious disease reporting operates through collaborations at multiple levels. At the local level, public health officials maintain communication with reporting sources and use disease reports to initiate prevention and control measures (e.g., chemoprophylaxis of close contacts and outbreak investigation). States' organizational structures vary, but state health departments generally support local surveillance activities and consolidate notifiable disease reports from city, county, or district public health agencies and directly from reporting sources. Since 1925, all states have voluntarily transmitted notifiable diseases data to the U.S. Public Health Service; the CDC currently oversees the National Notifiable Diseases Surveillance System (NNDSS). The CDC disseminates the NNDSS data from the states, territories, and large metropolitan areas via the *Morbidity and Mortality Weekly Report* (*MMWR*; http://www.cdc.gov/mmwr) and yearly summaries of notifiable diseases.

With few exceptions,[19] notifiable disease surveillance systems collectively encompass the United States in its geographic entirety. The systems link public health agencies to healthcare providers who may be the first to become aware of problems in the surveillance system's jurisdiction. For example, the disease that came to be known as acquired immunodeficiency syndrome (AIDS) was first reported in the United States by clinicians with ties to the Los Angeles County

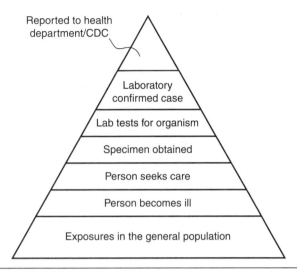

Figure 15.2   CDC's Burden of Illness Pyramid: Underascertainment of Food-Borne Illness in Notifiable Diseases Surveillance
Source: Adapted from Centers for Disease Control and Prevention. FoodNet Surveillance–Burden of Illness Pyramid. Available at: http://www.cdc.gov/foodnet/surveillance_pages/burden_pyramid.htm.

Department of Public Health.[20] The notifiable disease reporting approach also has recognized weaknesses. Reporting completeness varies considerably because many diseases are treated empirically without etiologic diagnosis (e.g., community-acquired pneumonia) and because systems often rely on voluntarily reporting by participants.[21,22] The CDC's burden of illness pyramid illustrates how reported cases of food-borne illnesses are a small fraction of the total number of illnesses under surveillance (**Figure 15.2**). Reporting is the culmination of a series of conditional events (e.g., laboratory confirmation, laboratory testing). Because each event is dependent on preceding events, absent or delayed events imply that receipt of morbidity and mortality reports will also be absent or delayed.

Sentinel Surveillance

Sentinel surveillance commonly refers to convenience sampling of data that are designed to characterize the magnitude of a public health problem in a larger population. Two components of influenza surveillance in the United States demonstrate how sentinel reporting can be useful.[23] The U.S. Influenza Sentinel Providers Surveillance Network monitors weekly morbidity through state-based networks of clinicians who report age group–specific counts of influenza-like illness (ILI) and corresponding denominators (i.e., total number of clinic visits). Proportions of patient visits for ILI have been a useful surrogate for reporting of confirmed influenza cases. The CDC compiles these morbidity data weekly, monitoring influenza activity regionally and nationally by tracking deviations from baseline levels. The CDC tracks weekly influenza mortality via the 122 Cities Mortality Reporting System. By reporting the number of deaths due to pneumonia and influenza and the total number of deaths occurring in 122 cities and metropolitan areas, sentinel data are used to monitor mortality patterns and assess the severity of circulating influenza virus strains.

The generalizability of the sentinel reporting data depends on how closely the populations served by the sentinel providers represent the general population. Public health agencies can increase generalizability by selecting participants who serve diverse geographic and demographic population strata. Although population-based incidence and prevalence rates cannot be obtained, sentinel surveillance may provide timely and cost-effective data. Sentinel networks can also facilitate acquisition of clinical specimens and isolates, which has been particularly valuable for infectious disease programs. Applications in the United States have included tracking drug-resistant gonorrhea, determining relatedness and relative frequencies of tuberculosis (TB) strains, and matching annual influenza vaccines to circulating viral subtypes.

Sentinel surveillance has another form. A sentinel health event refers to a disease or condition for which the occurrence of even a single case warns that improvements in preventive measures are warranted.[1,24] Sentinel health events include illness or injury considered avoidable, death deemed "untimely," and rare disease with a known, specific risk factor. In the United States, a single case of polio or a maternal death are sentinel events that warrant close scrutiny. The CDC's National Institute for Occupational Safety and Health (NIOSH) uses sentinel surveillance to monitor the occurrence of selected serious injuries, exposures, illnesses, and deaths in the workplace.[25] The sentinel health event approach shares the timeliness and cost-effectiveness advantages of sentinel reporting, but also requires motivated reporters. As with notifiable disease reporting, sentinel health reporting can trigger public health investigations.

Syndromic Surveillance

A primary aim of **syndromic surveillance** has been early outbreak detection, which can create the opportunity for rapid intervention to interrupt infectious disease transmission and prevent morbidity and mortality. Rather than monitor specific clinical diagnoses (the essence of notifiable disease reporting), syndromic surveillance is intended to identify early signals of increased illness frequency within a population. A syndromic surveillance system may track behavioral data (e.g., absenteeism, over-the-counter medicine purchases) or prediagnostic, clinical data (e.g., emergency department chief complaints, requests for laboratory testing). The term *syndromic surveillance* originates here: many syndromic systems tally sets of signs and symptoms into defined syndromes (e.g., gastrointestinal, respiratory, and neurologic illnesses). Syndromic surveillance is based on the notion that patients' signs and symptoms, such as fever, cough, and fatigue, will manifest and cluster in data captured by the system, triggering a public health investigation before a subset of patients with rapid symptom onset following infection are diagnosed and reported (**Figure 15.3**).[26] This rationale also recognizes that infectious diseases are frequently treated without assigning etiologic diagnoses (a noted weakness of notifiable disease reporting).[27] In fact, syndrome surveillance has been used for many years in settings where laboratory diagnosis is not generally sought.

Like all surveillance approaches, syndromic surveillance requires collection, processing, analysis, and interpretation of health indicator data.[28] Each step has alternatives, so syndromic

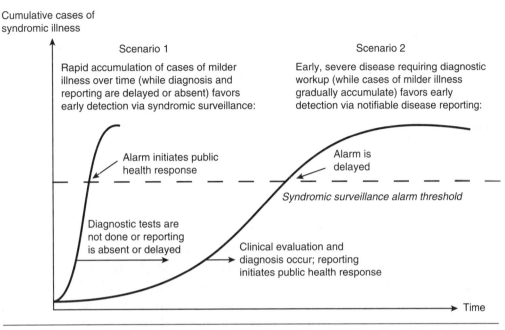

Figure 15.3   Number of Cumulative Cases of Syndromic Illness by Time for a Hypothetical, Unrecognized Infectioius Disease Outbreak; Two Scenarios for Early Detection
Source: Adapted from Buehler JW, Berkelman RL, Hartley DM, Peters CJ. Syndromic surveillance and bioterrorism-related epidemics. *Emerg Infect Dis.* 2003;9:1197–1204.

surveillance systems are diverse in form. Technology has made automated data transfer and real-time monitoring of electronic health information a hallmark of many syndromic surveillance systems. Connecting information systems, however, requires expertise, stakeholder support, and privacy and security safeguards. Processing indicator data often entails consolidation of data sources and standardization of data elements. The analyst focuses on detection of aberrations, which exist when the frequency of observed events differs statistically from an expected frequency; analysis and aberration detection are frequently aided by mapping and graphical display of the data. Event frequencies that exceed a statistical threshold within a defined time period, geography, or time and space are deemed significant, and sound an "alarm." Interpretation of the alarm may require further analysis before initiating an investigation. In other words, a true outbreak may or may not be occurring when an aberration is detected.

Federal funding, including CDC cooperative agreements for state and local bioterrorism preparedness, as well as technology-driven opportunities to transport and manipulate large amounts of health-related data,[29] have contributed to a proliferation of syndromic surveillance systems in the United States. Meanwhile, the relative merit of this surveillance approach has been disputed. Calibrating statistical thresholds to detect outbreaks with sensitivity, while reducing false alarms, has been a major challenge facing operational systems. Other concerns include the costs and resource diversions associated with implementing and maintaining syndromic surveillance when alternatives for enhancing infectious disease surveillance exist,[30] the large number of factors that influence how a covert attack of bioterrorism would initially be detected (e.g., natural history of the disease),[26] and the need for more critical research and evaluation.[31] Syndromic surveillance systems have detected naturally occurring outbreaks (e.g., diarrheal illness), have provided assurance that outbreaks are not occurring, and may be useful for monitoring known outbreaks. The growing collective wisdom of established systems (e.g., http://www.syndromic.org) and innovation invested in these systems have brought the field closer to real-time, integrated public health surveillance.[29]

Registries

Disease registries are often a rigorous and resource-intensive surveillance approach by which all cases of a disease, or type of disease, are ascertained for a defined population (typically a geographic area). By compiling information from multiple sources and linking data for individuals over time, registries can produce useful, detailed information. This feature has been valuable for supporting efforts to increase childhood immunization in the United States, where cumbersome and often incomplete paper-based vaccination records are being replaced by electronic childhood immunization registries.[32] States can enter children into a registry at birth (often by linkage with electronic birth records) and registry records are updated each time healthcare providers deliver an immunization. Registries are also valuable tools for chronic disease control programs, allowing disease stages (e.g., diagnosis, treatment) and outcomes (e.g., survival, mortality) to be tracked over time for individuals.[33] For example, the National Cancer Institute's Surveillance, Epidemiology, and End Results (SEER) Program and the CDC's National Program of Cancer Registries (NPCR) monitor cancer incidence throughout the U.S. population.[34] In addition to detailed data collection for several geographic areas, the SEER program shares data with and supports the NPCR state registries. The NPCR registries are similar to notifiable disease reporting systems in that state-level reporting requirements exist. Because immediate public health action is infrequently needed, however, clinical facilities and their healthcare providers report to centralized, statewide registries. The national network of central cancer registries produces an annual publication of cancer incidence and mortality for the United States.[35] Cancer registries are also a key data source for epidemiologic and health services research.[36]

Mandatory data recorded at the time of birth, death, marriage, divorce, and fetal death are a form of registration known as vital statistics. In the United States, the National Vital Statistics System tracks these vital events through contractual agreements between the National Center for Health Statistics (NCHS) at the CDC and states' vital registration systems, which have statutory authority to record these events.[37] These agreements are the foundation for data sharing; NCHS collects and disseminates national vital statistics (e.g., race-specific vital rates). Agreements also facilitate standardization of systems' data-collection procedures and mechanisms across jurisdiction (e.g., revision of birth, death, and fetal death certificates). Like other registries, near complete coverage of the population and the ability to calculate rates are primary advantages offered by vital statistics. Although vital records are available at local, state, and national levels, time may be needed for the compilation and release of population-based data. In addition, the validity and reliability of these data are often a concern. Despite these limitations, vital records are a key data source for surveillance in several areas, such as maternal and infant mortality, birth defects, and cause-specific mortality (e.g., cancer).

Health Surveys

Health surveys that periodically or continuously collect information can serve as a surveillance mechanism, providing data on health conditions, risk factors, or health-related knowledge, attitudes, and behaviors for the time period in which the surveys are conducted. Although other surveillance approaches are population-based (e.g., notifiable disease reporting) or may not be representative (e.g., sentinel surveillance), sampling is usually a key consideration for the design and use of health surveys. Probability sampling, where survey participants are chosen via a random selection process, allows the survey results to be extended to the larger population from which the participant sample was drawn. To target specific groups for intervention, such as racial or ethnic minority groups experiencing health disparities, survey designs are often complex (i.e., oversampling via stratification and multiple stages).[38]

In the United States, the NCHS sponsors several surveys and data-collection systems. By traveling with a mobile examination center (a moving medical clinic), the National Health and Nutrition Examination Survey (NHANES) has periodically combined data from physical exams and diagnostics with personal interviews for a random sample of noninstitutionalized Americans.[39] NHANES results have been vital in monitoring a number of health and nutrition issues. The survey has evolved and now collects data continuously for a wide range of public health areas.

The Behavioral Risk Factor Surveillance System (BRFSS) is the world's largest telephone survey,[40] continuously monitoring American adults' health-related behaviors by using a random-digit dialing protocol. The system is state-based and designed to have flexible content. Questionnaires have multiple components (sets of questions) that allow certain topics to be tracked nationally in a "core component," while other components are either designed by the CDC and optionally added by states or directly designed and added by the state when the topic is of particular importance for a state. **Table 15.1** shows another application of BRFSS, that has previously been used to measure progress toward *Healthy People* targets.

Combined Approaches

A combination of surveillance methods and data sources may be required to obtain a complete picture of health conditions. Veterinary surveillance and its application to monitoring of human health illustrate a combined surveillance approach. Following the emergence of West Nile virus (WNV) in the Western Hemisphere in 1999, for example, public health agencies began tracking its spread across the United States by monitoring avian, equine, and human disease. Surveillance for WNV in trapped mosquitoes also has been an important indicator of WNV activity, suggesting the potential for WNV-related human disease locally. One requirement makes this combined approach exceptional; experts from several disciplines (e.g., entomology, geography, veterinary medicine) have collaborated in surveillance efforts.

Table 15.1   Assessment of Progress Toward *Healthy People 2010* Targets Using Behavioral Risk Factor Surveillance System (BRFSS) Data for Selected Indicators

Objective[§]	State-Specific Median Proportion (Range)			Target for Year 2010
	1992/1993[±]	1996/1997[±]	2002	
Current cigarette smoking by adults (aged 18 years)	23.0% (15.7–30.7%)	23.2% (13.8–30.7%)	23.1% (16.4–32.6%)	<12%
Adults (aged 18 years) who engage in no leisure-time physical activity	27.4% (17.1–48.1%)	27.8% (17.1–51.4%)	24.4% (15.0–33.6%)	<20%
Adults (aged 18 years) who engaged in binge drinking in the preceding month	14.3% (5.4–24.5%)	14.5% (6.3–23.3%)	16.1% (7.9–24.9%)	<6%

[§]Respondents were classified as current smokers if they had smoked 2,100 cigarettes during their lifetimes and reported smoking every day or some days during the 12 months preceding the survey. Leisure-time physical activity was measured by the respondent's indication of any participation in exercise, other than their regular job, during the preceding month. Binge drinking was defined as having five or more drinks on at least one occasion during the preceding month.
[±]Physical activity data are for 1992 and 1996; cigarette smoking and binge drinking are for 1993 and 1997.
Source: U.S. Centers for Disease Control and Prevention. *MMWR Surveill Summ:* past volumes. Available at: http://www.cdc.gov/mmwr/sursumpv.html. Accessed January 27, 2006.

Surveillance for chronic diseases demonstrates how data on multiple risk factors and outcomes are brought together.[10] In 1996, the CSTE recommended for the first time nationwide surveillance of an avoidable risk factor, adult cigarette smoking. This action raised awareness of the need for a standardized approach to chronic disease surveillance across states. States' chronic disease program directors have worked with the CDC and the CSTE to develop and revise 92 chronic disease surveillance indicators.[41] States monitor these indicators as a means of evaluating disease-control programs and measuring progress toward national health priorities. The suggested indicators are drawn from the entire range of surveillance data sources, including BRFSS and the Youth Risk Behavior Surveillance System (a BRFSS analogue focusing on adolescents), U.S. Census Bureau labor statistics, state-level data on tobacco use and prevention and control, the U.S. Renal Data System, cancer registries, hospital discharge data, and death certification systems. Eventually, the surveillance system may include community-level indicators reflecting environmental and policy changes associated with chronic disease control, such as the number of miles of walking trails, sales volumes for fruits and vegetables, and proportion of restaurants with nonsmoking areas.[42]

While individual-level data may be available to a surveillance program, many of the indicators described earlier are summary measures of demographic or geographic groups. The distinction is noteworthy because investigations involving group-level units of analysis are ecologic, which implies that data cannot be linked at the individual level. Ecologic investigations are subject to an important inference constraint: Only associations at the ecologic level can be correctly examined.[43] For example, suppose a state's summary of vital statistics contains substantial chronic liver disease mortality and BRFSS data indicate that heavy alcohol use among adults in the state is prevalent. Whether the deceased themselves were heavy drinkers, and the extent to which chronic liver disease mortality in the state can be attributed to alcohol use alone and not other contributing risk factors (e.g., infection with hepatitis B or C viruses), remain unknown. On the other hand, demonstrating an ecologic association may be of primary importance. A rapid decrease in average alcohol consumption would likely be accompanied by a substantive decrease in liver cirrhosis mortality in a relatively short time.[44] Furthermore, a multilevel analysis (or hierarchical model) that examines individual-level and group-level determinants of morbidity and mortality simultaneously may be accomplished through a combined surveillance approach.[45]

Linkage of individual-level data from two or more discrete sources, or record linkage, is a combined surveillance approach that has several applications for surveillance. Examples can be found when expansion of existing data is necessary (e.g., generating comprehensive databases of healthcare services), when longitudinal data are of primary interest (e.g., creating reproductive histories), when exposures or outcomes are related (e.g., linking AIDS and TB registries), when individuals are related or the same (e.g., linking of birth and fetal death certificates), and when independent data are used to evaluate surveillance systems (e.g., completeness of disease-reporting studies). Although manual linkage of smaller datasets may be possible, electronic linkage methods are typical. The success of a linkage project depends on the availability, completeness, accuracy, and discriminatory power of the overlapping, identifying information (matching variables). Combinations of name, birth date, and record numbers are commonly used, but coding algorithms can also convert text data into more useful forms. When available matching variables are complete and accurate, a deterministic approach would assign linkages exactly, as all or none. Frequently, data sources' identifiers are not entirely complete or accurate. In these situations, linkages may be assigned probabilistically. Linkage decisions are based on a total "weight" (i.e., a score obtained from the sum of functions of variables' match probabilities) and a cut-off weight is assigned for the linkage decision.

Surveillance System Design and Operations

This section reviews key steps in the design and operation of surveillance systems. Based on system objectives, managers select and define health-related events and a source population during the system design phase. To implement a surveillance system, managers must consider mechanisms for collection, analysis, interpretation, and dissemination of surveillance data. Training for surveillance personnel, attention to evolving data standards, and periodic evaluations to strengthen the surveillance system are important maintenance requirements. General oversight responsibilities and management-related decisions that affect surveillance activities are described throughout the section.

Establish System Objectives

Surveillance system design begins with the specification of system objectives. In the United States, surveillance policies and practices are established through intergovernmental alliances at the federal, state, and local levels. The CDC distributes recommendations for the development of national disease-control strategies that include the collection and use of specific forms of surveillance data. State health departments then receive financial support from federal grants to establish surveillance mechanisms in compliance with CDC guidelines. Close collaboration is required among the different tiers for this system to be successful in achieving disease-control objectives. Surveillance requirements need to be sufficiently systematized across jurisdictions for data to be comparable and meaningful at the national level. At the same time, reporting requirements should be flexible enough to permit adaptation to local public health priorities.

Within this context, planners at the state and local levels must delineate the purposes they expect the system to serve. As part of establishing a surveillance system, it is recommended that one engage stakeholders—that is, the data suppliers and eventual data users. A common approach is to form an advisory committee to guide the implementation and operation of the surveillance system. Intended consumers of information, particularly those represented on the advisory committee, should be consulted when surveillance system objectives are being established to help ensure that surveillance data will be used appropriately and optimally. Typically, surveillance data will serve one or more of the following objectives:[11,46]

- Monitor the frequency and distribution of a health problem in a community.
- Describe the clinical and epidemiologic features of a disease.
- Examine the source causes of morbidity and mortality.
- Generate etiologic hypotheses.
- Assess healthcare delivery, quality, and safety.
- Assess the effects of changes in healthcare practice.
- Direct the development, implementation, and evaluation of interventions and policies.
- Prioritize resource allocation.
- Project future trends.
- Identify and support clinical and epidemiologic research needs.

Because surveillance systems are intended to produce information to support public health action, the process of delineating system objectives must include careful consideration of the expected follow-up activities. The public health manager can play an important role in ensuring that the agencies or individuals expected to use surveillance data will actually use them in public health planning and programming.

Select and Define Health Events to Be Monitored

Each step of surveillance implementation requires substantial resources, and the total cost of surveillance rises incrementally with each additional event that is monitored. Consequently, the selection of health-related events to be tracked by the surveillance system must involve prioritization in order to meet the surveillance objectives of primary public health importance. Various criteria have been proposed for assessing the relative importance of health-related events to be included in a system.[11,46,47] Criteria (and examples of their corresponding indices) include the following:

- Morbidity (case counts, prevalence and incidence rates)
- Mortality (case fatality ratio, mortality rates, and potential years of life lost)
- Risk (transmission modes, communicability)

- Severity (bed-disability days, hospitalization and disability rates)
- Preventability (preventable fraction, existing prevention measures)
- Catastrophic potential (societal costs, vulnerability)
- Direct and indirect economic costs (loss of productivity, healthcare expenditures)
- Public interest (media attention) and stakeholder opinion (consensus)

The World Health Organization (WHO) has collaborated with the World Bank and the Harvard School of Public Health to estimate the Global Burden of Disease (http://www.who .int/en/).[48] The project uses relevant, available data plus assumption and inference to calculate disability-adjusted life years (DALYs), a single measure that summarizes population health. DALYs measure the difference between a perfect health scenario, where the entire population lives disease free until old age, and the populations' actual life with years lost to disability and premature mortality. DALYs are available for grouped and specific causes of morbidity and mortality and are stratified by geographic region, age group, and sex. Thus, the project offers a metric for prioritizing health events internationally. A notable limitation of the metric is that the health effects of socioeconomic disruption following civil wars, disasters, and epidemics (e.g., severe acute respiratory syndrome [SARS]) are not included.

Different surveillance approaches result from selection of health-related events for monitoring. Data produced by each surveillance approach may have the strengths and weaknesses described in the previous section. Where capacity exists, compatible surveillance data sources can track a group of health-related events to gain a comprehensive understanding of the larger public health problem. The aforementioned chronic disease indicators illustrated how behaviors (e.g., prevalence of smoking among adults, cigarette sales) and disease stages (e.g., cancer diagnosis, hospitalization, death) can be correlated through combined approaches. Alternatively, a public health agency may only monitor an antecedent of disease or a specific disease stage. It has been suggested, for example, that vital event registration is the most important form of public health surveillance that a developing country can add to its health statistics.[49]

For many forms of surveillance, a **case definition** must be developed to clarify the health-related event being monitored and improve the comparability of reports from different data sources.[11] A case definition may have several components, including clinical (e.g., signs and symptoms, diagnostic results), epidemiologic (e.g., person, place, and time), and behavioral (e.g., risk factors) information. Case definitions may also distinguish between confirmed, probable, and suspect occurrences according to their degree of conformity with the event of interest. If the clinical presentation of a disease is indeterminate (such as viral hepatitis, cancer), laboratory confirmation is often a necessary case definition component. In the United States, the CDC works with the CSTE to publish "Case Definitions for Infectious Conditions Under Public Health Surveillance,"[17] which define the nationally notifiable infectious diseases via clinical, epidemiologic, and laboratory criteria.

The development and revision of a surveillance case definition has important considerations. Components of the definition must be devised with attention to both the system's objectives and the utility of data to be collected. A broad definition will be more sensitive, increasing the probability that the system ascertains the event when it occurs, but may require effort in discerning true cases from false positives.[46] A relatively sensitive definition might be appropriate when completeness of reporting is important or when reporting of false positives does not detract from the system's objectives.[1] The influenza-like illness monitored by sentinel providers in the United States uses a simple, broad case definition (temperature of 100°F plus either a cough or a sore throat). Although other respiratory diseases produce these signs and symptoms, the system is useful. A narrower definition, on the other hand, is generally more specific. Specificity increases the probability that the events detected by the system are true events of interest, the predictive value positive. A relatively specific definition might be appropriate when complete case ascertainment is not necessarily important or when valid diagnostics, such as laboratory tests, are available for inclusion in the case definition. Notably, when laboratory tests or other diagnostic procedures are included as components of the case definition, the sensitivity and specificity of the tests or procedures themselves impact the sensitivity, specificity, and predictive value of the surveillance case definition. U.S. surveillance for influenza-associated pediatric mortality has required laboratory confirmation of influenza because data from precise case ascertainment are needed to identify pediatric groups at risk for severe influenza and any consequent revision of vaccination policies.

Increased scientific understanding, availability of new diagnostics or therapies, and changing information needs may prompt case definition revisions. These definitions may, in turn, affect surveillance sensitivity and specificity. For example, in 1982 the CDC initiated AIDS surveillance in the United States using a set of opportunistic diseases, that were diagnosed in the absence of other known causes of immunodeficiency.[50] With the availability of HIV-antibody testing, surveillance specificity improved and a wider spectrum of HIV-related disease was recognized. The CDC revised its case definition in 1987 to include these diseases, which were presumptively diagnosed in persons testing positive for HIV infection.[51] As further knowledge was gained, the CDC changed its case definition again in 1993 to include direct evidence of immunodeficiency. Individuals who were HIV-positive and had CD41 T-lymphocyte counts less than 200 cells/mm^3 (or a CD41 proportion under 14%) were "counted" as having AIDS.[52] This change immediately impacted U.S. AIDS case counts; case reports increased 111% in 1993.[53] In contrast, many developing nations initially relied on clinical diagnoses of AIDS (e.g., weight loss) because laboratory capacities were inadequate.[54] Clinical diagnosis was simple and universally applicable, but surveillance specificity was low. Until the late 1990s, most developing countries' case definitions for AIDS relied less on the HIV test because testing was not widely conducted. Although HIV surveillance has begun in many parts of the world, surveillance is not satisfactory for following trends in health outcomes, since most persons are asymptomatic and do not seek HIV testing. Serosurveys (serologic surveys) have been implemented in part to monitor transmission patterns.

Establish the Population Under Surveillance

Although public health surveillance relies on records of individuals, the unit of interest is the population. Therefore, how the population is targeted for surveillance must be explicitly defined. Health surveys and sentinel surveillance sample the population; notifiable disease reporting and registries are population-based methods (i.e., they relate to the general population, often as defined by a geographic area).

Surveillance activities may focus on populations defined at geographic levels, which can range from a neighborhood to a nation or the entire world. Within a geographic domain, surveillance may be specifically directed toward an entire population or toward special subgroups that share demographic characteristics or risk factors for disease. Often the case definition reflects the population under surveillance. Residency within a geographic public health jurisdiction, for example, may be incorporated into a case definition to help define the surveillance population. Surveillance systems with populations delineated by geography have a special consideration. A decision to include cases based on where health-related events occurred or to include cases based on residency must be made.[1] When residency data are not readily available from reporting sources, inclusion based on where events occurred is a simple alternative if reports originate directly from eligible source locations. Diagnoses reported by a hospital located within the geographic area are an example. However, this approach will count events among nonresidents who are diagnosed in the area and may miss events among residents diagnosed outside the area.

Establish Reporting Procedures

Surveillance programs must delineate specific types of data that should be collected, recognizing that different information types may require different forms of surveillance. Health surveys, for example, may be the only source of data on knowledge, attitudes, and behaviors. Clinical events typically occur in the context of health care, so corresponding data are likely to be obtainable through health information systems or directly from healthcare providers. Depending on the event of interest and setting where care or services are likely to be provided, a variety of surveillance approaches may be appropriate.

Laboratory-based surveillance systems seek information from clinical laboratories where testing of samples or specimens is necessary to establish or confirm a diagnosis. In the United States, the emerging infections programs (EIPs) have created surveillance networks within 11 geographically defined sites (states, metropolitan areas, or counties).[55] The EIPs maintain ongoing communication with microbiology laboratories, where invasive bacterial diseases and food-borne illnesses that require culture confirmation for diagnostic and surveillance purposes can be tracked. The CDC also coordinates PulseNet, which is a laboratory-based network for molecular subtyping of food-borne bacterial pathogens (e.g., *E. coli* O157:H7, *Salmonella*).[56] The program uses a standardized pulsed-field gel electrophoresis (PFGE) methodology across a network of laboratories in state and local health departments as well as federal public health and food regulatory agencies. Using PFGE, pathogens' DNA "fingerprints" (patterns obtained from genetic material) can be electronically uploaded to a database for comparison amongst PulseNet participants. This molecular epidemiology capacity has been particularly helpful in identifying geographically dispersed, common-source outbreaks.

Systems and procedures for obtaining data also must be established. Depending on the application, a data-collection form may be simple or complex and can exist either on paper or electronically. Often forms use a standardized coding system to increase the efficiency of data collection, entry, and storage. Manual (paper-based) data collection can be implemented relatively quickly and easily, but may be labor intensive and unsustainable in the long term. Electronic reporting procedures have multiple applications for public health surveillance; investments in surveillance information technology are well worth consideration. In the United States, progress has been made in two areas: developing systems for automated, electronic laboratory reporting (ELR) and Internet-based case reporting.[57] ELR systems can greatly improve completeness and timeliness of notifiable disease reporting. In 1998, Hawaii implemented the first statewide automated laboratory reporting system.[58] By establishing data-transmission linkages with three commercial laboratories that provided approximately two-thirds of all laboratory-based notifiable disease reports, the state health department more than doubled the number of *Giardia, Salmonella, Shigella,* invasive *S. pneumoniae,* and vancomycin-resistant *Enterococcus* reports relative to the conventional (paper-based) system. Electronic reports were received 3.8 days earlier, and 12 of 21 data fields (57%) were significantly more likely to be complete when transmitted electronically. In the Netherlands, Internet-based case reporting has fully replaced the paper-based system for data transmission from municipal public health services to national public health authorities.[59] The change resulted in a 9-day improvement of median reporting timeliness and an 11% increase in the completeness of data fields. **Figure 15.4** is a screen capture of the initial data entry screen for another Internet-based, notifiable disease case reporting system, the State Electronic Notifiable Disease Surveillance System (SendSS) at the Georgia Division of Public Health.

Reporting an epidemic of communicable disease is often critical. **Table 15.2** presents an overview of select surveillance networks for detecting and responding to outbreaks and public

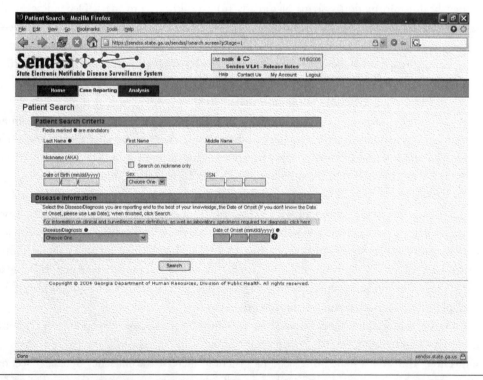

Figure 15.4 Initial Screen for Internet-Based Notifiable Disease Case Reporting to the State Electronic Notifiable Disease Surveillance Systems (SendSS), Georgia Division Public Health
Source: Georgia Department of Human Resources, Division of Public Health.

Table 15.2   Select Surveillance Systems for Detection and Reporting of Infectious Disease Outbreaks in the United States and Globally

Name	Sponsor	Objectives	Scope	Description
BioSense	U.S. Centers for Disease Control and Prevention	Early detection of public health emergencies, including naturally occurring outbreaks and bioterrorism, by federal, state, and local officials	Visits at federal medical facilities, national laboratory test orders, and over-the-counter retail in major metropolitan areas in the United States	National syndromic surveillance system, compiles data from various electronic sources
Enter-net	European Commission	Detect clusters of enteric pathogens, research antimicrobial resistance, standardize data collection and laboratory protocols	National reference laboratories and surveillance programs in European Union countries and beyond (Australia, Canada, Japan, and South Africa)	International surveillance network for salmonellosis and Vero cytotoxin-producing E. coli (VTEC) O157
Epidemic Information Exchange (Epi-X)	U.S. Centers for Disease Control and Prevention	Secure communication between public health officials, share preliminary information on health investigations, peer discussions, assistance, and coordination	Over 3,900 users at all levels of U.S. public health agencies in 2006	Secure Internet-based communication system for public health
Global Outbreak Alert and Response Network (GOARN)	World Health Organization and partners	Coordination in investigating, tracking, and responding to international disease outbreaks	WHO member countries, government and nongovernment organizations, scientists and technical experts worldwide	Global partnership for detection and response to internationally significant outbreaks
Global Public Health Intelligence Network (GPHIN)	World Health Organization/Health Canada	Identify possible infections disease outbreaks and other significant public health events	Worldwide media and Internet information sources in multiple languages	Software searches Internet-based sources globally for possible outbreaks
Laboratory Response Network (LRN)	U.S. Centers for Disease Control and Prevention	Enhance laboratory infrastructure and capacity, including tests for identifying biological and chemical agents	Public health, military, and international laboratories conducting specialized testing from human, veterinary, and environmental sources	Integrated network of public health and clinical laboratories
National Electronic Disease Surveillance System (NEDSS)	U.S. Centers for Disease Control and Prevention	Integrated, interoperable surveillance systems; efficient, confidential, and secure data transmission	U.S. public health agencies and surveillance partners	Development of architecture and data standards for Internet-based surveillance

Sources: U.S. Government Accountability Office. Emerging infectious diseases: review of state and federal disease surveillance efforts. Available at: http://www.gao.gov/htext/d04877 .html. Accessed December 16, 2005; Fisher I. The Enter-net International Surveillance Network—how it works. *Euro Surveill.* 1999;4:52–55; and systems' websites.

health emergencies both in the United States and globally. The objectives, scope, and reporting procedures of these and other systems vary widely. ProMED, for example, facilitates worldwide dissemination of information on human, veterinary, and plant disease outbreaks via moderated, daily email communications in multiple languages (www.promedmail.org). Information from any source is eligible for inclusion, which is both a strength and a weakness of the system. The emergence of severe acute respiratory syndrome (SARS) was first publicly reported in ProMED in 2003. The WHO/Health Canada Global Public Health Intelligence Network (GPHIN) also detected early signs of the SARS epidemic. GPHIN software scans the Internet to identify infectious disease outbreaks through media and other electronic sources. The WHO investigates and verifies potential epidemics detected through the system (Table 15.2). To further strengthen epidemic surveillance, the WHO adopted revised International Health Regulations (IHR) in 2005, which provide a legal basis for sharing of critical epidemiologic data across borders.[60] The revised IHR legally obligate reporting and verification of "all events that may constitute a public health emergency of international concern" by WHO member and nonmember states that agree to be bound by the IHR. Compliance with the regulations can protect against international spread of disease while minimizing impediments to travel and trade.

Optimizing completeness of reporting and maintaining a consistent flow of accurate data are major challenges for surveillance programs;[21] incomplete, inconsistent, or inaccurate data can introduce case ascertainment and information biases within surveillance data.[47] For example, cases detected in public-sector facilities may be more likely to be reported to health authorities than cases diagnosed by private clinicians, leading to higher reporting completeness for individuals seeking care in public clinics. Data on the incidence of sexually transmitted diseases tend to be more accurate in states with laws requiring that positive tests be reported.[61] Even at a single time and place, surveillance data can be biased. For example, respondents' faulty recall or reluctance to disclose stigmatizing conditions can lead to underreporting in surveillance surveys that rely on self-reporting.[62] Thus, surveillance system managers should be keenly aware of the potential for bias, assess its possible influence when detecting patterns of health-related events, and strive to base analyses on data sets that are as complete, comparable, and representative as possible. National programs often define minimally acceptable standards for data collection and processing. Funds for the field work associated with the operation of an active surveillance system (e.g., for quality control reviews, case-finding audits) are sound investments for a reliable surveillance database.

To maintain healthcare professionals' participation in surveillance activities, a multifaceted approach may be needed. The surveillance program manager must provide necessary support for meeting reporting responsibilities. Clinicians may be greatly aided by procedural manuals that specify the list of notifiable conditions, case definitions, information-recording requirements, and reporting schedules. Other ideas for encouraging reporting compliance include simplifying reporting procedures, conducting seminars or onsite visits to emphasize reporting, and providing multiple reporting modalities (e.g., 24-hour, toll-free numbers and Internet-based case reporting systems).[22,33]

Efforts to obtain surveillance data can be described along a spectrum of activities, ranging in intensity from passive to active. In the case of passive surveillance, public health officials rely on healthcare providers to report the occurrence of a health-related event voluntarily, as mandated by state law. With active surveillance, health officials routinely contact reporting sources to inquire about occurrences and review medical and laboratory reports to identify unreported occurrences. Relative to passive surveillance, active surveillance generally achieves more complete and accurate reporting (i.e., surveillance sensitivity is increased), but active surveillance is more resource intensive for the public health agency.

Analyze and Interpret Surveillance Data

Before investing in the analysis and interpretation of surveillance data, the analyst needs to be oriented to the surveillance system itself. Intricacies arise from the specifics of how health-related events and the underlying population are defined and, in particular, from how the data are reported.[63] Knowledge of how various factors have influenced reporting may become relevant when findings from the analysis are interpreted (e.g., when and why a case definition was revised, diagnostic and reporting procedures were changed, or media attention fluctuated).

Analysis of surveillance data should start simple.[63] The basic epidemiologic parameters of person, place, and time provide a framework. Depending on the specific objectives of the surveillance activities, an epidemiologist can apply a variety of analytic techniques that focus on one or more of these descriptors. Surveillance approaches that use sampling may lend themselves to statistical testing, which may be used for testing hypotheses and addressing random variation from the sample. Data from surveillance systems that ascertain all events in the population of interest may be directly described since observed variation is what has occurred in the population.

Descriptions of the persons experiencing the event under surveillance are frequently organized by demographic (e.g., age group, sex, race, and ethnicity) and epidemiologic (e.g., mode of transmission, disease type) characteristics. Analysis could begin by tabulating event frequency distributions for each relevant characteristic. Interactions between these characteristics also may need to be assessed. When stratified by race, for example, vital statistics data for the 1990s indicate that two minority populations, American Indians/Alaska Natives and African Americans, experienced higher mortality rates from traumatic brain injury (TBI) than other racial groups (**Figure 15.5**).[64] External cause-of-injury codes ("E codes"), which provide circumstantial and environmental information on injury causes, showed that motor vehicles were involved in half (49%) of the TBI deaths among American Indians/Alaska Natives and firearms were involved in half (49%) of the TBI deaths among African Americans.

Analyses by place can be based either on where health-related events occurred or based on residency of those experiencing the events (though this decision may have been made while establishing the population under surveillance).[1] Simple comparisons and displays of event counts by geographic areas (e.g., neighborhoods, cities, nations) can be useful, particularly when the area's population size is sufficient to yield stable estimates of event frequencies. Event rates allow for comparisons of frequency for a given time period across areas with varying population sizes. Depending on the event under surveillance, a variety of rates (e.g., disease attack rate, birth rate, cause-specific mortality rate) can be obtained by carefully specifying the numerator, denominator, and time interval. Within a defined area, the first step is to divide the number of

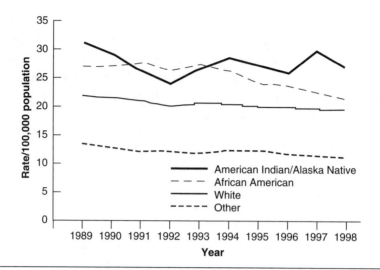

Figure 15.5   Age-Adjusted Traumatic Brain Injury Mortality Rate (Per 100,000 Population), by Race and Year–United States, 1989–1998
Source: U.S. Centers for Disease Control and Prevention. Surveillance for traumatic brain injury deaths–United States, 1989–1998. *MMWR Surveill Summ.* 2002;51:1–16.

events for a designated time interval (numerator) by an estimate of the population at risk during the same time interval (denominator).[63] Often this yields a fraction that is difficult to interpret. Suppose 2 maternal deaths in the year 2000 were recorded in a state's vital statistics for 78,123 live births. Two divided by 78,213 equals 0.0000256. The next step is to multiply this fraction by some factor of 10, where the choice of an appropriate factor may depend on the frequency of the event, the size of the population at risk, and convention. In the example, a rate of 2.56 maternal deaths per 100,000 live births (0.0000256 × 100,000) helps characterize the frequency of maternal deaths in the state. This rate also can be compared to maternal death rates in other states (using the same 100,000 multiplier). Most epidemiology texts discuss rates in general and standardization of crude rates to control for confounding bias.

The high concentration of stroke mortality in the Southeastern United States (the so-called "stroke belt") during the 1990s is readily apparent in **Figure 15.6**. In this choropleth map, degree of shading corresponds to quantitative information (stroke mortality rates) for specific areas (U.S. counties). The map exemplifies how rates help make comparisons across the counties' populations. Annual rates are averaged and categorized for the time period. Standardization allows for comparing rates after accounting for differences in the populations' age structures. Geographic Information Systems (GIS) applications are another important tool for spatial analyses of surveillance data. By geocoding (locating latitude and longitude from street address), precise event locations can be correlated with other area attributes. Maps can display these correlations by layering events and attributes.

Time is significant because surveillance systems often monitor temporal trends within defined geographies. An analysis might begin simply by comparing the number of events in

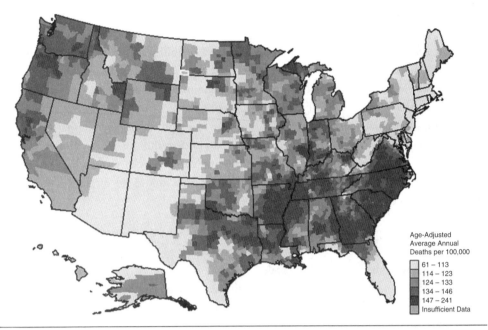

Figure 15.6   United States Total Population Ages 35+, Stroke Death Rates, 1991–1998
Source: U.S. Centers for Disease Control and Prevention. Heart disease and stroke maps: interactive state maps. Available at: http://www.cdc.gov/cvh/maps/statemaps.htm. Accessed January 25, 2006.

one time period to those of an equivalent time interval (e.g., season, year, week) in the past. Event counts could be tabulated for a table or graphically displayed, with time on the X axis. Building on findings from simpler analyses, a number of more complex methodologies are available for detecting aberrations, whether temporal, spatial, or in time and space.[8,63] For outbreak detection systems, such as syndromic surveillance, specialized statistical methods are described in other texts.[7,8]

Analyses involving time can either use dates when health-related events were reported or dates when health-related events occurred.[1] If reporting delays are considerable, report date may be an imprecise measure of when events actually occurred. The use of dates closer to the occurrence of the health event, such as diagnosis date, also needs to be interpreted carefully. When tracking chronic diseases with long latency periods, recent disease counts may underrepresent the current disease frequency. If either reporting delay or timeliness of diagnosis varies systematically, temporal imprecision may be differential across strata of the population under surveillance.

Disseminate and Apply Surveillance Findings

Reporting of surveillance findings to appropriate stakeholders, including health authorities, policy makers, clinicians, and the general public, is a critical component of surveillance activities. Individuals and agencies that contribute data to the surveillance system are most compliant with reporting requirements when they see the value of data produced by the surveillance program. Ongoing feedback is a particularly important incentive for the clinicians who participate in surveillance activities. Clinicians are motivated by the availability of information on local health conditions, especially in forms that are useful for patient care. In Germany, practicing physicians most often (85%) cited information related to infectious disease outbreaks when surveyed on preferences for feedback of notifiable disease–reporting data.[65]

Depending on what merits emphasis, a number of graphical display alternatives (graphs, tables, and maps) are available to help the audience to understand the data and appreciate their significance. If, for example, proportions are important, then a pie chart might be a good format for displaying surveillance data. General recommendations for visual display of quantitative information include the following:[63]

- Explain the graphic in the title, including when and where data were collected.
- Explain variables by labeling rows and columns (tables) or axes (graphs), including how variables were measured and the scale.
- Provide pertinent summary measures for the reader (e.g., row or column totals).
- Use a legend or a key to make categories or codes explicit.
- Define abbreviations with footnotes.
- If data are excluded or qualified, describe accordingly with footnotes.

A good rule of thumb is to imagine the table or figure alone (without accompanying text) and assess whether it remains self-explanatory to a reader who is unfamiliar with the data. Other references provide detailed considerations for how to display data effectively.[66]

A variety of mechanisms exist for publicizing surveillance findings and releasing surveillance datasets. In the United States, the CDC and its partners publish national data from a multitude of surveillance systems (http://www.cdc.gov/mmwr/mmwr_ss/ss_cvol.html). At the state and local levels, public health agencies also disseminate information via newsletters, electronic bulletins, press releases, news conferences, and public meetings. Frequently, surveillance programs (e.g., disease registries, health surveys) publish a concise report and then periodically publish a more detailed report with extensive analysis and interpretation.

The dissemination strategy must correspond to the purpose of the surveillance activities. Particular attention should be focused on establishing a message that is readily comprehensible and relevant for the intended audience. Effective communication may be accomplished during public hearings or small group discussions with key individuals. The media can also be an ally for information distribution by judicious use of prepared statements and carefully planned content. Public health managers are encouraged to keep lines of communication with the media open in times of "no news" in order to promote broader, less sensational messages such as cancer screening. Wherever possible, system managers should target informed reporters (e.g., scientific writers) for directed information releases. Cultivating credibility is always a sound policy.

To balance the principles of access to data with confidentiality, surveillance systems must establish protocols and procedures to make determinations on requests for information for scientific research.[67] The data-release protocol should include a clearly defined prioritization scheme to promote equal treatment of data requestors and data providers, expedite the release process, and encourage the release of a broad spectrum of data elements without compromising confidentiality.[68] Many states have legislated mandates to establish advisory boards or scientific review committees to oversee the use of surveillance data. Committee membership should include experts from appropriate disciplines who are experienced in the analysis of health data, disease coding, registry operations, and bioethics.

The ultimate objective of public health surveillance is to collect information for action. Therefore, surveillance data should be transformed into useful information concerning the prevalence of risk factors and healthy behaviors, the effects of interventions, and the direction of trends in disease and other health outcomes.[2] Accordingly, public health officials must determine the implications of their surveillance data; often these determinations are made on a regular basis. A committee composed of agency consultants (e.g., clinicians, academic epidemiologists, policy experts) can be formed to support an analysis of the data and assist with the formulation of and support for public health recommendations. Thresholds for public health action can be set so that unusual distributions of health events are identified and appropriate interventions can be implemented. Just as surveillance activities have expanded into various public health domains, the needs for interpretation of surveillance data have diversified as well. The National Program of Cancer Registries, for example, recommends that states allocate resources for epidemiologic guidance, especially for interpreting and applying cancer registry data. Similarly, greater attention has been placed on the interpretation and use of data derived from vital records for monitoring interventions aimed at reducing infant mortality and ensuring children's access to health care.

Maintain and Evaluate Operations

The public health manager must provide ongoing support to ensure consistent and effective surveillance operations. To do so, surveillance programs require trained personnel, attention to evolving standards for use and management of surveillance data, and periodic evaluation to strengthen the surveillance system itself.

Public health administrators must ensure effective communication and collaboration across the diverse disciplines that contribute to surveillance systems. Epidemiologists and statisticians frequently manage surveillance programs. Typically they compile, analyze, report, and interpret results from surveillance systems as well as design and refine systems that support valid, reliable, and relevant results. Other important professionals often include database programmers and persons with expertise in database design, linkage, and maintenance. Maintaining a qualified staff is an important consideration for good surveillance. For example, advances in information technology, including increased availability and standardization of electronic health information and expanding applications of the Internet, require a modern surveillance manager to be technologically savvy. The U.S. progress in electronic reporting described earlier (reporting procedures) requires knowledge of controlled vocabularies, particularly Health Level Seven (HL7) to apply syntax to data, Logical Observation Identifiers, Names, and Codes (LOINC) to describe tests, and Systematized Nomenclature of Medicine (SNOMED) for test results.[69] Funds for continuing education and professional organization memberships for professional development are important budget considerations for surveillance programs.

Surveillance programs and their personnel have ethical standards and legal requirements to maintain. Ethical responsibilities associated with public health practice include seeking information for devising policies and programs that assure health, while protecting the privacy and confidentiality of information, which, if released, could bring harm to an individual or community.[70] In fact, public health has a long history of safeguarding the privacy and confidentiality of individuals' health information while accomplishing their duties.[71] At the same time, legal and ethical responsibilities evolve and public health managers should be aware of necessary measures for compliance as well as the implications of legislation for their surveillance data sources (e.g., use of hospital discharge databases). For example, the Privacy Rule of the Health Insurance Portability and Accountability Act (HIPAA) provided the first national Standards for Privacy of Individually Identifiable Health Information. (Individually identifiable health information is also known as protected health information, or PHI.) Although HIPAA privacy directly relates to "covered entities" (health plans, healthcare providers, and healthcare clearinghouses with PHI), public health authorities work with covered entities to ensure that surveillance activities are allowed to continue and may be considered covered entities themselves. Sharing of PHI for public health is expressly permitted by HIPAA privacy law.[71]

Surveillance programs at the local level require personally identifying information for a number of functions, including public health follow up and investigation and identification of duplicate reports.[1] The CDC recommendations for security and confidentiality of HIV/AIDS surveillance data are a particularly useful resource.[72] Examples of these minimum standards include encryption during electronic data transfer, removal of identifying information with data transfer, record storage in physically secure areas with computer encryption and coded passwords, restricting data access to authorized staff who have signed confidentiality agreements that include penalties for data disclosure, and reporting for statistical purposes in formats that do not permit direct or indirect identification of individuals. This CDC resource has additional practices that can also be applied.

The distinction between public health research versus practice often arises.[73] Surveillance is a cornerstone of public health practice. As its primary intent is not to produce generalizable knowledge, typically it is not considered research as defined by federal laws for the protection of human research participants (known as the Common Rule).[74] However, distinguishing research and practice from among surveillance-related activities with multiple objectives can be ambiguous. A generic example is when surveillance identifies a public health problem; questions that may be considered research often can emerge from investigating the problem.

Public health surveillance systems require periodic monitoring and evaluation to ensure that desired objectives are being met and operations are efficient and effective. An evaluation begins by identifying and engaging stakeholders in the evaluation process itself.[75] In doing so, the evaluation results are more likely to be both useful and credible to the persons most invested in the surveillance system. Next, a process of describing the systems' objectives and operations can help clarify expectations, increase understanding of the system's nuances, and guide the evaluation through subsequent steps. Several resources offer guidelines for evaluating surveillance systems, including systems focusing on early outbreak detection.[11,31,47,76] The resources include sets of system attributes—criteria with which to assess the utility, efficiency, and effectiveness of the system. The following are common criteria for evaluating surveillance system performance:

- Sensitivity—Likelihood that health-related events under surveillance are identified when they occur
- Predictive value positive—Likelihood that events identified are true events under surveillance
- Representativeness—Degree to which characteristics of persons experiencing identified events are distributed consistently with characteristics of all persons experiencing events in the population
- Data quality—Completeness, reliability, and validity of information
- Timeliness—Duration of time intervals between event occurrence, event reporting, and report completion as well as information analysis, interpretation, and dissemination
- Simplicity—Ease of use for persons participating in all steps of system operation
- Flexibility—Adaptability of the system to changing objectives and circumstances

Evaluation culminates in the formulation of recommendations for system-strengthening interventions. To assess the utility of surveillance functions, evaluators are also encouraged to verify that surveillance activities are integrated into the overall public health system and verify that their results are routinely received, understood, and applied by appropriate policy makers.[11]

Future Outlook

Surveillance is a primary mechanism for generating and processing information in the cycle of formulating public health objectives, implementing interventions, measuring program impact, and refining interventions. Evaluation should assess whether the information produced by the surveillance system is useful for public health programming and policy making. The science and technology in this area continues to evolve at a rapid pace. Likewise, the global capacity in this area is expanding as many organizations around the planet work together in increasingly coordinated efforts. Surveillance systems are now more robust than ever and will continue to be the cornerstone to public health and health security.

Discussion Questions

1. Discuss why surveillance is central to the effectiveness of public health.
2. Give examples of surveillance accomplishments, such as disease prevention.
3. Go to the CDC website and become familiar with the wide range of diseases and health challenges under surveillance.
4. Describe the role of local and federal agencies in disease surveillance.
5. What do you see as needed improvements in the current surveillance system in the United States? In the world?

References

1. Buehler JW. Surveillance. In: Rothman KJ, Greenland S, eds. *Modern Epidemiology*. Philadelphia: Lippincott-Raven Publishers; 1998:435–57.
2. Stroup DF, Brookmeyer R, Kalsbeek WD. Public health surveillance in action. In: Brookmeyer R, Stroup DF, eds. *Monitoring the Health of Populations: Statistical Principles and Methods for Public Health Surveillance*. New York: Oxford University Press; 2004:1–35.
3. Halperin W, Baker E, eds. *Public Health Surveillance*. New York: Van Nostrand Reinhold; 1992.
4. Menck H, Smart C, eds. *Central Cancer Registries: Design, Management and Use*. Chur, Switzerland: Harwood Academic Publishers; 1994.
5. Fritz AG, Hutchison CL, Roffers SD, eds. *Cancer Registry Management: Principles and Practice*. Dubuque, IA: Kendall/Hunt Publishing Co; 1997.
6. Teutsch SM, Churchill RE, eds. *Principles and Practice of Public Health Surveillance*. New York: Oxford University Press; 2000.
7. Brookmeyer R, Stroup DF, eds. *Monitoring the Health of Populations: Statistical Principles and Methods for Public Health Surveillance*. New York: Oxford University Press; 2004.
8. Lawson AB, Kleinman K, eds. *Spatial and Syndromic Surveillance for Public Health*. Chichester, England: John Wiley & Sons; 2005.
9. Thacker SB. Historical development. In: Teutsch SM, Churchill RE, eds. *Principles and Practice of Public Health Surveillance*. New York: Oxford University Press; 2000:1–16.
10. Remington PL, Goodman RA. Chronic disease surveillance. In: Brownson RC, Remington PL, Davis JR. *Chronic Disease Epidemiology and Control*. Washington, DC: American Public Health Association; 1998:55–76.
11. U.S. Centers for Disease Control and Prevention. Updated guidelines for evaluating surveillance systems: recommendations from the guidelines working group. *MMWR Recomm Rep*. 2001;50:1–35.
12. U.S. Centers for Disease Control and Prevention. Outbreak of *Salmonella* serotype *muenchen* infections associated with unpasteurized orange juice—United States and Canada, June 1999. *MMWR*. 1999;48:582–5.
13. U.S. Renal Data System Coordinating Center. Researcher's Guide. Available at: http://www.usrds.org/research.htm. Accessed March 1, 2013.
14. U.S. Renal Data System. *USRDS 2005 Annual Data Report: Atlas of End-Stage Renal Disease in the United States*. Bethesda, MD: National Institute of Diabetes and Digestive and Kidney Diseases; 2005.
15. Parrish RG, McDonnell SM. Sources of health-related information. In: Teutsch SM, Churchill RE, eds. *Principles and Practice of Public Health Surveillance*. New York: Oxford University Press; 2000:30–75.
16. Council of State and Territorial Epidemiologists. NNDSS Assessment 2004. Available at: http://www.cste.org/nndssmainmenu2004.htm. Accessed November 28, 2005.
17. U.S. Centers for Disease Control and Prevention. Case definitions for infectious conditions under public health surveillance. *MMWR Recomm Rep*. 1997;46:1–55.
18. Roush S, Birkhead G, Koo D, et al. Mandatory reporting of diseases and conditions by health care professionals and laboratories. *JAMA*. 1994;282:164–70.
19. Kaufman JA, Reichard S, Walline A. Survey of HIV, sexually transmitted disease, tuberculosis and viral hepatitis case reporting practices in tribally operated and urban Indian health facilities. Council of State and Territorial Epidemiologists. Available at: http://www.cste.org/publications.asp. Accessed December 1, 2005.
20. U.S. Centers for Disease Control and Prevention. First report of AIDS. *MMWR*. 2001;50:429.
21. Doyle TJ, Glynn KM, Groseclose SL. Completeness of notifiable infectious disease reporting in the United States: an analytical literature review. *Am J Epidemiol*. 2002;155:866–74.
22. Silk BJ, Berkelman RL. A review of strategies for enhancing the completeness of notifiable disease reporting. *J Public Health Manag Pract*. 2005;11:191–200.
23. U.S. Centers for Disease Control and Prevention. Overview of influenza surveillance in the United States. Available at: http://www.cdc.gov/flu/weekly/pdf/flu-surveillance-overview.pdf. Accessed March 1, 2013.

24. Seligman PJ, Frazier YM. Surveillance: the sentinel health event approach. In: Halperin W, Baker E, eds. *Public Health Surveillance*. New York: Van Nostrand Reinhold; 1992:16–25.

25. Rustein DD, Berenberg W, Chalmers TC, et al. Measuring the quality of medical care: a clinical method. *N Engl J Med*. 1976;294:582–8.

26. Buehler JW, Berkelman RL, Hartley DM, et al. Syndromic surveillance and bioterrorism-related epidemics. *Emerg Infect Dis*. 2003;9:1197–204.

27. Reingold A. If syndromic surveillance is the answer, what is the question? *Biosecurity Bioterrorism: Biodefense Strat Pract Sci*. 2003;1:1–5.

28. Mandl KD, Overhage JM, Wagner MM, et al. Implementing syndromic surveillance: a practical guide informed by early experience. *J Am Med Inform Assoc*. 2004;11:141–50.

29. Koo D. Leveraging syndromic surveillance. *J Public Health Manag Pract*. 2005;11:181–3.

30. Hopkins RS. Design and operation of state and local infectious disease surveillance systems. *J Public Health Manag Pract*. 2005;11:184–90.

31. U.S. Centers for Disease Control and Prevention. Framework for evaluating public health surveillance systems for early detection of outbreaks. *MMWR Recomm Rep*. 2004;53:1–11.

32. U.S. Centers for Disease Control and Prevention. Immunization information system progress—United States, 2003. *MMWR*. 2005;54:722–4.

33. Birkhead GS, Maylahn CM. State and local public health surveillance. In: Teutsch SM, Churchill RE, eds. *Principles and Practice of Public Health Surveillance*. New York: Oxford University Press; 2000: 253–86.

34. U.S. Centers for Disease Control and Prevention. Cancer registries: the foundation for cancer prevention and control. Available at: http://www.cdc.gov/cancer/npcr/about2004.htm. Accessed December 5, 2005.

35. U.S. Cancer Statistics Working Group. *United States Cancer Statistics: 2002 Incidence and Mortality*. Atlanta, GA: Centers for Disease Control and Prevention, National Cancer Institute; 2005.

36. Sankila R, Black R, Coebergh JW, et al. *Evaluation of Clinical Care by Cancer Registries* (IARC Technical Publication No. 37). Lyon, France: International Agency for Research on Cancer; 2003.

37. U.S. Centers for Disease Control and Prevention. National Vital Statistics System. Available at: http://www.cdc.gov/nchs/nvss.htm. Accessed March 1, 2013.

38. Kalsbeek WD. The use of surveys in public health surveillance: monitoring high-risk populations. In: Brookmeyer R, Stroup DF, eds. *Monitoring the Health of Populations: Statistical Principles and Methods for Public Health Surveillance*. New York: Oxford University Press; 2004:37–70.

39. U.S. Centers for Disease Control and Prevention. National Health and Nutrition Examination Survey. Available at: http://www.cdc.gov/nchs/nhanes.htm. Accessed March 1, 2013.

40. U.S. Centers for Disease Control and Prevention. Behavioral Risk Factor Surveillance System. Available at: http://www.cdc.gov/brfss/. Accessed March 1, 2013.

41. U.S. Centers for Disease Control and Prevention. Indicators for chronic disease surveillance. *MMWR Recomm Rep*. 2004;53:1–6.

42. Meriwether R. Blueprint for a national public health surveillance system. *J Public Health Manag Pract*. 1996;2:16–23.

43. Greenland S. Ecologic inference problems. In: Brookmeyer R, Stroup DF, eds. *Monitoring the Health of Populations: Statistical Principles and Methods for Public Health Surveillance*. New York: Oxford University Press; 2004:315–40.

44. Berkelman RL, Buehler JW. Public health surveillance of non-infectious chronic diseases: the potential to detect rapid changes in disease burden. *Int J Epidemiol*. 1990;19:628–35.

45. Bingenheimer JB, Raudenbush SW. Statistical and substantive inferences in public health: issues in the application of multilevel models. *Annu Rev Public Health*. 2004;25:53–77.

46. Teutsch SM. Considerations in planning a surveillance system. In: Teutsch SM, Churchill RE, eds. *Principles and Practice of Public Health Surveillance*. New York: Oxford University Press; 2000:17–29.

47. Romaguera RA, German RR, Klaucke DN. Evaluating public health surveillance. In: Teutsch SM, Churchill RE, eds. *Principles and Practice of Public Health Surveillance*. New York: Oxford University Press; 2000:176–93.

48. Murray CJL, Lopez AD, eds. *The Global Burden of Disease: A Comprehensive Assessment of Mortality and Disability from Diseases, Injuries, and Risk Factors in 1990 and Projected to 2020.* Cambridge, MA: Harvard University Press; 1996.

49. White ME, McDonnell SM. Public health surveillance in low- and middle-income countries. In: Teutsch SM, Churchill RE, eds. *Principles and Practice of Public Health Surveillance.* New York: Oxford University Press; 2000:287–315.

50. U.S. Centers for Disease Control and Prevention. Current trends update on acquired immune deficiency syndrome (AIDS)—United States. *MMWR.* 1982;31:513–4.

51. U.S. Centers for Disease Control and Prevention. Revision of the CDC surveillance case definition for acquired immunodeficiency syndrome. *MMWR Supplement.* 1987;36:1S–15S.

52. U.S. Centers for Disease Control and Prevention. 1993 revised classification system for HIV infection and expanded surveillance case definition for AIDS among adolescents and adults. *MMWR Recomm Rep.* 1992;41:1–19.

53. U.S. Centers for Disease Control and Prevention. Current trends update: impact of the expanded AIDS surveillance case definition for adolescents and adults on case reporting—United States, 1993. *MMWR.* 1994;43:167–70.

54. World Health Organization. AIDS and HIV case definitions: overview of internationally used HIV/AIDS case definitions. Available at: http://www.who.int/hiv/strategic/surveillance/definitions/en/. Accessed March 1, 2013.

55. Pinner RW, Rebmann CA, Schuchat A, et al. Disease surveillance and the academic, clinical, and public health communities. *Emerg Infect Dis.* 2003;9:781–7.

56. Swaminathan B, Barrett TJ, Hunter SB, et al. PulseNet: the molecular subtyping network for foodborne bacterial disease surveillance, United States. *Emerg Infect Dis.* 2001;7:382–9.

57. U.S. Centers for Disease Control and Prevention. Progress in improving state and local disease surveillance—United States, 2000–2005. *MMWR.* 2005;54:822–5.

58. Effler P, Ching-Lee M, Bogard A, et al. Statewide system of electronic notifiable disease reporting from clinical laboratories: comparing automated reporting with conventional methods. *JAMA.* 1999;282:1845–50.

59. Ward M, Brandsema P, van Straten E, et al. Electronic reporting improves timeliness and completeness of infectious disease notification, The Netherlands, 2003. *Euro Surveill.* 2005;10:27–30.

60. World Health Organization. International Health Regulations (IHR). Available at: http://www.who.int/csr/ihr/en/. Accessed March 1, 2013.

61. Cates W. Estimates of the incidence and prevalence of sexually transmitted diseases in the United States. *Sex Trans Dis.* 1999;26:S2–S7.

62. Anderson JE, McCormick L, Fichtner R. Factors associated with self-reported STDs: data from a national survey. *Sex Trans Dis.* 1994;21:303–8.

63. Janes GR, Hutwagner L, Cates W, Jr., et al. Descriptive epidemiology: analyzing and interpreting surveillance data. In: Teutsch SM, Churchill RE, eds. *Principles and Practice of Public Health Surveillance.* New York: Oxford University Press; 2000:112–167.

64. U.S. Centers for Disease Control and Prevention. Surveillance for traumatic brain injury deaths—United States, 1989–1998. *MMWR Surveill Summ.* 2002;51:1–16.

65. Krause G, Ropers G, Stark K. Notifiable disease surveillance and practicing physicians. *Emerg Infect Dis.* 2005;11:442–5.

66. Tufte ER. *The Visual Display of Quantitative Information.* Chesire, CT: Graphics Press; 1983.

67. Storm HH, et al. *Guidelines on Confidentiality for Population-based Cancer Registration* (IARC Internal Report No. 2004/03). Lyon, France: International Association of Cancer Registries; 2004.

68. Havener LA, ed. *Standards for Cancer Registries. Vol III. Standards for Completeness, Quality, Analysis, and Management of Data.* Springfield, IL: North American Association of Central Cancer Registries; 2004.

69. Wurtz R, Cameron BJ. Electronic laboratory reporting for the infectious diseases physician and clinical microbiologist. *Clin Infect Dis.* 2005;40:1638–43.

70. American Public Health Association. Principles of the ethical practice of public health. Available at: http://www.apha.org/NR/rdonlyres/1CED3CEA-287E-4185-9CBD-BD405FC60856/0/ethics brochure.pdf. Accessed March 1, 2013.

71. U.S. Centers for Disease Control and Prevention. HIPAA Privacy Rule and Public Health. *MMWR Suppl.* 2003;52:1–24.

72. U.S. Centers for Disease Control and Prevention. Guidelines for national human immunodeficiency virus case surveillance, including monitoring for human immunodeficiency virus infection and acquired immunodeficiency syndrome. *MMWR Recomm Rep.* 1999;48:1–28.

73. Council of State and Territorial Epidemiologists. Public health practice vs. research: a report for public health practitioners including cases and guidance for making distinctions. Available at: http://www.cste .org/publications.asp. Accessed December 14, 2005.

74. Office for Human Research Protections. Public welfare: protection of human subjects, 2005. [45 CFR 46]. Available at: http://www.hhs.gov/ohrp/humansubjects/guidance/45cfr46.htm. Accessed December 14, 2005.

75. U.S. Centers for Disease Control and Prevention. Framework for program evaluation in public health. *MMWR Recomm Rep.* 1999;48:1–40.

76. European Commission. Protocol for the evaluation of EU-wide surveillance networks on communicable diseases. Available at: http://ec.europa.eu/health/ph_projects/2002/com_diseases/fp_commdis _2002_frep_18_en.pdf. Accessed March 1, 2013.

Strategic Planning in Public Health

James H. Stephens and Gerald R. Ledlow

LEARNING OBJECTIVES

- To describe the planning process and how decision making and resource allocation are related to leading and managing the strategic planning process in a public health organization
- To summarize the sequential steps in the planning process from situational analyses and strategy development to action planning and progress reporting
- To apply a strategy and associate goals, objectives, and action steps for a public health organization program or area of responsibility
- To differentiate the levels or components of the planning process and distinguish each level or component from the other within the hierarchy of a public health organization
- To plan and design a strategy and a strategic planning process for a public health organization based on a program or area of responsibility
- To compare and contrast two strategic plans from health-related organizations, noting the quality of the planning process, the ability to implement the plan, and the ability to conduct progress reporting

---

Chapter Overview

Strategic planning is essential in order to successfully navigate the situational and organizational changes that public health professionals face today. "Strategic processes encompass a wide range of topics including analysis, planning, decision making and many aspects of an organization's culture, vision and value system."[1] The art and science of planning must be embedded in the culture of the public health organization in order to positively impact population health status and meet health challenges at the local, state, regional, national, and even global levels. From a national perspective, *Healthy People 2000, 2010,* and *2020* are, in essence, strategies and goals developed as part of a strategic planning effort. Although most public health professionals focus on local, regional, or state responsibilities, the planning process—coupled with artful utilization of relationships and scientific utilization of planning tools—is salient at any level and for any type of public health organization.

Planning is a critical factor for success today. Of immediate concern, strategic planning is required for public health accreditation for county/district public health operations and also to comply with the federal mandate for implementing preparedness programs at the state and local jurisdictional levels in accordance with the Centers for Disease Control and Prevention (CDC) and the Assistant Secretary for Preparedness and Response under the Department of Health and Human Services. From this assessment, in essence a situational analysis of the public health environment, building and maintaining a culture of planning will be a critical and embedded component of successful public health operations and management into the future.

This chapter presents strategic planning as a fundamental function of leadership and management, from which all other outcomes are achieved; planning must become part of the organizational culture. Leaders in public health organizations utilize a strategic system of leadership and management. Much of the literature uses the phrase, "strategic management system." However, because people are led and resources are managed, a more appropriate name for this system is "strategic system of leadership and management." Human resources are "managed" within the context of a strategic human resources system that considers job analysis, job design, and the like. But people should be *led* rather than *managed.*

A useful metaphor for understanding strategic planning and leadership is "planning as roadmap or journey." In this light, strategy development and implementation are a journey that must be planned, and the organization's vision is the idealized destination. Many paths, stops, and issues will arise along the way. Leaders are critical in determining the optimal route (goals and objectives) to ensure that the organization reaches the intended destination (vision).

This chapter presents some working definitions of planning, discusses planning as a process and outcome, and explores the role of leaders in planning. It describes strategic thought and development of a strategic plan, the process and tools used to assess the external and internal situation, and the tactical action involved in implementing the plan. Although these processes and steps are presented linearly, in reality, they are iterative and often carried out in tandem. Many of the concepts and terms have been borrowed from the healthcare industry, where strategic planning has long served an important role. It is hoped that public health professionals, who increasingly are being called upon to employ strategic planning in a more systematic way, will benefit from the experience of healthcare leaders.

Planning

Planning is vital to the survival of the organization. Creating a plan is an investment of resources committed to improving the organization. Improvement is realized through internal acceptance, change, and evolution. Developing the organization to best meet the needs and demands of the community and other stakeholders is at the heart of planning. Because the environment, technology, information, people, financing, and governmental policies and laws constantly change, the organization must change in order to survive, succeed, and prosper.

A set of basic definitions will assist in understanding some distinctions among several types of planning:

1. **Planning** is a process that uses macro and micro environmental factors and internal information to engage stakeholders to create a framework, template, and outline for section, branch, or organizational success; planning can be strategic or operational or a combination of both.

2. **Strategic planning** is concerned with finding the best future for your organization and determining how the organization will evolve to realize that future; it is a *stream of organizational decisions* focused in a specific direction based on organizational values, strategies, and goals. The focus is on external considerations and how the organization can best serve the external markets' expectations, demands, and needs.

3. **Operational planning** is about finding the best methods, processes, and systems to accomplish the mission/vision, strategies, goals, and objectives of the organization in the most effective, efficient, and efficacious way possible. Operational planning focuses on internal resources, systems, processes, methods, and considerations.

Planning as Process and Outcome

Recall that planning can be thought of as a journey or a roadmap. The journey must have a destination. The journey must be planned. It is a planned journey forward in time. In that light, planning includes both a process (developing and achieving goals and objectives) and an outcome (the plan itself). Planning as a process involves moving an organization along a predetermined path based upon the organization's values. Similar to deciding what road to take, what stops to make, and who will drive, the process involves deciding upon what goals are most important to the organization and what objectives must be met to reach those goals. Planning can be described as an ongoing process of thinking and implementing at multiple levels. General and President Eisenhower said that the plan is important but the process of planning is even more important; the team building, achievement, and success orientation that a culture of planning and implementation bring to an organization are invaluable.

Planning also has an outcome. Effective planning will pave the way toward the organization's vision—a better future state based on organizational values and the external environment. Improving effectiveness, efficiency, efficacy, customer satisfaction, employee satisfaction, community satisfaction, and financial performance will move the organization to the next level, making it possible to realize the vision.

The Public Health Leader's Role in Planning

Planning is an essential leadership skill that requires knowledge about planning, the ability to structure and develop a system of planning, and the capacity to shape and lead a planning culture. Effective planning and consistent leadership practice are vital to linking clinical, policy, and administrative domains.[2] Planning is a key step in decision making.[3] Moreover, planning is a cultural imperative and a method for leaders to guide the organization to be more effective, efficient, and efficacious.[4,5] Public health leaders who can understand, apply, and evaluate planning will have advantages over those who haphazardly plan or fail to plan.

Public health leaders plan at all levels of an organization. Each leader will have a vision for his or her tasks or responsibilities. This importantly includes planning the operational actions necessary within each area of responsibility to implement the senior leadership team's strategic or operational plans. At each level, public health leaders are directing, staffing, organizing, controlling, and rewarding. These five elements are crucial as leaders embrace the foundations and functions of planning. In planning, leadership should come from within the organization at all levels.

Most people look for leaders who have a vision and can direct them along the path of the mission. Morris[6] and Senge[7] call strategists, in this case health organization strategists, *pathfinders* in that they provide a vision, determine the approaches to take to realize the vision and provide a clear methodology to implement and succeed. Health leaders are clearly in the pathfinder role for their organizations. Health leaders provide structure, process, macro direction, a shared outcome with all stakeholders, motivation, accountability, influence, obstacle removal, resources, and persistence in the overall effort of *directing, staffing, organizing, controlling, and rewarding.* The morale of the organization can sometimes fall into the hands of the visionaries of the organization: Staff members of the organization look to the visionaries to lead by example, and the effort should be exciting such that followers are excited to follow.

Embedding a strategic and operational planning structure and process (with feedback loops) into the organizational culture is paramount for organizations to survive in dynamic conditions. Regardless of organizational type, industry, or size, strategic systems are required. As complexity increases, strategic systems become more critical, as long as leaders consistently apply these systems in accordance with organizational values. Without effective leaders ensuring a well organized planning process, poor plans might be implemented or great plans might fail.

Strategic Thought and Planning

All organizations require the leaders' understanding and wise use of strategic thought and planning. Public health leaders should utilize a strategic and operational planning process to derive the organization's mission, vision, strategies, goals, objectives, and action steps. These elements are then used to transform and guide the organization, to develop and maintain an effective, efficient, and efficacious organizational culture, and to focus the collective energy of the health organization where people are led and resources are managed. "Strategy-making processes are organizational-level phenomena involving key decisions made on behalf of the entire organization."[8, p. 3]

Leaders must be ever cognizant to be consistent in the development of a mission statement and a vision statement and to embrace the values the health organization holds as important. Values are the beliefs and attitudes that an organization holds that guide day-to-day decision making, behavior, and actions. Yukl suggests that leaders use mission and vision to transform organizations by developing and articulating a clear and appealing strategic vision, by developing a strategy or strategies to attain the vision, and by focusing on the core mission(s) of the organization.[3] Schein argues that organizational mission, vision, and strategies are essential for adapting to the expectations of the external environment.[9] Senior leadership must be committed to and involved in the process of mission and vision statement development but must involve their subordinates and staff in the process as well.[10]

Mission, vision, and values are guideposts[4] that leaders utilize to focus the health organization's collective energy and resources. Strategic planning—including development of strategies, goals, objectives, and action steps—is how the organization intends to achieve its goals. Each element of strategic and operational planning is discussed in rational groupings.

Vision

Vision is an aspiration of what the organization intends to become. It is the shared image of the future organization that places the organization in a better position to fulfill its mission. In essence, vision is the dream of what the organization can become. Health leaders

> acquire vision from an appreciation of the history of the organization, a perception of the opportunities present in the environment, and an understanding of the strategic capacity of the organization to take advantage of these opportunities. These factors work together to form an organization's hope for the future.[10, p. 198]

The vision provides the motivational guidance for the organization and typically is defined and promoted by senior leadership.[11] The healthcare leader must energize his followers to "buy in" to the vision in order for the organization to begin its strategic journey on the correct path. However, public health leaders must understand that implementing strategic plans is quite difficult if the vision goes against the grain of the organization's culture. The strategic vision must be tested and retested to ensure buy in from all stakeholders, including external and internal. A vision may require many drafts and revisions to ensure that the needs of all stakeholders are met.

"The purpose of a vision statement is to provide a group, organization, or community with a shared image of its direction over the long term. … the vision should be stated in the form of concrete ideals rather than generalizations, should directly link the organizational values and culture to the future direction of the organization, and should communicate a unique future to stakeholders."[12]

"Vision statements should:

1. Describe an organization's big picture and project its future
2. Be grounded in sound knowledge of the business
3. Be concrete and as specific as practical
4. Contrast the present and the future
5. Stretch the imaginations and creative energies of people in the organization
6. Have a sense of significance"[13]

The following is an example of a well-written public health vision statement for the city of Chicago, Illinois:

> The Chicago Partnership's vision for local public health is: A responsive, sustainable public health system that, through cooperative efforts, planning and policy development, a broad focus on health promotion and disease prevention, and shared leadership and accountability, is positioned to respond to current and future public health challenges, and protects and promotes the health and wellbeing of all Chicago communities, residents, and visitors, particularly the most disadvantaged.[14]

Once an organizational vision is developed, intent must be established. Intent describes the impact to the organization if change does not occur. Organizational leaders must outline how these impacts or crises could potentially impact the viability of the organization. Examples of crises include market changes, technological advances causing older technology to become obsolete, personnel shortages, and decreased reimbursement from payers. Revisiting the roadmap analogy, failing to establish intent would be like driving the wrong direction without a roadmap to help correct course.

Mission

Mission defines where the organization currently exists in terms of what its purpose is and how it intends to accomplish that purpose. Mission is why the organization exists, what business it is in, whom it serves, and where it provides its products or services. The **mission statement** identifies the organization's reason for being. The mission statement also provides guidance in decision making, ensuring that the organization stays on the track that its leaders have predetermined. From the mission, strategies to achieve the mission and, ultimately, the vision are devised.

A health organization's mission is tied to its purpose. Purpose defines what the organization does every day to meet the needs and demands of the external environment and stakeholders and to deliver its outputs to a community in some competitive way (effective, efficient, efficacious, and accessible). Stakeholders are individuals or groups, such as patients, customers, staff members, suppliers, members of the community, and companies, that interact with the organization. Stakeholders can directly and indirectly influence the success of the organization. An extension of purpose is a health organization's mission.

Mission statements must be written using language that allows any member within the organization to fully understand and articulate it to others. The mission statement must answer three questions:

1. *Who* are they?
2. *What* do they want to accomplish?
3. *How* are they going to accomplish it?

The following are characteristics of mission statements:

1. "Mission statements are broadly defined statements of purpose;
2. Mission statements are enduring;

3. Mission statements should underscore the uniqueness of the organization; and

4. Mission statements should identify the scope of operations in terms of service and market."[10, pp. 191–2]

The following is an example of a well-written mission statement from the American Cancer Society:

> The American Cancer Society is the nationwide community-based voluntary health organization dedicated to eliminating cancer as a major health problem by preventing cancer, saving lives, and diminishing suffering from cancer, through research, education, advocacy, and service.[15]

Strategies

Strategies, goals, and objectives are the sequential building blocks of planning to successfully achieve the mission but also to strive to achieve the vision of the health organization. In some ways, "mission, vision, values, and strategic goals are appropriately called directional strategies because they guide strategists when they make key organizational decisions."[10, p. 187] Strategies follow "a decision logic of development."[10, p. 227] Directional strategies lead to adaptive strategies, market-entry strategies, and competitive strategies; each strategy should also have an implementation strategy.[10, p. 227]

The Strategic Plan

Once the vision, mission, and strategies have been established, the strategic plan needs to be developed. The strategic plan includes goals, objectives, and action steps in a hierarchical order. This multilevel approach focuses and narrows effort for each section within the health organization. From the roadmap perspective, the quickest, most efficient route must be drawn to the final destination (i.e., the vision). One can assume that a good plan will lead to an effective outcome. That outcome is achieving the vision while reporting progress along the way.

Goals

"Strategic goals are those overarching end results that the organization pursues to accomplish its mission and achieve its vision."[10, p. 187] Goals are broad statements (sometimes aspirations) of direction that come from strategies, and are hierarchically above objectives. They further refine the broad strategies by focusing organizational resources to achieve the vision and the mission. They are expected to be general, observable, challenging, and untimed.[16] Of note, different strategic frameworks sometimes switch goals with objectives and objectives with goals. Whatever framework you select for your organization, try to be consistent. It is not important if goals are at a higher level than objectives or vice versa; what does matter is that a planning and execution culture grows and matures in your health organization.

Objectives

Objectives fall hierarchically under goals. They are specific statements that align organizational resources to meet the stated goals. Objectives should be measurable, assigned to a responsible person or agent or owner, have timelines for completion, and be frequently reviewed by the health organization leadership for progress and resource sufficiency. The focus should be to develop objectives within the "SMART" framework; to be SMART, objectives must be specific, measurable, attainable, rewarding, and timed.

Action Steps

Establishing and implementing action steps or tactics follows the establishment of the vision, mission, and strategic including goals and objectives. Action steps or tactics represent a final level of planning and provide the most specific approach to describing who, what, when, where, and how activities will take place to accomplish an objective. Action steps (or action plans) are created to produce a step-by-step or task-level implementation sequence for each objective. Each task in the action steps (or plan) has a responsible person(s) or owner, a time range for accomplishment, and sometimes a measureable variable as well. Action step owners report to the objective owner who reports to the goal owner who ultimately reports to the leadership team; the senior leadership team directs the organization at the strategy level.

The Situational Assessment

Strategic planning can be described as an organizational planning process that analyzes the current situation of an organization and forecasts how an organization will change or evolve over a specified period of time. In all public health organizations, departmental restructuring, implementation of new technologies, health threat dynamics, and demographic changes may indicate a need for an organization to develop a strategic plan to support the overall plan of the organization. A crucial step in strategic planning is to conduct a situational assessment, which includes assessing the environment and the internal organization, after which the vision, mission, strategies, goals, objectives, and action steps are developed. Without this structure and sign posts as first steps, the organization cannot move forward. All public health leaders must be able to conduct a situational assessment, which would incorporate an assessment of the internal and external environments. A situational assessment must be an objective and honest look at the numerous diverse factors that could impact the public health organization's success in achieving its vision, mission, strategies, and goals and, importantly, meeting federal, state, and local governmental mandates.

One tool commonly used for the external and internal assessment is the SWOT analysis, which investigates internal *s*trengths and *w*eaknesses and external *o*pportunities and *t*hreats.[17] The purpose of a SWOT analysis is to measure whether an organization is prepared to perform effectively in a challenging and competitive environment. The SWOT analysis offers insight into the internal and external factors that will have an effect on an organization's performance and success.

Assessing the External Environment

Continuous environmental scanning is crucial for organizations to survive in the dynamic public health and healthcare industries. A leader's and leadership team's responsibility is to remain current and relevant to situational and environmental change that can or will impact the organization. Forces that contribute to the health industry's rapid and dynamic environment are varied but are cumulative and thus have a cumulative impact on the industry. "Technology, demography, economics, and politics drive change, not only as individual factors but interacting to make the rate of change faster."[18, p. 1]

Every organization needs more information about the environment than just its potential opportunities and threats. Choo reports that it is important to obtain information about relationships, trends, and information in the external environment; health leaders need to know what is impacting the industry and the economy.[19] A focused environmental scan concentrates on specific information, such as how many consumers bought a particular product or service in the last year. External scanning, whether focused or more general, is essential for planning and forecasting the organization's performance into the future.

Another approach is to look at the dynamic environment as macro-environmental forces and health as micro-environmental forces. Validated over the 2 decades since 1992, Rakich, Longest, and Darr[20] provided categories for this approach that give leaders categories to scan (environmental scanning) to keep current and relevant in the industry:

1. Macro-Environmental Forces
   a. Legal, ethical forces;
   b. Political forces;
   c. Cultural, sociological forces;
   d. Public expectations;
   e. Economic forces; and
   f. Ecological forces.
2. Health Environmental [micro-environmental] Forces
   a. Planning, public policy forces;
   b. Competitive forces;
   c. Healthcare financing, governmental funding;
   d. Technology forces;
   e. Health research and education;
   f. Health status and health promotion; and
   g. Integration with other health disciplines such as primary, secondary and
      tertiary care and other public health forces.[18, p. 17]

The Rand Corporation suggests that the immense pressure of cost containment and speed of change are the leading factors in the health industry at this time.[21] Multiple forces cumulatively contribute to change in the health industry. If one compares the health organizations of the 1960s or 1970s to those of today, there is a vast difference between the two temporal organizations. The speed of that change in a mere 40 to 50 years is astonishing, and so is the success of healthcare delivery systems to diagnose, treat, and rehabilitate patients who present with health needs. In public health, consider the life expectancy of people living in the 1960s compared to today. "Between 1961 and 1999, average life expectancy in the U.S. increased from 66.9 to 74.1 years for men and from 73.5 to 79.6 for women."[22] Trends in aging are also tied to life expectancy but have profound impact on health services.[23] The dynamic whirlwind, often called "white water change," frames a picture of the world the health leader must navigate.

Although there have been tremendous successes, public health leaders must continue to use the dynamic nature of the industry to challenge their organizations, groups, teams, and individuals to become more efficient, effective, and efficacious while under significant cost-containment pressure. Consider the number of natural, man-made, and terrorism-related disasters, threats, and challenges faced by our nation in the past 3 decades to get a perspective on the importance of situational assessment. From a practical viewpoint, Kotter suggests eight steps to transform organizations in dynamic situations:

1. Establishing a sense of urgency;
2. Forming a powerful guiding coalition;
3. Creating a vision;
4. Communicating the vision;
5. Empowering others to act on the vision;
6. Planning for and creating short-term wins;
7. Consolidating improvements and producing still more change; and
8. Institutionalizing new approaches.[24, p. 7]

Kotter's eight steps are a sequence of leader actions and are cybernetic (there is a feedback loop from the last step back to the first step). Leaders of public health organizations should consider the changes in the macro and micro environment against the *cost, quality,* and *access* health assessment constructs for community members they serve. The leader must stay attuned to the macro and micro forces of change; professional associations and societies can assist greatly in this continuous effort.

Understanding the Internal Environment

Understanding the internal environment of the health organization is vital to strategic thinking, planning, and implementation. Roney suggests internal assessment is a basic component of any comprehensive plan.[25] Internal scanning, monitoring, and assessment of the health organization are vital leadership activities. Research consistently points to active and ongoing leadership emphasis in this area.

To understand the internal health organization's environment, attention should be focused on systems such as human resources management, supply chain, technology, information, and culture and subcultures. The salient theme is integrated synergy among all the health organization's systems. Specific areas of scanning, monitoring, and assessing for the health leader are: 1) competitive advantage and the unique or distinctive competencies the organization possesses (e.g., centers of excellence); 2) strengths and weaknesses of the organization; 3) functional strategies for implementation of strategies that are supported by goals, objectives, and action steps; 4) operational effectiveness, efficiency, and efficacy; and 5) organizational culture (i.e., whether the culture aligned with the organization's direction).

Health leaders must create a well thought out approach to internal scanning, monitoring, and assessing the organization against the current strategic and operational plans (that focus effort toward the organization's vision and mission) and the fit with the external environment. How the health leader conducts internal scanning, monitoring, and assessment depends on the viewpoint or paradigm or context. Leaders develop assumptions and constraints that are internally oriented to achieve understanding of the internal environment. Assumptions in this context are internal (rooted in organizational circumstances) and are characterized by a situation or state that exists now or in the future that guides thinking. Constraints are a current condition that may prevent strategies or goals from being pursued in striving to meet the organizational vision. Constraints are rooted in existing rules, traditions, habits, policies, social norms, or laws that set parameters on what an organization or individual can do.

Tactical Action to Implement the Strategic Plan

Strategic thought and planning are followed by tactical action, which includes commitment, execution, and accountability. In health, we define these as the feelings, practices, and metrics for changing the future state of the organization.[12] If strategic thought is the plan for the journey to reach the final destination, tactical action is the journey itself, including the mechanism for getting there. Tactical action requires commitment within the organization, execution of the plan, and finally, accountability within organizational leadership.

Commitment

Commitment, like the strategic vision, involves buy in by the organization and its internal and external stakeholders. It involves a relationship between organizational leaders and followers whereby each party has a clear understanding of the strategic vision and his or her role in reaching the vision. Without commitment on all levels, it is impossible to achieve the strategic vision effectively and efficiently. The responsibility of successfully implementing the strategic vision is assigned to all members of the organization, whether they are management or staff. From a leadership perspective, a leader can foster commitment within his or her team by serving as a model and demonstrating a strong commitment to the plan and vision. A leader cannot expect buy in from followers if he or she has not fully committed to the vision.

Execution

The execution phase of the strategic plan involves each team member performing his or her assigned duty. Without a strong, unified commitment, execution of the plan will be a dismal failure. It is the leader's responsibility to enhance motivation and maintain commitment within the team, particularly when facing obstacles. The health leader must be supportive of his or her team members, enabling them with the skills, equipment, and materials to effectively carry out their role in the plan.

Accountability: Measurement and Feedback

Public health leaders must remember that what is measured gets done; all planning objectives and action steps must be measureable, assigned to an accountable and responsible person, and be set within a specific time period. Leaders and followers require consistent feedback about performance during execution of the plan. It will be necessary for measures to be in place to gauge successes or lack thereof during this time. Periodic progress reviews (monthly or quarterly) are essential to see the movement toward success. Successes should be acknowledged between leaders and followers, because employees desire to know that a plan is working. Public health leaders also should publically praise success and reward those who achieve predetermined action steps, objectives, and goals. On the other hand, lack of success should be treated as an opportunity for improvement. Leaders must analyze the execution of the plan to identify inconsistencies and make appropriate modifications.

Future Outlook

As highlighted in the beginning of the chapter, planning is required for accreditation of public health organizations as well as for meeting federal mandates for public health preparedness programs in all states, territories, and consularies of the United States. Creating a planning culture is essential for success. An example is provided using the Public Health Emergency Preparedness (PHEP) program, which is managed by the Centers for Disease Control and Prevention (CDC), and the Healthcare/Hospital Preparedness Program (HPP), managed by the Assistant Secretary for Preparedness and Response (both are subordinate to U.S. Department of Health and Human Services). **Figure 16.1** provides a "mental map" of the planning process in action. The

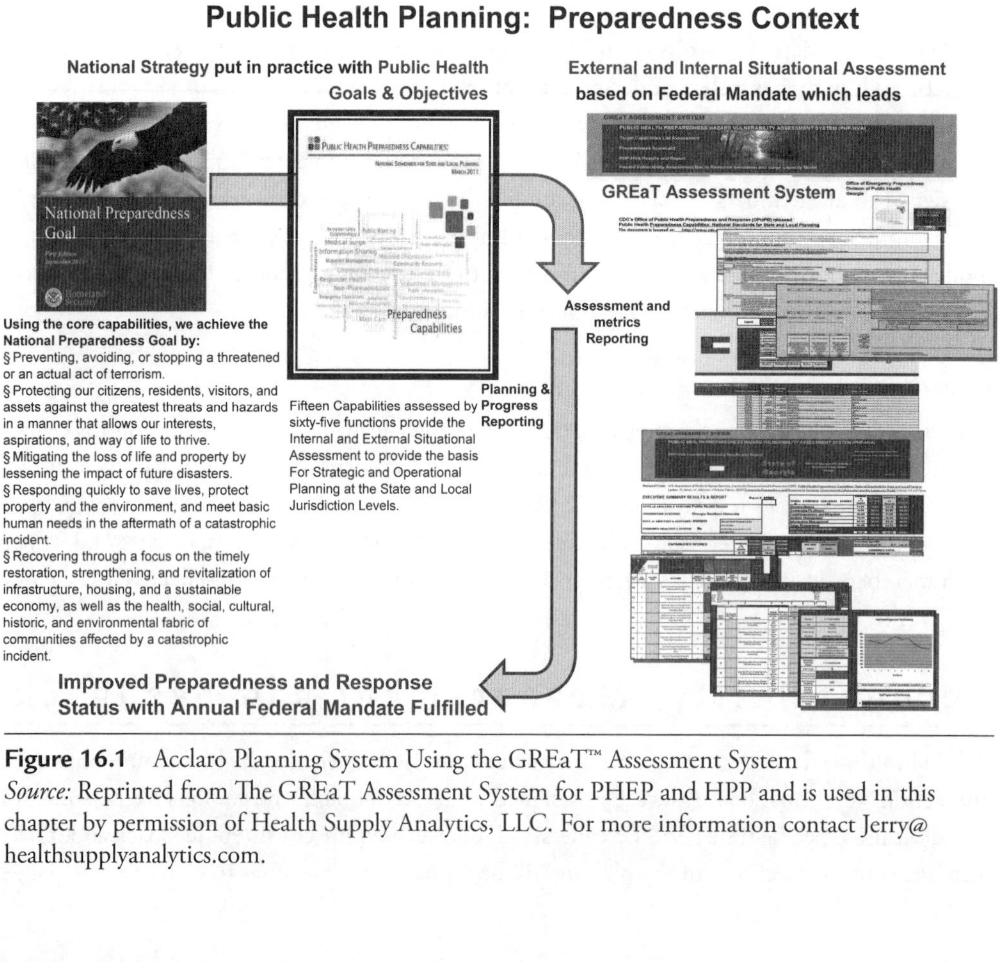

Figure 16.1 Acclaro Planning System Using the GREaT™ Assessment System
Source: Reprinted from The GREaT Assessment System for PHEP and HPP and is used in this chapter by permission of Health Supply Analytics, LLC. For more information contact Jerry@ healthsupplyanalytics.com.

GREaT Assessment System provides the basis for the required assessment of 15 capabilities and 65 functions for the PHEP program and 8 capabilities and 29 functions of the HPP program.[i]

In the future, planning will lead to improvement of public health practices, disaster and terrorism preparedness and response, and, ultimately, improvement in community health status. In all that public health does, planning will be an essential part of the culture in the ongoing effort to improve health and quality of life for our nation and world.

Discussion Questions

1. Describe the process of developing a strategic plan and its core key element for a public health organization.
2. How would a public health executive compare and differentiate two strategic plans from public health–related organizations?
3. Outline the difference between goals and objectives when designing a strategic plan for a public health organization.
4. Describe how decision making and resource allocation are important to managing a strategic planning process in a public health organization.
5. What are the sequential steps in the planning process from situational analyses and strategy development to action planning and progress reporting?

References

1. Hart S. An integrative framework for strategy-making processes. *Acad Manag Rev*. 1992;17:327–51.
2. Granda-Cameron C, Lynch MP, Mintzer D, et al. Bringing an inpatient palliative care program to a teaching hospital: lessons in leadership. *Oncol Nurs Forum*. 2007;34(4):772–6.
3. Yukl G. *Leadership in Organizations*. 3rd ed. Englewood Cliffs, NJ: Prentice Hall; 1994.
4. Ledlow G, Cwiek M. The Process of Leading: Assessment and Comparison of Leadership Team Style, Operating Climate and Expectation of the External Environment. Global Business and Technology Association Proceedings Volume, Lisbon, Portugal, July 2005.
5. Ledlow G, Cwiek M, Johnson J. Dynamic culture leadership: effective leader as both scientist and artist. In: Delener N, Chao C, Eds. Proceedings of Global Business and Technology Association International Conference, *Beyond Boundaries: Challenges of Leadership, Innovation, Integration and Technology*. 2002; 694–740.
6. Morris GB. The executive: a pathfinder. *Org Dynamics*. 1988;16(2):62–77.
7. Senge P. The leader's new work. *Sloan Manag Rev*. 1990;21(1):8.
8. Dess GG, Lumpkin GT. Emerging issues in strategy process research. In: Hitt MA, Freeman RE, Harrison JS, Eds. *The Blackwell Handbook of Strategic Management*. Malden, MA: Blackwell Publishing; 2005.
9. Schein EH. *The Corporate Culture Survival Guide: Sense and Nonsense About Culture Change*. San Francisco, CA: Jossey-Bass; 1999.
10. Swayne LE, Duncan WJ, & Ginter PM. *Strategic Management of Health Care Organizations*. 5th ed. Malden, MA: Blackwell Publishing; 2006.
11. *The Bible*, Proverbs 29:18.
12. Eicher JP. (2006). Making strategy happen. *Performance Improvement*. 2006;45(10):31–48.

---

[i] The GREaT Assessment System for PHEP and HPP is used in this chapter by permission of Health Supply Analytics, LLC. For more information contact Jerry@healthsupplyanalytics.com.

13. Lerner H. Vision statements. *Principal's Report*, 2003;3(12):2. As cited in Swayne LE, Duncan WJ, & Ginter PM. *Strategic Management of Health Care Organizations*. 5th ed. Malden, MA: Blackwell Publishing; 2006.

14. NACCHO. Sample Vision Statements. Available at: http://www.naccho.org/topics/infrastructure/mapp/visionsamples.cfm. Accessed March 25, 2013.

15. ACS Mission Statements. Available at: http://www.cancer.org/aboutus/whoweare/acsmissionstatements. Accessed March 25, 2013.

16. Higgins J. *The Management Challenge*. 2nd ed. New York: Macmillan; 1994.

17. Van der Werff TJ, CMC. Strategic Planning for Fun and Profit. Available at: Global Future http://www.globalfuture.com/planning9.htm. Accessed July 27, 2009.

18. Griffith JR. *The Well-Managed Healthcare Organization*. 4th ed. Chicago: Health Administration Press; 1999.

19. Choo CW. Environmental scanning as information seeking and organizational learning. *Information Research*. 2001;7(1).

20. Rakich J, Longest B, Darr K. Man*aging Health Services Organizations*. Baltimore, MD: Health Professions Press; 1992.

21. Brook RH. Changes in the healthcare system: goals, forces, solutions. *Pharmacoeconomics*. 1998;1:45–8.

22. Harvard University School of Public Health. Life expectancy worsening or stagnating for large segment of the U.S. population. Available at: http://www.hsph.harvard.edu/news/press-releases/2008-releases/life-expectancy-worsening-or-stagnating-for-large-segment-of-the-us-population.html. Accessed March 8, 2013.

23. Centers for Disease Control and Prevention. Public Health and Aging: Trends in Aging—United States and Worldwide. *MMWR*. 2003;52(06):101–6. Available at: http://www.cdc.gov/mmwr/preview/mmwrhtml/mm5206a2.htm. Accessed March 8, 2013.

24. Kotter JP. Leading change: why transformation efforts fail. In: *Harvard Business Review on Change*. Boston, MA: Harvard Business School Press; 1998:1–20.

25. Roney CW. *Strategic Management Methodology: Generally Accepted Principles for Practitioners*. Westport, CT: Praeger Publishers; 2004.

Performance Management in Public Health

Leslie M. Beitsch, Laura B. Landrum, Bernard J. Turnock, and Arden S. Handler

LEARNING OBJECTIVES

- To understand the challenges faced by public health practitioners related to performance at the many different levels of the public health system
- To appreciate the historical trends that resulted in the development of public health standards and measures
- To describe and explain the elements of performance management as developed by Turning Point: performance standards, performance measures, reporting of progress, and quality improvement process
- To explain the meaning and use of performance measures and standards
- To develop an understanding of the "10 Essential Public Health Services" as a foundation for the National Public Health Performance Standards (NPHPS), the "Operational Definition of a Functional Local Health Department," and the new Public Health Accreditation Board accreditation program standards
- To understand the integration of national public health performance standards into the community assessment process, and why it improves public health infrastructure and capacity
- To discuss the development of the nascent Public Health Accreditation Board accreditation program and how it may improve public health performance

Chapter Overview

Many public health organizations use performance management efforts to track the work they produce and the results they achieve. Additionally, organizations rely on performance measurement activities to achieve internal quality improvement goals and to demonstrate accountability to external stakeholders. Public health organizations have begun to focus on using performance measures to actively manage complex public health processes. Performance management integrates an organization's use of standards, measurement, and performance improvement to change institutional capacities, processes, and priorities and to more effectively address the needs of the communities they serve. A growing array of practical tools is available to assist organizations in carrying out performance management activities on a routine basis. The recently launched voluntary national health department accreditation program reinforces the trend toward greater deployment of quality improvement to strengthen health department performance and ensure public accountability.

Public health leaders and managers face issues related to performance at many levels of the public health system, including the performance of individuals, programs, agencies, interorganizational collaborations, and the public health enterprise itself. Although these levels represent different aspects of public health performance, each can be assessed using common approaches that focus on the work produced and the results achieved. Performance measurement is an important management tool with an impressive record of improving performance throughout the public and private sectors. These accomplishments derive from fundamental principles of the improvement science field: to improve something we must be able to control it; to control it we must be able to understand it; and to understand it we must be able to measure it.[1] The increasing ability of public health practitioners to link performance measurement and performance improvement provides a context for understanding the lessons and implications of performance measurement efforts in public health since the early 1990s. This chapter examines these lessons, as well as various applications using performance standards to improve the performance of public health organizations and systems, including the accreditation of public health agencies.

This chapter also describes the initial development of a performance management framework for use in public health organizations and systems as an early effort to link the various practices that have evolved in performance measurement, performance standards, and quality improvement.

The Elements of Performance Management

Drawing on a growing body of literature and new resources on performance standards, performance measures, and quality improvement, the Turning Point Performance Management National Excellence Collaborative in 2002 articulated the key elements of managing public health performance.[2,3] The collaborative defined performance management as the active use of performance data in making management decisions. The four quadrants of performance management are the following:

- Performance standards—various direction-setting practices, including goal setting, development of desired performance targets, benchmarking of levels of excellence in the field, a generally accepted expectation of what should be achieved

- Performance measures—the quantitative assessment of actual performance, particularly as it relates to relevant performance standards
- Reporting of progress—studies of performance trends, comparing actual to desired levels, and the distribution of these results to program managers, organizational leaders, and others who need to learn about and understand public health practice
- Quality improvement process—the use of standards, measurement, and performance reports in an action-oriented change-management process to revise program strategy and tactics and program and public policies and procedures to better attain desired performance results

The performance management model illustrated in **Figure 17.1** integrates elements of public health practice into a coherent model for understanding and directing complex public health programs, organizations, and systems. The framework also ties together more conceptual and elusive issues in public health policy, such as accountability, effectiveness, and benchmarking, incorporating

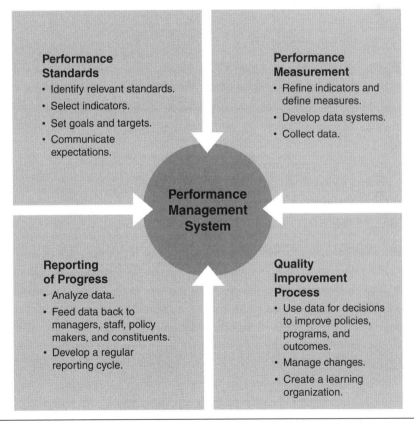

Figure 17.1   The Performance Management Model
Source: Reprinted from Turning Point National Office. *From Silos to Systems: Using Performance Management to Improve the Public's Health.* Seattle, WA: Turning Point; 2003. Copyright Robert Wood Johnson Foundation. From Turning Point, a national program of the Robert Wood Johnson Foundation from 1996–2006. Used with permission from the Robert Wood Johnson Foundation.

them into a practical and feasible model. The forerunner of this thinking about managing performance began with public health activities focused on performance measurement.[3,4]

Defining Performance Measurement

Performance measurement, performance monitoring, and performance improvement are topics that are extensively addressed in the literature.[5–7] **Performance measurement** is the selection and use of quantitative measures to reflect critical aspects of activities, including their effect on the public and other public health customers. Stated simply, it is the regular collection and reporting of data to track work that is performed and results that are achieved.

An effective performance measurement process incorporates stakeholder input; promotes top leadership support (enhancing organizational quality improvement [QI] culture); creates a clear mission statement; develops long-term goals and objectives; formulates short-term goals and interim measures; devises simple, manageable approaches; and provides support and technical assistance to those involved in the process. In this light, performance measurement serves several important purposes, providing information concerning the capacity to perform, results of current efforts, and effectiveness of current performance. Potential organizational benefits from measuring performance include the following:

- Clear goals and objectives
- Identification of strengths and weaknesses
- Opportunities for collaborative approaches internally and externally
- Clearer lines of accountability
- Improved quality
- Better tracking of progress over time
- More effective communication
- Better resource allocation and deployment
- Strengthened organizational effectiveness

Performance measurement focuses on what is occurring, but it does not extensively address why or how. Evaluative research (often called program evaluation) provides more in-depth assessment of the conceptualization, design, implementation, and utility of social interventions of the underlying activities being measured.[8] Performance measurement can be viewed as one component of a comprehensive evaluation, but its primary purpose is to inform managers so that changes can be instituted within the lifecycle of a set of activities. In sum, performance measurement is a management and oversight tool to facilitate positive change and improvement in performance.

The terminology used in performance measurement is often inconsistent and confusing; the definitions used in this chapter are adapted from several sources.[9,10] More recently, definitions specific to public health have been adopted.[11,12] In general, a performance measure is the specific quantitative representation of a capacity, process, or outcome that is deemed relevant to the assessment of performance. Similar to the concept of prevention, performance measurement requires an object. It is critical to specify what activity or performance is being measured. In public health, performance measurement most frequently occurs within the context of a particular program (e.g., childhood immunizations or retail food safety). However, the performance of an agency (e.g., a state or local health department), partnership, or community public health system is also an appropriate subject of performance measurement. Because the primary focus of this chapter is on measuring and improving performance in organizations and complex public health systems, the term *performance measurement* means the selection and use of quantitative measures of public health system capacities, processes, and outcomes to inform public health leaders and managers and the public about critical aspects of the public health system.

Performance measures that are used to determine whether or to what extent a performance standard is achieved are often called performance indicators. For example, a performance standard might call for a comprehensive community health assessment to be completed every 3 years. Performance indicators for this standard could take one of several forms. The administrator of the local public health agency could be asked whether this standard was met, or more objectively a review team might look for a completed assessment at the time of a site visit as empirical evidence. The agency administrator's response (yes or no) and the actual document are both performance indicators in this example that serve as evidence to determine whether the standard has been achieved. Standards and measures are used in precisely this manner with the National Public Health Performance Standards Program and the new voluntary national accreditation program. This interplay between performance standards and performance measures also conforms with the first two quadrants of the Turning Point model framework described earlier.

The definition of performance measurement acknowledges critical dimensions of performance, including capacities, processes, and outcomes. It is important to consider the meaning of the following terms as they relate to performance measurement for public health organizations and public health systems:

- Capacities refer to the resources and relationships necessary to carry out the important processes of public health; the capacity to perform is made possible by the maintenance of the basic infrastructure of the public health system, and by specific program resources.
- Processes refer to what is done to, for, with, or by defined individuals or groups to identify and address community or population-wide health problems. The performance of key processes (e.g., monitoring health status, investigating health hazards, and building constituencies) leads to the development of other processes that can also be viewed as "outputs." In public health practice, these outputs take the form of interventions (e.g., policies, programs, and services) intended to achieve outcomes that are important to the system. Established in 1994, the *Public Health in America* statement articulates the general outcomes and the key processes of public health practice; it is presented in **Exhibit 17.1**.[13] Its formulation, known as the "Essential Public Health Services," embodies these key processes and outputs of public health practice and is in common use today as a framework for organizing public health activities.
- Outcomes reflect the immediate and long-term changes (or lack of change) experienced by individuals and populations as a result of the processes. Measures of outcome reflect the magnitude and direction of the effect of processes on health status, risk reduction, social functioning, or consumer satisfaction outcomes.

Exhibit 17.1   Links Between the *Public Health in America* Framework and Performance Measurement

Public Health in America Elements	Usefulness for Performance Measurement Activities
Healthy People in Health Communities Promote physical and mental health and prevent disease, injury, and disability	Vision Statement Mission Statement *Useful for formulating vision and mission statements*
Public health: • Prevents epidemics and the spread of disease • Protects against environmental hazards • Prevents injuries • Promotes and encourages healthy behaviors	Broad categories of outcomes affected by public health activities; sometimes viewed as what public health does
• Responds to disasters and assists communities in recovery • Ensures the quality and accessibility of health services	*Useful for developing performance measures for public health outcomes*
Essential public health services: 1. Monitor health status to identify community health problems 2. Diagnose and investigate health hazards in the community	Processes of public health practice that affect public health outcomes; sometimes viewed as how public health does what it does
3. Inform, educate, and empower people about health issues 4. Mobilize community partnerships to identify and solve health problems 5. Develop policies and plans that support individual and community health efforts. 6. Enforce laws and regulations that protect health and ensure safety 7. Link people with needed personal health services and ensure the provision of health care when it is otherwise unavailable 8. Ensure a competent public health and personal healthcare workforce 9. Evaluate effectiveness, accessibility, and quality of personal and population-based health services 10. Research for new insights and innovative solutions to health problems	*Useful measures for public health processes; these can be linked with capacity measures for more comprehensive assessment of public health performance*

Source: Data from Public Health Functions Steering Committee. *Public Health in America*. Available at: http://www.health.gov/phfunctions/public.htm. Accessed March 11, 2013.

Performance measures provide useful information concerning the capacity to perform, process performance (including outputs), and ultimate results (impact/outcomes). Useful individually, performance measures provide richer information when multiple dimensions are measured and related to each other. For example, relating capacities to outcomes (e.g., the cost-effectiveness or cost per case of disease prevented) is a common approach to assessing effectiveness of an activity or intervention. Similarly, measures relating capacities to processes (e.g., the cost per unit of service delivered) provide useful insights into efficiency. Ideally, measuring and relating measures for all of these dimensions provide the most useful information for improving performance.

Performance measurement and performance improvement initiatives proliferated in the public sector in the final decades of the 20th century, fueled in part by the potential for improving the quality of public programs and services. Federal agencies have been subject to the Government Performance and Results Act since the mid-1990s; state and local governments have adopted a variety of accountability systems.[6,9] Likewise, performance measurement has gained widespread acceptance in the health sector, both public and private. Similarly, accreditation programs based on principles of performance measurement are in place for a wide variety of healthcare organizations and settings, including community networks providing health services.

Paralleling these developments, specific interest in performance measurement within the public health system matured steadily during the 20th century, especially after the Institute of Medicine's (IOM's) sentinel 1988 report, *The Future of Public Health.*[14] This interest was advanced by aspirations of improving quality, enhancing accountability, and strengthening the science base of public health practice, embracing the challenge set forth in *The Future of Public Health.*[15–17] Yet earlier in the 1900s, strong foundations for this progress were laid. The pioneering work of our predecessors is described in greater detail in **Box 17.1**. A timeline of critical events is displayed in **Exhibit 17.2**.

Box 17.1   Measuring Public Health Performance Before 1988

Over the past century, efforts to measure public health performance have ranged from simple accounting to more sophisticated strategies in which performance is judged against already established expectations or standards.[1] Much of the early activity focused on local public health practice, although the very earliest attempt targeted state health departments. In that 1914 effort, Charles Chapin completed a survey of state health agencies for the American Medical Association (AMA) in order to describe the services of those agencies and their role in fostering the development of local health departments, or local public health agencies (LPHAs). Chapin's report concluded that state public health agencies were "mostly ill-balanced. Much of what is done counts little for health and much is left undone which would save many lives."[2, p. 96] He proposed the use of relative values for various preventive services and rated the state agencies on each service and in the aggregate. This quantitative approach was later incorporated into local public health practice appraisal initiatives orchestrated by the American Public Health Association (APHA).

In 1921, the first report of APHA's Committee on Municipal Health Department Practice called for the collection of information on local public health practice to provide the basis for the development of standards of organization and achievement for LHDs serving the nation's largest municipalities.[3,4] The committee concluded that "few standards are available to the health officers who would pattern their departments after those which predominate in American practice or achieve most satisfactory results."[3, p. 7] A survey instrument was developed and applied to 83 cities through site visits involving various committee members, including public health giants Winslow (committee chairman), Chapin, and Frost.

The committee soon saw the need to examine local public health practice more broadly, and in 1925 the committee was reconstituted as APHA's Committee on Administrative Practice. The new committee developed an appraisal form to be used as a self-assessment tool by local health officers.[5] Strengths and weaknesses of this initiative are apparent in its aspirations:

> The idea was to measure the immediate results attained—such as statistics properly obtained and analyzed, vaccinations performed, infants in attendance at instructive clinics, physical defects of school children discovered and corrected, tuberculosis cases hospitalized, laboratory tests performed—with the confidence that such immediate results would inevitably lead on to the ultimate end of all public health work, the conservation of human life and efficiency.[5, p. 1]

(continues)

Box 17.1   Measuring Public Health Performance Before 1988 (continued)

Successive iterations of the appraisal form appeared throughout the 1920s and 1930s; these were well received by LHDs, although there were occasional concerns that quantity was being emphasized over quality.[6] Using these forms, local health officers were able to compare their ratings with other agencies and submit their assessment to the Health Conservation Contest and its successor, the National Honor Roll. The basis for comparison was a numerical rating score based on aggregated points awarded across key administrative and service areas. Comparative ratings were to be used to improve health programs, advocate for resources, summarize health agency activities in annual reports, and engage other health interests in the community.[5] Agency ratings often attracted considerable media interest, resulting in both good and bad publicity for local agencies. Despite the initial intent to emphasize "immediate results," the major focus of the ratings remained on measuring public health capacity and the intervention or output aspects of public health processes.

In 1947, a new and still voluntary instrument, the evaluation schedule, which included capacity, process, and outcome measures and was scored centrally by the APHA Committee on Administrative Practice, replaced the appraisal form.[6,7] No longer was the focus on good or bad scores; results were presented for health agencies of varying size and type so that individual LHDs could directly compare their performance in meeting community needs with that of their peers. The use of these tools lost momentum in the 1950s when APHA's interest in public health performance and its measurement diminished.[8]

Prior to 1990, there were several other efforts to assess public health performance across the entire national public health system. One focused primarily on capacity factors, such as the presence or absence of an LHD in a jurisdiction and the full- or part-time availability of health officers.[9] The Emerson report in 1945 advanced several national standards, including one calling for complete coverage of the population by full-time LHDs (meaning those with full-time health officers).[10] Several other targets established in the Emerson report also provide interesting insights into the capacity of the national public health system at the time. For example, the committee concluded that the nation had 64% of the public health personnel and 63% of the financial resources needed to ensure full coverage of the population with six basic public health services (vital statistics, communicable disease control, environmental sanitation, public health laboratory services, maternal and child health services, and public health education).[10]

Another of these efforts provided extensive information on state health agencies. The Association of State and Territorial Health Officials (ASTHO) established a national public health reporting system, which functioned throughout much of the 1970s and 1980s. Although useful in terms of expenditures and programs for the official state health agencies, these reports had very little information on the public health activities of LHDs. Information on state-level environmental protection, substance abuse, and mental health services was also incomplete regarding whether these services were the responsibility of agencies other than the official state health agency.

In retrospect, a major limitation of the public health performance measurement activities before 1990 was the lack of emphasis on the more fundamental processes of public health practice (e.g., building constituencies and assessing and prioritizing community health needs), and the inability to link measures of capacities, processes, and outcomes in order to understand their relationships to performance. The lack of a conceptual framework that delineates these relationships was the root cause for this limitation. As a result, the basic assumption expressed in the appraisal form that "immediate results would inevitably lead on to the ultimate end of all public health work, the conservation of human life and efficiency"[5, p. 1] remained largely unrealized.

1. Turnock BJ, Handler AS. From Measuring to Improving Public Health Practice. *Annu Rev Public Health*. 1997;18:261–82.

2. Vaughan HF. Local health services in the United States: the story of CAP. *Am J Public Health*. 1972;62:95–108.

3. American Public Health Association. Committee on Municipal Health Department Practice, First Report, Part 1. *Am J Public Health*. 1922;12(2):7–15.

(continues)

Box 17.1   Measuring Public Health Performance Before 1988 (continued)

4. American Public Health Association. Committee on Municipal Health Department Practice, First Report, Part 2. *Am J Public Health*. 1922;12(2):138-347.

5. American Public Health Association Committee on Administrative Practice. Appraisal form for city health work. *Am J Public Health*. 1926;16(1):1-65.

6. Walker WW. The new appraisal form for local health work. *Am J Public Health*. 1939;29(5): 490-500.

7. Halverson WL. A twenty-five year review of the work of the committee on administrative practice. *Am J Public Health*. 1945;35(12):1253-9.

8. American Public Health Association. *Evaluation Schedule for Use in the Study and Appraisal of Community Health Programs*. New York: American Public Health Association; 1947.

9. Krantz FW. The present status of full-time local health organizations. *Public Health Rep*. 1942;57:194-6.

10. Emerson H, Luginbuhl M. *Local Health Units for the Nation*. New York: Commonwealth Fund; 1945.

Measuring Public Health Performance After 1988

The 1988 IOM report identified the three core functions of public health as assessment, policy development, and assurance.[14] The concepts and critique set out in this report prompted a series of initiatives to facilitate the implementation of the core functions framework. *Healthy People 2000* included, for the first time ever, a national health objective for coverage of the population by an effective local public health presence. *Healthy People 2000* objective 8.14 called for 90% of the population to be served by an LHD that was effectively carrying out public health's core functions in that community.[18] Despite little consensus as to what was meant by "effectively" addressing the core functions of public health, it was clear that the performance of key public health processes in public health organizations and systems was the focus of this new objective. Much of what is known concerning current public health performance in the United States has been developed within the context of various initiatives inspired by the IOM report. Unfortunately, many of these experiences were unpublished. However, more than a dozen reports on various aspects of public health performance were published during the 1990s. Although these studies used somewhat different panels of performance measures, their contribution to public health performance measurement largely resides in their focus on performance measures for key processes related to the public health core functions and essential public health services. Based on a variety of field tests and performance studies completed in the early 1990s, a consensus set of 20 practice performance measures (**Box 17.2**) was established by leading researchers in the field. Other investigators have also used these performance measures in published reports, and more than a dozen states have examined public health performance within their state–local public health system using these measures. These studies consistently demonstrate suboptimal performance of key public

Exhibit 17.2   Public Health Performance Management Timeline

1914
- Charles Chapin assessment of state health departments for the American Medical Association

1921
- First report of American Public Health Association (APHA) Committee on Municipal Health Department Practice

1925
- APHA Committee on Administrative Practice self-assessment appraisal form

1947
- APHA Committee on Administrative Practice voluntary evaluation instrument with capacity, process, and outcome measures

1988
- Institute of Medicine report: *The Future of Public Health,* introducing public health core functions, while finding public health in disarray

1994
- Development of core function–related public health practice standards
- Development of the "10 Essential Public Health Services" within *Public Health in America*

2001
- Launch of Mobilizing for Action through Planning and Partnerships (MAPP)
- Launch of the National Public Health Performance Standards

2003
- Institute of Medicine report: *The Future of Public's Health in the 21st Century,* calling for an examination of accreditation

2005
- National Association of County and City Health Officials (NACCHO) *Operational Definition of a Functional Local Health Department*
- Funding of *Multi-State Learning Collaboratives for Quality Improvement* by the National Network of Public Health Institutes/Robert Wood Johnson Foundation (RWJF)

2005
- National Network of Public Health Institutes/RWJF *Multi-State Learning Collaborative* initiate first round of funded projects

2007
- Public Health Accreditation Board (PHAB) is incorporated

2009
- Definition of quality improvement in public health is developed and published

2011
- PHAB publishes final accreditation standards and measures
- Voluntary national accreditation program is launched

Box 17.2   Core Function–Related Measures of Local Public Health Practice Effectiveness Developed Collaboratively by University of North Carolina and University of Illinois–Chicago Investigators, 1995

Assessment

1. For the jurisdiction served by your local public health agency, is there a community health needs assessment process that systematically describes the prevailing health status and needs of the community?
2. In the past 3 years in your jurisdiction, has the local public health agency surveyed the population for behavioral risk factors?
3. For the jurisdiction served by your local public health agency, are timely investigations of adverse health events, including communicable disease outbreaks and environmental health hazards, conducted on an ongoing basis?
4. Are the necessary laboratory services available to the local public health agency to support investigations of adverse health events and meet routine diagnostic and surveillance needs?
5. For the jurisdiction served by your local public health agency, has an analysis been completed of the determinants and contributing factors of priority health needs, adequacy of existing health resources, and the population groups most impacted?
6. In the past 3 years in your jurisdiction, has the local public health agency conducted an analysis of age-specific participation in preventive and screening services?

Policy Department

7. For the jurisdiction served by your local public health agency, is there a network of support and communication relationships, which includes health-related organizations, the media, and the general public?
8. In the past year in your jurisdiction, has there been a formal attempt by the local public health agency at informing elected officials about the potential public health impact of actions under their consideration?
9. For the jurisdiction served by your local public health agency, has there been a prioritization of the community health needs that have been identified from a community needs assessment?
10. In the past 3 years in your jurisdiction, has the local public health agency implemented community health initiatives consistent with established priorities?
11. For the jurisdiction served by your local public agency, has a community health action plan been developed with community participation to address community health needs?
12. During the past 3 years in your jurisdiction, has the local public health agency developed plans to allocate resources in a manner consistent with the community health action plan?

Assurance

13. For the jurisdiction served by your local public health agency, have resources been deployed, as necessary, to address the priority health needs identified in the community health needs assessment?
14. In the past 3 years in your jurisdiction, has the local public health agency conducted an organizational self-assessment?
15. For the jurisdiction served by your local public health agency, are age-specific priority health needs effectively addressed through the provision of/or linkage to appropriate services?
16. In the past 3 years in your jurisdiction, has there been an instance in which the local public health agency has failed to implement a mandated program or service?
17. For the jurisdiction served by your local public health agency, have there been regular evaluations of the effect that public health services have on community health status?
18. In the past 3 years in your jurisdiction, has the local public health agency used professionally recognized process and outcome measures to monitor programs and to redirect resources as appropriate?
19. For the jurisdiction served by your local public health agency, is the public regularly provided with information about current health status, healthcare needs, positive health behaviors, and healthcare policy issues?
20. In the past year in your jurisdiction, has the local public health agency provided reports to the media on a regular basis?

Source: Adapted from Turnock BJ, Handler AS, Miller CA. Core function-related local public health practice effectiveness. *J Public Health Manag Pract.* 1998;4(5):28.

health practices and considerable variability in the performance of specific measures. A snapshot of study findings from the early 1990s indicates:

- Based on surveys of LHDs conducted by the National Association of County and City Health Officials (NACCHO)[19,20] for 48 questions associated with the three core functions, mean LHD performance was 50%.
- Studies using practice measures based on the core functions reported performance scores of 57% performance for 14 LHDs in 1992, 56% for 370 LHDs in 1993, and 50% for 208 LHDs in 1993.[21–25] When similar performance measures were used on a statewide basis in Iowa in 1995, the overall performance score was 61%.[26]
- Using 20 the consensus measures of public health practice with a random sample of 298 LHDs stratified by population size and type of jurisdiction, an effort was made to assess the extent to which the U.S. population in 1995 was being effectively served by public health core functions.[27] Performance for these 20 measures ranged from 23 to 94%. The most frequently performed measures were investigating adverse health events, maintaining necessary laboratory services, implementing mandated programs, and maintaining a network of relationships. The least frequently performed measures were assessing the use of preventive and screening services in the community, conducting behavioral risk factor surveys, and regularly evaluating the effect of services on the community. The overall weighted mean performance score for all 20 measures was 56%. City- and county-based LHD jurisdictions with populations greater than 50,000 performed these measures more frequently (65%) than other local public health jurisdictions in this study.
- Another study conducted in 1998 using the same 20 measures found similar levels of performance (65%) in 356 jurisdictions with populations of 100,000 or more.[28] Although the performance of the more populous jurisdictions was somewhat higher than the combination of large and small jurisdictions included in the 1995 national study, both the relative rankings and the population size–specific scores were quite similar in these two studies.

Although the various studies conducted throughout the 1990s used somewhat different methods and measures, they consistently demonstrate practice (process and outputs) performance in the 50–70% range and paint a picture of less than optimal functioning of the public health system nationally and in many states. Notably, this range is consistent with conclusions of the Emerson report 50 years earlier as to effective public health coverage of the nation based on an assessment of capacity factors (see Box 17.1). Although the precise status is not known, it is clear that the United States fell well short of its *Healthy People 2000* target of having 90% of the population residing in jurisdictions in which public health's core functions are being effectively addressed. Two studies of practice performance conducted nationally in the 1990s concluded that only approximately one-third of the U.S. population in the 1990s was effectively served.[25,27]

These efforts to measure core function performance have served several important purposes. By providing information on key processes and outputs of public health practice, many state and local systems have initiated public health practice improvement strategies. These efforts also provide the opportunity for measures of public health practice performance to be linked with measures of capacity and outcomes, furthering the understanding of the relationships among these key dimensions of the public health system.

The relationship between capacity and process performance (including outputs) has also been examined. One study linked practice performance measures from a 1993 national survey with NACCHO profile information for 264 LHDs.[25,29] Capacity factors linked to higher levels of practice performance included having a full-time agency head, larger annual LHD expenditures, greater number of total and part-time staff, budgets derived from multiple funding sources, private health insurance as a significant budget component, and female agency heads.

A 1998 study of LHDs in the most populous jurisdictions identified several capacity factors associated with higher levels of practice performance.[28] These were population size, presence of a local board of health, existence of mixed or shared arrangements with a state health agency, and participation in public health activities by managed care plans and universities. This study also documented the substantial contribution (one-third of the total effort) to practice performance made by parties other than the governmental health agency in these jurisdictions, strengthening the case for more focused attention to measuring the outputs of public health systems. The most important public health system contributors to process performance were state agencies, hospitals, local governmental agencies, nonprofit organizations, physicians and medical groups, universities, federally funded community health centers, managed care plans, and federal agencies.

The link between key processes and programs/services (outputs) offered by LHDs has also been examined. One study linked higher levels of performance of key processes with a greater percentage of services being directly provided, as well as the provision of the following specific services: personal prevention and treatment, maternal and child health, chronic disease personal prevention, health education, injury control, dental health, case management services, and human immunodeficiency virus (HIV)/acquired immune deficiency syndrome (AIDS) testing.[29] In another study, only the provision of behavioral health services was linked with higher levels of performance of key public health processes.[28]

Lessons from 20th-Century Efforts

During the 85-year period from 1914 to 1999 (see Box 17.1 and Exhibit 17.2), several lessons are demonstrated. The first is that measurement for the sake of measurement was never the purpose of these activities. The intent has consistently been to gather information that would be useful for the improvement of local public health practice. However, the early instruments—including the appraisal form and evaluation schedule—placed considerable emphasis on the performance of specific services (outputs) rather than on more basic public health processes, such as community assessment or constituency building. None of these efforts has comprehensively examined the links between capacity, processes, and outcomes and their relationship to an effective governmental public health presence. Through more than 8 decades of efforts, it has been easier to measure specific aspects of the public health system than to

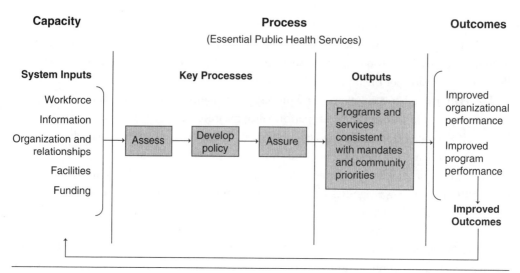

Figure 17.2 Framework for Measuring Public Health System Performance

develop a consensus about what these measurements tell us about overall public health performance.

Although these efforts included outcome measures, most failed to link capacity and process measures to these health outcomes. Prior to 1990, there was no significant effort to do so, but after 1990 it became more commonplace. One study attempted to relate LHD practice performance levels to some general community health status indicators.[30] No clear links were found, in part because the study did not focus on health outcomes that were directly targeted by community health assessments. It is now possible to perform such an examination in environments where practice performance has been tracked over time and where community health assessments have led to interventions for high-priority community health problems. Various levels of practice performance can now be related to changes in key outcome measures in order to identify the effectiveness of the various practices. As suggested by the framework depicted in **Figure 17.2**, performance measurement in the public health system can now begin to measure capacities, processes, and outcomes in ways that allow for changes in one to be linked with changes in others.

Standards and Measurement Based on Essential Public Health Services

Public health performance standards, when used prior to 1990, primarily related to capacities and outputs of public health practice rather than the key processes necessary to carry out the public health core functions. Standards, or performance expectations, for public health practice developed after 1990 focused on key processes and outputs and had a wide variety of beneficial applications, including agency self-assessment for capacity building, measures of state and local public health systems performance, and state and national surveillance regarding *Healthy People*

2000 and *2010* objectives. The paragraphs that follow summarize the evolution of standards development and their potential for current application.

The 1990s witnessed many public health organizations conducting organizational self-assessments, identifying strengths and weaknesses, and channeling this information into organizational capacity-building plans. The panel of performance expectations for local public health practice in the Assessment Protocol for Excellence in Public Health (APEXPH) served as an early blueprint for many public health agencies seeking to focus and strengthen their roles in their communities.[31] APEXPH adoption and implementation experience was substantial, although not universal. Where APEXPH was implemented widely, public health practice performance was found to be substantially higher than areas where it was less frequently used. Evidence from the most extensive implementation of an APEXPH derivative on a statewide basis showed actual performance nearly doubling in Illinois over a 2-year timeframe.[32] Despite its strengths, APEXPH lacked a strategic planning component and a focus on community public health systems, thus limiting its potential impact. A 1997 survey found that nearly 90% of the states reported some level of involvement in local public health performance assessment, although only half had an active and ongoing process.[33] Frameworks based on the core functions or essential public health services were used as the basis for these assessments in 22 states. However, few states use these assessments to allocate state funds across program areas and local jurisdictions, inform budget-appropriation decisions made by the state legislature, or evaluate public health programs.[33] The 1997 study also found that some states are using various combinations of capacity and process (including outputs) standards as a way to improve performance. In the intervening years, even more state and local health departments have been performing assessments and updating improvement plans.[34–39]

Although the 1990s saw only modest progress toward the establishment of a framework for continuous quality improvement in public health, the beginnings of a new focus on performance began to formulate. The overall lack of uniformity and consistency among various state and local efforts reflected the different needs, values, and circumstances of the relatively autonomous state and local public health networks across the United States. This diversity and the lack of consistency in public health efforts across the nation were significant factors in the U.S. Centers for Disease Control and Prevention's (CDC) Public Health Practice Program Office's shift to promote the development of innovative new public health products for state and local public health agencies and systems interested in improving their effectiveness through systems collaborations. These applications include: 1) Mobilizing for Action through Planning and Partnerships (MAPP), a new strategic approach to community health improvement; 2) performance standards for use in state and local public health systems and local governing boards; and 3) exploring the feasibility of accreditation of public health organizations.[40] By 2000, this evolving interest in performance measurement, quality improvement, and strategic effectiveness spawned several new tools and resources for strengthening public health practice.[41]

In 1997, increased interest in performance measurement and improvement in public health resulted in expanded community-driven and state-level collaborations focused on improving public health practice. Notable examples of this trend were the local and state partnerships initiated under *Turning Point: Collaborating for a New Century in Public Health*. Turning Point was inspired partly by the enhanced community health improvement process outlined by the IOM in its 1997 report on performance monitoring to improve community health, promoting the use of performance measures and performance monitoring to link accountable partners to community improvement efforts.[17] Funded by the Robert Wood Johnson Foundation (RWJF) and the W. K. Kellogg Foundation, Turning Point emerged from the foundations' concern about the capacity of public health systems to respond to emerging challenges of the 21st century. The Turning Point program funded 21 state and 41 local public health jurisdictions to develop multisectoral partnerships to strengthen and transform the public health mission and practice of public health through the collective efforts of systems partners. Core strategies employed by Turning Point grantees were innovative collaborations for the public's health, increased capacity for effective policy development, and alternative structures for improving community health. Underlying the widespread work of state and local public health jurisdictions in Turning Point projects was the recognition that governmental public health alone will not be able to achieve important public health goals in the 21st century, rather public health systems were required.[42]

Another prime example of the turn of the century trend toward strategic effectiveness was the evolution of APEXPH into MAPP, with its increased emphasis on local public health systems rather than on community public health agencies alone.[43] MAPP, launched in 2001, is a community-wide strategic planning tool promoting broader community health improvement efforts that link public and private community partners to specific performance expectations for addressing priority health needs in the community.[44] Emphasizing the values of strategic planning, systems thinking, and community empowerment, MAPP is a structured but flexible process that at its best produces collective action at the community level to improve health.

The MAPP process represents an important transition from more traditional or categorical health planning approaches to a model that is grounded in strategic planning concepts. The complex challenges facing public health dictate a strategic decision-making framework that includes several different analytic phases. The MAPP model supports the identification of strategic community health issues by the findings of four assessments: the community health status assessment, a forces of change assessment (an environmental scan), a community themes and strengths assessment, and a local public health systems assessment. The assessment of the local public health system anchors MAPP in systems development to stimulate systems changes that link to needed improvements in community health. This is accomplished by integrating the application of the local public health systems performance standards into the community assessment process, a major step forward in the examination and ultimate improvement of public health infrastructure and capacity.[45]

The National Public Health Performance Standards Program (NPHPSP) is a CDC-led partnership of national public health organizations—ASTHO, NACCHO, the National Association of Local Boards of Health (NALBOH), the Public Health Foundation, the American Public Health Association (APHA), and the National Network of Public Health Institutes—to improve public health systems through the development and application of local- and state-based performance standards. Launched in 2002, the NPHPSP consists of three performance self-assessment instruments, one for state public health systems, one for local public health systems, and one for local governing bodies. The state and local performance standards are designed for voluntary use by systems partners representing key organizations in the public, private, and voluntary sectors to assess systems strengths and weaknesses as part of a performance improvement process. The NPHPSP standards have undergone validity studies and have been found to have face and content validity as a basis for measuring public health system performance.[46–49]

The NPHPSP standards are framed as optimal standards using the "10 Essential Public Health Services" framework, and as such constitute a unique resource to examine public health system expectations and measure current performance.[50] **Exhibit 17.3** provides examples of performance standards and measures for local and state public health systems used in NPHPSP assessments. Now in its third iteration, the local NPHPSP instrument includes 30 local model standards for local public health systems, focusing on specific types of activities that should be conducted in all local jurisdictions to carry out each essential service. The state NPHPSP instrument establishes 40 state model standards, with performance measures for key state-level

---

Exhibit 17.3   Excerpts from the National Public Health Performance Standards

Essential Public Health Service 3: Inform, Educate, and Empower People about Health Issues
Local Public Health System Assessment (LPHSA) Model Standard 3.1: Health Education and Promotion

The local public health system (LPHS) designs and puts in place health promotion and health education activities to create environments that support health. These promotional and educational activities are coordinated throughout the LPHS to address risk and protective factors at the individual, interpersonal, community, and societal levels. The LPHS includes the community in identifying needs, setting priorities, and planning health promotion and education activities. The LPHS plans for different reading abilities, language skills, and access to materials.

To accomplish this, members of the LPHS work together to:

- Provide policymakers, stakeholders, and the public with ongoing analyses of community health status and related recommendations for health promotion policies
- Coordinate health promotion and health education activities to reach individual, interpersonal, community, and societal levels
- Engage the community in setting priorities, developing plans, and implementing health education and health promotion activities

State Public Health System (SPHS) Model Standard 3.4: Public Health Capacity and Resources

SPHS partner organizations effectively invest in and utilize human, technology, information, organizational, and financial resources to inform, educate, and empower people about health issues. Coordinated use of system assets is grounded in the alignment of organizational strategic plans around collective efforts in health education, promotion, and communication. The state public health agency enhances the capacity of the SPHS by its leadership activities in this service. The workforce of SPHS partner organizations coordinates collective system-wide activities. These investments in informing and educating people by all SPHS partner organizations are essential for a well functioning system capable of empowering people to gain knowledge and act to reduce their health risks.

To accomplish these results, the partner organizations in the SPHS:

- Commit adequate financial resources to informing, educating, and empowering people about health issues
- Align organizational relationships to focus statewide assets on health communication and health education and promotion services
- Use a competent workforce skilled in developing and implementing health communication and health education and promotion interventions

Source: Centers for Disease Control and Prevention. National Public Health Performance Standards Program.

functions within each essential service; these four key state functions are planning and imple-mentation, state–local relationships, performance management and quality improvement, and public health capacity and resources. The governance NPHPSP instrument examines one gov-ernance model standard for each essential service, examining the oversight functions of boards of health in assuring appropriate legal authority, resources, policy base, community collabora-tion, and accountability for local public health.[51] The version three standards have undergone an extensive reengineering process that is intended to reduce the workload related to the system assessment, while retaining the overall value derived.

The NPHPSP is a national leadership effort to improve public health system-wide perfor-mance. The use of its standards by state and local public health jurisdictions and local governing bodies has modeled a noncategorical approach to the examination and management of public health performance. Focused on capacity and processes, the standards enable user jurisdictions to examine key infrastructure elements of their system, identify strengths and weaknesses in their performance and capacity, establish priorities, and, through an improvement process, agree on future collective action.[51] A variety of salutary effects has been cited by the NPHPSP as potential benefits of a nationwide public health performance standards initiative. These include quality improvement in the user jurisdiction; improved accountability; enhanced capacity building for community, state, and national public health systems; widespread use of best practices; and an improved science base for public health practice.[52]

Although the National Public Health Performance Standards represent real progress in estab-lishing optimal expectations of the performance and capacity of public health systems, their use has not been universal. Issues related to incorporating these innovations into routine practice are:

- The voluntary nature of the use of the standards has slowed their adoption. Without financial or regulatory incentives, state and local public health agencies, the natural leaders of these systems-oriented processes, have tended not to consider the use of the standards as an urgent or compelling need when confronted by the tyranny of everyday priorities.
- Although users of the NPHPSP report positive results in systems development and strate-gic planning, achieving those results has been a time-intensive process requiring collabora-tive leadership skills. Since the launch of the NPHPSP, the time and resources of many public health leaders have been devoted to crisis preparedness and other emerging prob-lems and not overall organization or systems-wide performance assessment and improve-ment. More recently, severe economic downturns have also blunted NPHPSP uptake.
- Although the NPHPSP is incorporated into the MAPP process as the local public health sys-tems assessment, MAPP is not in consistent local use. State NPHPSP users have also strug-gled to develop strategic planning processes as vehicles for using NPHPSP results. Currently, a state-level version of MAPP is under development. The lack of strategic planning capacity in public health agencies has been a barrier to effective quality improvement activities.[53]

Despite its importance to achieving public health results, developing multisectoral partner-ships at the state and local levels is labor intensive and typically lacks dedicated financial support. Similarly, Turning Point projects demonstrated many impressive systems changes, but the state and local collaborative projects have faced numerous sustainability challenges.[54]

Performance Measurement and Improvement After 2000

Until recently there have been limited attempts to use performance standards and measures to examine the public health system on a nationwide basis.[25,27,28] Scant attention was paid to whether the nation achieved its *Healthy People 2000* national health objective calling for 90% of the population to be effectively served by an LHD with capacity to carry out the core functions of public health. As a result, the potential for a nationwide performance measurement system to serve as a stimulus for reengineering and system-wide improvement was underemphasized. The specific national objective related to effective LHDs was dropped in *Healthy People 2010*, in lieu of an extensive panel of national health objectives addressing public health infrastructure (**Exhibit 17.4**).[55] The infrastructure objectives have been retained in *Healthy People 2020*.

In 2001, the Turning Point Performance Management National Excellence Collaborative (PMC) studied performance management practices in state public health agencies. The PMC found that nearly every reporting state public health agency has some form of performance management process in place and more than three-quarters of states reported that their performance management efforts have resulted in improved performance.[56] State public health agencies in 2001 most frequently measured, reported, and used performance data related to health status, not focusing on other organizational or systems performance measures. In addition, few state agencies reported having a process to conduct quality improvement or to carry out changes based on performance data for the state public health agency or local public health agencies.[2]

Several recent studies have continued to track progress of state and local health department implementation of quality improvement and performance management.[37,38,57] The Public Health Foundation is presently refreshing the performance management model first developed by the PMC (see Figure 17.1), as a result of their study of state health departments.

Critical Issues for Success

Several major issues challenge efforts to improve performance within the public health system through a national public health performance standards initiative. Resolution of these issues will require consensus on the purpose or purposes of the effort, the definition and components of quality, and the ability to effect widespread change. Another major consideration in terms of improving quality is whether performance measurement will be limited or widespread. If limited implementation of quality improvement and performance management tools leads to only scattered local data or piecemeal state and national information, there will be only minimal opportunities to improve quality. It is important to consider mechanisms and incentives for performance standards and measures to be widely used. This may require expanded system-building efforts at the state and local levels, involving greater use of mandates via requirements in statutes and rules or through inclusion in federal grant deliverables. Other incentives, such as grants in aid and direct financial support, or the establishment of professional standards of practice and accreditation initiatives may also be necessary to build sufficient infrastructure and capacity.

Exhibit 17.4 *Healthy People 2020* Objectives: Public Health Infrastructure

Workforce

PHI-1   Increase the proportion of federal, tribal, state, and local public health agencies that incorporate Core Competencies for Public Health Professionals into job descriptions and performance evaluations.

PHI-2   (Developmental) Increase the proportion of tribal, state, and local public health personnel who receive continuing education consistent with the Core Competencies for Public Health Professionals.

PHI-3   Increase the proportion of Council on Education for Public Health (CEPH)–accredited schools for public health, CEPH-accredited academic programs, and schools of nursing (with a public health or community health component) that integrate Core Competencies for Public Health Professionals into curricula.

PHI-4   Increase the proportion of 4-year colleges and universities that offer public health or related majors and/or minors.

PHI-5   (Developmental) Increase the proportion of 4-year colleges and universities that offer public health or related majors and/or minors that are consistent with the core competencies of undergraduate public health education.

PHI-6   Increase the proportion of 2-year colleges that offer public health or related associate degrees and/or certificate programs.

Data and Information Systems

PHI-7   (Developmental) Increase the proportion of population-based *Healthy People 2020* objectives for which national data are available for all major population groups.

PHI-8   Increase the proportion of *Healthy People 2020* objectives that are tracked regularly at the national level.

PHI-9   (Developmental) Increase the proportion of *Healthy People 2020* objectives for which national data are released within 1 year of the end of data collection.

PHI-10   Increase the number of states that record vital events using the latest U.S. standard certificates and report.

Public Health Organizations

PHI-11   Increase the proportion of tribal and state public health agencies that provide or assure comprehensive laboratory services to support essential public health services.

PHI-12   (Developmental) Increase the proportion of public health laboratory systems (including state, tribal, and local) that perform at a high level of quality in support of the "10 Essential Public Health Services."

PHI-13   Increase the proportion of tribal, state, and local public health agencies that provide or assure comprehensive epidemiology services to support essential public health services.

PHI-14   Increase the proportion of state and local public health jurisdictions that conduct a public health system assessment using national performance standards.

PHI-15   Increase the proportion of tribal, state, and local public health agencies that have implemented a health improvement plan and increase the proportion of local health jurisdictions that have implemented a health improvement plan linked with their state plan.

PHI-16   (Developmental) Increase the proportion of tribal, state, and local public health agencies that have implemented an agency-wide quality improvement process.

PHI-17   (Developmental) Increase the proportion of tribal, state, and local public health agencies that are accredited.

Source: U.S. Department of Health and Human Services. *Healthy People 2020.* Available at: http://www.healthypeople .gov/2020/default.aspx. Accessed March 11, 2013.

Without these kinds of system incentives, goodwill alone may be insufficient to improve overall quality in the public health enterprise.

A useful definition of performance improvement is positive change in the capacity, process, and outcomes of public health organizations and public health systems (public, private, and voluntary organizations that collectively contribute to the health of the public). This definition utilizes the concepts established earlier in this chapter to provide a balanced framework for the basic elements of change in public health. The elements of structural capacity, processes, and outcomes were outlined in 2001 as essential components of examining the work of public health systems.[58] These concepts have been used in NACCHO's efforts to develop its "Operational Definition of a Local Public Health Agency" (**Exhibit 17.5**).[59] This landmark project to develop an operational definition of local public health departments describes specific functions of county, municipal, and other local governmental public health agencies and reflects shared opinions about how local public health departments serve their communities.

Exhibit 17.5　Local Health Department (LHD) Standards

1. Monitor health status and understand health issues facing the community.
   a. Obtain and maintain data that provide information on the community's health (e.g., provider immunization rates; hospital discharge data; environmental health hazard, risk, and exposure data; community-specific data; number of uninsured and indicators of health disparities, such as high levels of poverty, lack of affordable housing, limited or no access to transportation, etc.).
   b. Develop relationships with local providers and others in the community who have information on reportable diseases and other conditions of public health interest and facilitate information exchange.
   c. Conduct or contribute expertise to periodic community health assessments.
   d. Integrate data with health assessment and data collection efforts conducted by others in the public health system.
   e. Analyze data to identify trends, health problems, environmental health hazards, and social and economic conditions that adversely affect the public's health.
2. Protect people from health problems and health hazards.
   a. Investigate health problems and environmental health hazards.
   b. Prevent, minimize, and contain adverse health events and conditions resulting from communicable diseases; food-, water-, and vector-borne outbreaks; chronic diseases; environmental hazards; injuries; and health disparities.
   c. Coordinate with other governmental agencies that investigate and respond to health problems, health disparities, or environmental health hazards.
   d. Lead public health emergency planning, exercise, and response activities in the community in accordance with the National Incident Management System, and coordinate with other local, state, and federal agencies.
   e. Fully participate in planning, exercises, and response activities for other emergencies in the community that have public health implications, within the context of state and regional plans and in a manner consistent with the community's best public health interest.
   f. Maintain access to laboratory and biostatistical expertise and capacity to help monitor community health status and diagnose and investigate public health problems and hazards.
   g. Maintain policies and technology required for urgent communications and electronic data exchange.

(continues)

Exhibit 17.5 Local Health Department (LHD) Standards (continued)

3. Give people information they need to make healthy choices.
   a. Develop relationships with media to convey information of public health significance, correct misinformation about public health issues, and serve as an essential resource.
   b. Exchange information and data with individuals, community groups, other agencies, and the general public about physical, behavioral, environmental, social, economic, and other issues affecting the public's health.
   c. Provide targeted, culturally appropriate information to help individuals understand what decisions they can make to be healthy.
   d. Provide health-promotion programs to address identified health problems.

4. Engage the community to identify and solve health problems.
   a. Engage the local public health system in an ongoing, strategic, community-driven, comprehensive planning process to identify, prioritize, and solve public health problems; establish public health goals; and evaluate success in meeting the goals.
   b. Promote the community's understanding of, and advocacy for, policies and activities that will improve the public's health.
   c. Support, implement, and evaluate strategies that address public health goals in partnership with public and private organizations.
   d. Develop partnerships to generate interest in and support for improved community health status, including new and emerging public health issues.
   e. Inform the community, governing bodies, and elected officials about governmental public health services that are being provided, improvements being made in those services, and priority health issues not yet being adequately addressed.

5. Develop public health policies and plans.
   a. Serve as a primary resource to governing bodies and policymakers to establish and maintain public health policies, practices, and capacity based on current science and best practices.
   b. Advocate for policies that lessen health disparities and improve physical, behavioral, environmental, social, and economic conditions in the community that affect the public's health.
   c. Engage in LHD strategic planning to develop a vision, mission, and guiding principles that reflect the community's public health needs, and to prioritize services and programs.

6. Enforce public health laws and regulations.
   a. Review existing laws and regulations on a regular basis and work with governing bodies and policymakers to update them as needed.
   b. Understand existing laws, ordinances, and regulations that protect the public's health.
   c. Educate individuals and organizations of the meaning, purpose, and benefit of public health laws, regulations, and ordinances and how to comply.
   d. Monitor, and analyze over time, the compliance of regulated organizations, entities, and individuals.
   e. Conduct enforcement activities.
   f. Coordinate notification of violations among other governmental agencies that enforce laws and regulations that protect the public's health.

7. Help people receive health services.
   a. Engage the community to identify gaps in culturally competent, appropriate, and equitable personal health services, including preventive and health-promotion services, and develop strategies to close the gaps.
   b. Support and implement strategies to increase access to care and establish systems of personal health services, including preventive and health-promotion services, in partnership with the community.
   c. Link individuals to available, accessible personal healthcare providers (e.g., a medical home).

(continues)

Exhibit 17.5   Local Health Department (LHD) Standards (continued)

8. Maintain a competent public health workforce.
   a. Recruit, train, develop, and retain a diverse staff.
   b. Evaluate LHD staff members' public health competencies,* and address deficiencies through continuing education, training, and leadership development activities.
   c. Provide practice- and competency-based educational experiences for the future public health workforce, and provide expertise in developing and teaching public health curricula through partnerships with academia.
   d. Promote the use of effective public health practices among other practitioners and agencies engaged in public health interventions.
   e. Provide the public health workforce with adequate resources to do their jobs.
9. Evaluate and improve programs and interventions.
   a. Develop evaluation efforts to assess health outcomes to the extent possible.
   b. Apply evidence-based criteria to evaluation activities where possible.
   c. Evaluate the effectiveness and quality of all LHD programs and activities and use the information to improve LHD performance and community health outcomes.
   d. Review the effectiveness of public health interventions provided by other practitioners and agencies for prevention, containment, and/or remediation of problems affecting the public's health, and provide expertise for those interventions that need improvement.
10. Contribute to and apply the evidence base of public health.
   a. When researchers approach the LHD to engage in research activities that benefit the health of the community:
      i. Identify appropriate populations, geographic areas, and partners.
      ii. Work with them to actively involve the community in all phases of research.
      iii. Provide data and expertise to support research.
      iv. Facilitate their efforts to share research findings with the community, governing bodies, and policymakers.
   b. Share results of research, program evaluations, and best practices with other public health practitioners and academics.
   c. Apply evidence-based programs and best practices where possible.

*As defined by the core public health competencies developed by the Council on Linkages Between Academia and Public Health Practice.

Source: National Association of County and City Health Officials (NAACHO). Operational Definition of a Functional Local Health Department. Available at: http://www.naccho.org/topics/infrastructure/accreditation/OpDef.cfm. Accessed March 11, 2013.

More recently, a specific definition of public health QI has been developed:

> Quality improvement in public health is the use of a deliberate and defined improvement process, such as Plan-Do-Check-Act, which is focused on activities that are responsive to community needs and improving population health. It refers to a continuous and ongoing effort to achieve measurable improvements in the efficiency, effectiveness, performance, accountability, outcomes, and other indicators of quality in services or processes which achieve equity and improve the health of the community.[60]

This definition tracks well with the foundations laid previously, and emphasizes capacity, processes, and outcomes.

Additional work to define reasonable performance expectations for governmental public health agencies has been occurring in states. Extensive use of standards, performance measures, and performance improvement processes has been done in Washington, Illinois, Missouri, North Carolina, Michigan, Florida, New Jersey, and other states. The growing record of experience in these states has stimulated nationwide interest in accreditation of state and local public health agencies as a vehicle to improve public health performance.

Accreditation of Public Health Agencies

Interest in strategies to accredit public health organizations is longstanding and has arisen from several sources.[61] The 2003 IOM Report, *The Future of the Public's Health in the 21st Century*, calls for careful study of the feasibility of creating a national voluntary public health agency accreditation system.[62] This recommendation stems from the fact that public health organizations are among only a few health-related entities that are not subject to national standards and review from an external accrediting body. In fact, credentialing of both individuals and organizations has become such an accepted means of fostering quality improvement and accountability throughout the health sector that its absence from the public health system is noteworthy. Indeed, this fact has not escaped the notice of policymakers and funders.

Accreditation of educational and healthcare organizations generally involves several steps. Initially, major stakeholders develop an independent entity that establishes the standards and review process to be applied. For example, the Joint Commission was developed through the efforts of organized medicine and the hospital industry. Institutions of higher learning saw accreditation as a means to facilitate transferring credits earned at one institution to be used toward a degree at another. The Council on Education in Public Health (CEPH) now operates as a collaboration between the APHA and the Association of Schools of Public Health.

In fact, just such an effort has occurred regarding public health accreditation. Following the recommendation of the IOM report, and the well traveled pathway of successful predecessors like the Joint Commission, the CDC and the RWJF joined forces to fund an exploration of public health agency accreditation. They convened a national gathering of key public health organizational stakeholders in 2004 to gather input and consider whether a voluntary accreditation process was indeed feasible given the environment. Consensus was achieved regarding the merit of further study. As a result, the CDC and the RWJF agreed to fund a joint ASTHO/ NACCHO–staffed study of accreditation for public health agencies. The Exploring Accreditation Project (EAP) was a yearlong endeavor, with its planning committee led by APHA and NALBOH in concert with NACCHO and ASTHO. Guidance for the EAP activities emanated from the steering committee that comprised these key public health organizations. As a result of the EAP findings and recommendations, the Public Health Accreditation Board (PHAB) was formed in 2007.

In general, across most fields of endeavor, accreditation activities commence with a self-study or self-assessment by the entity seeking to be accredited. The self-assessment document is submitted to the accrediting body and examined by staff and experts who then perform a site visit of the applicant in order to verify conformance with the standards. Decisions as to full or conditional accreditation are based on the extent to which standards are addressed. Finally, the results are made public. If plans of correction are required, these are generally reviewed on an interim basis or examined at the time of the next review. The key elements in this process are the standards and the reviewers. Accreditation is not inexpensive for the applicant organization, which pays a fee to the accrediting body and absorbs the substantial costs of preparation, on-site review, and follow up. Preparation for most organizations is an intensive endeavor and accounts for fully 80% of accreditation costs, mostly in the form of staff time commitment.[63]

Although accreditation is considered to be voluntary, in many industries it is anything but that. Hospitals and schools of public health, for example, perceive accreditation as essential to doing business. Accreditation has its greatest demand where there are multiple parties that value or require it. Third-party payers and governmental regulatory agencies require accreditation of hospitals. A variety of federal grants and contracts can only be awarded to accredited schools of public health. Creating similar incentives to act as drivers for voluntary accreditation may pose a formidable challenge for the public health system, which may create unintended consequences. Such concerns were recognized and addressed by the EAP and continue to be monitored by PHAB.

Concurrent with the Exploring Accreditation Project, the RWJF also funded a Multi-State Learning Collaborative for Performance and Capacity Assessment or Accreditation of Public Health Departments (MLC). The National Network of Public Health Institutes and the Public Health Leadership Society comanaged this effort to advance the innovations of states already conducting accreditation and accreditation-like programs within their health departments and to identify and disseminate best practices to the broader public health practice community. The long-term goal is to maximize the effectiveness and accountability of governmental public health agencies.[64] Five states were selected to participate in the first round of the MLC: Illinois, Michigan, Missouri, North Carolina, and Washington. A fundamental intent underlying the project design was for the learning of the MLC to be available to inform the deliberations of the EAP. Subsequent rounds of MLC grants ultimately included 16 states. Although continuing to emphasize public health accreditation, quality improvement was given equal importance. Ultimately more than 160 quality improvement projects were conducted by more than 230 health departments participating in mini-collaboratives encompassing 10 target areas.[65,66]

The inspiration for PHAB accreditation has derived from pioneering state programs and the development of standards discussed previously. Several MLC states have functioned as the laboratories for the study of public health accreditation, with many having embarked upon accreditation or similar processes. Typically, the LHD has been the focal point. Nonetheless, similar emphasis on state health departments is likewise warranted and is included in the PHAB accreditation program.

Accreditation programs often must strike a fine balance between minimal and optimal standards. State standards programs and similar initiatives often favor optimal rather than minimal standards. This was certainly the case with respect to the standards adopted in the State of Washington public health standards program, which were designed to "stretch" the capacity and performance of local and state public health departments.[67,68] Accreditation and standards programs prefer to focus on clearly accountable entities (e.g., a local public health agency rather than a community public health system).[69] Beyond financial incentives that may be in place, organizations pursuing accreditation must perceive internal value emanating from the process. This was, indeed, reported to be the case in many of the LHDs undertaking accreditation in MLC states.

Experiences in other fields also suggest that the value of accreditation is related to how extensively the credential is accepted and used by external stakeholders.[63] For accreditation to be successful, there must be short- and long-term benefits. Public health goals for a healthier population reflect appropriate long-term benefits. PHAB has expressed that the benefits of accountability and organizational excellence are embedded in the accreditation process. Moreover, the stated purpose of accreditation is to strengthen organizational performance and promote quality improvement. Short-term and measurable benefits of accreditation to public health organizations must also be articulated, if for no other reason than to provide a reasonable counterbalance to the cost in time, dollars, and political energy needed for the effort.[70] Other potential benefits might include ability to compete directly for federal funds, contracting advantages with Medicaid and other state agencies, a market advantage in competition when directly contracting with the private sector for some services, and participation in a dedicated learning community of public health organizations. However, even when examining results of accreditation across a number of fields, to date there is limited research data available demonstrating that it improves organizational performance.[63] For public health accreditation to be sustainable, a solid research and evaluation enterprise must be built that is able to conclusively demonstrate value and improvement through the process. In fact, a standing PHAB Research and Evaluation Committee was formed early on to accomplish these objectives, and a research agenda has been developed and disseminated.

The PHAB accreditation program development has been an intensive iterative process building upon the strong foundations of the previous work described in this chapter. Fundamental to this effort was the development of standards and measures. This was accomplished through the dedicated work of experts and practitioners from the field, complemented by the participation of national practice organizations and academic partners. An alpha field test was conducted in a small number of state and local health departments of varying size and structure, validating the standards. Following revision based upon feedback from the alpha test, public comment was solicited, with thousands of inputs received and analyzed.

Concurrently, an assessment process was drafted by another workgroup.[71] A seven-step process was conceived as follows: 1) pre-application phase, 2) application, 3) evidence selection and submission, 4) site visit, 5) accreditation determination, 6) annual reporting, and 7) reaccreditation. There are three prerequisites for PHAB accreditation. Applicants must have completed a community/state health assessment, a community/state health improvement plan, and an agency strategic plan within the previous 5 years. Pre-application is the readiness assessment and preparation stage of accreditation. Once the application is submitted with the fee, the clock begins to tick. Each health department seeking accreditation selects a site coordinator who attends specific training in this phase. Evidence in the form of documentation is submitted electronically to PHAB and made available to site visitors for review. The site visit is conducted by an external peer team selected with expertise related to the health department to be visited. A PHAB accreditation review committee will render accreditation decisions quarterly. Accreditation is for a 5-year term, and accredited health departments are expected to maintain conformance with PHAB standards throughout the accreditation cycle. Regular annual reports will enable PHAB to monitor conformance and quality improvement activities.

The improved standards and measures with the assessment process were put to a more extensive beta test by 30 representative state, local, and tribal health departments during late 2009 and 2010. Again, valuable feedback resulted in modifications of the process and standards. All standards apply equally to state, local, and tribal health departments, although measures may vary somewhat. Version 1.0 of the PHAB accreditation standards (see **Exhibit 17.6**) containing 12 domains was released followed by publicly launching the accreditation process in September 2011.[72]

Exhibit 17.6   PHAB Domains and Standards

Assess

Domain 1: Conduct and disseminate assessments focused on population health status and public health issues facing the community

Standard 1.1: Participate in or conduct a collaborative process resulting in a comprehensive community health assessment

Standard 1.2: Collect and maintain reliable, comparable, and valid data that provide information on conditions of public health importance and on the health status of the population

Standard 1.3: Analyze public health data to identify trends in health problems, environmental public health hazards, and social and economic factors that affect the public's health

Standard 1.4: Provide and use the results of health data analysis to develop recommendations regarding public health policy, processes, programs, or interventions

Investigate

Domain 2: Investigate health problems and environmental public health hazards to protect the community

Standard 2.1: Conduct timely investigations of health problems and environmental public health hazards

Standard 2.2: Contain/mitigate health problems and environmental public health hazards

Standard 2.3: Ensure access to laboratory and epidemiologic/environmental public health expertise and capacity to investigate and contain/mitigate public health problems and environmental public health hazards

Standard 2.4: Maintain a plan with policies and procedures for urgent and nonurgent communications

Inform and Educate

Domain 3: Inform and educate about public health issues and functions

Standard 3.1: Provide health education and health-promotion policies, programs, processes, and interventions to support prevention and wellness

Standard 3.2: Provide information on public health issues and public health functions through multiple methods to a variety of audiences

Community Engagement

Domain 4: Engage with the community to identify and address health problems

Standard 4.1: Engage with the public health system and the community in identifying and addressing health problems through collaborative processes

Standard 4.2: Promote the community's understanding of and support for policies and strategies that will improve the public's health

Policies and Plans

Domain 5: Develop public health policies and plans

Standard 5.1: Serve as a primary and expert resource for establishing and maintaining public health policies, practices, and capacity

Standard 5.2: Conduct a comprehensive planning process resulting in a tribal/state/community health improvement plan

Standard 5.3: Develop and implement a health department organizational strategic plan

Standard 5.4: Maintain an all hazards emergency operations plan

(continues)

Exhibit 17.6 PHAB Domains and Standards (continued)

Public Health Laws

Domain 6: Enforce public health laws

Standard 6.1: Review existing laws and work with governing entities and elected/appointed officials to update as needed

Standard 6.2: Educate individuals and organizations on the meaning, purpose, and benefit of public health laws and how to comply

Standard 6.3: Conduct and monitor public health enforcement activities and coordinate notification of violations among appropriate agencies

Access to Care

Domain 7: Promote strategies to improve access to healthcare services

Standard 7.1: Assess healthcare capacity and access to healthcare services

Standard 7.2: Identify and Implement strategies to improve access to healthcare services

Workforce

Domain 8: Maintain a competent public health workforce

Standard 8.1: Encourage the development of a sufficient number of qualified public health workers

Standard 8.2: Assess staff competencies and address gaps by enabling organizational and individual training and development

Quality Improvement

Domain 9: Evaluate and continuously improve processes, programs, and interventions

Standard 9.1: Use a performance management system to monitor achievement of organizational objectives

Standard 9.2: Develop and implement quality improvement processes integrated into organizational practice, programs, processes, and interventions

Evidence-Based Practices

Domain 10: Contribute to and apply the evidence base of public health

Standard 10.1: Identify and use the best available evidence for making informed public health practice decisions

Standard 10.2: Promote understanding and use of research results, evaluations, and evidence-based practices with appropriate audiences

Administration and Management

Domain 11: Maintain administrative and management capacity

Standard 11.1: Develop and maintain an operational infrastructure to support the performance of public health functions

Standard 11.2: Establish effective financial management systems

Governance

Domain 12: Maintain capacity to engage the public health governing entity

Standard 12.1: Maintain current operational definitions and statements of the public health roles, responsibilities, and authorities

Standard 12.2: Provide information to the governing entity regarding public health and the official responsibilities of the health department and of the governing entity

Standard 12.3: Encourage the governing entity's engagement in the public health department's overall obligations and responsibilities

Source: Public Health Accreditation Board. *PHAB Standards Overview 1.0.* Available at: http://www.phaboard.org/wp-content/uploads/PHAB-Standards-Overview-Version-1.0.pdf. Accessed March 11, 2013.

Voluntary accreditation of public health organizations could lead to greater interest in the possibility of credentialing various segments of the public health workforce. In one form or another, there are already credentials for some public health workers, including sanitarians, health educators, and public health administrators, with New Jersey licensing local public health administrators and Illinois maintaining an independent competency-based certification program for public health administrators working in a variety of public and private agencies. More recently, graduates of accredited public health schools and programs are eligible to take a national public health certification exam offered by the National Board of Public Health Examiners. Viewed collectively, these burgeoning credentialing initiatives, when combined with the ongoing accreditation efforts described earlier, hold the potential to produce high-performing public health organizations with a competent workforce, consistently capable of providing the essential services of public health while achieving health outcome goals.

Future Outlook

Performance management leading to performance improvement initiatives were undertaken in many different settings during the 1900s, including the public sector, where they were applied to improving governmental processes, programs, and services. Although only undertaken in a few locales, its application to improving the performance of public health core functions has been largely positive, suggesting that a national public health performance standards program based on the essential public health services framework could be successful. "What gets measured gets done," is the performance measurement analogy for what is known in research as the Hawthorne effect.[73] Its lesson for the public health community is that the measurement process itself influences the credibility and consistent performance of that which is measured. What we are better able to measure, we will be better able to manage and improve.

With interest increasing inside the public health community and broader participation in public health improvement efforts evolving in many states and localities, the opportunity for more rigorous use of performance standards and measurement, emphasizing performance management and quality improvement strategies, has never been greater. Although a national accreditation system for public health has become a reality, there will nonetheless remain a continuing need for concerted efforts to improve the performance of public health agencies and systems, bolstering the efforts of the accreditation process. Utilizing the Turning Point Performance Management framework and tools such as MAPP, NPHPSP, community health improvement processes linked to *Healthy People 2020* objectives, and leading health indicators in conjunction with performance standards will enable motivated organizations to achieve desired goals.[74,75] Success may also be predicated upon reform of state and local public health systems, organizing them around the core functions and essential public health services rather than categorical programs and services. It is only within this larger context that accreditation initiatives for organizations and credentialing for individuals will be valued and meaningful, especially when reinforced by grant funding linked to the performance of essential public health services, performance reporting, and commitment to evaluative research activities.

In sum, performance management activities that include performance standards, measurements, public accountability, and quality improvement will boost quality if they focus on all aspects of the public health system—its capacity, its processes, and the links between them and important community health outcomes—and if the public health community accepts, values, and uses these standards. Early attention to and consensus around these issues will determine the quality and relevance of public health practice in the 21st century.

Discussion Questions

1. What tools can public health leaders and managers use to address performance challenges at many different levels of the public health system, including the performance of individuals, programs, agencies, interorganizational collaborations, and the system-wide enterprise itself?

2. Define *performance management* and its elements.

3. Most public health agencies do not yet have fully developed performance management systems. Describe the status of performance management in health departments with which you are familiar. What are the elements of performance management? How can their introduction be facilitated?

4. How is a performance measure different from a performance standard?

5. How have community assessment tools such as MAPP advanced community health assessment and improvement?

6. Explain the role of the "10 Essential Public Health Services" in the development of other important tools and frameworks.

7. What role might accreditation have in improving performance in health departments?

References

1. Harrington HJ. *The improvement process: How America's Leading Companies Improve Quality.* New York: McGraw-Hill; 1987.

2. Turning Point Program National Office. *Performance Management in Public Health: A Literature Review.* Seattle, WA: Turning Point; 2002.

3. Turning Point Program National Office. *From Silos to Systems: Using Performance Management to Improve the Public's Health.* Seattle, WA: Turning Point; 2003.

4. Landrum LB, Baker SL. Managing complex systems: performance management in public health. *J Public Health Manag Pract.* 2004;10(1):13–8.

5. Wholey JS, Hatry HP. The case for performance monitoring. *Public Admin Rev.* 1992;52(6):604–10.

6. Wholey JS, Newcomer K. Clarifying goals, reporting results. *New Direct Eval.* 1997;75:91–8.

7. Trott C, Baj J. *Building State Systems Based on Performance: The Workforce Development Experience, A Guide for States.* Washington, DC: National Governors Association; 1996.

8. Rossi P, Freeman H. *Evaluation: A Systematic Approach.* Thousand Oaks, CA: Sage Publications; 1994.

9. Perrin E, Durch J, Skillman SM, et al. *Health performance measurement in the public sector: principles and policies for implementing an information network.* Washington, DC: National Academies Press; 1999.

10. Joint Commission. *Primer on Indicator Development and Application: Measuring Quality in Health Care.* Oakbrook Terrace, IL: JCAHO; 1990.

11. Riley WJ, Moran JW, Corso LC, et al. Defining quality improvement in public health. *J Public Health Manag Pract.* 2010;16(1):5–7.

12. U.S. Department of Health and Human Services. *Consensus Statement on Quality in the Public Health System.* Available at: http://www.hhs.gov/ash/initiatives/quality/quality/phqf-consensus-statement.html. Accessed March 12, 2013.

13. Public Health Functions Steering Committee. *Public Health in America.* Available at: http://www.health.gov/phfunctions/public.htm. Accessed March 11, 2013.

14. Institute of Medicine. *The Future of Public Health.* Washington, DC: National Academies Press; 1988.

15. Perrin E, Koshel J, eds. *Assessment of Performance Measures for Public Health, Substance Abuse, and Mental Health.* Washington, DC: National Academies Press; 1997.

16. Northwest Prevention Effectiveness Centern. *Enabling Performance Measurement Activities in the States and Communities*. Seattle, WA: University of Washington; 1998.

17. Institute of Medicine, Committee on Using Performance Monitoring to Improve Community Health, Durch J, et al. *Improving Health in the Community: A Role for Performance Monitoring*. Washington, DC: National Academies Press; 1997.

18. U.S. Public Health Service. *Healthy People 2000: National Health Promotion and Disease Prevention Objectives*. Washington, DC: U.S. Government Printing Office; 1990.

19. National Association of County and City Health Officials. *1990 National Profile of Local Health Departments*. Washington, DC: NACCHO; 1992.

20. National Association of County and City Health Officials. *1992–1993 National Profile of Local Health Departments*. Washington, DC: NACCHO; 1995.

21. Miller CA, Moore KS, Richards TB, et al. A screening survey to assess local public-health performance. *Public Health Rep*. 1994;109(5):659–64.

22. Miller CA, Moore KS, Richards TB, et al. A proposed method for assessing the performance of local public-health functions and practices. *Am J Public Health*. 1994;84(11):1743–9.

23. Richards TB, Rogers JJ, Christenson GM, et al. Assessing public health practice: application of ten core function measures of community health in six states. *Am J Preve Med*. 1995;11(6):36–40.

24. Richards TB, Rogers JJ, Christenson GM, et al. Evaluating local public health performance at a community level on a statewide basis. *J Public Health Manag Pract*. 1995;1(4):70–83.

25. Turnock BJ, Handler A, Hall W, et al. Local health department effectiveness in addressing the core functions of public health. *Public Health Rep*. 1994;109(5):653–8.

26. Rohrer JE, Dominguez D, Weaver M, et al. Assessing public health performance in Iowa's counties. *J Public Health Manag Pract*. 1997;3(3):10–5.

27. Turnock BJ, Handler AS, Miller CA. Core function-related local public health practice effectiveness. *J Public Health Manag Pract*. 1998;4(5):26–32.

28. Mays GR, Halverson PK, Baker EL, et al. Availability and perceived effectiveness of public health activities in the nation's most populous communities. *Am J Public Health*. 2004;94(6):1019–26.

29. Handler AS, Turnock BJ. Local health department effectiveness in addressing the core functions of public health: essential ingredients. *J Public Health Policy*. 1996;17(4):460–83.

30. Schenck SE, Miller CA, Richards TB. Public health performance related to selected health status and risk measures. *Am J Prev Med*. 1995;11(6):55–7.

31. National Association of County and City Health Officials. *An Assessment Protocol for Excellence in Public Health*. Washington, DC: NACCHO; 1990.

32. Turnock BJ, Handler A, Hall W, et al. Capacity-building influences on Illinois local health departments. *J Public Health Manag Pract*. 1995;1(3):50–8.

33. Mays GP, Halverson P, Miller CA. Assessing the performance of local public health systems: a survey of state health agency efforts. *J Public Health Manag Pract*. 1998;4(4):63–78.

34. National Association of County and City Health Officials. *2005 National Profile of Local Health Departments Report*. Available at: http://www.naccho.org/topics/infrastructure/profile/upload/naccho_report_final_000.pdf. Accessed March 12, 2013.

35. National Association of County and City Health Officials. *2008 National Profile of Local Health Departments*. Available at: http://www.naccho.org/topics/infrastructure/profile/resources/2008report/upload/NACCHO_2008_ProfileReport_post-to-website-2.pdf. Accessed March 12, 2013.

36. Association of State and Territorial Health Officials. *ASTHO Chartbook of Public Health*. Available at: http://www.astho.org/Display/AssetDisplay.aspx?id=4888. Accessed March 12, 2013.

37. Madamala K, Sellers K, Beitsch LM, et al. Quality improvement and accreditation readiness in state public health agencies. *J Public Health Manag Pract*. 2012;18(1):9–18.

38. Leep C, Beitsch L, Gorenflo G, et al. Quality Improvement in local health departments: progress, pitfalls, and potential. *J Public Health Manag Pract*. 2009;15(6):494–502.

39. Beitsch LM, Leep C, Shah G, et al. Quality improvement in local health departments: results of the NACCHO 2008 survey. *J Public Health Manag Pract*. 2010;16(1):49–54.

40. Centers for Disease Control and Prevention. *National Public Health Performance Standards: State Public Health System Performance Assessment Instrument.* Available at: http://www.cdc.gov/od/ocphp/nphpsp/TheInstruments.htm. Accessed February 22, 2012.

41. Lenihan P. MAPP and the evolution of planning in public health practice. *J Public Health Manag Pract.* 2005;11(5):381–6.

42. Nicola R, Berkowitz B, Lafronza V. A Turning Point for public health. *J Public Health Manag Pract.* 2002;8(1):iv–vii.

43. National Association of County and City Health Officials. *Mobilizing for Action through Planning and Partnerships.* Washington, DC: NACCHO; 2001.

44. Corso LC, Wiesner PJ, Lenihan P. Developing the MAPP community health improvement tool. *J Public Health Manag Pract.* 2005;11(5):387–92.

45. Salem E, Hooberman J, Ramirez D. MAPP in Chicago: a model for public health systems development and community building. *J Public Health Manag Pract.* 2005;11(5):393–400.

46. Beaulieu JE, Scutchfield FD. Assessment of validity of the National Public Health Performance Standards: the local public health performance assessment instrument. *Public Health Rep.* 2002;117(1):28–36.

47. Beaulieu JE, Scutchfield FD, Kelly AV. Content and criterion validity evaluation of national public health performance standards measurement instruments. *Public Health Rep.* 2003;118(6):508–17.

48. Beaulieu JE, Scutchfield FD, Kelly AV. Recommendations from testing of the National Public Health Performance Standards instruments. *J Public Health Manag Pract.* 2003;9(3):188–98.

49. Scutchfield FD, Knight EA, Kelly AV, et al. Local public health agency capacity and its relationship to public health system performance. *J Public Health Manag Pract.* 2004;10(3):204–15.

50. Bakes-Martin R, Corso LC, Landrum LB, et al. Developing national performance standards for local public health systems. *J Public Health Manag Pract.* 2005;11(5):418–21.

51. Centers for Disease Control and Prevention. National Public Health Performance Standards Program. Available at: http://www.cdc.gov/od/ocphp/nphpsp/overview.htm. Accessed February 18, 2012.

52. Turnock BJ. Can public health performance standards improve the quality of public health practice? *J Public Health Manag Practice.* 2000;6(5):19–25.

53. Madamala K, Sellers K, Pearsol J, et al. State landscape in public health planning and quality improvement: results of the ASTHO survey. *J Public Health Manag Pract.* 2010;16(1):32–8.

54. Mays GP. From collaboration to coevolution: new structures for public health improvement. *J Public Health Manag Pract.* 2002;8(1):95–7.

55. U.S. Department of Health and Human Services. *Healthy People 2010: Understanding and Improving Health.* Available at: http://www.healthypeople.gov/2010/. Accessed March 12, 2013.

56. Turning Point Program National Office. *From Silos to Systems: Using Performance Management to Improve the Public's Health.* Available at: http://www.turningpointprogram.org/Pages/pdfs/perform_manage/Silos_to_Sytems_FINAL.pdf. Accessed March 12, 2013.

57. Beitsch LM, Leep C, Shah G, et al. Quality improvement in local health departments: results of the NACCHO 2008 survey. *J Public Health Manag Pract.* 2010;16(1):49–54.

58. Handler A, Issel M, Turnock B. A conceptual framework to measure performance of the public health system. *Am J Public Health.* 2001;91(8):1235–9.

59. National Association of County and City Health Officials. *Operational Definition of a Functional Local Health Department.* Available at: http://www.naccho.org/topics/infrastructure/accreditation/OpDef.cfm. Accessed March 12, 2013.

60. Riley W, Moran J, Bialek R, et al. Defining quality improvement in public health. *J Public Health Manag Pract.* 2010;16(1):5.

61. Turnock BJ, Handler AS. From measuring to improving public health practice. *Annu Rev Public Health.* 1997;18:261–82.

62. Institute of Medicine. *The Future of the Public's Health in the 21st Century.* Washington, DC: National Academies Press; 2003.

63. Mays G. *Can Accreditation Work in Public Health? Lessons from other Service Industries.* Little Rock, AR: UAMS College of Public Health; 2004.

64. National Network of Public Health Institutes. Multi-State Learning Collaborative for Performance and Capacity Assessment or Accreditation of Public Health Departments. Available at: http://www.cdc.gov/nceh/ehs/ephli/Resources/MLC_Performance_and_Capacity.pdf. Accessed March 12, 2013.

65. Beitsch L, McKeever J, Pattnaik A, et al. The QI Story Behind the Storyboards: Lessons Learned from the Multi-State Learning Collaboratives (A Synthesis of 162 QI Projects Conducted by 234 Health Departments). Unpublished manuscript.

66. Beitsch L, Carretta H, McKeever J, et al. The quantitative story behind the QI storyboards: a synthesis of QI projects conducted by the multi-state learning collaborative. *J Public Health Manag Pract.* 2013; Feb 6. [Epub ahead of print].

67. Thielen L. *Exploring Public Health Experience with Standards and Accreditation.* Princeton, NJ: Robert Wood Johnson Foundation; 2004.

68. Beitsch L, Thielen L, Mays G, et al. The multistate learning collaborative, states as laboratories: informing the national public health accreditation dialogue. *J Public Health Manag Pract.* 2006;12(3):217–31.

69. Schyve PM. Joint Commission perspectives on accreditation of public health practice. *J Public Health Manag Pract.* 1998;4(4):28–33.

70. Greenberg EL. How accreditation could strengthen local public health: an examination of models from managed care and insurance regulators. *J Public Health Manag Pract.* 1998;4(4):33–7.

71. Public Health Accreditation Board. Available at: http://www.phaboard.org/. Accessed April 18, 2009.

72. Public Health Accreditation Board. Standards and Measures. Available at: http://www.phaboard.org/accreditation-process/public-health-department-standards-and-measures/. Accessed March 12, 2013.

73. Roethlisberger F, Dickson W. *Management and the Worker.* Cambridge, MA: Harvard University Press; 1947.

74. Baker EL, Melton RJ, Stange PV, et al. Health reform and the health of the public—forging community-health partnerships. *JAMA.* 1994;272(16):1276–82.

75. Harrell J, Baker E. The essential services of public health. *Leadership Public Health.* 1994;3:27–31.

Engaging Communities and Building Constituencies for Public Health[*]

Michael T. Hatcher and Ray M. Nicola

LEARNING OBJECTIVES

- To describe how organizational management of four process sets forms the community and constituency engagement practice
- To discuss four strategies and the potential uses when undertaking community and constituency engagement initiatives
- To explain the roles of community and constituency engagement in population-based health interventions
- To identify tools and resources that support constituent involvement in population-based health interventions
- To discuss opportunities to apply community and constituency engagement in emerging health system reform initiatives

---

[*]**Disclaimer:** The findings and conclusions in this chapter are those of the authors and do not necessarily represent the views of the Agency for Toxic Substances and Disease Registry and the Centers for Disease Control and Prevention.

Chapter Overview

In order to achieve improvements in population health, communities and constituents must be engaged. Generally, health improvement interventions use behavioral, systems, or environmental change strategies. For any of these approaches to succeed, there must be behavior adoption, policy compliance, or environmental change acceptance. Understanding that intervention must result in individual and community adoption, compliance, or acceptance makes clear the importance of community and constituency engagement. Based on this understanding, considerable attention has been given to activities and processes of engaging communities and constituents to address health issues. Within the construct of the Essential Public Health Services (EPHS), this work is described within EPHS 4: Mobilize Partnerships to Identify and Solve Health Problems.[1] Specific attributes of EPHS 4 are:[2]

- Organization and leadership to convene, facilitate, and collaborate with partners to identify public health priorities and create effective solutions to solve state and local health problems
- Building of partnerships to collaborate in the performance of public health functions and essential services in efforts to utilize the full range of available human and material resources to improve health status
- Assistance to help partners and communities organize and undertake actions to improve health

One important point in this description is the building of a partnership to collaborate in the performance of public health functions and essential services. This recognition indicates that community and constituency engagement is required in performing most of the other EPHS.

The Public Health Accreditation Board (PHAB) describes the same work with the domain heading: "Engage with the Community to Identify and Address Health Problems." This domain description aligns with EPHS 4: Mobilizing Partnerships. The PHAB description recognizes the importance of community partners to identify and solve public health issues while leveraging community knowledge and resources.[3]

This chapter outlines an organizational practice framework for managing community and constituency engagement to achieve and sustain improvements in population health. Within this framework, public health and preventive medicine leaders identify their constituencies explicitly and broadly, delineate constituent participation factors, develop and manage effective interactions with constituency groups, and apply models for evaluating and improving the engagement of constituencies in population health issues. Each of these tasks requires explicit analytic and management strategies for linking constituency engagement activities and processes to community health improvement. This framework and these task processes are discussed later in this chapter.

Leadership Challenges in Engaging Communities and Constituents

The goal of community and constituency engagement is to achieve dialogue, develop shared constituent leadership in determining health improvement actions, and gain shared ownership in achieving community health improvement objectives.

Shared leadership is demonstrated by active participation in bidirectional communication among partners who collectively make community-level decisions and take actions based on mutual trust and collective benefits that contribute to achieving community health objectives. Shared ownership is the commitment and investment of tangible (e.g., cash, facilities, and volunteers) and nontangible assets (e.g., time, energy, and commitment to the cause) that individuals or groups contribute to collaborative actions that achieve an agreed upon goal or aspiration.

The history and experience of the community and the convening organization in collective decision making will influence the initial level of shared leadership and ownership that may be possible.[4] It is likely that a convening organization will have some collaborative experience and trust with some but not all segments of the community they serve. It is also likely that there will be segments of the community where participation is needed but the convening organization has little or no history of collaboration with those community groups. Understanding this, a convening organization will need to apply different approaches to achieve participation from all community constituents potentially impacted by the proposed community health improvement initiative. The Community Engagement Continuum (**Figure 18.1**)[5] defines five levels of increasing participation and leadership. This continuum provides convening organizations with insight on engaging constituent groups based on the history of the convening organization with each constituent group. Within this continuum the five levels of input and community participation are outreach, consultation, involvement, collaboration, and shared leadership. These community involvement levels demonstrate how increasing involvement can impact trust, leadership and ownership of community health improvement activities.[5]

Public health and preventive medicine leaders who are engaged in population health improvements are challenged to develop effective relationships with the complex constellation of constituents who are involved in or affected by community health issues. An effective community and constituency engagement practice enables these leaders to develop relationships that facilitate community health improvement. Leaders effectively applying this organizational practice identify public health constituents, delineate participation factors, develop and manage effective interactions with constituency groups or populations, and apply strategies for evaluating and improving community and constituency engagement in health improvement initiatives. Each of these tasks requires explicit analytic and organizational management strategies and capacities to apply constituency engagement processes to community health improvement actions.[6]

Public health and preventive medicine leaders operate within increasingly complex institutional environments that include many types of constituents. The consumers of public health and preventive medicine services in any given community are many and diverse, as are the

Outreach	Consult	Involve	Collaborate	Share Leadership
Some Community Involvement	More Community Involvement	Better Community Involvement	Community Involvement	Strong Bidirectional Relationship
Communication flows from one to the other, to inform.	Communication flows to the community and then back, answer seeking.	Communication flows both ways, participatory form of communication.	Communication flow is bidirectional.	Final decision making is at the community level.
Provides community with information.	Gets information or feedback from the community.	Involves more participation with community on issues.	Forms partnerships with community on each aspect of project from development to solution.	Information is codeveloped with the community.
Entities coexist.	Entities share information.	Entities cooperate with each other.	Entities form bidirectional communication channels.	Entities have formed strong partnership structures.
Outcomes: Optimally, establishes communication channels and channels for outreach.	**Outcomes:** Develops connections.	**Outcomes:** Visibility of partnership established with increased cooperation.	**Outcomes:** Partnership building, trust building.	**Outcomes:** Broader health outcomes affecting broader community. Strong bidirectional trust built.

Figure 18.1 Increasing Level of Community Involvement, Impact, Trust, and Communication Flow. There is a continuum for community engagement as mentioned earlier. In the early literature it was described by looking at levels of how action was taken from social action (outside experts making plans and implementing programs based on their expert insight), social reform with community representation in planning and program development, to empowerment where planning and program development are driven by the community.

Here is a model of that type of interaction, involvement, and influence.

This model provides a way to think about engagement planning across community population segments that allows you to specify level of communications and outcomes. Segments of the community will fall in each of these levels and you will need to plan for the level of involvement needed overtime.

individuals and organizations involved in producing these services. Improving health within communities and populations requires coordinated decision making and problem solving by all of these constituents. Such problem solving occurs most readily and successfully when constituents are actively engaged in addressing health issues that matter to them.[4]

Problem solving in public health rarely occurs through spontaneous consensus. In a democratic society, change is produced through the tensions of multiple interests and asymmetrical power relationships demonstrated through opinions and actions of differing societal segments. These population segments seeking action or inaction on community health issues represent constituency challenges for public health and preventive medicine leaders initiating engagement processes for improving community health. All too frequently, these leaders rely on a false dichotomy in developing relationships with constituents—they approach each constituent as either an adversary or an ally. Adversarial situations stimulate defensive responses that stagnate progress. These situations often arise because communication is limited to debate and entrenched positions instead of dialogue, negotiation, and solution development. On the flip side of this dichotomic coin, leaders focus on attracting and sustaining the attention of allies and other uninvolved constituents on health issues requiring community-based decisions and actions. Allies are typically sought among individuals and organizations that pursue similar missions and that engage in similar types of activities to improve public health. However, this dichotomous approach to constituency engagement can severely limit the actions and outcomes that public health and preventive medicine organizations achieve. An analytic and management framework for linking constituency building with community health improvement goals can transcend this false dichotomy and enable leaders to approach relationship building with the purpose of creating problem-solving opportunities and agreement on how to collectively improve health.[6–9]

The constituency engagement framework, presented in **Figure 18.2**, offers an approach.[7–9] It begins with the understanding that people need a reason to invest their energy in processes that address community health. If people and the community they are a part of are not motivated and ready to participate, action will not occur. The second aspect of the framework is focused on managing the constituency engagement processes and factors for constituent involvement. This segment of the framework addresses the responsibility to manage and enable effective constituent engagement. The third aspect of the framework focuses on approaches or models that facilitate constituent and community engagement and lead to intervention actions. The fourth aspect of the framework includes use of evidence-based public health and preventive medicine

Know		Do			Produce	
Constituent Participation Factors	Organizational Practice Elements	Constituent Involvement Approaches	Public Health Interventions	Health Impacts	Health Outcomes	Quality-of-Life Improvements
• Community Attachment • Motivations • Readiness	• Know the Community • Develop Positions and Strategies • Build and Maintain network Linkages • Mobilize for Action	• *Healthy People 2020* Tools • MAPP • Healthy Cities and Communities	• Clinical • Behavioral • Systems • Environmental	• Clinical • Behavioral • Systems • Environmental	• Decreased Morbidity • Decreased Mortality	• Physical • Mental • Social • Spiritual • Environmental

Figure 18.2   Linking Constituent Engagement to Community Health Improvement

interventions to produce population health improvements. The remaining portion of the framework demonstrates how community and constituent actions are linked to producing behavioral, systems, and environmental impacts, which in turn produce desired health outcomes and quality-of-life improvements.[7-9] This chapter address the first three aspects of this framework and identifies how community and constituency engagement is managed and applied to achieve effective use of evidence-based health interventions that result in desired population health outcomes.

Who Is Public Health's Constituency?

A **constituency**, in addition to the meaning of a body of voters, is: 1) a group of supporters or patrons, and 2) a group served by an organization or institution; a clientele.[10,11] By definition, therefore, people who benefit from public health actions and people who support improved health of the public are the constituency. Because public health serves the entire population, everyone in the country is part of the public health constituency. There are, however, certain groups in the constituent population who are in a special position to influence public health outcomes; these include public health and preventive medicine workers, policymakers, business leaders, and others.

Building on the concepts of supporters and clients, an operational definition of constituency engagement can be established. For the purposes of this chapter, constituency engagement is the art and science of establishing an organization's relationships with the public it serves, the governing body it represents, and other health-related organizations in the community. Relationships are established to generate solution-seeking debate, dialogue, decisions, and actions among constituent groups in addressing community health issues. Key points of this definition acknowledge that sciences such as political science, interpersonal communications, media advocacy, and others can be applied to building linkages and relationships with constituents. Applying the appropriate science at the right time, however, requires artful application. Complicating the simplicity of this definition is the fact that people and organizations are often members of multiple constituencies, and their movement between groups is fluid and frequently based on alignment of issues within groups.[4,12] Due to the fluid nature of constituent alignment on community health issues, leaders in public health and other organizations must develop a strategic understanding of individual and organizational values, missions, and assets held by constituents affected by or having influence over decisions and actions required to address community health concerns. Such influence may be constituted through an asymmetrical position of power that shapes opinions and directs organizations, controls resources and information, or possesses key technology. Such an understanding is critical in managing constituency relationships.

Incentives for Constituency Participation

An understanding of why people participate in community activities provides the first guidance for constituency building. Factors include the sociopolitical environment; community needs, attitudes, and beliefs; and existing leadership and organizational structures in the community.[12] The literature from various fields of study and authors including Wandersman, Brown, Butterfoss, Mattessich, Staley, and others offers insight into the motivations that move people to act.[12-18] For example, people participate when they feel a sense of community, see their involvement and the issues as relevant and worthy of their time, believe that the benefits of participation outweigh the cost, and view the process and organizational climate of participation as open and supportive of their right to have a voice in the process.[4] Constructs for assessing community readiness to act have been researched and applied. One construct, developed by Chilenski and colleagues, includes community and individual characteristics and investigates community attachment, initiative, efficacy, and leadership.[18] Chavis and colleagues also offer support in learning about community readiness factors with the Sense of Community Index II.[19]

The issues themselves also influence participation. People are motivated to work for change when conditions of an issue are no longer acceptable to them. The readiness of constituents to take action can be determined by understanding the perception of, and support for, the issue within the community. For example:

- Are there perceptions that a problem or threat that affects health exists?
- Is the issue perceived to be important, achievable, and deserving of community action?
- Is there a science base to resolve the issue?
- Is community collaboration likely due to political and public interest?
- Is there a history of community leadership and collaboration?
- Are resources available for action?
- Is the political and social climate supportive of the constituency's goals?
- Is there a community infrastructure to sustain interest and community action?

Answers to these and related questions are necessary to help public health and preventive medicine leaders determine constituent readiness and the level of action that may be possible.[20,21] Leaders who understand the motives for constituent participation and the attributes of readiness can stimulate action with appropriate information and public processes that fulfill individual and group needs for participation.

Organizational Management for Effective Constituency Interaction

Leaders who seek constituent participation on a community health issue can design organizational structures and management processes within their agencies or organizations that facilitate and direct interactions with constituents, for purposes of:[6–9]

- Knowing the community and its constituents
- Establishing positions and strategies that guide the organization's interaction with constituents
- Building and sustaining formal and informal networks necessary for maintaining relationships, communicating messages, and leveraging resources
- Mobilizing constituencies for community-based decision making and action

Performance of the organizational practice community and constituency engagement is accomplished through four process-related practice elements noted in this bulleted list. The processes of this practice are likely to be shared across an organization, with specific roles delegated to organizational units such as an assessment and planning unit, an education and outreach group, and a senior management and policy group. The organizational structures or units tasked with creating or delegating the management and performance of these processes are dependent on existing forms and functions within the governmental agency, community-based organization, or coalition partnership.

By managing these processes, engagement leaders can consistently address factors that produce effective constituent involvement, including:[7–9,18–21]

- The clarity of initiative goals
- The defined roles for constituent involvement
- Constituent ownership of both initiative process and outcome
- The design of capacity-building elements incorporated into processes and structures used to facilitate individual and group constituent actions
- The overall feeling of satisfaction and community attachment, rather than frustration, a process achieves in fulfilling a constituent's reasons for participating in community activities

Knowing the Community and Its Constituents

Knowing the community and its constituents is more than an epidemiologic assessment. It involves coordinating and directing activities that are necessary to identify constituent groups, analyzing group characteristics and factors that generate constituent involvement, and assessing current and potential assets (including fiscal, physical, informational, organizational, and human resources) that constituents and their organizations can direct toward resolving community health issues. The tasks involved in constituent identification and analysis of group characteristics include demographic groupings; individual and organizational beliefs, values, missions, and goals; and organizational and leadership structures of constituent groups as well as their history of working with others. Through this assessment, it is possible to determine the roles and type of support (political, financial, manpower, etc.) constituents can reasonably provide to a public health initiative, as well as possible conflicts of interest that may arise among groups.[22–25]

To be most effective, engagement leaders must determine which constituents are affected by specific issues, assess their probable response to addressing these issues, and use the most effective methods to involve each constituent group in appropriate activities. Constituent skills should match those needed for resolving the public health issue for which the engaging organization is facilitating dialogue and action. If the skills do not match, a determination must be made concerning training and education necessary to increase constituent involvement. In identifying and recruiting a constituent base for population health, the engaging organization must have policies, structures, resources, and leadership to assess community engagement efforts and assist in developing human and other constituency resources for population health action. Mechanisms that enable the identification and analysis of the engaging organization's constituent base provide essential information concerning potential collaborators on health issues. From a leadership perspective, knowing the community is essential because social programs tend to fail when there is a lack of appropriate management and an oversimplified view of constituent motivations.[6]

Establishing Positions and Strategies to Guide Interaction with Constituents

The second element within the community and constituency engagement practice is focused on organizational decision making leading to establishment of positions and strategies for bringing health issues before constituents. The purpose of this decision making and planning is to initiate constituent dialogue that leads to action. Engagement leaders must make their decisions based on understanding of multiple domains of influence on health such as social, epidemiologic, behavioral, environmental, ecologic, and political factors.[24–26] Through such analysis in decision making, engagement leaders are better equipped to consider the position options available and weigh each option's effect on different constituencies. Specific attention should be given to the perceived needs of customers served (including social determinants of health and environmental justice considerations), attitudes of policy-making bodies, application of population health science, population health delivery system capabilities, and appropriate community health data needed to formulate the organization's position. A position is established against this pool of competing interests. Through this practice element, the agency prepares itself to participate in the democratic process of decision making with constituents. The result is stimulation of debate, dialogue, and involvement around solution development by the community to address health issues and a determination of the community's expectations regarding resolution of the health issues. This internal organizational position development is not intended to exclude constituent input. Instead, it provides a starting point for dialogue with constituents and enables the engagement leader to communicate clearly.

Once an organization's position has been reached, strategy options can be evaluated and selected based on the best chance for achieving dialogue and action. Four organizational strategy types—authoritative, competitive, cooperative, and disruptive—can be considered:[27]

1. The authoritative strategy applies rules and regulations to require a desired action. It is used when an organization has control over its environment. Successful authoritative strategies require an organization's ability to monitor and enforce its directives. This strategy was used effectively by the National Highway Traffic Safety Administration in the early 1980s when it announced that airbags would be required in automobiles unless a specified percentage of the U.S. population was subject to mandatory seatbelt laws requiring occupant restraint use. This prompted policy debate and the passage of state vehicle occupant protection laws across the nation. More current authoritative strategies have occurred in regulating smoking in public places, legislation for graduated teen driver licenses, and dietary regulations applied to retail food services requiring reductions in trans-fats and salt and also menu labeling.[28]

2. Competitive strategies attempt to make an organization's position more desirable and attractive to constituents. The successfully competitive organization attracts adequate support to accomplish its purpose and avoids pressures from others that promote actions that are incongruent with the desired public health goals. Public health and other organizational

leaders often apply this strategy when funding is sought and there is competing interest for the same dollars. Success is won by demonstrating why the proposed program spending is needed, the quality and impact of the program over others, and external support for the program. Public health actions associated with public policy referendums also employ a competitive strategy to influence decisions on issues such as alcohol sales, tobacco product taxation, and support for public bond sales to make health and safety infrastructure improvements like building sidewalks, installing street lighting, and upgrading sewage systems.

3. Cooperative strategies establish agreements that offer mutual benefits to constituents and their organizations. An organization may use one of three cooperative strategy forms: 1) contracting, which is a negotiated agreement between two parties for exchanging resources or services; 2) coalition, which is a pooling of resources by several organizations for a joint venture; or (3) co-optation, which is the absorption (or conversion) of representatives from key (opposition or competitive) constituent groups into the leadership or policy-making structure of an organization in order to moderate or avoid opposition or competition. The use of coalitions, consortia, and federations are types of cooperative organizations employed to improve public health and healthcare delivery.[14,29] The list of local, state, and national coalitions is abundant with coalitions working to address single and multiple disease prevention and health promotion concerns like those targeted by *Healthy People 2020*.

4. Disruption strategies are "the purposeful conduct of activities which threaten the resource-generating capacities" of an adversary.[27] The most visible public health example of this strategy over the past decade is anti-tobacco media campaigns that promote tobacco use as socially unacceptable. Such action intends to limit tobacco sales and the customer base of tobacco companies by preventing children from purchasing tobacco and motivating them to adopt nonsmoking behaviors.

Throughout the position and strategy development process, it is essential to focus on the needs and interests of the organization's constituency. The question of when to engage direct constituent involvement is of critical concern. Is constituent input advisable during the problem analysis phase or as strategy and objectives are being weighed? Although early constituent engagement is usually indicated, organizational time and resource constraints may dictate that constituents are most appropriately engaged during the intervention implementation phase. Some considerations in determining the time most appropriate for involving constituents are the following:

- Operating timeframe: How much time is there to achieve the goal?
- Level of constituent knowledge: How much education will constituents need?
- Constituent commitment: How much of a time commitment are constituents willing to make?

Whatever the judgment on a point of entry for constituent engagement, clear positions and supportive strategies must be established to guide interaction and communication with constituents acting on important community health issues.

Building and Sustaining Networks

Network development is the third process area public health and preventive medicine leaders must consider in the organization's operations. Developing networks is focused on establishing and maintaining relationships, communication channels, and exchange systems that promote linkages, alliances, and opportunities to leverage resources among constituent groups. Effective performance results in open bidirectional channels of communication with constituents, enables active and ongoing collaborative interactions, and accelerates resource commitment and community engagement efforts for new or ongoing service delivery and policy issues. If organizational leaders view networking as an ongoing and essential activity in its operations, constituency engagement can be productive and require little special effort. If organizational leaders only communicate with constituents as a crisis management technique, they may find that communication channels that were once useful no longer exist.

The challenge for public health and preventive medicine organizations is establishing ties with a network of diverse constituency supporters impacted by and responsive to an array of public health issues. Key to successful networking is identifying and assessing the network structures in place and understanding the effect of structure on the availability of resources for population-level health improvement. Organizations have access to formal and informal constituent groups. The formal groups or organizations have recognized stability and influence in the community; informal groups may represent less structured and influential constituents, but they are often very resourceful when challenged. Each group brings with it important considerations that engagement leaders need to be aware of if true networking potential is to be realized.[23] Thus, the ability of engagement leaders to develop and direct networking activities relies heavily on identifying and assessing the existing networking structure.

Assessment methods and tools to conduct network analysis examine items like the number of interactions and value of each partner linkage, quality and trust of partner relationships, and partner functions within the network. Through such assessments, critical questions can be answered about quality and effectiveness of interactions, ability to leverage resources across the network, and where network connections and functions can be improved.[24,25] Developing this type of understanding will enable engagement leaders to maintain and strengthen constituent interactions, flow of information and resources, coordination of service delivery, and leverage of individual and organization influence within the constituency network to shape policy decisions. A lack of ties with diverse constituency groups in the community may impede organizational outreach, performance, and community health outcomes. Effective engagement leaders understand the value and return on investment made through maintaining, strengthening, and using network connections wisely.

Mobilizing Constituencies

Mobilizing constituencies for community-based decision making and social action is the fourth process area or element in the community and constituency engagement practice. Through community engagement and mobilization, community interest on health issues is stimulated, constituents are prepared to act, and, if necessary, constituents are assisted to develop capacity to respond in resolving the community health issue. Organizational engagement leaders support mobilization by assembling resources needed to collectively take agreed upon actions. Resources may include operating structure, physical facilities and equipment, fiscal resources, and a range of information resources that may include demographic data, analysis methods, and evidence-based intervention approaches needed to resolve the community health issue. If constituents are not prepared for undertaking the intended actions, the engaging organization must provide or leverage technical capacities to prepare constituents for those actions.[6]

Key questions to answer in selecting a mobilization approach are:

- Who are the constituents and stakeholders within the community?
- Does the community believe itself capable of affecting its environment?
- Will the community hear and absorb the information that is supplied about the health issue?
- Does the community have the capability to mount a response?

The answers to these and other questions provide the framework that the agency can use to analyze its engagement and mobilization options. The mobilization option chosen to bring dialogue and action on a public health issue must support the agency position and be consistent with the strategy selected so as to guide constituent interaction and the constituents' capacity to act. Specific models for mobilization are discussed later in this chapter.

Assessing the Effectiveness of Constituencies to Act

Assessing the capabilities of public health constituency actions is focused on the constituents' health beliefs and attitudes and their ability to assess information, enter into dialogue on community health issues, participate in drawing conclusions from available information, and participate in needed actions to address community health concerns. In the case of mobilizing for community health improvement, effectiveness means taking actions that have clarity and are evidence based. Clarity must be a goal in each step of the health improvement action from the population health objectives to its political appeal and the intervention science used to achieve the health objectives.

Political appeal is one factor in determining health improvement actions. Political appeal is measured against any competing actions that are proposed to achieve the same objective. If the competing actions are equally effective at accomplishing the objective, and one does not cost more than the other, a compromise rather than opposition is appropriate. If the competing action is not built on good public health science, then opposition may be necessary, though unfortunate, because all involved in a fight become injured. Given the choice between compromise and opposition, it is necessary to apply a competitive strategy to raise the appeal for an advocated action.

Clarity of science is achieved with selection and use of effective interventions and mobilization approaches. Appropriate use of science enables identification of measures to establish objective targets and evaluate collaborative actions and intervention outcomes. The health objectives and outcomes require an adequate assessment of the community's health status. Although this chapter is not focused on assessment tools, many approaches described in the following sections are useful in assessing health status. Some of the resources available to aid in establishing objective targets and monitoring progress are *Healthy People 2020*, the National Committee for Quality Assurance's Healthcare Effectiveness Data and Information Set (HEDIS), and the National Center for Health Statistics' (NCHS) leading health indicators.[30–32]

Intervention Guidance to Support Constituent Action

Once there is an understanding of the participation "drivers" of constituents and knowledge of the organizational factors that contribute to effective constituency interactions, it is time to move to action. Population health constituencies become stronger by taking effective action to improve the public's health; that is, the success of reaching group goals provides reinforcement of constituency engagement.

Many tools are available for use that provide guidance for public health and preventive medicine interventions on specific diseases and social conditions contributing to disease. The Guide to Clinical Preventive Services provides the evidence base for clinical preventive medicine intervention.[33] Similarly, the Guide to Community Preventive Services provides the evidence base for the effectiveness of interventions directed at populations in a community setting.[34] Several broad, cross-cutting interventions are available that facilitate constituent engagement in planning for health actions; examples of these are described in the next section.

Tools to Mobilize Constituents for Public Health Action

Public health and preventive medicine practitioners at local, state, federal, and global levels have developed tools and initiatives to assist in achieving long-term health improvements in populations. Examples of these approaches include *Healthy People 2020*, Centers for Disease Control and Prevention's (CDC) Healthy Communities Program, Mobilizing for Action through Planning and Partnership (MAPP), and Turning Point,[30,35–37] all of which facilitate constituent involvement.

Resources to Guide Community and Constituency Engagement

Principles of Community Engagement

The body of knowledge supporting public health constituency engagement continues to grow as does collaboration between population health leaders and the communities they serve. This growth is reflected throughout the literature review in the second edition of *Principles of Community Engagement*[6,38] (published in 2011, 14 years after the first edition); it provides an in-depth look at the social and behavioral science and examines the practical experiences of public health practitioners and researchers in public health and health care. From this review, the principles of community engagement were reaffirmed. A relationship between the principles and the community and constituency engagement practice elements can be drawn from this text; these linkages are presented in **Table 18.1**.[6]

PARTNER

The Program to Analyze, Record, and Track Networks to Enhance Relationships (PARTNER) is a tool that offers one analytic approach to performance of the community and constituency

Table 18.1   Relationship Between Principles of Community Engagement and Community and Constituency Engagement Practice Elements

Principles of Community Engagement	Community and Constituency Engagement Practice by Elements			
	Know the Community	Establish Positions and Strategies	Build and Sustain Networks	Mobilize Communities
1. Be clear about the populations/communities to be engaged and the goals of the effort		X		
2. Know the community, including its economic condition, political structure, norms, history, and experience with engagement efforts	X			
3. Go into the community to build trust and relationships and seek commitments from formal and informal leadership			X	
4. Accept that collective self-determination is the responsibility and right of all community members		X		X
5. Partnering with the community is necessary to create change and improve health				X
6. Recognize and respect community cultures and other factors affecting diversity when designing and implementing engagement approaches	X	X		X
7. Sustainability results from mobilizing community assets and developing capacities and resources for community health decisionmaking and actions	X		X	X
8. Be prepared to release control to the community and be flexible enough to meet its changing needs		X		X
9. Community collaboration requires long-term commitment	X	X	X	X

Source: Hatcher MT, Warner D, Hornbrook M. Managing organizational support for community engagement. In: *Principles of Community Engagement*. 2nd ed. Washington, DC: U.S. Department of Health and Human Services (NIH Pub #: 11-7782); 2011: 94-9. Available at: http://www.atsdr.cdc.gov/communityengagement/pdf/PCE_Report_Chapter_4_SHEF.pdf. Accessed March 12, 2013.

engagement practice.[24] It is a social network analysis tool designed to measure and monitor collaboration among people and organizations. The tool is free (sponsored by the Robert Wood Johnson Foundation) and designed for use by collaboratives/coalitions to demonstrate how members are connected, how resources are leveraged and exchanged, levels of trust, and outcomes of the collaboration processes.

The tool includes an online survey that you can administer to collect data and an analysis program that analyzes these data. By using the tool, you can:

- Evaluate how well your collaborative is working in terms of identifying the "right" partners, leveraging resources, and strategizing for how to improve the work of the collaborative.
- Demonstrate to partners, stakeholders, evaluators, and funders how your collaborative is progressing over time and why working together is making tangible change.
- Engage in strategic collaborative management to develop action steps and implement change to reap the benefits of social networking.[24]

Developing Public Health Constituencies Within Accreditation

In September 2011, the Public Health Accreditation Board (PHAB) began accepting applications from local, state, and tribal public health agencies for voluntary accreditation by meeting a set of standards developed over several years by the board and large numbers of practitioners. In order to meet the accreditation standards, public health agencies must measure outcomes and demonstrate documentation of achievements. The accreditation standard domains cover the essential public health services plus a domain on administrative and management capacity and one on governance.[3] Many domains require a close working relationship with community groups and constituencies. In order to meet accreditation standards, public health agencies will need to document partnerships throughout the community, with nonprofit organizations, other governmental entities, and citizen groups. Written agreements and minutes from meetings, for example, can form the basis of documentation.

Resources to Engage Constituents in Health Improvement Initiatives

Healthy People 2020 *Tools*

Healthy People 2020 is the latest preventive health agenda for the nation and provides direction for state and local health initiative leaders to identify and set priorities and develop health objective targets.[30] The *Healthy People 2020* framework builds on earlier *Healthy People* initiatives that have been pursued since the early 1980s. Like its predecessors, *Healthy People 2020* was developed through a broad consultation process characterized by inter-sectorial collaboration and community participation. *Healthy People 2020* offers the Healthy People Consortium Toolkit, which is designed to support state and local leaders in establishing their priority health objectives. The second resource is "MAP-IT: A Guide to Using *Healthy People 2020* in Your Community," which offers guidance on mobilizing partners, assessing the needs of your community, creating and implementing a plan to reach *Healthy People 2020* objectives, and guidance to track your community's progress.[39]

The Community Tool Box

The Community Tool Box, developed by the University of Kansas, is a free online resource with extensive how-to guidance on engaging and organizing communities to plan and implement interventions to achieve *Healthy People 2020* goals.[21]

CDC's Healthy Communities Program

CDC's Healthy Communities Program represents decades of experience conducting community engagement initiatives to reduce chronic diseases. This program builds on the foundation of the 1983 Planned Approach to Community Health (PATCH) mobilization and planning model. More recent initiatives described in the Healthy Communities Program offer tools to works with communities through local, state, territory, and national partnerships to improve community leaders' and stakeholders' skills and commitments for establishing, advancing, and maintaining effective population-based strategies that reduce the burden of chronic disease and achieve health equity. Communities create momentum that assists people in making healthy choices where they live, learn, work, [worship], and play through sustainable changes that address the major risk factors—tobacco, physical inactivity, and unhealthy eating. [35]

Numerous tools and resources are available to address chronic disease interventions.

MAPP

Under the leadership of the National Association of County and City Health Officials (NAC-CHO) and the CDC, the Mobilizing for Action through Planning and Partnership (MAPP) tool was developed.[36] MAPP provides local health department and community leaders with a robust tool to guide creation of a local health system that ensures the delivery of services essential to protecting the health of the public. The MAPP tool offers interrelated features for assessment and planning for public health systems and community health improvement. One feature provides indicators to measure community capacity for providing essential public health services. This MAPP feature adopts the local health system measures used by the CDC's National Public Health Performance Standards Program. A second MAPP feature presents and supports strategic planning. The community health assessment feature in MAPP provides guidance in the traditional health status assessment on environmental health, behavioral risk factor data, and health-related, quality-of-life indicators.

Healthy Cities and Communities

The Association for Community Health Improvement (ACHI),[40] a program of the American Hospital Association's Health Research and Educational Trust, is a well established national association for community health, community benefit, and healthy communities professionals. It offers many useful resources including a Community Health Assessment Toolkit. It presents a six-step assessment framework and provides practical guidance drawn from experienced professionals and a variety of proven tools that examine health data sources, community benefit models, a healthy community's processes, and prevention strategies.[40]

Turning Point

Turning Point was an initiative of the Robert Wood Johnson Foundation and the W. K. Kellogg Foundation that operated between 1997 and 2006.[37] Its mission was to transform and strengthen the public health system in the United States by increasing capacity for community-based collaborations to respond to emerging challenges in public health, specifically the system's capacity to work with people from many sectors to improve health status in an equitable manner. Turning Point created a network of public health partners consisting of 21 states and 43 communities that took collective health improvement actions. Resource materials developed through these collaborative continue to offer guidance to inform current community health improvement initiatives.[37]

Principled Engagement

The guiding principles of community engagement presented earlier in this chapter underscore the ethics of collaborative engagement and the importance of principles in maintaining trust. Just as it is important for an organization to know its community, the community must know and trust the public health and preventive medicine organizations. Thus, community engagement is bidirectional and there is importance in knowing constituency groups and being known and positively viewed by constituency groups within a community. This consideration must be included in establishing constituent engagement plans within a health organization. Building constituencies is neither an automatic nor an intuitive process for public health and preventive medicine leaders to undertake. Nonetheless, effective constituencies can be formed and sustained through explicit managerial strategies combined with sound evaluation tools. Because constituent interaction is critical for effective organizational performance and community health improvement, community and constituency engagement cannot be overlooked as a strategic action for public health and preventive medicine leaders and their organizations.[22]

Future Outlook

Looking to the future for insights about community and constituency engagement requires no crystal ball. Challenges faced within the health system will require collective problem solving at every governance level among public, nonprofit, and private sector health services organizations. Those skilled in community and constituency engagement will help lead the way in formulating collective actions to create and respond to health system changes demanded by critical societal issues. The underlying societal issues demanding this health system response are:

- Changes in U.S. demographics, including increasing population diversity and a growing older segment of the population that will increase demand for health services
- The systemic healthcare financing issues demanding new business and care models focused on preventive care and health promotion
- The structural and professional changes that will be required to reintegrate public health and health care that are needed to create a seamless preventive care and health-promoting delivery system

Finding and implementing acceptable solutions will demand engagement across diverse populations with differing interests. Solutions that are not acceptable to those served, those providing service, and those paying for service will not implement well. Engagement of these competing interests will provide greater opportunity for give and take in solution development.

One set of initiatives may shape and inform solution development. Community and constituency engagement is woven into each of these initiatives. These initiatives are reviewed to increase awareness and to encourage engagement.

Community Benefit and Community Health Assessment

Community benefit is the term used to describe the hospital activities required to receive tax-exempt (nonprofit) status under Internal Revenue Service (IRS) Revenue Ruling 69-645, 1969-2.C.B.117. In order to comply with federal requirements in the Patient Protection and Affordable Care Act (Public Laws 111–148 and 111–152), a tax-exempt hospital must: 1) conduct a community health needs assessment every 3 years, 2) adopt an implementation strategy to meet the community needs, and 3) report how it is addressing the needs identified in the community health needs assessment.

PHAB completed a set of national standards and measures in 2011 that requires state, local, and tribal health departments to ensure that the services they offer meet community need, improve community health, and are continuously improved to recognize changes in the community.[3]

The overlap between the PHAB standards and IRS requirements for hospitals demonstrate a similarity of goals and activities that can be most effectively leveraged with collaborative efforts.[41] The American Public Health Association, Association of Schools of Public Health, Association of State and Territorial Health Officials, National Association of County and City Health Officials, National Association of Local Boards of Health, National Network of Public Health Institutes, and Public Health Foundation, in a consensus statement, developed a set of principles and recommendations on implementing community health needs assessments (CHNA):[42]

- The goal of CHNA and implementation strategies should be to ensure maximum impact of hospital community benefits on the health of people in communities.
- Governmental public health agencies are key partners and resources for CHNA and health improvement planning.
- The benefit to communities can also be maximized through use of public health expertise.
- CHNA and implementation strategies should aim to increase health equity through consideration of social determinants of health.
- CHNAs and implementation strategies should address the needs of underserved and low-income populations.
- Community engagement is a key element of meaningful and effective CHNA and community health improvement planning.

The associations recommend that hospitals consult with public health experts and with state and local health departments, and ask for input from community representatives. They recommend that the community defined by hospitals include medically underserved and low-income populations and that implementation strategies address all identified needs, include evaluation measures, and be widely available to the public. The associations urge that hospitals be allowed to conduct CHNA with others and to use resources to support the needed assessment work.[42]

Local health departments can take initiative by meeting with hospital executives to offer leadership in coordinating a needs assessment process that effectively describes the health needs throughout the jurisdictions that align with hospital service areas.

Primary Care and Public Health Integration

A 2012 Institute of Medicine report explores better integration of primary care and public health to improve overall population health.[43] The report identifies a set of core principles for successful integration: a common goal of improving population health; involvement of the community in defining and addressing its needs; strong leadership to bridge disciplines, programs, and jurisdictions; sustainability; and the collaborative use of data and analysis. It urges federal agencies to join forces to support the integration of primary care and public health: it calls for the CDC and the Human Resources and Services Administration to create research and learning networks that disseminate best practices and for the Centers for Medicare and Medicaid Services to focus on improving community health and to find regulatory options for graduate medical education funding.[43]

A fundamental challenge for healthcare reform in the United States is to expand access to all residents, while improving the delivery system to raise quality and lower cost. Success will require a shift in emphasis from fragmentation to coordination and from highly specialized care to primary care and prevention. The patient-centered medical home (PCMH) model was described by the primary care professional organizations in 2007 and endorsed by a broad coalition of healthcare stakeholders, including all of the major national health plans, most of the Fortune 500 companies, consumer organizations and labor unions, the American Medical Association, and 17 specialty societies. Multistakeholder demonstration pilot projects are underway in 14 states.[44]

Health Reform

The Patient Protection and Affordable Care Act created a number of prevention programs, including the National Prevention Council, the National Prevention and Health Promotion Strategy, and the Prevention and Public Health Fund. These programs will allow jurisdictions to meet the health needs of their populations by using the strategies described earlier in this chapter. Programs with a community focus are funded from the Prevention and Public Health Fund as follows:

- Community Transformation Grants support evidence-based community public health interventions
- "Healthy Aging, Living Well" pilot grants fund states to provide community-based interventions and clinical preventive services to individuals 55–64 years of age
- A demonstration program provides an "individual wellness plan" to at-risk individuals seeking care from Federally Qualified Health Centers

- An education and outreach campaign promotes public awareness of available clinical preventive benefits
- Grants support school-based health centers, among others[45]

In summation, these initiatives and others yet to be framed will require acceptance and collaborative problem solving to implement. Those skilled in community and constituent engagement have a critical role in these and future efforts that call for collaborative innovation to serve the public's health needs.

Discussion Questions

1. Why is community and constituency engagement important in initiatives to improve health status and health systems?
2. Why is a practice framework for performing and managing community and constituency engagement important for organizations?
3. How do the four strategies presented in this chapter prepare organizations to plan community and constituency engagement initiatives?
4. How do the engagement practice elements "know your community" and "develop and maintain networks" guide implementation of population-based health interventions?
5. As the health system is reformed to improve population health through integrated preventive services and health promotion, what challenges will face organizational leaders in their management of community and constituency engagement?
6. How will you, as a future health system leader, address the identified community and constituency engagement challenges?

References

1. Core Public Health Functions Steering Committee. *10 Essential Public Health Services.* Atlanta, GA: Centers for Disease Control and Prevention; 1994. Available at: http://www.cdc.gov/nphpsp/essential Services.html. Accessed March 12, 2013.
2. National Public Health Performance Standards Program. *State public health system performance standards, Essential public health service 4.* Atlanta, GA: Centers for Disease Control and Prevention; 2002. Available at: http://www.cdc.gov/nphpsp/documents/statemodelstandardsonly.pdf. Accessed March 12, 2013.
3. Public Health Accreditation Board. *Standards and measures: version 1.0.* Available at: http://www .phaboard.org/wp-content/uploads/PHAB-Standards-and-Measures-Version-1.0.pdf. Accessed March 12, 2013.
4. CDC/ATSDR Committee on Community Engagement. *Principles of community engagement.* Atlanta, GA: Centers for Disease Control and Prevention; 1997. Available at: http://www.cdc.gov/phppo/pce/ part2.htm. Accessed March 12, 2013.
5. McCloskey DJ, McDonald MA, Cook J, et al. Community engagement: definitions and organizing concepts from the literature. In: *Principles of Community Engagement.* 2nd ed. Washington, DC: U.S. Department of Health and Human Services (NIH Pub #: 11-7782); 2011: 5–7. Available at: http:// www.atsdr.cdc.gov/communityengagement/pdf/PCE_Report_Chapter_1_SHEF.pdf. Accessed March 12, 2013.
6. Hatcher MT, Warner D, Hornbrook M. Managing organizational support for community engagement. In: *Principles of Community Engagement.* 2nd ed. Washington, DC: U.S. Department of Health and

Human Services (NIH Pub #: 11-7782); 2011: 94–6. Available at: http://www.atsdr.cdc.gov/communityengagement/pdf/PCE_Report_Chapter_4_SHEF.pdf. Accessed March 12, 2013.

7. Nicola RM, Hatcher MT. A framework for building effective public health constituencies. *J Public Health Manag Pract.* 2000;6(2):1–10.

8. Hatcher MT, Nicola RM. Building constituencies for public health. In: Novick LF, Morrow CB, Mays GP, eds. *Public Health Administration: Principles for Population-Based Management.* 2nd ed. Sudbury, MA: Jones and Bartlett Publishers; 2008:443–58.

9. Hatcher MT, Nicola RM. Building constituencies for public health. In: Novick LF, Mays GP, Eds. *Public Health Administration: Principles for Population-Based Management.* Gaithersburg, MD: Aspen Publishers; 2001:510–20.

10. *The American Heritage Dictionary of the English Language.* 5th ed. Boston: Houghton Mifflin Harcourt Publishing Company; 2011. Available at: http://ahdictionary.com/word/search.html?q=constituency. Accessed March 12, 2013.

11. *Merriam-Webster Online Dictionary.* Constituency. Available at: http://www.merriam-webster.com/dictionary/constituency. Accessed March 12, 2013.

12. Brown ER. Community action for health promotion: a strategy to empower individuals and communities. *Int J Health Serv.* 1991;21(3):448–51.

13. Wandersman A, Florin P, Friedmann R, et al. *Who Participates, Who Does Not, and Why? An Analysis of Voluntary Neighborhood Organizations in the United States and Israel.* New York: Springer; 1987.

14. Butterfoss FD, Kegler MC. Toward a comprehensive understanding of community coalitions. In: DiClemente RJ, Crosby RA, Kegler MC, eds. *Emerging Theories in Health Promotion Practice and Research: Strategies for Improving Public Health.* 1st ed. San Francisco: Jossey-Bass; 2002:117–77.

15. Butterfoss FD. Process evaluation for community participation. *Annu Rev Pulb Health.* 2006;27:325–330.

16. Mattessich PW, Murray-Close M, Monsey BR. *Collaboration: What Makes It Work: A Review of Research Literature on Factors Influencing Successful Collaboration.* 2nd ed. St. Paul, MN: Amherst H. Wilder Foundation; 2004:7–30.

17. Staley K. *Exploring Impact: Public Involvement in NHS, Public Health and Social Care Research.* East Leigh, UK: INVOLVE; 2009:48–88.

18. Chilenski SM, Greenberg MT, Feinberg ME. Community readiness as a multidimensional construct. *J Community Psychol.* 2007;35(3):347–65.

19. Chavis DM, Lee KS, Acosta JD. The sense of community (SCI) revised: The reliability and validity of the SCI-2. Paper presented at the 2nd International Community Psychology Conference, Lisboa, Portugal; 2008. Available at: http://www.communityscience.com/pdfs/Sense%20of%20Community%20Index-2(SCI-2).pdf. Accessed March 12, 2013.

20. Edwards RW, Jumper-Thurman P, Plested BA, et al. Community readiness: research to practice. *J Community Psychol.* 2000;28(3),302–5.

21. Work Group for Community Health and Development. *The Community Toolbox: Community Readiness.* Available at: http://ctb.ku.edu/en/tablecontents/section_1014.aspx. Accessed March 12, 2013.

22. CTSA Task Force on the Principles of Community Engagement. Principles. In: *Principles of Community Engagement.* 2nd ed. Washington, DC: U.S. Department of Health and Human Services; 2011:44–53. (NIH Pub #: 11-7782) Available at: http://www.atsdr.cdc.gov/communityengagement/pce_principles_starting.html. Accessed March 12, 2013.

23. Varda D, Shoup JA, Miller S. A systematic review of collaboration and network research in the public affairs literature: Implications for public health practice and research. *Am J Public Health.* 2012;102(3):564–71.

24. Varda D, Retrum JH. Program to analyze, record, and track networks to enhance relationships (PARTNER). Robert Wood Johnson Foundation. Available at: http://www.partnertool.net/. Accessed April 30, 2012.

25. Tscheschke S. *Utilizing Network Analysis to Transform a Community Collaborative.* Available at: http://www.partnertool.net/wp-content/uploads/2011/08/Utilizing-Network-Analysis-to-Transform-a-Community-Collaborative.pdf. Accessed March 12, 2013.

26. Green LW, Kreuter MW. *Health Program Planning: An Educational and Ecological Approach.* 4th ed. New York: McGraw-Hill; 2005.

27. Hasenfeld Y. *Human service organizations*. Englewood Cliffs, NJ: Prentice-Hall; 1983.

28. Mello MM. Health law, ethics, and human rights: New York City's war on fat. *N Engl J Med*. 2009;360:2015–20.

29. D'Aunno TA, Zuckerman HS. A life-cycle model of organizational federations: The case of hospitals. *Acad Manag Rev*. 1987;12(3):534–45.

30. U.S. Department of Health and Human Services. *Healthy People 2020*. Available at: http://www.healthypeople.gov/2020/about/default.aspx. Accessed March 12, 2013.

31. National Committee for Quality Assurance. Summary table of measures, product lines and changes. HEDIS-health plan employer data. Available at: http://www.ncqa.org/LinkClick.aspx?fileticket=O-31v4G27sU%3d&tabid=1415. Accessed March 12, 2013.

32. Centers for Disease Control and Prevention, National Center for Health Statistics. *Health, United States, 2010*. Available at: http://www.cdc.gov/nchs/hus.htm/. Accessed March 24, 2012.

33. U.S. Department of Health and Human Services, Agency for Healthcare Research and Quality. *Guide to Clinical Preventive Services*. Available at: http://www.ahrq.gov/clinic/pocketgd.htm. Accessed March 12, 2013.

34. Task Force on Community Preventive Services. *Guide to community preventive services*. Available at: http://www.thecommunityguide.org/default.htm. Accessed March 13, 2013.

35. U.S. Department of Health and Human Services. CDC's Healthy Communities Program. Available at: http://www.cdc.gov/healthycommunitiesprogram/communities/index.htm. Accessed March 24, 2013.

36. National Association of County and City Health Officials. Mobilizing for action through planning and partnership. Washington, DC: NACCHO; 2000. Available at: http://www.naccho.org/topics/infrastructure/mapp/framework/mapppubs.cfm. Accessed March 12, 2013.

37. Robert Wood Johnson Foundation, W. K. Kellogg Foundation. *Turning Point*. Available at: http://turningpointprogram.org. Accessed March 12, 2013.

38. Institute of Medicine. *The Future of the Public's Health in the 21st Century*. Washington, DC: National Academies Press; 2002.

39. U.S. Department of Health and Human Services. *Healthy People 2020 MAP-IT*. Available at: http://www.healthypeople.gov/2020/implement/MapIt.aspx. Accessed March 12, 2013.

40. Association for Community Health Improvement. *American Hospital Association, Health Research and Educational Trust*. Available at: http://www.communityhlth.org/communityhlth/about/mission.html. Accessed March 12, 2013.

41. Scutchfield FD, Evashwick CJ, Carman AL. Commentary: public health and hospital collaboration: new opportunities, new reasons to collaborate. *J Public Health Manag Pract*. 2011;17(6),522–3.

42. Consensus Statement from American Public Health Association, Association of Schools of Public Health, Association of State and Territorial Health Officials, National Association of County and City Health Officials, National Association of Local Boards of Health, National Network of Public Health Institutes, and Public Health Foundation. *Maximizing the Community Health Impact of Community Health Needs Assessments Conducted by Tax-Exempt Hospitals*. Available at: http://www.apha.org/NR/rdonlyres/78190210-F339-4511-9C0E-EC678B206F55/0/CHNAConsensus031312FINAL.PDF. Accessed March 12, 2013.

43. Institute of Medicine, Committee on Integrating Primary Care and Public Health Board on Population Health and Public Health Practice. *Primary Care and Public Health: Exploring Integration to Improve Population Health*. Washington, DC: National Academy of Sciences; 2012. Available at: http://www.iom.edu/~/media/Files/Report%20Files/2012/Primary-Care-and-Public-Health/PCPH_rb.pdf%20on%204/29/2012. Accessed March 12, 2013.

44. Rittenhouse DR, Shortell SM. The patient-centered medical home: will it stand the test of health reform? *JAMA*. 2009;301(19):2038–40.

45. Senate Democrats. The Patient Protection and Affordable Care Act: Detailed summary. Available at: http://dpc.senate.gov/healthreformbill/healthbill04.pdf. Accessed April 30, 2012.

Evaluation of Public Health Programs

L. Michele Issel and Michael C. Fagen

LEARNING OBJECTIVES

- To understand the distinction between evaluating health programs and evaluating health or medical care services
- To understand the health program planning and evaluation cycle
- To understand the three main evaluation phases: formative assessment, process evaluation, and outcome evaluation
- To understand program, professional, and evaluation accountability
- To understand the relationship between evaluation, quality assurance, and quality improvement activities
- To understand the relationship between evaluation and performance measurement
- To understand the distinction between research and evaluation
- To understand important trends in health evaluation

Chapter Overview

This chapter is focused on the key issues health administrators are likely to face when planning or evaluating health programs, as distinct from health or medical care services. The first section gives definitions to clarify that distinction. The next section describes the health program planning and evaluation cycle, with attention to the feedback loops likely to occur during a cycle, and briefly describes each stage in the overall cycle.

A more in-depth overview of the three key stages in the cycle focuses on the type of evaluation conducted at those stages. The first stage entails an assessment evaluation, which examines the community health needs, the feasibility of conducting a subsequent program evaluation, and the extent to which the health needs are being met by existing services. The next stage in the cycle broadly includes the planning and the implementation of the health program. Attention is given to the development of measurable objectives about the implementation process and the desired effects of the program. The last stage to be discussed is the evaluation of the effect of the health program, both the short-term outcomes and the long-term impacts.

Administrative oversight of health programs will likely be concerned with accountability. Accountability is examined from several perspectives, with attention to the administrative actions associated with each. Given that health professionals will be employed to deliver the health program, issues around professional accountability are also highlighted. Also included in this chapter is an overview of the distinctions and interface among program evaluation, quality improvement processes, performance measurement, and research. The chapter concludes by addressing the future outlook for health program planning and evaluation, with an emphasis on paradigmatic shifts and novel approaches applicable throughout the planning and evaluation cycle.

Terminology: Health Programs, Projects, and Services

Before beginning the discussion of evaluation, the distinctions between what constitutes a program, a project, and a service need to be understood. In general, a *program* connotes a structured effort to provide a set of services or interventions, usually over an extended timeframe. In contrast, a *project* refers to a very specific set of activities accomplished over a specific and limited timeframe. Thus, Medicare is a program but preparing for accreditation is a project. A *service* is the transitory interaction between a provider and client during which something of intangible value is provided. What is provided is not specified in this definition of service, which allows for making distinctions between services provided through a program and a medical service. Thus, a *health program* is the organized structure designed to provide fairly discrete, health-focused interventions that are designed for a specific target audience. Health programs tend to provide educational services, have a prevention focus, and may be delivered to individuals but are more likely to be delivered to groups and populations. In contrast, *health or medical care services* are the organizational structures through which providers interact with patients in order to assess, diagnose, and treat health problems of patients. Keeping the distinction between health programs and health services in mind makes it easier to identify the specific planning and evaluation needs of each.

The Planning and Evaluation Cycle: A Model

Planning and evaluation constitute a cyclical process despite commonly being described in a linear sequential manner. The activities comprising program planning and program evaluation are cyclical and interdependent (**Figure 19.1**), with activities occurring more or less in stages that flow almost seamlessly from one into the next. The learning, insights, and ideas that result

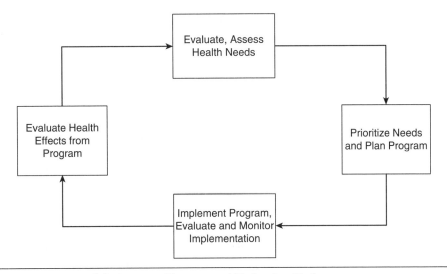

Figure 19.1   Figure of the Program Planning and Evaluation Cycle
Source: Issel LM. *Health Program Planning and Evaluation: A Practical, Systematic Approach.* 2nd ed. Sudbury, MA: Jones and Bartlett Publishers; 2009.

at one stage can influence the available information for the next stage and thus affect the decision making and actions of subsequent stages. Interdependence of activities and stages results from information and data feedback loops that connect the stages. Naturally, not all of the possible interactions among program planning, implementation, and evaluation are shown in Figure 19.1. In practice, the cyclical and interactive nature of health program planning and evaluation exists in varying degrees. The planning and evaluation cycle can be affected by external influences. This requires that program planners and evaluators remain flexible and be creative in responding to those influences while remaining true to the intent of the planning and evaluation of the health program.

A prioritization process is then used to select the health issue or issues to be addressed by a health program. There are several standardized approaches to conducting the needs assessment from a public health perspective,[1] such as the Mobilizing for Action through Planning and Partnerships (MAPP) model,[2] and to the prioritization process.[3,4] The planning phase includes identifying an evidence-based intervention to address the health problem, and then being explicit on the connection between the program and its recipients. The planning stage also includes an assessment of the organizational and infrastructure resources that can be utilized to implement and sustain the program. A key activity embedded in program planning is setting goals and objectives that are measurable and will guide the evaluations.

Program implementation begins after the resources have been secured and the program intervention activities have been explicated. The logistics of implementation include marketing the program to the target audience of potential recipients, training program personnel, establishing management processes, and providing the intervention as planned. Throughout the implementation of the program, evaluation activities focus on the extent to which the program is provided as planned; this is called the process or implementation evaluation. It occurs in real time while the program is being delivered. The data and findings from this evaluation are used as feedback in the planning and evaluation cycle, leading to adjustments to or revisions in how the program is delivered.

At some point in time after the recipients have received the health program interventions, they ought to experience an effect—whether a stabilization or improvement in their health. This applies regardless of whether the recipients of the program were individuals or a community or an entire population. The evaluation for the presence of those anticipated and hoped for effects can be immediate and closely causally linked programmatic effects. This type of effect evaluation is often referred to as an **outcome evaluation**. In contrast, an impact evaluation focuses on the more temporally and causally distal effects of the program. Both types of evaluations provide information useful in subsequent program planning, often about how to improve the program intervention. The effect evaluation findings also can be used in the next cycle of assessments of the need for future or other health programs.

Evaluation Types Across the Cycle

Across the planning and evaluation cycle, different types of activities are sometimes called evaluations. Each of the different evaluation types has a specific focus and purpose, with an associated set of skills. The types of evaluations are introduced here as an overview of the field of planning and evaluation. First, the concepts of goals and objectives are briefly reviewed.

Program Goals and Objectives

Goals and *objectives* are terms that are widely used in program planning and evaluation. Strictly speaking, goals are broad statements about the impact to be achieved by the program, whereas objectives are specific statements given in measurable terms about specifics related to the program. The terms *objectives* and *goals* are not used in a consistent manner, making it imperative to focus on the intent of the statement and keeping in mind the distinction. Understanding the distinction between goals and objectives is the basis for subsequently making the distinctions between short-term outcomes and long-term impacts of the program, and for having metrics to assess the program's implementation and effects.

Evaluate the Need: Assessment

Usually something triggers the beginning of the cycle, such as heightened awareness of a health problem, a recent strategic planning effort, or a new grant opportunity. This trigger event stimulates the collection of data about the extent of various health problems, the characteristics of those affected by the different health problems, perceptions about the health problem, and availability of health and human resources related to the health problem. This **needs assessment** of the healthcare needs and barriers launches the cycle. The needs assessment, as an evaluation of the current state of health and care systems, provides the data on the breadth, severity, and seriousness of the health problems. These data constitute a community needs and assets assessment, and are used to prioritize the problems and their solutions. This forms the basis for the subsequent program development stage.

Most local and state public health agencies engage in a needs assessment and prioritization process on a periodic basis. These needs assessments are used to make choices in funding programs and developing new health programs to address the newly identified health needs. Similarly, healthcare organizations undertake market and community health assessments, which are then used for developing services or product lines rather than health programs. As a result, many needs assessments are based on existing (secondary) data such as the incidence, prevalence, or age-adjusted mortality rate of certain health conditions or diseases. These data are often presented using standard epidemiological tools such as odds ratios or confidence intervals. Geographic information systems (GIS) and mapping data are increasingly being used to graphically represent the location of health-related assets, resources, and disease concentrations. Sometimes, employing original (primary) data collection techniques such as interviews with program-related stakeholders is necessary in order to provide a complete needs assessment.

Evaluate the Doing: Process/Implementation/Monitoring

At the program implementation phase of the cycle, evaluations focus on that implementation. The terminology used for evaluations includes formative, process, monitoring, and implementation evaluations. A *formative evaluation* is conducted early in the implementation of the program and focuses on the implementation to date and the preliminary outcomes. Formative evaluations are more likely for a new or experimental program. More typically, the *process evaluation* is conducted, which focuses on assessing the extent to which the program is being implemented as planned.

Process (TAAPS) Objectives

The assessment of the implementation uses the process objectives as the standard against which to assess the implementation. Process objectives ought to have the following elements: *t*imeframe, *a*mount of what *a*ctivities done by which *p*articipants/program *s*taff (TAAPS). TAAPS objectives address the key and essential actions or activities of the program staff or of participants, which are specific to delivering the program or doing the interventions. A suggested format for writing TAAPS objectives would be: "by when, which staff/participant will do what, to what extent." For example, "After attending three educational sessions, 90% of program participants will walk for 20 minutes three times per week." TAAPS objectives focused on program staff would be:

1. During each session, 100% of the program staff will correctly and completely follow the curriculum for that session.
2. One week before the first session, the program assistant will have sent reminders to 100% of potential program participants.

As these examples demonstrate, the objectives are sufficiently specific so that the data can be collected to reveal the extent to which the objective is met.

Process Evaluation Findings and Actions

A common implementation problem identified through process evaluation concerns the extent to which the program is reaching the target number of eligible participants, referred to as coverage. *Undercoverage*, not reaching the targeted number of eligible participants, can have several causes, such as being a small program addressing a big problem or insufficient marketing. TAAPS objectives relating to marketing of the program ought to be reviewed for having been met. If those TAAPS objectives were not met, the plan ought to be reviewed and perhaps revised based on the process evaluation data. Alternatively, undercoverage might be related to cultural appropriateness, and thus the cultural acceptability of the program ought to be reviewed.

For programs with a long history, decreases in attendance and efficiency need to be considered as warning signs, possibly requiring a fine-tuning of the program.[5] The fine-tuning and updating may require updating the needs assessment in order to have more current and accurate numbers for those in need of the program. The program objectives would also be revised to reflect current health intervention practices and a renewed marketing strategy. The precise nature of the fine-tuning depends upon the process evaluation data and the interpretations given to those data.

The process evaluation provides data on the quality and fidelity of delivering the interventions. Such data can help develop corrective actions. Suppose that a child immunization clinic is scheduled for Wednesdays in the early morning. Attendance records indicate few mothers come with their infants. Staff members learn that mother–baby classes are given at that same time by the park district. Putting together the low attendance, the TAAPS objective of having at least 100 infants immunized at each clinic session, and the conflicting program, changing the day or time for the clinic along with increased marketing efforts could help achieve the objectives. This would not require changing the objectives or the participant eligibility criteria. This scenario shows that much of the revision to the implementation process is common sense. Although a change in the day of the immunization clinic is a simple solution, it may not be simple to implement because of other constraints and organizational factors. So, a simple solution may require considerable effort to make the change.

Managing Group Processes

The purpose of conducting a process evaluation is to assure complete and accurate implementation of the program, especially of the programmatic interventions. Thus, the process evaluation data identify which aspects of the implementation need improvement, modification, refinement, or change. Having this understanding is only useful to the extent that the program staff can then be motivated to make the changes. Two considerations for program managers will surface: anticipating the reactions of individuals and groups to being evaluated and having the corresponding skills to address their reactions.

When the program manager brings recommendations to the program staff for making delivery improvements, staff may interpret this as having received a poor performance evaluation. A natural reaction is to become defensive. As with managing any staff, the approach taken to introduce the needed changes and to gain support from the program staff for those changes can influence or determine the success in making the changes. The approach taken will be more successful if skills related to managing groups are used.

Group process skills applicable to program management include communication, motivation, purpose and direction setting, setting group norms, understanding stages of group formation, and cooperation building. In addition, program managers may use a wide range of strategies to assure the quality and fidelity of program implementation. For example, drawing on network theory, a program manager may focus on creating an ally of a staff member who is central to the network of program staff. By doing so, the program manager can indirectly influence the broader network of staff. Alternatively, a program manager may interpret the program issues in terms of the stages of group formation (forming, storming, norming, performing). If a program has brought together a new group of employees to implement the health program, the implementation problem may still be in an artifact of the forming stage. Alternatively, if the program staff members are knowledgeable and highly motivated, a program manager can allow the staff to evolve in ways that enhance the quality and fidelity of the program. Such an approach would stem from the self-organization principle of complexity theory. Whichever approach the program manager uses, the action path must fit with the program, characteristics of the program staff, and the nature of change needed to have an optimally delivered program.

A different approach is to engage the program staff throughout the process evaluation. Often a report describing how the process data were collected and connections between the data and the TAAPS objectives is an output of the process evaluation. Sharing the report, or portions of it, with program staff, funding agencies, and other stakeholders can be an effective approach to improving the program delivery. Such a report would identify factors contributing to meeting the TAAPS objectives and lead to discussion of reasons for not meeting the objectives and aspects of the program that are amenable to managerial intervention. Equally important, sharing the process evaluation data with staff gives them an opportunity to express their views, issues, and challenges in completely and accurately meeting the intervention specifications. Staff involvement will also have an overall positive effect on morale.

Evaluate the Effect: Outcome/Impact/Summative

The evaluation of the effect of the heath program goes by various names. *Outcome evaluation* assesses the effects of the program interventions that occur most immediately and most directly. In contrast, an *impact evaluation* assesses the effect of the program interventions in the long term and thus less directly attributable to the program. *Summative evaluation* is a term that refers to a comprehensive assessment of a program at its conclusion, and thus might include process and effect evaluation elements. These evaluations are conducted later in the cycle, once the program has been implemented sufficiently and for a long enough time that health effects can be measured. The data from the effect evaluation can be used to revise the program intervention as well as to substantiate the continuation of the health program as is.

Effect (TREW) Objectives

All programs need to have clearly stated expected benefits for the program participants; these are called *effect objectives*. Effect objectives have the following elements: in what *t*imeframe, what portion of *r*ecipients experience what *e*xtent *w*hich type of change (TREW). As with the process objectives, TREW objectives can be written in the general format of: "After how much intervention, how many recipients will experience what extent of which type of change." Extent refers to how much or what degree of change (effect, benefit) is anticipated as result of having received a sufficient dosage of the intervention. In writing the extent portion of the objective, two approaches can be used to determine the extent. One approach is to write the objective in terms of increasing or reducing the level of a certain outcome, but it must be done in comparison to a benchmark level. For example, "After attending 95% of the Safe Sex Program sessions, 100% of the adolescent male participants will have a 20% lower sexually transmitted infection (STI) rate compared to adolescent males not participating." This TREW objective uses non-participants as the comparison—that is, the benchmark. The challenge with writing a TREW objective using words like "increase" or "decrease" is that the extent of difference will need to be very specific and measurable. An alternative approach is to state the extent as a target value the program seeks to achieve. Modifying the previous objective accordingly, it would look like this: "After attending 95% of the Safe Sex Program sessions, 100% of the adolescent male participants will have zero STIs for at least 6 months after completing the program."

The other element of the TREW objective that deserves attention is the timeframe. The timeframe needs to be linked to a quantity of dosage (amount of intervention received through the program). The timeframe is critical for having received the intervention and for that intervention to have taken effect. Well stated TREW objectives that include these elements act as a blueprint for designing the evaluation of program effect.

Conducting Effect Evaluations

In short, conducting effect evaluations relies on utilizing research skills and knowledge. The various types of evaluation designs are the same as would be used to conduct experimental, quasi-experimental, and observational studies. The choice of an effect evaluation design is influenced by a wide range of considerations, such as whether a comparison group exists, whether members of the comparison group can be randomly assigned to receive the program, and whether the effect variable can be measured before the start of the program.[1]

The approaches used to collect data on the effects are also the same methods as would be used in research. Data collection methods can consist of any combination of questionnaires, observations, interviews, existing data from medical records, or biological measures. The data collection method is selected based on the TREW objectives and what is specified as needing to be measured. The data analysis approach and the choice of the statistical analysis depend upon the type or types of data collected and the number of groups for which data exist. A savvy program evaluator will keep handy a favorite textbook on research and statistics for quick reference.

Conducting a scientifically rigorous effect evaluation can be expensive, depending upon the design and data collection method. For example, an effect evaluation of a program to screen for diabetes could be designed to track over several years and interview individuals who were and were not screened. The costs of such an evaluation would be much higher than for an evaluation that uses two groups, but only collects data once using a brief survey. In many cases, an effect evaluation is limited by available funds or by grant requirements, thus the effect evaluation must be designed with the cost limitations in mind. The best time to develop and negotiate the budget for the implementation and effect evaluations is during the program planning stage.

Accountability and Health Programs

Health programs are based in a wide range of types of healthcare organizations, including federal agencies such as Centers for Disease Control and Prevention (CDC), state and local health departments, not-for-profit and for-profit health systems, community-based not-for-profit organizations, church-affiliated organizations, and international relief and assistance organizations such as the Red Cross. Many of these organizations are subject to the same legal constraints and grant-reporting obligations. Meeting these legal requirements and other obligations requires accountability and responsibility, cornerstones of program implementation. Being *accountable* means being held answerable for what is done and the resulting successes or failures of the program. In contrast, being *responsible* means being charged to assure that the correct things are done and done correctly. Program managers have accountability for the program's implementation and responsibility for how the program is implemented. More specifically, program managers are accountable for the program implementation and are accountable professionally.

Program Accountability

Rossi, Freeman, and Lipsey proposed that program managers are accountable for the program in six areas.[5] Five of these six relate to the process of delivering the health program. Having a clear sense of the distinctions among these areas of accountability enables the program manager to more thoughtfully anticipate and possibly avoid implementation problems.

Accountability areas can be defined as follows:

- *Fiscal accountability*, as the name implies, denotes the need for accurate accounting with complete documentation of expenses and sources of revenues.
- A related accountability, *efficiency accountability*, focuses on delivering the program with efficient use of the resources.
- Efficiency is related to coverage, and thus, *coverage accountability* addresses whether the program reached the intended recipients.
- The last process-related accountability is *services delivery accountability*—the extent to which the intervention is provided as planned. Demonstration of this accountability is done through showing the number of units of service provided, as well as the transparent disclosures regarding how often the program intervention protocol was not followed and how frequently the intervention was changed.
- Assuring that staff members act in accordance with local, state, and federal laws and within their professional licensure limits comprises *legal accountability*.

The one type of accountability related to the program effect is *impact accountability*. This is concerned with being answerable for the extent to which the program had an outcome and impact on those who received the program intervention. Impact accountability can be demonstrated, but only through metrics and data tailored to capture and reflect achieving the intended theory of the program.

Professional Accountability

Health programs very likely involve health professionals, with state licenses and professional norms. Therefore, program managers need to be cognizant of **professional accountability**. Professional accountability of an individual from a health profession includes being bound by professional norms and codes and any moral and ethical codes related to serving the public. In health care, professional accountability exists for the individual in terms of performing according to professional standards and ethics and for the entire program in terms of addressing disparities and social justice. For program managers, individual professional accountability is addressed through the usual personnel management that might require the involvement of personnel or human resources. In contrast, the program-level professional accountability can be more difficult to achieve. With tight and shrinking program budgets, program eligibility criteria may become such that individuals in need of the program are not accepted into the program. This situation has the potential to create an ethical dilemma that puts professional accountability at odds with the program limitations.

Evaluation Accountability

The last type of accountability concerns the evaluation itself. The American Evaluation Association established the four standards of evaluation: utility, feasibility, propriety, and accuracy.[6] Meeting all four of these standards helps assure that the evaluators are answerable to those using the evaluation. The utility standard for evaluations specifies that the evaluation must be useful to those who requested the evaluation. An evaluation would be considered useful if it reveals ways to make improvements to the intervention itself or to increase the efficiency of the program. The feasibility standard refers to the ability to conduct the evaluation, and recognizes that an ideal evaluation may not be practical to implement. If an evaluation is too complex or costly, it will not be carried out by programs with limited capabilities and resources. Another standard, propriety, concerns conducting the evaluation in an ethical and politically correct manner. This standard acknowledges that some evaluations can invade privacy or might be harmful to program participants or program staff. The propriety standard holds evaluators accountable for upholding all of the other standards. Lastly, the accuracy standard is achieved through scientific rigor.

Distinctions

Evaluation Complements Quality Assurance and Quality Improvement Activities

With the widespread adoption of quality improvement approaches as an adjunct to the older and still very important quality assurance, the question becomes: how do they interface with program evaluation? **Quality assurance** refers to meeting a minimum acceptable requirement for a process or output as the criteria for taking corrective action if that minimum is not met.

For example, specific equipment and procedures must be followed to obtain an accurate blood pressure. Quality assurance checks verify that the equipment is used according to the protocol. Quality assurance, as it relates to health programs, can be used to assure that program interventions are delivered as planned and according to the program protocols. Quality assurance teams typically look for errors and then take steps to bring the processes into compliance. Because quality assurance stresses following procedures, it does not foster overall improvement but only maintains a minimum standard.

Quality improvement refers to a set of techniques used to make changes to a set of processes or a system to make sustainable changes that enhance the delivery of services. Healthcare organizations adopted continuous quality improvement (CQI)[7] and total quality management (TQM)[8] as tools to reduce costs while improving the quality of services. CQI and TQM focus on examining organizational processes using statistical and other scientific tools. CQI and TQM are based on two premises: 1) that problems, flaws, and mistakes are best addressed through looking at the system as a whole; and 2) that employees are the best source of possible solutions to make corrections. By the 1990s, both approaches had became popular means of enhancing organizational effectiveness and commonplace in healthcare organizations.[9]

CQI and TQM have evolved into a generic ongoing process for assessing the inputs into key organizational processes that influence the use of resources and of patient outcomes. As ongoing organizational processes, quality improvement efforts are conducted by standing quality improvement committees that include employees who are directly involved in the processes being addressed. Seven basic tools are used by improvement committees to statistically control the processes. The tools rely on some basic statistical analyses and graphic displays of the numerical information. **Table 19.1** shows the seven tools, with examples of corresponding graphs. Each of the tools is relatively easy to use and requires minimal statistical knowledge. The tools include the following:

- PERT charts involve diagramming the sequence of events against a specific timeline and thus shows when tasks need to be accomplished.
- Fishbone diagrams, or cause diagrams, represent sequential events and major factors at play at each stage.
- Control charts show whether a variable is within the acceptable parameters based on using an average, with upper and lower confidence intervals and standard deviations. Control charts emphasize setting and staying within parameters for a select set of outcome indicators.
- A histogram is a simple bar graph showing the frequency of a value for one variable.
- A Pareto chart uses a bar graph to identify the major source of a problem.
- A scatter diagram plots the relationship between two variables and readily shows the direction of the relationship.
- A flowchart diagrams the sequence of activities from the beginning through to the last step.

Other approaches have gained usage in healthcare organizations and nearly all use data as the base for making improvement decisions. Six Sigma is a process to reduce variation in clinical and business processes[10] that are attributed to defects that deviate from the specified product, where

Table 19.1   List of Quality Improvement Tools with Graphic Examples

Tools	What the Tool Does	Visual Example*
Cause-and-effect diagram, Ishikawa or fishbone chart	Identifies many possible causes for an effect or problem, sorts contributing causes into sequenced and useful categories	
Check sheet	Form for collecting and analyzing data	**Check Data to Be Reviewed and Analyzed** • ✓ Name recorded • ✓ Age recorded • ✓ Visit at recommended interval • ✓ Attended health-promotion class
Control charts	Graph shows values relative to upper and lower control limits set at 3 sigma for one variable either across individuals as shown or across time (not shown)	
Histogram	Shows frequency distributions for one variable (used age of 20 women in the Neural Tube Defects Prevention Program)	

(continues)

Table 19.1   List of Quality Improvement Tools with Graphic Examples (continued)

Tools	What the Tool Does	Visual Example*
Pareto chart	Bar graph to help identify the few "problem" individuals or variables that create the majority of the nonconformity to the process (0 = no screening, 1 = yes screened to understand who exceeds the recommended 20 minutes)	
Scatter diagram	Graph shows relationship between pairs of numerical data with one variable on each axis (used age and number of minutes of counseling)	
Flow chart	Shows separate process steps in sequential order, with connections between processes and end points	

*The control chart, historgram, Pareto chart, and scatter diagram were developed using SPSS© v.15 (http://www.spss .com/), whereas the fishbone and flow charts were developed using Chartist © v.4 (http://www.novagraph.com/).

Source: Reproduced from Issel LM. *Health Program Planning and Evaluation: A Practical, Systematic Approach.* 2nd ed. Sudbury, MA: Jones and Bartlett Publishers; 2009.

the product can be a service or a tangible item. The Balanced Score Card (BSC), developed by Kaplan and Norton[11,12] is another widely adopted approach. The BSC integrates financial performance measures with measures of customer satisfaction, internal processes, and organizational learning. Although developed for business, the BSC approach has been adapted to the not-for-profit sector[13] and the British National Health Service.[14]

The presence of CQI/TQM can affect evaluations in several ways. In organizations engaged in CQI /TQM employees will already be sensitized to the use of data that may affect the evaluation.[15] These employees will have had an introduction to data-analysis methods, and will be accustomed to participating in analytic and change activities. In addition, staff with exposure to being on CQI/TQM teams may expect to be involved in the development of a program and its evaluation. Staff members with training and knowledge of techniques, especially PERT charting, fishbone diagramming, and the use of control charts, can be very useful in program planning, as they will be able to articulate and diagram underlying program processes. The presence of CQI/TQM does not preclude the need for program evaluations, especially outcome or impact evaluations. Process improvement approaches differ from evaluation with regard to the underlying philosophy, the purposes, who does the activity, and the methods used (**Table 19.2**).

Evaluation and Performance Measurement

Performance measures are standardized indicators of process, output, or outcomes. Since passage of the Government Performance and Results Act of 1993, emphasis on performance measures has grown considerably. The Act requires that each federal governmental agency "express the performance goals for a particular program activity in an objective, quantifiable, and measurable form."[16] This requirement led federal agencies that fund health programs to develop performance measures that are used to hold grantees accountable. The emphasis on standardized testing and use of evidence in education has affected the practice of evaluation.[17] The common wisdom is

Table 19.2   Comparison of Improvement Methodologies and Program Process Evaluation

	Process Improvement Methodologies	Program Process Evaluation
Philosophy	Organizations can be more effective if they use staff expertise to improve services and products	Programs need to be justified in terms of their effect on participants
Purpose	Systems analysis and improvement are focused on identified problem areas from the point of view of customer needs	Determine whether a program was provided as planned and if it made a difference to the participants (customers)
Approach	Team-based approach to identifying and analyzing the problem	Evaluator-driven approach to data collection and analysis
Who does it	Staff—employees from any or all departments, mid-level managers, top-level executives	Evaluators and program managers, with or without the participation of employees or stakeholders
Methods	Engineering approaches to systems analysis	Scientific research methods

Source: Reproduced from Issel LM. *Health Program Planning and Evaluation: A Practical, Systematic Approach.* 2nd ed. Sudbury, MA: Jones and Bartlett Publishers; 2009.

that requiring reporting on performance measures leads to attention of what is measured. However, the evidence in support of this premise is equivocal. Even marginal or small improvements in outcomes that result from attention to performance measurement are improvements that may contribute to a significant improvement in health status outcomes.

A good set of performance measures includes the following features:[18]

- Useful in improving patient outcomes by being evidence based
- Interpretable by practitioners and actionable by improvement committees
- Rigorous measure design that includes validity and reliability
- Denominator and numerator specification
- Feasible measurement implementation

Performance measures, including those approved by the federal Office of Management and Budget (OMB), will have these highly specific characteristics. The list of performance measure characteristics reveals a similarity to program objectives. Therefore, when developing TAAPS process and TREW outcome objectives, it may be useful to align objectives with performance measures on which the program needs to report. Program planners, managers, and evaluators would need to communicate early in the planning process regarding this and work out data-sharing agreements to help minimize redundancies in what processes and outcomes are being tracked and measured. Lastly, the program evaluator needs to be able to articulate and explain the connection between performance measures and the program evaluation.

Evaluation and Research

The last distinction that deserves attention is between evaluation and research. Both use similar methods and both seek rigor in applying those methods. Both also must address the protection of human research subjects, particularly if the evaluation findings will be published. The major differences are found in their purposes and implementation. Research's primary purpose is creating knowledge. For example, a large body of research, much of it conducted using randomized controlled trial (RCT) designs, has generated the knowledge that obesity is a risk factor for diabetes. Evaluation, though often used to generate knowledge, is primarily focused on utility and action. Given the known association between obesity and diabetes, an evaluation might assess the development, implementation, and effects of a diabetes prevention program. Since RCTs are often impractical to implement in community- or organization-based settings, this evaluation's design might use a comparison (rather than a control) group. The evaluation's desired outcome would be a health program that fits well in an organization, can be delivered by its staff, and serves to forestall or prevent diabetes among program participants.

Future Outlook

Evaluators working in health care will experience a continual adoption of more current approaches to improve the processes and outcomes of healthcare organizations. Because such methodologies direct attention toward solving problems, program evaluators need to be sensitive to how current process-improvement approaches might influence program development and implementation and, hence, the evaluation.

For example, the current emphasis on accountability in health care has several implications for evaluation. First, it is likely that performance measures will continue to be emphasized by government and regulatory agencies, accreditation bodies, and funders. As a result, health evaluators will need to familiarize themselves with the many approaches to performance measurement. Since performance measures are often used to assess program implementation, process evaluation skills will be increasingly important in the health domain.

The current accountability focus also highlights the importance of evidence-based public health.[19] Public health administrators are being asked to implement evidence-based programs or demonstrate that their initiatives are designed and implemented based on credible research. In either scenario, administrators will need evaluation skills, either to assess the fit of evidence-based programs within their organizational environments or to evaluate available research evidence when developing new initiatives.

Relatedly, a final implication of the health domain's accountability focus will be the emphasis on sound program development. Whether adapting an evidence-based program or creating a new initiative, administrators will face increasing pressure to "get it right the first time." In this environment, careful program development that emphasizes organizational fit, maximum staff efficiencies, and well articulated program objectives becomes increasingly important. One emerging approach to carefully designing and assessing programs is developmental evaluation, where program administrators, staff, and evaluators work together throughout the planning and evaluation cycle.[20] In developmental evaluations, public health administrators will likely play leadership or facilitation roles.

Overall, the outlook for public health administrators with evaluation skills is bright. Such administrators will be steeped in the planning and evaluation cycle, understand accountability and performance measurement, and be adept at translating evidence-based programs into practice. With these skills in hand, administrators will be poised to make meaningful contributions to their public health organizations.

Discussion Questions

1. Discuss the relationship between the three major phases in the planning and evaluation cycle. Is any one phase likely to be prioritized by public health administrators? Why or why not?

2. What is the most important form of accountability in a healthcare organization that you are familiar with? How does this form of accountability relate to evaluation?

3. How are quality assurance and quality improvement similar? How are they different? How do they relate to performance measurement?

4. Provide examples of specific performance measures that might be emphasized in a particular type of healthcare organization. Given current trends in health evaluation, how might these measures change over time?

5. In addition to the health evaluation trends discussed in this chapter, what do you see as the most important evaluation trends for public health administrators?

References

1. Issel LM. *Health Program Planning and Evaluation: A Practical, Systematic Approach.* 2nd ed. Sudbury, MA: Jones and Bartlett Publishers; 2009.
2. National Association of County and City Health Officials. MAPP Network: MAPP in the News. Available at: http://mappnetwork.naccho.org/page/mapp-in-the-news. Accessed October 24, 2011.
3. National Association of County and City Health Officials. First Things First: Prioritizing Health Problems. Available at: http://www.naccho.org/topics/infrastructure/accreditation/upload/Prioritization-Summaries-and-Examples.pdf. Accessed March 13, 2013.
4. Neiger BL, Thackeray R, Fagen MC. Basic priority rating model 2.0: current applications for priority setting in health promotion practice. *Health Promotion Pract.* 2003;12(2):166–71.
5. Rossi PH, Freeman HE, Lipsey ML. *Evaluation: A Systematic Approach.* 6th ed. Thousand Oaks, CA: Sage Publications; 1999.
6. American Evaluation Association. The Program Evaluation Standards. Available at: http://www.eval.org/EvaluationDocuments/progeval.html. Accessed March 13, 2013.
7. Juran JM. *Juran on Leadership for Quality: An Executive Handbook.* New York: The Free Press; 1989.
8. Deming WE. *Quality, Productivity, and Competitive Position.* Cambridge, MA: MIT Press; 1982.
9. Shortell SM, Jones RH, Rademaker AW, et al. Assessing the impact of total quality management and organizational culture on multiple outcomes of patient care for coronary artery bypass graft surgery patients. *Medical Care.* 2000;38:207–17.
10. Lazarus IR, Neely C. Six Sigma: raising the bar. *Managed Healthcare Executive.* 2003;13:31–3.
11. Kaplan RS, Norton DP. The balanced scorecard—measures that drive performance. *Harvard Bus Rev.* 1992;70:71–9.
12. Kaplan RS, Norton DP. *The Balanced Scorecard: Translating Strategy into Action.* Boston: Harvard Business School Press; 1996.
13. Urrutia I, Eriksen SD. Application of the balanced scorecard in Spanish private health care management. *Measuring Bus Excellence.* 2005;9(4):16–26.
14. Radnor Z, Lovell B. Success factors for implementation of the balanced scorecard in the public sector. *J Corporate Real Estate.* 2003;6(1):99–108.
15. Mark MM, Pines E. Implications of continuous quality improvement for program evaluation and evaluators. *Eval Pract.*1995;16:131–139.
16. Government Performance and Results Act of 1993, United States Senate and House of Representatives Office of Management and Budget. Available at: http://www.whitehouse.gov/omb/mgmt-gpra/gplaw2m.html. Accessed March 13, 2013.
17. Berry T, Eddy RM. *Consequences of No Child Left Behind for Educational Evaluation: New Directions for Evaluation Number 117.* Indianapolis, IN: Wiley; 2008.
18. Krumholz HM, Anderson JL, Brooks NH, et al. ACC/AHA clinical performance measures for adults with ST-elevation and non-ST-elevation myocardial infarction: a report of the American College of Cardiology/American Heart Association Task Force on Performance Measures. *J Am Coll Cardiol.* 2006;4(1):236–65.
19. Brownson RC, Gurney JG, Land GH. Evidence-based decision making in public health. *J Public Health Manag Pract.* 1999;5(5):86–97.
20. Fagen MC, Redman SD, Stacks J, et al. Developmental evaluation: building innovations in complex environments. *Health Promotion Pract.* 2011;12(5):645–50.

Advancing Public Health Systems Research

Leiyu Shi

LEARNING OBJECTIVES

- To distinguish public health systems research from other types of health research
- To appreciate current knowledge and acknowledge gaps in research regarding public health and social determinants of health
- To identify the priorities necessary for public health systems research
- To propose a course of action to enhance public health systems research
- To appreciate the challenges in carrying out public health systems research

Chapter Overview

This chapter summarizes what is known and unknown regarding the relationship between public health systems performance and core areas such as social determinants of population health and public policy, based on the research being carried out in these domains. As there is a lack of knowledge in many of these areas, topics for further research will also be identified. Finally, a course of action is recommended to implement public health systems research for better public health outcomes.

Defining Public Health Systems Research

Public health systems research (PHSR) has been defined as "a field of study that examines the organization, financing and delivery of public health services in communities, and the impact of these services on public health."[1] Studies within this field are designed to produce evidence essential to key public health decision makers to illustrate public health systems issues and the solutions needed to improve the effectiveness and efficiency of these systems. PHSR differs from other types of health research primarily in its focus on systems, and not just individuals or populations (see **Figure 20.1**). Two highly influential Institute of Medicine reports greatly contributed to the beginnings of the PHSR field: The first is the classic 1988 report, *The Future of Public Health*,[2] and the second is the 2002 follow-up report focused on public health systems.[3] The 1988 report was a landmark in the field of public health, particularly for first recognizing as necessary new federal investment in public health: "Governmental roles of assessment, policy development, and assurance became the new public health mantra; and many changes in the practice of public health and the public health system occurred as the result of the report's recommendations."[4] The 2002 IOM report went even further in acknowledging the importance of PHSR and found that this emerging field needed to expand considerably to address the current and future need for evidence in public health practice:

> Research is needed to guide policy decisions that shape public health practice. …CDC [Centers for Disease Control and Prevention], in collaboration with the Council on Linkages between Academia and Public Health Practice and other public health system partners, should develop a research agenda and estimate the funding needed to build the evidence base that will guide policy making for public health practice.[3]

The first federal response to the earlier IOM report came in 1990, in which the Department of Health and Human Services included a goal in their *Healthy People 2000* report that "by 2000 at least 90% of the population would be served by a public health department that effectively carries out the IOM's core functions."[5] In 1994, credited to be a direct result of the 1988 IOM report, the CDC became involved in strengthening the public health system, founding the Public Health Practice Program Office (PHPPO), designed to help "monitor and encourage efforts to improve delivery of public health services and cut across disease-specific categorical funding" in order to achieve the newly defined list of 10 essential public health services (monitoring health status in the community, diagnosing/investigating community health issues, informing/

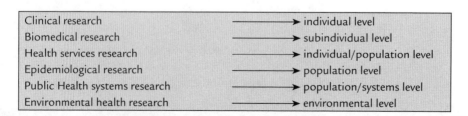

Figure 20.1   Types of Health-Related Research and Level of Focus

educating people about health issues, mobilizing community partnerships for addressing health issues, developing policies that support individual and community health, enforcing health-protective laws and regulations, making sure people know how to receive health services and ensuring need is met, making sure the public health workforce can meet community demand and issues, research to evaluate community health care, and research for novel solutions to health problems).[6,7] The PHPPO administered this National Public Health Performance Standards Program, with the help of several partners involved in public health practice, in an effort to conduct research on how organization and management issues would influence public health infrastructure broadly and the specific delivery of the 10 essential services.[6] Although the PHPPO could be characterized as "small, under-resourced and now defunct," much of the PHSR literature between 1994 and 2004—"the early work by the pioneers in the field—is clearly the result of the efforts catalyzed by the 1988 report" and the early funding provided by the PHPPO.[8] It is this time period, during which federal backing and a concrete list of issues to be addressed were generated, that most consider the birth of PHSR.[8]

This first period of PHSR came to an end as the initial investments through the CDC began to deplete and, eventually, the PHPPO office was closed.[8] However, in 2004, the Robert Wood Johnson Foundation (RWJF) began a 10-year investment in PHSR.[9] The RWJF has become one of the biggest names in PHSR through their continued and generous funding of this fledgling research, because as put by Scutchfield et al., "Funding of this research makes a difference. Academicians and researchers are expert practitioners of the Sutton Principle. If there is funding, there will be research; with no funding, no research."[8] This RWJF funding has led to a second "boost in production" for PHSR after the loss of CDC funding.[8] Today, the RWJF funds a significant portion of all PHSR in the United States, including efforts to promote idea sharing and discussion by convening state representatives working on PHSSR (beginning in 2006); the 2007 award to the University of Kentucky, providing more than $2.8 million to create the first major public health systems research center; and supporting the AcademyHealth interest group, which provides "programs and services that support the development and use of rigorous, relevant and timely evidence to increase the quality, accessibility, and value of health care, to reduce disparities, and to improve health."[10]

Also importantly, the RWJF has funded research to assess the current state of PHSR, further define the field, identify strengths, and overcome challenges. A study published in 2011 with RWJF funding found that half of their identified PHSR community members (academics, public health practitioners, and others with an interest and role in the field) became involved after 2004, when the foundation originally entered the arena. Additionally, the study found that 107 out of the 652 total self-identified community members had received RWJF funding in the last 3 years, making the foundation the most prominent supporter of PHSR in the country, above the CDC (79 members), the National Institutes of Health (NIH; 33 members), and the Human Resources and Services Administration (HRSA; 30 members).[9] The study found that PHSR strengths include good collaboration between researchers (even in different disciplines), a mix of different background specialties and professional experiences, and high levels of resource sharing between individuals and organizations.[9] However, there was also concern expressed over PHSR's reliance on few organizations for most of their funding, significant problems in trying to translate their research expertise into public health practices, and some ongoing inability to efficiently distribute new research and knowledge. Overall, studies like this are continuing to define the field of PHSR and help set an agenda for moving forward.

Current Public Health Systems Research

As PHSR is still evolving, current research encompasses a broad range of subjects and methods. A short overview of current PHSR gives a more complete view of the field to date and the future steps for PHSR.

As referenced in the previous section, a 2011 study supported by the Robert Wood Johnson Foundation and conducted by Merrill et al. found that 652 of the persons were contacted due to their involvement with the AcademyHealth PH Systems Research Interest Group or from attendance at a PHSR meeting/event self-identified as being a part of the PHSR community.[9] They also identified a small core group of the 133 most productive, most active public health systems researchers, who tended to have been involved with the PHSR community longer and to a greater extent (providing more mentoring, attending more meetings, receiving more funding, and presenting more research).[9] These community members come from a variety of backgrounds; 40% have a master of public health (MPH) degree, and the most commonly reported areas of expertise include health policy management (52%), quality improvement/outcome evaluation (48%), social and behavioral sciences (44%), public health practice (43%), and epidemiology (30%). About 51% are employed within academia, 20% are public health practitioners, 12% work for associations or nonprofit organizations, and 18% report working for a foundation/healthcare organization/advocacy group/non-healthcare background/media/other. The authors believe that although they had no better method with which to identify members of the PHSR community, it is likely that this survey is quite representative of the community as a whole. If so, this research demonstrates the wide variation between PHSR practitioners that makes the field a vibrant and multidisciplinary community, and helps explain the conceptual and methodological differences in their work.[9]

Some of these methodological differences are examined in a 2012 review by Harris et al., which finds that of the 327 eligible (original data analysis conducted domestically) PHSR articles available from the Public Health Services and Systems Research (PHSSR) library developed by the University of Kentucky Center for Public Health Services and Systems Research (CPHSSR) research pieces, 68.5% used quantitative methods, 13.8% were qualitative, and 17.7% used mixed methods.[5] The most common quantitative design was a cross-sectional study (80.9% of the 282 studies classified as quantitative or mixed method), while the most common qualitative design was case study (46 total studies, 52.9%). Additionally, only 59 of the 228 cross-sectional studies used multiple points of observation, meaning that a vast majority (74.1%) of these studies are based on information collected at a single time. The most common collection method was through surveys and questionnaires and collected data on individuals, followed by collection of data at the local health department level (often supplemented by secondary data from the National Association of County and City Health Officials [NACCHO]). The large percentage of mixed methods studies can be interpreted as a positive (can provide complementary information about different aspects of a subject) or negative (trying to draw conclusions about a single phenomena from two irreconcilable perspectives). Therefore, while the authors found the huge growth in PHSR to be exciting, both in number of studies and the breadth of research ("The empirical PHSSR examined here varied from surveillance studies of influenza and other infectious and chronic diseases, to quantitative and qualitative studies examining how public health agencies, workforce, and educational programs rate according to standards, to research on how public policy influences health and how PHSSR can influence policy."), they also acknowledge that this discipline still must mature, recommending a greater use of multiple points of measurement, probability samples, and advanced statistical analysis.[5]

PHSR today is also taking place in a variety of settings. A review done using the primary organization affiliation of the first author of PHSR research "indicates that published systems research has been indexed for ~20 foundations and institutes, 10 government agencies, and more than 62 universities in the United States and abroad and represents the work of hundreds of authors, coauthors, and collaborators," in addition to public health practitioners at the local or state level who contribute to PHSR.[4] However, as previously discussed, the funding for PHSR continues to come from very few sources (most notably the RWJF).[4]

So, today, PHSR continues to encompass a large area and bring together many disciplines. For instance, in an October 2009 special issue of *Health Services Research* on PHSR, the articles ranged from "Applying Health Services Research to Public Health Practice" and "Geographic Variations in Public Health Spending: Correlates and Consequences," to "Public Health Systems: A Social Networks Perspective" and "Public Health Emergency Preparedness at the Local Level."[11] In 2010, the National Coordinating Center for PHSSR commissioned "systematic reviews of the PHSSR literature in four broad areas: the public health workforce, quality improvement, organization and structure, and technology, data and methods"; a more complete report was also commissioned by the Altarum Institute, the findings of which were used to create a new list of PHSR priorities.[12] Also in 2009, the CPHSSR prepared a report for the NIH's Health Services Research and Public Health Information Programs on the PHSR workforce. This report found that, overall, there is still considerable confusion about the function and the composition of the public health workforce in the United States, a situation that must be remedied for if PHSR "is to be successful in investigating the dynamics of the public health system, and how the system impacts communities, developing a greater understanding of the role and makeup of the public health workforce will be a cornerstone of these efforts."[13] Other current PHSR comes from the approximately $50 million in public health emergency preparedness funding given to the CDC through the Pandemic and All-Hazards Preparedness Act of 2006, which led to the establishment of research centers at seven schools of public health throughout the country (Emory University Rollins School of Public Health, Johns Hopkins Bloomberg School of Public Health, University of Minnesota School of Public Health, Harvard School of Public Health, University of North Carolina at Chapel Hill Gillings School of Global Public Health, University of Pittsburgh Graduate School of Public Health, and the University of Washington School of Public Health); "This funding represented the largest single award for PHSR by any organization."[4]

The field will continue to evolve, but some areas of attention identified include the need to develop databases to store and provide centralized information for PHSR; the development of new skills by current and future PHSR researchers, such as systems thinking, which "includes concepts such as supporting dynamic and diverse networks, inspiring integrative learning, using systems measures and models, fostering systems planning and evaluation, showing potential of systems approaches, exploring systems paradigms and perspectives, utilizing systems incentives, and expanding cross-category funding"; and the improvement of the public health system in general to better reflect the results of this and other areas of research.[4] While PHSR is still a young field, its contributions to public health foundation and practice are already great.

Knowledge Gaps and Research Priorities

In order to address the existing public health services research gaps, we must first summarize the current knowledge regarding social determinants of population health, the role of public health in influencing population health determinants, the relationship between public policy and public health, the relationship between public health performance and governance structure, and the relationship between public health performance and preparedness. Next, we must use this knowledge to identify further health services research priorities.

Social Determinants of Population Health

There has been extensive literature regarding the social determinants of population health. In order to help explain and categorize this relationship, a variety of frameworks for modeling the determinants of population health can be used. Commonly identified determinants include distal factors (political, legal, institutional, and cultural) and proximal factors (socioeconomic status, physical environment, living and working conditions, family and social network, lifestyle or behavior, and demographics). These models can be used to depict the trajectories or pathways through which these determinants affect population health.

However, there is a general lack of knowledge about the relative magnitude or effect of these determinants on population health. Knowledge of the relative effects could help us focus on key determinants and streamline funding priorities when faced with limited resources. In this situation, the overriding population health determinants question becomes relatively straightforward: What is the optimal balance of investments (e.g., dollars, time, policies) in the multiple determinants of health (e.g., behavior, environment, socioeconomic status [SES], medical care, genetics) that will maximize overall health outcomes and minimize health inequities at the population level? While this question may be straightforward, the answer is far from simple.

Furthermore, little is known about how specifically these determinants affect population health disparities, although such knowledge is a prerequisite to developing strategies that eventually overcome health inequalities. General population health is greatly influenced by population health disparities; therefore, to ultimately improve population health, reducing and eliminating population health disparities is crucial.

Public Health and Population Health Determinants

In the United States, public health has been highly influential in shaping the environmental and behavioral determinants of population health. Through environmental interventions, public health has contributed to the reduction and elimination of diseases or deaths that result from interactions between people and their environment, in particular infectious diseases. Through behavioral interventions, public health has greatly contributed to the prevention and reduction of risk factors that are connected to chronic diseases, the present-day leading causes of death. Great progress continues to be made in these areas through effective public health research and programs.

However, public health, at least in the United States, has not been successful in addressing the socioeconomic determinants of health. U.S. health policy does not have the broad mandate necessary to address major health determinants such as income, education, and employment. Current policies do not pay adequate attention to traditional and emerging public health issues and functions, let alone promote novel research in new, multidisciplinary arenas. For instance, the importance of SES to health has been recognized in Europe since the early 1900s when mortality statistics were first reported according to occupation; the United States, however, has been slower to adopt this practice. In 1976, the U.S. Department of Health and Human Services (HHS) released its first report on the nation's health, which revealed substantial differences in mortality and morbidity according to SES.[14] Since that time, though, little actual progress has been made. Further research is needed to summarize the successful experiences of other industrialized countries and to explore how public health strategies can be developed in the United States to better address and change the socioeconomic determinants of population health.

Likewise, studies are needed to examine how policies and strategies can be developed to reduce SES disparities among and between subpopulations. The United States has much greater income inequality than most developed countries; of the 20 countries ranked highest in human development in the 2010 Human Development Report published by the United Nations, the United States had the greatest inequality (a Gini index coefficient of 40.8).[15] Israel had the second greatest inequality (39.2), followed by New Zealand with a Gini coefficient of 36.2. Denmark and Japan had the lowest levels of inequality with Gini coefficients of 24.7 and 24.9 respectively.[15] While the United States is ranked highly for human development with a human development index (HDI) score of 90.2% (the fourth highest in the world), taking inequality into account using the international HDI scale, which "captures the HDI of the average person in society, which is less than the aggregate HDI when there is inequality in the distribution of health, education and income,"[15] causes the United State's score to drop to 79.9% (a ranking of 13th). An unequal society faces serious issues, because "the chance to lead a meaningful life depends on the conditions people face, including the distribution of advantages in their society."[15] Because socioeconomic status influences population health, countries with greater income inequality (like the United States) can also be expected to experience greater inequality in health and life outcomes. Research into the social determinants of health must seek to address these underlying inequalities if health parity is to be achieved.

Public Policy and Public Health

The significant relationship between public policy and public health is well known. Countries who choose to use broad, far-reaching public policy to achieve their goals of improving population health are more likely to direct this effort at the social determinants of health, including income, education, employment, housing, and healthcare services. Countries with the more narrow, simplistic public policy goal of treating individual-level illnesses are more likely to direct their public health efforts at medical aspects or risk factors, rather than using health policy to address broader social problems.

While these distinctions in the use of public policy obviously exist, there is a lack of research that systematically examines why and how certain countries embrace broad public health policy goals while others embrace more narrow ones. What are the facilitators and barriers shaping decisions to adopt broad public policy goals for public health improvement, and how can strategies be developed to enhance the facilitators and reduce the barriers? Cross-country comparisons are necessary for this type of inquiry; case studies of other countries can provide valuable lessons for the United States as it attempts to broaden its public policy to focus on population health and improve the health of its citizens.

Public Health Performance and Governance Structure

There is clear agreement that public health performance is related to the governance structure of an institution. However, it is less clear exactly how that relationship works. The public health systems literature tends to focus on the deficiencies of the current U.S. public health system, including discrepancies between missions and funding level, the limitations of categorical funding, the lack of leadership and shared vision, discrepancies between expanding roles and old infrastructure, structural variability, inadequate workforce, and inconsistent information technology. However, focusing only on these deficiencies does not promote innovation or improvement.

Therefore, further studies are needed to examine how the public health system (including its structure, processes, and performance) can be redesigned to fulfill the mission of improving population health and reducing health disparities at the national, regional, state, and local levels. Specifically, studies need to develop indicators that capture and quantify achievements in the improvement of population health and the reduction of health disparities, develop and assess the essential services needed to lead to the intended improvements, and develop and assess the structure (including governance, organization, financing, workforce, and information system) necessary to provide these essential services. These studies need to be performed at the national, regional, state, and local levels, all of which must be a part of any public health solution. Moreover, these studies should standardize common features, allowing all participants and studies to identify results that are relevant to specific levels of government or types of communities. **Table 20.1** summarizes these research priorities in relation to public health systems research.

Table 20.1   Public Health Systems Research Priority Areas

- Social determinants of population health
  - The relative magnitude/effect of different social determinants on population health
  - The pathways/trajectories through which social determinants affect population health disparities
- Public health policy and population health determinants
  - How to develop public health strategies to influence socioeconomic determinants of population health
  - How policies and strategies can be developed to reduce SES disparities among subpopulations
- Public policy and public health
  - Examples of broad public policies that focus on population health
  - Facilitators and barriers for broad public policies that focus on population health
- Public health performance and governance structure
  - Which public health strategies, efforts, services, and programs are needed to fulfill the mission of improving population health and reducing health disparities
  - How the public health system (including its structure, process, and performance) can be designed at the national, regional, state, and local levels to carry out these services and programs and therefore fulfill the mission of improving population health and reducing health disparities
    - Develop indicators to measure improvement of population health and the reduction of health disparities
    - Develop and assess the essential services needed to lead to better performance
    - Develop and assess the structure (including governance, organization, financing, workforce, and information systems) necessary to provide these essential services

Course of Action to Implement Public Health Systems Research

The following course of action will help promote the research priorities necessary to improving public health systems.

1. Develop Logic Models on How Public Health Efforts Improve Population Health and Reduce Health Disparities

Although there is a large body of evidence proving that public health contributes to population health and that it often does so by modifying social determinants of health, we know very little about how public health can practically be used to address health disparities. There is little consensus about the ideal role of public health systems and officials at the federal, state, and local levels. A clearer conceptual understanding of these issues is critical, serving as the foundation for concerted efforts toward further research and practice. Therefore, theoretical logic models need to be developed, clearly explaining how public health improves population health and reduces health disparities at all levels.

One way to accomplish this objective would be to convene a joint expert panel and stakeholder meeting where draft logic models are proposed, discussed, and refined after incorporating inputs from all participants. The refined models could then be circulated within the public health community and among public health systems researchers for further comments and refinement. Providing a well-known theoretical framework for public health interventions' effect on population health can help health systems researchers establish a common basis for future work and demonstrate cooperation within the field. Over time, these models may be updated as new evidence is gathered.

2. Develop Indicators to Measure Public Health Performance at the National, State, and Local Levels

Once consensus is reached regarding the proper role of public health for improving population health and the related logic models have been formulated, it will be necessary to develop indicators at the national, state, and local levels that measure public health performance, allowing the collection of evidence that shows, quantitatively, how public health can improve population health and reduce health disparities. A comprehensive national surveillance system for tracking these indicators consistently and over time must also be developed. Eventually, the system should track and measure inputs (resources, capacity, etc.) and core function–related processes (public health practices and services) and outcomes. One strategy to accomplish this indicator development is to encourage a joint expert panel and stakeholders to propose, discuss, and refine draft indicators (tied to the logic models) after incorporating inputs from all participants. The refined indicators, along with the logic models, are then circulated within the public health community for further comment and refinement. These indicators may also be updated periodically as new evidence is gathered.

In this scenario, states are likely to be primarily responsible for developing and implementing a tracking system that captures the public health performance indicators. Since not all states are equal in terms of readiness for running such a program, technical assistance will be needed to enable states to learn from each other and collect comparable information.

3. Conduct International Studies That Draw Lessons from Other Industrialized Countries

Case studies of public health systems in other industrialized countries that have similar political and economic systems and comparable cultural values would help the United States to learn from their experiences; the health systems research of other countries contains valuable lessons of successful and unsuccessful attempts to improve health systems performance. Indeed, many of the topics identified in the research priority areas can benefit from an international perspective. For example, international studies can help address and establish public health's relationship with population health determinants (such as how public health strategies can be developed to influence the socioeconomic determinants of population health, and how policies and strategies can be developed to reduce SES disparities among subpopulations), public policy and public health (examples of broad public policies that focus on population health, and facilitators and barriers toward broad public policies that focus on population health), and public health performance and governance structure (what public health strategies, efforts, services, and programs are needed to fulfill the mission of improving population health and reducing health disparities, and how the public health system can be designed to carry out these services and programs). One way to accomplish this is by using existing or newly commissioned studies that explore these issues for selected countries (e.g., Sweden, the United Kingdom, Canada, Australia). Public health professionals and experts from these countries could also be invited to attend an international symposium on public health systems performance and research with an emphasis on "lessons learned." The commissioned studies, presentations by local experts, and the discussions that follow could help promote a systematic understanding of other countries' experiences and lessons.

4. Advocate State Innovations to Improve Public Health Performance

Due to the political and institutional structures of the United States, and the diversity of local needs and resources, significant and meaningful reforms are most likely to happen at the state level. For this reason, the federal government needs to encourage state innovations to improve public health infrastructure and performance. One way to accomplish this is to fund and publish evaluations of states' innovative efforts at improving their public health systems infrastructure, practices, and performance. This information will be invaluable in refining structure and practices, helping to build an evidence base. It is also important to encourage states to address the major determinants of population health and health disparities by focusing on social and community factors, not just access to public health and medical care services for selected individuals. While it is much more difficult to influence social and economic determinants, public health officials must understand that it is necessary and beneficial to intervene much earlier in the process of poor health development. Since many of these distal social factors are the root causes of poor health, addressing them will be paramount to improving population health and resolving health disparities in the United States. Therefore, to promote and protect society's interest in health and wellbeing, public health must exert more influence on the social, economic, political, and medical care factors that affect health and illness.

For example, Turning Point was an initiative of The Robert Wood Johnson Foundation to transform and strengthen the public health system, operating from 1997–2006. The 23 states participating in this initiative developed multisector partnerships to produce public health improvement plans and chose one or more priorities for implementation.[16] Strategies employed for transforming public health systems include institutionalization within government, establishing "third-sector" institutions, cultivating relationships with significant allies, and enhancing communication and visibility among multiple communities. With this support, states were able to expand their health services research and activities in ways that promoted better population health and reduced health inequality.

5. Advance Community-Based Projects That Integrate Research and Practice

A plausible way to help address the research priorities developed earlier is to encourage more community-based projects that integrate research with practice. Community has been defined as individuals with a shared affinity, and perhaps geography, who organize around an issue, using collective discussion, decision making, and action,[17] or alternatively as a group of people who have common characteristics, defined by location, race, ethnicity, age, occupation, interest in particular problems or outcomes, or other common bonds.[17,18] For the purpose of promoting a public health perspective, community could be broadly defined as including all those individuals, organizations, and institutions situated in a defined geographic area with close political, social, or economic interactions.

Community-based projects should adhere to some fundamental principles. Community-based projects should foster collaboration between public health agencies and other entities that can contribute toward the goal of improving health. Improving the health of populations and reducing health disparities will certainly require the participation of traditional health agencies, but will also demand involvement from education, housing, environmental, criminal justice, and economic agencies and authorities. To achieve cross-agency collaboration, these agencies should create standing mechanisms for policy development between sectors and promote inter-departmental collaboration, along with creating networks among public and private agencies, and particularly with advocates, to openly study, evaluate, and disseminate policy options.

Community-based projects should stress multilevel integration of interventions. In the United States, for some vulnerable groups there are gaps in service provision and for others there are major duplications and waste. Building on the example of multiple risk factors, efforts could be made toward unifying services across agencies and organizations with common goals. Domestic and foreign public health initiatives have shown greater promise when utilizing the collective resources of different public and even private advocates. For instance, a 2011 report in the United Kingdom encouraged that vulnerable groups, such as the elderly or people suffering from multiple chronic conditions, could benefit from better integrated care; integration, in their view, must occur in the health and the social care sectors, and will involve diverse organizational actors. Regardless of these challenges, the authors still believe that integrated care's benefits will outweigh its costs.[19] Recognizing common goals encourages multisector alliances and minimizes partisan or other political barriers.

Community-based projects should stress participation and empowerment, characteristics that are regarded as critical components for intervention acceptance, success, and continuation. Greater community involvement and leadership in priority-setting and policy development would also be critical for any community-based program's ultimate success. In these cases, one of the best ways to include communities in decision making is to focus on and base programs on community strengths and resources rather than community deficits or problems. Communities should be seen as action centers for development, progress, and change. Community members and community leaders should have a central role in planning and managing initiatives. Through community mobilization, skill building, and resource sharing, communities can be empowered to identify and meet their own needs, making them stronger advocates for supporting the vulnerable populations within and across their community boundaries.

Community-based projects should also ensure feasibility, which is a critical component of success. Areas of feasibility to be considered include: technical feasibility (can the intervention plausibly solve or reduce the problem as defined?), economic feasibility (what are the costs and benefits of a given intervention from an economic standpoint?), political feasibility (will this intervention be considered politically acceptable?), and administrative feasibility (how possible would it be to implement the intervention given a variety of social, political, and administrative constraints?). Overall, achieving success through any program will depend on support from key officials, other stakeholders inside and outside of government, and, often, voters.

Community-based projects should also apply novel strategies for success. An approach that has been successful in Europe—restating a public health issue using different languages—may attract new attention to a problem not previously compelling to the public or policymakers. For instance, in the past, advocates have most often used a social justice argument to attempt to persuade the public that inequality in the United States should be eliminated. On the other hand, politicians in the Netherlands were more impressed by a discussion centering on "lost human potential" than inequality. Perhaps the same effect would be seen among Americans if the national conversation on public health was expanded to address concerns other than social justice.

Community-based projects should include a systematic evaluation component to encourage feedback and allow for programmatic refinement. Programs that are comprehensive in scope (addressing multiple risks) should be evaluated along multiple dimensions, but must also be evaluated using criteria that are feasible to obtain and interpret. In too many circumstances, health and social programs are judged on whether they directly impact the long-term health of their target population, even though the program is only funded for a short-term cycle (e.g., just 2 or 3 years). If these projects were implemented over a longer period, then programs may be held accountable to meeting the goals of improving population health.

6. Search for Innovative Ways of Funding Public Health Systems Research

Funding for public health systems research, which affects a large variety of people and institutions, ought to come from a variety of sources. In addition to traditional federal funding from the CDC, NIH, HRSA, and Agency for Healthcare Research and Quality (AHRQ), foundations can play a major role in shaping and fostering public health systems research. Foundations provide a unique avenue for promoting scientific and policy discussion of a public health issue, because in addition to providing the necessary financial resources to further explore issues such as disparity, foundations are able to influence public opinion through publications and media and the discourse it inspires. Many foundations are already involved in health systems research, including the Rockefeller Foundation through their "Transforming Health Systems" program[20] and the fellowships provided through the Robert Wood Johnson Foundation or the Commonwealth Fund for the purpose of supporting health services research and researchers.[21] In addition, the private sector should also be encouraged to engage in health services research, especially for funding community-based projects. These programs aim to improve community health and benefit all those residing in the community, including private businesses, their employees, and employees' families.

7. Develop New Methodologies and Analytic Tools

Much of the research and evaluation in this field will be unlike traditional medical research that relies on control groups, a large sample size, and a limited number of variables. In contrast, public health systems research typically involves a single community and multiple variables, without the ability to tightly control the behavior of the actors. Because there are still few evaluation methods developed specifically for health systems research, new methodologies and analytic tools must be tested to further this line of inquiry and advance the field. One way to facilitate this research could be through a retreat where experts in related fields (e.g., social scientists, health services researchers, public health researchers, methodologists, qualitative researchers, and practitioners) gather and discuss challenges facing PHSR and possible solutions/new processes. As a result, suggested approaches (methodological and analytic) to carry out public health systems research could then be summarized and promoted broadly.

8. Educate the Public and Enhance Dissemination

Education can be used as a tool to raise awareness about population health problems and to promote support for programmatic changes to help eliminate disparities. New technology has provided innumerable means for distributing information. A media campaign incorporating the Internet, television, radio, and print ads promoting a simple, readable, and galvanizing message could reach and motivate a broad segment of the population to support these new health policy goals. Policy analyses and research should also be well published in highly regarded academic publications in order to exert consistent political pressure on policymakers. In addition to increasing awareness of these issues, it is critical that the public and policymakers understand the severity of the problems we face. Policymakers are more likely to act when there is a clear public demand and when there is a perceived crisis. One way to demonstrate severity is the publication of international rankings on key health and healthcare indicators, on which the United States often performs far more poorly than the average citizen would expect. Taking advantage of national pride by highlighting an issue in which the United States performs poorly compared to other countries may motivate the public to take steps to improve their national ranking. This strategy has often been invoked to garner support for infant mortality interventions. The U.S. ranking as the country with the 9th highest infant mortality rate among Organisation for Economic Co-operation and Development (OECD) nations should continue to inspire outrage; 6.5 deaths per 1,000 live births shows that the country's prenatal and postnatal care leads to outcomes more closely related to Chile (7.8 deaths per 1,000 live births) and Hungary (5.6 deaths per 1,000 live births) than most developed European nations (Sweden has 2.5 deaths per 1,000 live births, Luxembourg only 1.8).[22] These rankings have contributed to the growing discontent that a country with so many resources does not ensure adequate care for its most vulnerable citizens.

Education can also be used to establish relevance. Although most Americans are concerned about the plight of vulnerable populations, relatively few consider these to be their own problems. Even fewer understand that it is actually to their economic advantage to better address the plights of vulnerable populations. A rational review of the costs and benefits associated with improving the health of vulnerable populations reveals the advantage of making such an investment; for example, in their 2010 study Milstein et al. found that "a strategy that also strengthens primary care capacity and emphasizes health protection would improve health status, reduce inequities, and lower costs."[23] The consideration of costs to the nation resulting from poor health status among the vulnerable cannot evade the public's attention much longer.

9. Engage the Policy Community

To elevate the status and urgency of public health and public health systems research, the policy community must be engaged. As discussed earlier, in the United States, there is a lack of political conviction for improving population health and reducing health disparities. This is reflected in the absence of a coherent public policy agenda for promoting population health and in the lack of authority and funding for public health. The federal government has six main areas in which it plays a role in population health: policy making, financing, public health protection, collecting and disseminating information about health and healthcare delivery systems, capacity building for population health, and direct management of services.[24] A more coherent public health policy can act in a more concerted manner, better utilizing all these capacities and governmental abilities. Indeed, events in recent years, including natural or human-created disasters, have presented a unique opportunity to strengthen the core capacity for delivery of the essential public health services and to strengthen public health. As McGinnis stated, "public policymakers need to begin thinking in terms of a health agenda rather than a health care agenda or—even more narrowly—a health care financing agenda."[25] Faced with evidence of emergency unpreparedness, the United States was spurred to better coordinate public health functions between agencies and departments, leading to a better overall health policy for the country.

The United States needs to develop a health agenda that reflects not just the impact of medical care on health, but more importantly, the impact of social and environmental factors on health. An examination of current health policy reveals that most debates center primarily on financing of health care rather than health outcomes or social determinants of health. The United States should expand this focus from just financing and issues of cost containment to make better use of "health impact assessments," a tool that can estimate the influence of social, economic, and healthcare policies on population health. Using this type of metric will give a more holistic view of how health policy influences population health than cost-centered analyses do, and can help demonstrate to the public the true value of public health interventions.

10. Form a National Center for Public Health Excellence That Coordinates National Efforts to Improve Public Health Performance

A National Center for Public Health Excellence could be formed to facilitate many of the research, evaluation, and service activities associated with promoting the public health systems research agenda. For example, the center could provide technical assistance to state- and community-based projects, including designing and collecting standard measures and providing training on models commonly used in community health development and evaluation projects. Examples of these theoretical models used in health services research include the Health Belief model; the Transtheoretical model (stages of change); the Planned Approach to Community Health (PATCH) model; the Predisposing, Reinforcing, and Enabling Constructs in Education/Environmental Diagnosis and Evaluation model, in conjunction with its implementation phase—Policy, Regulatory, and Organizational Constructs in Education and Environmental Development (PRECEDE-PROCEED); and the Multilevel Approach to Community Health (MATCH) model,[18] all of which offer important insights into the process of health services research and can be valuable for the people in charge of formulating and implementing public health research or intervention programs. The center could also help with the evaluation of projects implemented at the state or local level and help disseminate important findings.

Future Outlook

This chapter examines current knowledge regarding the relationships between public health, social determinants of health, and public policy; identifies the priority areas for further research and knowledge development; and recommends a course of action. The next step is for the public health practice and research community to deliberate and establish a consensus plan for improving public health through health systems research and program implementation and establish concrete priorities. With public health gaining attention and importance, there will be increased demand for research to guide the development of better public health services and spur the improvement of public health performance. The establishment of a shared understanding among all actors of the priority research areas and strategies for implementing evidence-based policy is paramount to advancing the field of public health research.

Discussion Questions

1. How do you distinguish public health systems research from other types of health research?
2. What are the current knowledge areas and gaps in research regarding public health and social determinants of health?
3. What are some research priorities in public health systems research?
4. What are the steps that need to be taken to enhance public health systems research?
5. What are the challenges in carrying out public health systems research?

References

1. Mays GP, Halverson PK, Scutchfield FD. Behind the curve? What we know and need to learn from public health systems research. *J Public Health Manag Pract*. 2003;9:179–82.
2. Institute of Medicine. *The Future of Public Health*. Washington, DC: National Academies Press; 1988.
3. Institute of Medicine. *The Future of the Public's Health in the 21st Century*. Washington, DC: National Academies Press; 2002.
4. Van Wave TW, Scutchfield FD, Honore PA. Recent advances in public health systems research in the United States. *Annual Rev Public Health*. 2010;31:283–95.
5. Harris JK, Beatty KE, Barbero C, et al. Methods in public health services and systems research: a systematic review. *Am J Prev Med*. 2012;42(5S1): S42–S57.
6. Scutchfield FD, Shapiro. RM. Public health services and systems research: entering adolescence? *Am J Prev Med*. 2011;41(1):98–9.
7. Mays GP, McHugh MC, Shim K, et al. Institutional and economic determinants of public health system performance. *Am J Public Health*. 2006;96:523–31.
8. Scutchfield FD, Marks JS, Perez DJ, et al. Public health services and systems research. *Am J Prev Med*. 2007;33:169–71.
9. Merrill J, Keeling JW, Wilson RV, et al. Growth of a scientific community of practice: public health services and systems research. *Am J Prev Med*. 2011;41(1):100–4.

10. AcademyHealth. AcademyHealth: What We Do. Available at: http://www.academyhealth.org/. Accessed March 13, 2013.

11. Robert Wood Johnson Foundation. *Health Services Research* (special issue). Available at: http://www.rwjf.org/content/rwjf/en/research-publications/find-rwjf-research/2009/10/foreword.html. Accessed March 13, 2013.

12. National Coordinating Center for PHSSR. Issue Brief: Setting the Agenda for Public Health Services and Systems Research. Available at: http://www.publichealthsystems.org/uploads/docs/PrePub_PHSSR Agenda_IssueBrief.pdf. Accessed March 13, 2013.

13. University of Kentucky Center for Public Health Systems and Services Research. Public Health Systems and Services Research Workforce Report: Recent and Future Trends in Public Health Workforce Research. Available at: http://www.nlm.nih.gov/nichsr/phssr/phssr_workforce.html. Accessed March 13, 2013.

14. Shi L, Stevens G. *Vulnerable Populations in the United States.* San Francisco: Jossey-Bass; 2005.

15. United Nations Development Program. Human Development Report 2010: The Advance of People. Available at: http://hdr.undp.org/en/reports/global/hdr2010/chapters/en/. Accessed March 13, 2013.

16. Robert Wood Johnson Foundation. Turning Point. Available at: http://www.turningpointprogram.org. Accessed March 13, 2013.

17. Labonte R. Health promotion: from concepts to strategies. *Healthcare Manag Forum.* 1988;1(3):24–30.

18. Brownson RC, Baker EA, Leet TL, et al., eds. Developing an action plan and implementing interventions. In: *Evidence-Based Public Health.* New York: Oxford University Press. 2003:169–93.

19. Goodwin N, Smith J, Davies A, et al. Integrated care for patients and populations: Improving outcomes by working together. The King's Fund and the Nuffield Trust. Available at: http://www.networks.nhs.uk/nhs-networks/common-assessment-framework-for-adults-learning/archived-material-from-caf-network-website-pre-april-2012/documents-from-discussion-forum/IntegratedCarePatients PopulationsPaper-KingsFundNuffieldTrust2011.pdf. Accessed March 13, 2013.

20. The Robert Wood Johnson Foundation. Transforming Health Systems: The Challenge. Available at: http://www.rockefellerfoundation.org/what-we-do/current-work/transforming-health-systems. Accessed March 13, 2013.

21. Health Services Research Information Central. Grants, Funding and Fellowships. Available at: http://www.nlm.nih.gov/hsrinfo/grantsites.html. Accessed March 13, 2013.

22. Organisation for Economic Co-operation and Development. OECD Fact Book 2011–2012. Available at: http://www.oecd-ilibrary.org/economics/oecd-factbook-2011-2012/infant-mortality_factbook-2011-105-en. Accessed March 13, 2013.

23. Milstein B, Homer J, & Hirsch G. Analyzing national health reform strategies with a dynamic simulation model. *Am Public Health.* 2010;100(5):811–9. doi: 10.2105/AJPH.2009.174490.

24. Lister SA. CRS Report for Congress—An Overview of the U.S. Public Health System in the Context of Emergency Preparedness. Available at: http://www.fas.org/sgp/crs/homesec/RL31719.pdf. Accessed March 13, 2013.

25. McGinnis JM. National priorities in disease prevention. *Issues Sci Technol.* 1989;5(2):46–52.

Social Marketing and Consumer-Based Approaches in Public Health

Moya Alfonso and Mary P. Martinasek

LEARNING OBJECTIVES

- To define two consumer-based approaches to creating social change
- To discuss the importance of "knowing the audience"
- To define and discuss social marketing's key concepts
- To discuss the importance of formative research in understanding the audience
- To differentiate between qualitative and quantitative research methods
- To define and discuss community-based prevention marketing
- To apply skills for communicating effectively with your target audience
- To discuss future directions of consumer-based approaches to social change and the importance of multilevel theories

Chapter Overview

Obesity is *the* modern-day epidemic, and, thus, the current number one public health priority. Obesity has reached alarming rates in recent years and has received national attention due to its adverse health outcomes. Persons classified as obese are more at risk for premature death and decreased quality of life.[1] More than one-third of adults and 17% of children and adolescents are considered obese.[2] Obesity can be defined as the accumulation of excess body fat to the extent that it adversely affects health.[1] Obesity is caused by lack of physical activity and unhealthy eating practices, the causes of which are multidetermined.[3] Childhood obesity is a delicate and urgent topic, and for the first time the United States is faced with a generation likely to live shorter lives than their parents.[4] Obesity during childhood is a major predictor of obesity during adulthood.[5] Individuals overweight as children are more susceptible to severe obesity as adults.[5] Children at or above a body mass index (BMI) in the 85th percentile are considered overweight, while children at or above the 95th percentile are considered obese.[5] Children classified as obese are more at risk for diabetes, hypertension, asthma, and low self-esteem.[6] Children who live in rural communities, live in poverty, or are African American show higher levels of obesity rates than any other subgroups.[6]

To bring about social changes that will result in improved health outcomes, including reductions in overweight/obesity among adults and youth, public health professionals must communicate effectively with their audience (i.e., consumers of public health information). Historically, public health as a field has struggled to communicate effectively to its audience. As scientific findings emerge, we bombard our audience with often conflicting information that leaves them unsure of what steps to take to change their behavior to meet healthy living guidelines. In addition, audiences may not be receptive to public health's message for many reasons, such as public health messages are often controversial,[7] lack of interest in health,[8] lack of match between the message and their cultural or worldview,[8] low literacy levels,[8] or a lack of trust and/or belief in scientific evidence.[8] The way public health professionals communicate with their audiences is often not audience centric or consumer based and can fail to provide simple explanations and interpretations that appeal to the audience, put the message into the context of prior information or recommendations, and limit the amount of information to avoid "overload."[8]

Consumer-based communication approaches are systematic processes that, when followed, have the power to engage the audience or consumer in creating social change, thereby increasing the odds of lasting change. The purpose of this chapter is to present two consumer-based planning models—social marketing and community-based prevention marketing (CBPM)—which are capable of bringing about social changes needed to address health outcomes, including obesity. The tools outlined in this chapter can aid public health professionals in communicating effectively with their audience, thereby avoiding confusion and creating lasting social and behavioral change. The foundation of consumer-based planning models is discussed first—knowing the audience. Then, overviews of social marketing and CBPM are provided with emphasis on key marketing concepts. Case studies specific to both approaches are provided. Specific principles on how to communicate effectively with consumers are detailed. Finally, the future outlook for consumer-based planning models is discussed.

The Importance of Knowing Your Audience

As discussed in the book *Social Marketing for the 21st Century*, the campaigns must be audience centered and must always begin with a thorough understanding of the target population that is to be influenced.[9]

An organization's consumer orientation manifests itself in how the organization approaches the exchange of benefits over costs and how it approaches the consumer. Andreasen discussed a number of characteristics that are typical of an organization-centered (rather than consumer-centered) mindset:[10]

- The organization's mission is seen as inherently good.
- Customers are seen as the problem (e.g., assuming they are not doing something they should be doing, rather than determining if in fact they are not doing something and, if so, how that could be fixed).
- Marketing is seen as communications (rather than a broader range of potential solutions).
- Marketing research has a limited role.
- Customers are treated as a mass.
- Competition is ignored.
- Staffers are drawn from those with product (the behavior itself) or communications skills.

In contrast, consumer-oriented organizations analyze the transaction from the consumer's point of view rather than the organization's. They define the "problem" in terms of what the priority population needs and wants, not what the organization would like to provide: "Their mission in life is to know who their customers are, what they want and need, and where and how to reach them."[11, p. 204] They do this by following a careful process of audience analysis, and then using this analysis to segment the audience along key dimensions, such as readiness or ability to change behavior. They then select audience segments and determine what is necessary to facilitate behavior change for each segment. In many instances, "fixing" a problem behavior involves much more than communicating with consumers about it. This may require changing any of the marketing variables—the product itself, the price, the experience of getting it, or communication concerning it.

Social Marketing

Social marketing is "the adaptation and adoption of commercial marketing activities, institutions, and processes as a means to induce behavioral change in a targeted audience on a temporary or permanent basis to achieve a social goal."[12, p. 151] The primary goal of social marketing is to bring about volitional behavior change. Successful uses of the social marketing technique include the U.S. Centers for Disease Control and Prevention's (CDC) VERB program, which garnered a 34% increase in weekly free-time physical activity sessions among 8.6 million children ages 9–10 years, and the Truth campaign, which contributed to reduced smoking among U.S. teenagers.[13,14] Since then, the social marketing framework has been employed in many behavior change campaigns throughout the world—for example, to redefine gender norms in Mexico, to prevent tuberculosis in Peru, to prevent obesity in Italy, to increase school meals in England, and to increase the use of mosquito nets in Nigeria.[15]

Social marketing has had a strong presence in health promotion and behavior change over the past several decades. Social marketing strategies have been successfully applied in areas such as public health, environmental protection, and health policy development. The broader use of marketing techniques in public health has helped to bring about policy development and/or change, strategy formulation by governments and the public sector, and increased support for public health as an institution. For example, the social marketing framework provided a strong foundation for many of the advocacy activities undertaken to support tobacco control and for efforts to preserve or increase public health funding.[16] Andreasen notes, "Structural and policy change at the broadest level will have to take place if long-term solutions are to be achieved."[9] More recently, there have been efforts to more fully integrate social marketing into public health institutions and use it as a way to approach social change. A prime example is the incorporation of social marketing into the *Healthy People 2020* goals.

Key Marketing Concepts

Social marketing can be distinguished from other approaches to influencing changes in individuals and in policies by its emphasis on the following concepts.

Exchange

Marketers believe that exchange is central to the actions people take: A person gives something in order to get something he or she values in return. Before entering into an exchange, a person weighs the benefits to be received against the costs (in money, time, or psyche). Only if the benefits are greater than the costs will the person make the exchange—hence the emphasis on creating, communicating, and delivering value as the essence of marketing in the standard definitions used in the marketing professions. It is important to understand that the only relevant costs and benefits are those that are important to the person contemplating the exchange. For individual health behaviors, these may or may not be health-related costs and benefits. Immediate tangible benefits usually are more compelling to people than longer term, intangible benefits. The field of behavioral economics is important to social marketers in how it has deposed the rational man model that typically underlies commercial marketing.[17]

Self-Interest

> In most situations, people act primarily out of self-interest; in commercial marketing, this self-interest clearly and consistently is acknowledged and pursued. . . . In public health and social issues, managers often ask members of the target market to behave in ways that appear to be opposite of that member's perception of self-interest and are often the opposite of the current manifestation of that self-interest as observed through the member's current behavior.[18, p. 26]

Self-interest can also play a role in education and policy, though in quite different ways. Educational efforts may include appeals to self-interest (e.g., "If you get 60 minutes of physical activity each day, you will have more energy"), whereas policy "offers a self-interested return by promising not to punish those who behave correctly."[18, p. 27] Understanding self-interest is critical to developing and delivering an exchange that target audience members will value.

The Four Ps: Product, Price, Place, and Promotion

> A successful marketing strategy includes the design of a marketing mix with the right combination of products, offered at the right price, in the right place, and then promoted in such a way that makes it easy and rewarding for the individual to change his or her behavior.[19]

Product, price, place, and promotion are the key combined elements that require an integrated understanding as they constitute the marketing mix—the center of social marketing. When combined, these elements provide guidance in planning and implementing a comprehensive social marketing behavioral change program.

The key principle *product* is often divided into three specific domains for an intervention: the *core product*, the *actual product*, and the *augmented product*. The core product refers to the benefits to the consumer of adopting the core product or behavior change and is discovered through formative research as not necessarily being a health benefit (e.g., peace of mind, bonding, increase in self-confidence). The actual product is the behavior that is being promoted (e.g., increased physical activity). The augmented product is the goods and services that enhance the adopted behavior. The augmented product is not necessary in every behavioral change campaign but may serve to facilitate ease of adoption for the consumer (e.g., toll-free hotline, pocket-sized monitoring kit). The product must provide a solution to consumer-identified problems and offer benefit the consumer values.[20]

Price refers to costs that are exchanged for the product benefits. Costs may be monetary; however, they can also constitute intangible costs (e.g., fear, time, perceived affordability). The determination of price as viewed by the consumer is uncovered in the formative research phase where key insights into the consumer are explored. Overcoming these discovered barriers is one of the key features aiding in adoption of the desired behavior.

Place can be viewed as either the physical location where behavior adoption would occur or the time of day when consumers would be most likely to perform the desired behavior. In addition, place can be viewed as the location where augmented products are distributed and where the individuals and organizations who can facilitate the behavior change process are located.

Understanding and utilizing the combination of the key principles is central to social marketing. **Exhibit 21.1** presents definitions for each variable and key questions that public health practitioners should answer as part of social marketing strategy and activities.

Two Other "P"s to Consider: Partners and Policy

Partners can be other organizations involved with a social change effort or serving as conduits to target audiences. Questions to ask about potential partners include the following:

- What other organizations are conducting activities addressing the social change?
- What organizations are credible to the target audience?
- What are the opportunities to work together with either type of organization?

Policy is important because policy changes often are necessary before behavior change can occur or they can support individual behavior change efforts. Two examples of the first situation

---

Exhibit 21.1   The Marketing Mix (as Applied in Social Change Settings)

Product

The behavior, good, service, or program exchanged for a price—ultimately, the behavior change sought

- What are the benefits of the behavior change to members of the target audience—what needs or wants do they have that the product (behavior change, program, or policy) can fulfill?
- What is the competition for the product?
- What legal, technological, and/or economic policy changes can facilitate individual behavior change?
- What accomplishments can reasonably be expected independent of policy changes?

Price

The cost to the target audience member, in money, time, effort, lifestyle, or psyche, of engaging in the behavior

- What will the behavior change cost each target audience?
- Do target audience members perceive the cost to be a fair exchange for the benefit they associate with the behavior change?
- How can costs be minimized?

Place

The channel(s) through which products are distributed—or situations in which behavior changes can be made

- What are target audience members' perceptions of place?
- What barriers (costs) does the place create, and how can they be overcome?

Promotion

Some combination of advertising, media relations, promotional events, personnel selling, and entertainment to communicate with target audience members about the product

- What is the current demand among target audience members for the behavior change?
- What messages can best influence demand?
- What promotional materials and activities are appropriate for the message?
- How can those materials and activities best be delivered to target audience members?

Source: Adapted from Siegel M, Lotenberg L. *Marketing Public Health: Strategies to Promote Social Change.* Sudbury MA: Jones and Bartlett Publishers; 2007:223.

---

are the child safety seat issue (discussed in more detail later) and exposure to secondhand smoke. Members of the public cannot reasonably avoid secondhand smoke in public places, such as restaurants, shopping malls, and airports, without policies that restrict smoking to confined areas. An example of a policy change that facilitates individual behavior changes is the U.S. Food and Drug Administration's (FDA's) rule mandating "Nutrition Facts" labels on most foods, which provide consumers with the information they need to select foods that are lower in fat or sugar. Restaurants that identify lower fat menu items provide a similar service.

Questions to ask about policy include the following:

- What policy changes are necessary for individuals to improve their health behaviors?
- What policy changes could support individuals in their efforts to improve their health behaviors?
- What policy changes can this organization bring about?

It is important to note that the type of intervention (education, policy change or, social marketing) is dependent on the priority populations' motivation, opportunity, and ability to act, which in turn determines how likely they are to be *prone, resistant*, or even *unable to change* their behavior.[9] When the consumer or priority population is prone to act then education may serve to be the most efficient and effective type of intervention. When the priority population is resistant or extremely reluctant to change their behavior even for societal good, then policy change should be explored as a more effective type of intervention. For those consumers who are unable to change their behavior due to lack of opportunity or lack of ability then social marketing may best facilitate behavior change. Andreasen notes, "these are the majority of the cases."[9, p. 86]

Social marketing, education, and policy change are not mutually exclusive and can be integrated to achieve successful behavioral change. However, the first step is to determine the specific characteristics of the priority population. Are they prone, resistant, or reluctant? Understanding the target audience of the social marketing campaign is key in determining the strategic approach that will best meet the consumer needs and reach those who are most likely to change their behavior. Tailoring the intervention to reach the goal of behavioral influence will achieve more progress than interventions that treat everyone as if they are the same.[9]

Behavior Change

> The bottom line of all marketing strategies and tactics is to influence behavior. Sometimes this necessitates changing ideas and thoughts first, but in the end, it is behavior change we are after. This is an absolutely crucial point. Some nonprofit marketers may think that they are in the "business" of changing ideas, but it can legitimately be asked why they should bother if such changes do not lead to action.[21, p. 110]

Depending on the situation in which a marketing approach is being applied, the behavior to be influenced may be colleagues' attendance at a meeting, at-risk individuals coming in for screening for sexually transmitted diseases, or policymakers' support of a new public health initiative. However, the end goal is always getting the audience to take an action, not merely increasing knowledge or changing attitudes. Marketers will increase knowledge to the extent that such activities are precursors to behavior change (e.g., parents are unlikely to get their children vaccinated unless they know they need to do so), but the focus is on identifying exactly what is necessary for the behavior change to take place.

Often a challenge is to select one specific behavior to change when a number of behaviors may lead to desired outcomes. Integral to this decision is selecting a behavior that is perceived as "doable" by target audience members. Sometimes this means focusing on one step toward the desired behavior. For example, in its early years the national 5 A Day campaign asked the target audience to add two servings of fruits and vegetables each day, even though the program goal was eating five servings each day. This decision was made because target audience members were already eating two to three servings a day, and adding an additional two was more reasonable to them.[22] Appropriate models and theories of behavior change can help practitioners make such decisions.

Competition

Competition can be defined as: "any environmental or perceptual force that impedes an organization's ability to achieve its goals."[23, p. 7] For a public health initiative, competition can be defined as anything that limits resources, diverts attention from the subject of the initiative, or calls for contrary behaviors. As noted by Kotler and Lee, there are three main sources of competition: existing behaviors, other behavior changes the audience would prefer, and organizations and individuals who project opposing messages to the behavior being promoted.[24, p. 164] Identifying competition allows planners to identify a niche in which to position a program or activity in regard to the competition. Sometimes, another organization—even a "friend"—may be promoting a product, service, or practice that is in conflict with the public health organization's goals. At other times, a commercial opponent may encourage the very behavior that public health practitioners are trying to stop, such as smoking or ownership of certain types of firearms. More often, commercial advertising, television programs, or magazines emphasize behaviors or choices that have negative health consequences if they are not moderated or balanced by other behaviors, such as having nonmonogamous sex without using condoms or eating only "junk" foods. Identifying and assessing the competition may be helpful in determining the segments to target and the product to promote.[20]

Selecting and Understanding Target Audiences

Marketers begin selecting target audiences by segmenting the population into groups and then studying each group to determine which one(s) would be the most appropriate target audience(s). The process begins with a heterogeneous population and ends with smaller homogenous segments that are most worth pursuing. The traditional, less effective approach consists of an undifferentiated audience that receives the same messages or recommendations and the same promotional strategies; whereas, in the social marketing model, everyone is considered different. Individuals have different experiences, personalities, and live in varied conditions. Because it would be impractical to design programs to meet every individual need, social marketers try to identify subgroups that share key characteristics and then select certain groups to approach and design a marketing mix to best meet their needs. This method produces better results as compared to the "one size fits all" approach of traditional models of behavior change. An example from the commercial marketing sector is Coca-Cola. The company knows that everyone differs in their tastes and needs; therefore, the company offers a variety of products to meet the needs of specific segments, such as those wanting to avoid calories versus those wanting the "real thing."

Given limited resources and the knowledge that people differ in behaviors, benefits, costs, barriers, and personal characteristics, social marketers must be strategic in selecting groups or segments to give the best return on investment. The most common methods of segmentation are based on current behavior, responsiveness, desired benefit, and personal characteristics.

One useful exercise is to compare "doers" (those who already engage in the behavior) with "nondoers" (those who do not) to see what other differences exist between the two groups.

Often, such an analysis provides insights into the determinants of each group's behavior. These determinants can then be addressed by the marketing initiative. For example, women who have mammograms every 5 years differ from those who have never received the exam. Therefore, motivating these two segments requires much different strategies based on formative research with each segment to understand their perceived and real barriers and benefits.[25] Another example of segmentation can be knowledge based: Perhaps the child safety seat initiative's program planners discovered that caregivers who install the safety seats properly know that they should not move more than 1 inch in any direction, and a large percentage of those who install them improperly do not have this knowledge.

Secondary sources may have the necessary variables for a behavioral segmentation; if not, a custom study needs to be conducted. Additional factors to consider when selecting target audience segments are shown in **Exhibit 21.2**.

It is important to consider the likelihood of progress toward the initiative's objectives when selecting audience segments. For example, the audience should be large enough that if a reasonable percentage of the members take action, noticeable progress will be made. Sometimes, practitioners want to choose the group that is most "in need" of a particular action (e.g., their current behavior is farthest from it). But this group may be least likely to respond; choosing a group closer to taking the action may require fewer resources, result in greater progress toward objectives, and positively influence the social norm regarding the behavior.

In the child safety seat example, if only occasional caregivers such as grandparents or babysitters who have a child safety seat in their vehicle infrequently were targeted, little progress would be made toward increasing the percentage of child safety seats that are properly installed. Yet this audience might seem to be a logical choice if they are least likely to be familiar with proper installation and therefore most "in need" of the knowledge. Careful selection of audience segments can be particularly critical when the audience is policymakers: Persuading those who are undecided, especially if many are, is likely to be far more productive than trying to reach those who are definitely opposed to a change.

Once target audience segments have been selected, they need to be profiled thoroughly to determine the best strategies to help or convince them to take action. In the child safety seat example, the planners took two courses of action: a policy change to improve the product (and therefore make the behavior easier), and education to give people the knowledge they need to

---

Exhibit 21.2   Factors Influencing the Selection of Target Audiences

- Audience size
- Extent to which the group needs or would benefit from the behavior change
- How well available resources can reach the group
- Extent to which the group is likely to respond to the program
- For secondary audiences, the extent to which they influence primary audiences

Source: Reprinted from Siegel M, Doner L. *Marketing Public Health: Strategies to Promote Social Change.* Gaithersburg, MD: Aspen Publishers; 1998:271.

engage in the behavior. Next, they needed to determine how to reach members of the target audience and persuade them to take the action of installing a safety seat correctly. To do this, they needed to understand the benefits and barriers the audience associates with the behavior, where and when to reach the audience, and the types of messages the audience would find compelling. Qualitative research is often used to help craft this understanding.

On the policy side, a consumer preference clinic (somewhat similar to a focus group) was conducted by U.S. and foreign vehicle manufacturers to assess consumer reactions to various technological changes that would enable child safety seats to attach to an anchorage designed specifically for them. All systems were strongly preferred over existing designs that used vehicle seat belts to attach the restraint to the vehicle. When making its final decision, the National Highway Traffic Safety Administration (NHTSA) considered the results of this research, the preferences of vehicle and safety seat manufacturers and other interested parties, cost implications of the various designs, and compatibility with the systems approved or likely to be approved in other countries.[26]

For example, when it became apparent that many child safety seats were improperly installed in the United States, the NHTSA and many local community and law enforcement agencies worked together to educate parents and caregivers about proper installation procedures and sponsored events where installation could be checked and corrected, if necessary.[26] A product usability study, however, revealed that many safety seats were installed incorrectly because of poor installation technology.[26] Therefore, NHTSA used its educational efforts as an interim approach while it used its policy-making ability to mandate a technological change: a standardized anchorage system in passenger vehicles and corresponding standardized attachments on child safety seats.[27]

Formative Research

"Formative research is foremost in understanding the wants, needs, and desires of the priority population. It provides more value for the effort than any other kind of research."[28, p. 63] Social marketers place great emphasis on formative research because it underpins how the problem is defined by the priority population and how strategies to address it are crafted (selection of audience segments, actions they should take, and the approaches that will be used to help them). If a strategy is wrong or incomplete, every tactic can be executed flawlessly, but program objectives are still unlikely to be accomplished. As a result, social marketers tend to allocate a large proportion of their research and evaluation dollars to studies that are conducted to understand the problem and the audience, and to develop and assess reactions to proposed strategies, including products, service-delivery approaches, messages, and materials.

Common Formative Research Methods

Social marketers tend to rely on a mixture of qualitative and quantitative research to better understand the target audience and for statistical segmentation. This mixture of qualitative and quantitative research is often referred to as mixed methods research and provides for a stronger study than either quantitative or qualitative research.[29] Mixed methods research can be sequential or concurrent. When qualitative data collection precedes quantitative data collection, this allows for improved survey development and a more robust interpretation of the factors that affect the consumer. When quantitative data collection precedes qualitative data collection, this allows for further explanation of the survey findings as well as clarification of unanticipated findings.[30]

Formative research is designed to make marketing decisions by gaining a better understanding of the consumers. Formative research can also be used to pretest concepts, product designs, or message designs with the target audience.[31] Strolla and colleagues used mixed methods research to develop tailored nutrition intervention materials to members of the target audience.[32] Common qualitative techniques, such as in-depth interviews, focus groups, and observations, typically support the planning and development stages; however, they can play important roles in process and outcome evaluation, and verification and interpretation of the quantitative research findings.[30] Qualitative research allows the identification of perceived benefits of and barriers to taking a particular action, as well as to create a vivid profile of the consumer. It is also a good forum for exploring target audience reactions to new or existing products and potential ways of framing messages. All of these methods provide valuable insight into understanding the consumer. For example, participant observation helps to understand the context of the situation and the behavioral patterns that exist. In-depth interviews allow the researcher to explore deeper into the feelings and attitudes of the consumer and aids in exploring complex subjects. Focus groups provide an opportunity to observe group interaction and help to generate ideas in an expedited fashion.

In contrast, quantitative techniques provide estimates or measures of how many members of a population have particular knowledge, engage in a particular behavior, or would be willing to take a specific action. They are particularly useful for obtaining baseline measures and segmenting and selecting audiences; they also can be used to test positioning and messages in some instances. Additionally, quantitative techniques help to identify determinants from a statistical standpoint and aid in evaluating impact of the behavior change campaign. Quantitative methods are most often some type of survey, although observational studies (e.g., observing people and counting how many engage in a particular behavior) or methods such as medical chart review can also fall in this category. Many types of surveys are available for development and their selection is based on accessibility to a priority population, resources such as time and personnel, the complexity of the questions, and the need for clarification or interviewer assistance. Examples of types of surveys include central intercept surveys, Internet surveys, mail surveys, door-to-door surveys, surveys administered through mobile technology such as smart phones, and telephone interviews.

Because of the cost and time involved in obtaining solid quantitative data, market researchers often look first to secondary data sources (information that has already been collected for some other purpose). Useful federal and/or state data sources can include the Behavioral Risk Factor Surveillance System (BRFSS), the Youth Risk Behavior Surveillance System (YRBSS), the National Health Interview Survey (NHIS), and the National Health and Nutrition Examination Surveys (NHANES). Useful commercial sources include the annual studies conducted by Mediamark Research & Intelligence (MRI) and Simmons Market Research Bureau. Some market research companies, such as Nielson SiteReports, provide geodemographic segmentation systems that allow neighborhoods to be categorized and mapped according to demographic and lifestyle characteristics. An example is provided in **Box 21.1**.

Box 21.1   Formative Research Case Study

Waterpipe tobacco smoking (hookah) has become a social staple among young adults throughout the United States. This form of communal smoking incorporates a long-stemmed pipe that houses a flavored tobacco and burning charcoal that bakes the tobacco. A dearth of research has been conducted on hookah smoking. As a part of the formative research process, researchers chose a sequential mixed methods approach (i.e., participant observation and intercept interviews, focus groups, online survey, and verification focus group). Participant observations took place in hookah bars/cafes surrounding a university—a location where it would be most likely to observe college students partaking in the behavior. The advantage of this technique is it allows the researcher to validate interview data and take notes during the observation.[26] Intercept interviews were conducted to explore normative and behavioral beliefs about hookah smoking. A total of 63 10–15 minute interviews were conducted with smokers and nonsmokers of hookah. The information gathered from the intercept interviews helped to inform the questions asked during the focus groups and to illuminate findings from the observations. Three focus groups were conducted with individuals who acknowledged smoking hookah. Focus groups stimulated a rich discussion of the factors that influence waterpipe smoking, clarified differences between students' perceptions of their behavior and practices observed in hookah bars, and provided wording for the online survey.[27,28] In the second phase of the research, an online survey was administered to a random sample of students. After the data were analyzed, a verification focus group was conducted with smokers and nonsmokers to clarify and verify the findings from the study. This mixed method approach to data collection proved valuable in exploring attitudes, beliefs, and behaviors of students who smoke hookah. Systematically triangulating qualitative and quantitative methods resulted in increased validity of study results.

When there is no previous research on the topic, social marketers may lean toward conducting only qualitative research. Qualitative research can be conducted when time and the budget are limited. This research will allow for future survey question development when time and budget allow.

Strategic Plan Development, Testing, Implementation, and Evaluation

As potential solutions (target audiences, the actions they should take, and the means of getting them to take these actions) are identified through formative research, a strategic plan can be assembled. Such a plan should be tailored to the situation but typically resembles the outline shown in **Figure 21.1**. If multiple approaches are being used (e.g., a policy change and individual behavior changes), then separate goals, objectives, target audiences, strategy, and components sections might be developed for each approach. The plan should be used to develop and assess tactics and implementation plans. Also, it (or the executive summary of it) can be shared with partners and other interested parties as a quick way of explaining what the organization is doing.

> In the final analysis, textbooks can offer little on implementation that will improve upon a good plan, an adequate budget, good organizational and policy support, good training and supervision of staff, and good monitoring in the process evaluation stage. . . . key to success in implementation beyond these six ingredients is experience, sensitivity to people's needs, flexibility in the face of changing circumstances, an eye fixed on long-term goals, and a sense of humor.[33, p. 205]

Executive summary

Background and mission

Challenges and opportunities

Goals

Objectives (measurable outcomes)

Target audiences

Core strategy

Components for implementing and monitoring strategy:

Product and/or service development

Managing perceived price

Improving access and channels of distribution (place)

Promotion (including communication strategy)

Partnerships

Evaluation

Figure 21.1   Outline of a Strategic Plan
Source: Adapted from Siegel M, Doner L. *Marketing Public Health: Strategies to Promote Social Change.* Gaithersburg, MD: Aspen Publishers; 1998:235.

Selecting Appropriate Tactics

Tactics are the short-term, detailed steps that are used to implement a strategy.[11] Changing a clinic's hours, holding a community event, or producing an ad are all tactics. Selecting tactics for a marketing effort involves considering the model of how change is expected to occur, the marketing strategy, available resources, and the initiative's timeline. Because different social change efforts employ a wide range of tactics, it is impossible to review all possible considerations here. However, the following list of questions can be used to help assess the appropriateness of each tactic:

- Is it on strategy? It may be a great idea, but if it doesn't fit with the strategy, save it for another program.
- To what degree does it complement and reinforce other tactics?
- Can it be created and implemented in a timeframe that works with the overall timeline and with other tactics that may need for it to be in place before they are put into place (e.g., training staff prior to implementing other program elements)?
- Will the tactic's contribution to achieving objectives be worth its cost?
- What will each promotional tactic contribute to reach and frequency? The goal should be to reach as many target audience members as possible as often as possible.
- Does it make sense for the organization to develop or sponsor this tactic, or would it be a better fit for one of the partner organizations?

With complex, multifaceted programs, it is important to have "reality check" meetings periodically to make sure that the various components will work together and reinforce each other conceptually, that nothing has drifted off strategy, that everything can be rolled out in a timeline that makes sense, and that each tactic will cost a reasonable amount relative to what it is expected to accomplish.

Pretesting

Before producing a new product, finalizing a new service, making changes in product or service delivery, or producing messages and materials, pretesting should be conducted with target audience members to ensure optimal results:

- *Products and services.* If a new product or service will be created, it is desirable to develop a prototype and conduct usability tests prior to production (or, for services, finalizing plans). Usability testing is also a good idea for websites. This process can reveal problems, some of which may need to be corrected through design changes; others can be addressed in accompanying instructions. It is wise to test accompanying instructions for any product or service (new or old) included in an initiative to ensure that directions for use are clear and understandable and that they address common questions and misperceptions.
- *Changes in product or service delivery.* When a new process for obtaining products or services has been designed or an old process has been streamlined, pretesting any forms and pilot testing the process itself can help to identify and resolve areas of confusion or bottlenecks prior to wider implementation.
- *Messages and materials.* Pretesting messages and materials (e.g., advertisements, message points, pamphlets, brochures, instructions, forms) will not ensure success, but it can identify potential misinterpretations and problems with executional details of materials (e.g., readability of typeface or type size, reactions to colors, music, voices, timing) and it can assess the extent to which materials are clear, true to the strategy, and understood by the intended audience. Details on designing, fielding, and analyzing pretests are available in other sources.[11,34]

Assessment

Evaluation is a critical aspect of marketing. However, marketers use evaluation to improve efforts, not just assess them. Beyond "How are we doing?", marketers expect evaluation data to help them answer, "How can we do better?"

Earlier in this chapter, formative research and evaluation were discussed, as was their importance in crafting successful intervention components. This section highlights two additional types of evaluation:

- Process evaluation "typically tracks and documents implementation by quantifying what has been done; when, where, and how it was done; and who was reached."[11, p. 449] This type of evaluation allows ongoing monitoring and refinement of implementation.
- Outcome evaluation (sometimes termed *impact* or *summative evaluation*) examines the degree to which an intervention achieved its objectives or had the effects it was planned to have.

Importance of Monitoring and Refinement

Marketers use process evaluation data to monitor and refine an intervention constantly once it is in place. Doing so allows tactics to be adjusted in response to changes in audience needs, competitive activities, or environmental factors, thereby maximizing progress toward objectives. Some form of process information should be available for each tactic included in a marketing effort. Ideally, these data will document what was done and also provide information on who was motivated enough to take action as a result. The best way to ensure that adequate monitoring information will be available is to build it into or set it up for each tactic from the beginning. Steckler and Linnan's *Process Evaluation for Public Health Interventions and Research* presents a range of process evaluations and is a useful source of ideas.[35]

Issues in Evaluating Outcomes

Evaluating the results of public health marketing efforts often is challenging for a number of the following reasons:

- Marketing efforts do not occur in isolation. Because other organizations and secular trends usually address the same social change, it is difficult, and often impossible, to attribute effects to a particular intervention.
- Standard evaluation techniques are not designed to assess interventions that are constantly being refined (e.g., tactics that are not working are altered or dropped, and new tactics may be introduced).
- Measuring statistically significant change may require unreasonable outcome expectations.

How, then, can you approach the need to evaluate and assess how well an intervention did or is doing? Consider the following questions when planning an intervention and its corresponding outcome evaluation.[11]

What Outcomes Are Reasonable to Expect?

The crucial word here is "reasonable." Often, public health marketing efforts are expected to attain unrealistically large effects. As Beresford and colleagues noted in discussing population-wide efforts to change eating habits:

> The public health model, or population strategy, consists of shifting the entire distribution of a risk factor, including the mean, down. The diminution in risk for a given individual is typically small and may not even be clinically important. Nevertheless, because the entire distribution is affected, the impact on morbidity and mortality can be substantial.[36, p. 615]

If large effects are expected, can the intervention be structured so that it is of sufficient intensity and duration to achieve this level of success? Sometimes expectations for large effects have been carried over from expectations for clinical studies. At other times, the power (or lack thereof) of the evaluation drives expectations. For population-wide efforts, measuring statistically significant change can be prohibitively expensive—affordable (smaller) sample sizes have larger margins of error, so larger effects are required before observed changes can be considered statistically significant.

Commercial marketers generally have far greater resources yet expect modest effects. As Fishbein remarked:

> Thus, while a condom manufacturer would be more than happy if an advertising campaign increased the company's share of the market by 3% or 4%, a public health intervention that increased condom use by the 3% or 4% probably would be considered a failure.[37, p. 1075]

One of the major factors influencing outcome expectations should be the type of intervention. Is it reasonable to expect slow, gradual changes or rapid, large changes? For most public health interventions, an expectation of slow, gradual changes is much more likely.[38] However, it is possible to see large, rapid changes in behaviors that are very easy to change and that result in sharply reduced risks of devastating events (e.g., preventing Reye's syndrome by using an aspirin substitute rather than aspirin, and reducing sudden infant death syndrome by putting babies to sleep on their backs rather than on their stomachs).[39]

What Type of Evaluation Design Is Most Appropriate for the Intervention Setting?

The gold standard is a randomized controlled trial. That is, target audience members are randomly assigned to treatment and control groups, outcome variables are measured to establish a baseline, the intervention is implemented (usually remaining constant through the implementation period), and outcome variables are measured again. In this way, any differences between the two groups can be attributed to the intervention. Quasi-experimental designs are similar, but assignment to each group is not random. Examples of quasi-experimental designs include community interventions where treatment and comparison communities are matched on key variables or populations within a community are divided into groups (this approach might be used with a school-based intervention).

For public health interventions, a frequent problem with any experimental or quasi-experimental approach is what has been termed "the fantasy of untreated control groups."[40, p. 76] With many public health initiatives employing communication, education, or marketing techniques, it is very unlikely that members of the control group are receiving no intervention. They may not be receiving a particular organization's intervention, but they are almost certainly receiving something. As Feinlieb observed:

> Science does not operate in a vacuum; the forces that operate to justify large, expensive community intervention studies also are operating among the general public to get them to accept the evidence and act on it even before the scientific establishment does.[41, p. 1697]

Alternatives to experimental and quasi-experimental designs are designs for full-coverage programs, or programs that are delivered to all members of a target population. Such designs include comparisons between cross-sectional studies (e.g., independent surveys taken at different points in time), panel studies or repeated measures designs (measuring outcomes multiple times among the same group of people), and time-series analyses (taking many measures of outcome variables prior to intervention, using those measures to project what would have happened without the intervention, and comparing the results to repeated measures taken after the intervention). See Hornik's *Public Health Communication: Evidence for Behavior Change* for examples.[42]

How Will Outcomes Be Measured?

Measures should be consistent with what an initiative attempted to accomplish. For example, if the child safety seat intervention was designed to get caregivers to attend a local event where the installation of the safety seat could be checked, the outcome measure should be what percentage of them did that, not what percentage of them have properly installed safety seats.

Measures also need to be sufficiently sensitive to capture progress toward outcomes. Commenting on a community intervention designed to increase safer sex that used as an outcome measure the proportion of young men who engaged in any act of unprotected anal sex, Fishbein wrote, "Was it fair to view a person who reduced unprotected sex acts from 100 to 0 as no more of a success than one who reduced such acts from 1 to none?"[37, p. 1076]

What Was Actually Implemented?

A surprising number of outcome evaluations conclude that an approach or program failed when in fact it was not adequately implemented or was not measured as implemented.[43] This disconnect between implementation and evaluation can occur when the evaluation and implementation teams are totally separate and do not communicate well, or when insufficient process evaluation data were collected, so it becomes impossible to determine the degree to which various tactics were implemented.

Community-Based Prevention Marketing

"CBPM is a program planning framework that blends social marketing techniques and community organization principles into a synergistic design to tailor, implement, evaluate, translate, and disseminate public health intervention among selected audience segments."[44, p. 333] CBPM is an amalgamation of the strengths of community organizing and social marketing. Community organization can be defined as the process through which community members receive help to take control over issues in their community.[45] Community organizing assumes that, with guidance, community groups can collectively identify problems, set goals, mobilize resources, develop strategies for meeting their goals, and implement and evaluate those strategies.[46] Social marketing, as defined earlier, is "the adaptation and adoption of commercial marketing activities, institutions, and processes as a means to induce behavioral change in a targeted audience on a temporary or permanent basis to achieve a social goal."[12, p. 151] In essence, the community organizing component of CBPM puts the power of commercial marketing strategies in the hands of the people, thereby increasing capacity to effect change in their community.

Once the community is organized and trained in the social marketing process, it must participate in the process of CBPM in order to be successful. CBPM requires high levels of participation, which can serve as a barrier to success.[47] Community members are expected to participate in each phase of the process from the development of a community profile to tracking and evaluation. In order to participate fully, community members must have the capacity (i.e., community infrastructure, skills, resources, power) to do so.[47,48] Another aspect related to capacity and participation is community readiness.[49] Communities have varying levels of readiness (e.g., awareness, leadership, resources) to address an issue. In some cases, where readiness is low, participation and capacity building may need to wait until the community is brought to a higher stage of readiness.[44,50]

CBPM has the potential to result in community empowerment and increased competence according to Bryant et al.[44] Perhaps the best example of this is the VERB Summer Scorecard (VSS) CBPM campaign developed in Lexington, Kentucky, by a community advisory board (CAB) with the assistance of Dr. Bryant.[44,51] As a result of being guided through the CBPM process when developing the VSS,[52] a now promising intervention is being disseminated nationally and the coalition has moved on to use CBPM to bring about additional community changes such as the elimination of soda machines from local schools.

CBPM Steps

There are nine steps in the CBMP planning process (see **Figure 21.2**), of which seven (i.e., Steps 2, 3, 5–9) stem from the traditional social marketing framework,[18] and two (i.e., Steps 1 and 4) stem from community organizing principles.[45,53]

The first step in the process, *Mobilize the Community*, involves creating the community-level structure to support the entire process. For example, in the Florida Prevention Research Center's (originators of the model) demonstration project, *Believe in All Your Possibilities* (i.e., an alcohol and tobacco prevention campaign), the community structure was formed from a prior community-based assessment.[54,55] A coalition had been formed and Step 2, *Develop Community Profile*, had already been carried out by the community.[54] This level of preparedness to take action represents a high level of community capacity and resulted in timely movement through the steps in the process.[55] The demonstration community, Sarasota, Florida, is known for having high levels of community capacity to create change. Other areas, such as rural areas with limited infrastructure, may need more assistance in organizing a community coalition. Either way, once the CAB is established, technical assistance is provided by those with expertise in CBPM, with the intent of transferring knowledge of the process to the coalition. The ultimate goal of the first step in CBPM is to put the power to bring about change in the hands of the community.[44,53,56,57]

Steps 2 and 3 in CBPM, as shown in Figure 21.2, are very typical in most social marketing frameworks. However, in CBPM the community is intimately involved with *developing the community profile*, because they know their community the best. As community insiders, they have knowledge of data sources and access to data that researchers may not have.[58] During this stage, community members work collaboratively to assemble what is known about the community specific to the issue under consideration (e.g., physical activity) and summarize what is known about potential target audiences.[44,58] Once existing data are summarized in the form of a community profile, the coalition, after reviewing the profile, *Selects Target Behaviors, Audiences, and Interventions* (see Figure 21.2). Researchers working with the coalition service as a process resource and ensure that coalition members make selections based on the data at hand.[44,58,59]

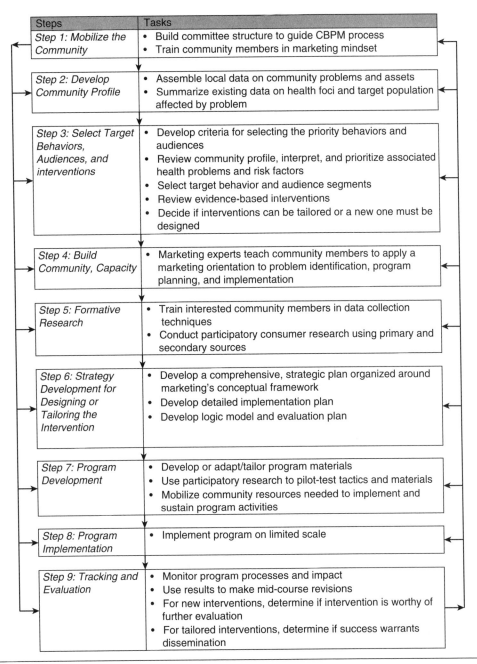

Steps	Tasks
Step 1: Mobilize the Community	• Build committee structure to guide CBPM process • Train community members in marketing mindset
Step 2: Develop Community Profile	• Assemble local data on community problems and assets • Summarize existing data on health foci and target population affected by problem
Step 3: Select Target Behaviors, Audiences, and interventions	• Develop criteria for selecting the priority behaviors and audiences • Review community profile, interpret, and prioritize associated health problems and risk factors • Select target behavior and audience segments • Review evidence-based interventions • Decide if interventions can be tailored or a new one must be designed
Step 4: Build Community, Capacity	• Marketing experts teach community members to apply a marketing orientation to problem identification, program planning, and implementation
Step 5: Formative Research	• Train interested community members in data collection techniques • Conduct participatory consumer research using primary and secondary sources
Step 6: Strategy Development for Designing or Tailoring the Intervention	• Develop a comprehensive, strategic plan organized around marketing's conceptual framework • Develop detailed implementation plan • Develop logic model and evaluation plan
Step 7: Program Development	• Develop or adapt/tailor program materials • Use participatory research to pilot-test tactics and materials • Mobilize community resources needed to implement and sustain program activities
Step 8: Program Implementation	• Implement program on limited scale
Step 9: Tracking and Evaluation	• Monitor program processes and impact • Use results to make mid-course revisions • For new interventions, determine if intervention is worthy of further evaluation • For tailored interventions, determine if success warrants dissemination

Figure 21.2   The Community-Based Prevention Marketing Process
Source: Reproduced from Bryant CA, McCormack Brown K, McDermott RJ, et al. Community-based prevention marketing: A new planning framework for designing and tailoring health promotion interventions. In: DiClemente RJ, Crosby RA, & Kegler MC. (eds.). *Emerging Theories in Health Promotion Practice and Research: Strategies for Improving Public Health.* 2nd ed. San Francisco: John Wiley & Sons, Inc.; 2009:331–356.

The next step, *Build Community Capacity*, stems from community organizing principles (see Figure 21.2). Communities must have the capacity required to effect change; thus, they must have community infrastructure and involvement, skills (e.g., ability to access resources), resources (e.g., funding, people power), and power (e.g., shared vision).[47,48] Some communities, such as Sarasota, Florida, have high levels of community capacity to effect change.[47] Others may need support to develop capacity in one or more of the components of community capacity (e.g., skills). Interestingly, *Build Community Capacity* is listed as the fourth step; however, in reality, capacity building occurs throughout every stage of the process. The role of the research partner is to recognize deficits in capacity and provide the training and resources needed to develop capacity in these areas. For example, during the formative research phase, CAB members most often need training in what options are available and how to select among them. The principles of community-based participatory research are helpful in this case.[45,53]

Step 5, *Formative Research*, is the next step in CBPM, but because it has been covered in depth in the social marketing section of this chapter, it will not be discussed in detail here. However, it is important to note what distinguishes formative research in the social marketing framework from how it is carried out in CBPM. In CBPM, researchers and community members collaboratively conduct formative research.[44] Ideally, community members are involved in each step of the research process from question formation to data reporting. At this stage, principles of community-based participatory research are followed, including:

- It is participatory.
- It is cooperative, engaging community members and researchers in a joint process in which both contribute equally.
- It is a co-learning process.
- It involves systems development and local community capacity building.
- It is an empowering process through which participants can increase control over their lives.
- It achieves a balance between research and action.[45, p. 9]

For example, in a study by Sharpe et al.,[60] community members recruited focus group participants, advised on the focus group process, and reviewed and interpreted focus group results. Involvement in the formative research process is vital, because it builds capacity for data-based decision making and buy-in throughout the rest of the process.[44,56,57]

The next step, *Strategy Development*, should flow naturally from formative research. Once the CAB has reviewed the formative research results, other key stakeholders in addition to the CAB are invited to a strategy session where key, data-based strategic decisions are made. This high level of participation in strategy selection increases buy-in and increases the odds that whatever is developed will be sustained over the longrun.[44,56] In fact, some communities take such ownership of the strategies developed during this session and resulting CBPM campaign that they may sustain the program for several years or more, as has happened with the *Believe in All Your Possibilities Campaign*, which has been institutionalized in Sarasota, Florida.

Once strategies are developed, CBPM concludes with Steps 7 through 9 (see Figure 21.2). Once strategies are selected and a marketing is plan developed, the CAB, with external support (e.g., media consultants), creates their CBPM campaign, pretests their messages and materials, and pilot tests the campaign. Capacity is again developed during this stage as the researcher trains the CAB in how to develop a campaign, pretest messages, and pilot test the campaign with a small sample for revision purposes.[44,56] Finally, once trained in evaluation, the CAB leads the development of a process and outcome evaluation plan. It is important that the CAB lead the design, because they know best which methods will work, who to gather information from, and when to gather it.[45,53] In some cases, CAB members or other community members with particular skills (e.g., Microsoft Excel data analysis) and interest may participate in data analysis and interpretation. At a minimum, CAB members should be informed of evaluation results in a timely manner and given opportunities to discuss results and provide feedback.[44,56] An example of the application of CBPM in a community setting is described in **Box 21.2**.

Box 21.2   Using CBPM to Culturally Tailor VERB™ Summer Scorecard in the Rural South

Georgia ranks second highest in the United States for childhood obesity. Rural areas possess unique challenges, as environmental factors such as county sprawl can be significant mediating factors of obesity. A recent review of the literature on the role of the built environment and obesity found substantial heterogeneity among results, suggesting the need for the development of new, multidisciplinary methods. The VERB Summer Scorecard (VSS) is an innovative community-based prevention marketing (CBPM) campaign designed to provide tweens with action outlets/opportunities and encourage them to try new types of physical activity. VSS has spread nationally and is promoted by the Centers for Disease Control and Prevention (CDC) as an intervention communities can adopt to increase physical activity and promote healthy outcomes among youth and ultimately prevent chronic disease. Core elements of the VSS include: 1) activities that are consistent with a tailored marketing plan (e.g., product strategy to give kids opportunities to have fun, spend time with friends, master new skills while being physically active); 2) targeting of "tweens"—kids between 8 and 13 years of age; 3) offering of a variety of action outlets or opportunities for tweens to be active that must comply with the marketing plan in order to allow them to try new things, be safe, and minimize competition and the chance for failure and embarrassment; 4) utilizing a method (e.g., paper or online card) to encourage tweens to monitor their physical activity during a designated period of time; and 5) planning and implementation by a community advisory board (CAB) that can facilitate offering of a variety of action outlets throughout the community.

Since fall 2010, Dr. Alfonso has developed a university–community partnership with key stakeholders (e.g., Boys and Girls Club, the health department, schools) with the intent of culturally tailoring VSS to work for rural, high-minority areas such as Bulloch County, GA. Conversations over the course of a year resulted in the joint application for foundation funds to support the use of CBPM to culturally tailor VSS to work for Bulloch County. Once funds were received, a CAB was organized to guide the process. The university in conjunction with CAB members conducted a community profile to inform the process. Formative research with African American parents, youth, and community leaders is being conducted to determine the aspects of VSS that would need to be modified to make it culturally appropriate for a rural, high-minority area (e.g., the provision of transportation to and from events). Once data are collaboratively analyzed and interpreted, CAB members and other key stakeholders will use the information to identify product, price, place, and promotion strategies that are tailored to the audience—rural, African American 8 to 13 year olds. Program development will occur with implementation slated for summer of 2012. The Reach Effectiveness Adoption Implementation Maintenance (RE-AIM, http://www.re-aim.org) evaluation framework will be used to evaluate campaign reach, effectiveness, adoption (by organizations in the community), implementation (i.e., implementation context and fidelity), and maintenance or the potential for sustainability. Once successfully culturally tailored for rural, African American communities, Dr. Alfonso and her colleagues will use social marketing strategies to disseminate the tailored program to rural communities throughout the state of Georgia.

The Principles of Effective Communication in Public Health

"Open and transparent communication is a crucial process in health promotion. Not so much because health promotion is about bringing useful health messages to the people, but more because social mobilization for health promotion needs effective communication strategies."[61] Effective communication is a staple in successful public health messages and campaigns. From the interpersonal level in conducting formative research with individuals regarding their personal health information to media advocacy to suggesting regulation changes, communication is vital to the profession. In order to reduce risk in disasters and disease outbreaks, the Centers for Disease Control and Prevention (CDC) developed an online resource for health communication and social marketing information.[62] Such resources aid the many public health professionals seeking to use communication to increase awareness in their target populations, help form beliefs or attitudes, stimulate interpersonal communications, generate self-seeking information, and, most importantly, change negative behaviors and promote healthy behaviors.

Communication among key stakeholders in health program planning begins at the outset with building a coalition and continues through final program evaluation. Not all health-promotion campaigns result in a program aimed at changing behavior. Through formative research it may be determined that educational messages are the first step in raising awareness. There are key strategies in disseminating information for a health-communication campaign: 1) Pick one straightforward vehicle to develop and maintain awareness; 2) pick one moderately complex vehicle to enhance motivation and change attitudes; 3) pick one substantial vehicle to carry major messages and testimonials; and 4) fit the message to the audience, objectives, and the situation.

However the messages are disseminated, there are several other "rules" in making for an effective communication campaign.

- Lesson 1: Keep it simple. Avoid jargon and confusing language when communicating to the target population. Pretest, pretest, pretest messages and gain insight into the effectiveness of the messages. In 2004, the Institute of Medicine (IOM) and the Agency for Healthcare Research and Quality (AHRQ)—two major players in U.S. health care—both issued health literacy reports, placing the importance of plain language for messaging at the forefront of the nation's health agenda.[63]
- Lesson 2: Be accurate and consistent. The CDC advocates for the STARCC principle in communication:
  - S = Simple
  - T = Timely
  - A = Accurate
  - R = Relevant
  - C = Credible
  - C = Consistent

- Lesson 3: No lecturing or blaming the victim. Acknowledge people's concerns and most importantly be respectful of their needs.
- Lesson 4: Give people something to do! Mobilizing the community and providing action items for them not only provides empowerment and a sense of control but also provides for skill pedagogy.

Future Outlook

Healthy People 2010 established health communication efforts as a critical piece of prevention efforts aimed at improving the people's health. Since then, funding and other efforts, including *Health People 2020*, have supported the development of a number of health communication campaigns and research into communication strategies that are effective in bringing about behavioral change.[64] So, what does the future hold for consumer-based approaches to social change? Given the evidence that behavior is in large part not individually determined, social marketing and CBPM approaches need to expand the focus to the societal level—not the individual level.[65] Spanning the level from individual to societal exemplifies the socioecological model, a key model utilized in public health efforts. Social marketing and CBPM have the capacity to make more pronounced changes. CBPM, in particular, has the capacity to increase social capital defined as the "norms, skills, or other individual characteristics and structures that facilitate groups of people working toward the collective or community good."[65, p. 597] Increasing social capital increases health in the community and makes programs more sustainable.[65] When communities are empowered and have the social capital they need to effect change, they can bring about changes that are far beyond the capabilities of teams of researchers divorced from the communities.

Related to the current obesity epidemic, our number one public health problem, Wymer[67] recommends changing the focus of social marketing from the individual to the policymaker and the corporation—two groups who have control over the food industry and, therefore, are large contributors to the obesity epidemic. Social marketing and CBPM offer tools to advocate for changes at the policy and organizational level that would have far greater impact on the obesity epidemic than programs geared toward individuals at risk.[44,66] By bringing about changes in the environment through using social marketing or CBPM to advocate for policy or system-level changes, individuals will demand communities that provide access to good nutrition and physical activity, rather than neighborhoods surrounded by fast-food restaurants and limited space and safety for physical activity.

To modify the focus of consumer-based approaches to societal change, public health students, health educators, program planners, and other public health stakeholders need to be trained in how to think of problems through the lens of social marketing or CBPM. For example, most of the public health theories are focused on individual behavior change (e.g., the Health Belief Model). Students should be taught more novel theories that capture the complex interaction between individual and environment that can be used in conjunction with consumer-based communication approaches. Then, once the thought process is changed, public health stakeholders need exposure to consumer-based approaches, such as social marketing and CBPM, that are capable of bringing about societal change. Along with exposure to consumer-based approaches to social change, public health stakeholders need examples of promising prevention campaigns, such as VSS—which focuses on modifying youth's environments to increase the number of physical activity outlets in the community so that it offers a better opportunity to increase physical activity and reduce obesity.[52]

Discussion Questions

1. How do consumer-based approaches to societal change differ from top-down planning approaches?
2. What are the strengths and limitations of consumer-based approaches to societal change?
3. If you were conducting formative research, would you prefer qualitative, quantitative, or mixed methods approaches? What are the advantages of each?
4. Which approach—social marketing or community-based prevention marketing—would be most relevant to your research? Why?
5. What are the best methods for measuring and evaluating societal change? What questions would you ask? Who would you ask? What methods would you use?

References

1. Georgia Department of Public Health. Obesity surveillance. 2012. Available at: http://health.state .ga.us/epi/cdiee/obesity.asp. Accessed March 20, 2013.
2. Centers for Disease Control and Prevention. U.S. obesity trends: national obesity trends. Available at: http://www.cdc.gov/obesity/data/trends.html. Accessed March 20, 2013.
3. Georgia Department of Human Resources, Division of Public Health. Overweight and Obesity in Georgia, 2005. (Publication Number: DPH05.023HW). Available at: http://health.state.ga.us/pdfs/ familyhealth/nutrition/Obesityrep.DPH05.023HW.pdf. Accessed January 19, 2012.
4. Olshansky SJ, Passaro DJ, Hershow RC, et al. A potential decline in life expectancy in the United States in the 21st century. *N Engl J Med*. 2005;352(11):1138–45.
5. Centers for Disease Control and Prevention. Basics about childhood obesity. Available at http://www .cdc.gov/obesity/childhood/basics.html. Accessed March 20, 2013.
6. Georgia Department of Community Health, Division of Public Health. 2010 Georgia data summary: obesity in children and youth. Available at: http://health.state.ga.us/pdfs/epi/cdiee/DPH.Epi.7-20-11 .pdf. Accessed March 20, 2013.
7. Schneider M. *Introduction to Public Health*. 3rd ed. Burlington, MA: Jones & Bartlett Learning; 2011.
8. Nelson DE. Understanding and reporting the science. In: Parvanta C, Nelson DE, Parvanta SA, et al., eds. *Essentials of Public Health Communication*. Burlington, MA: Jones & Bartlett Learning; 2011: 55–73.
9. Andreasen A. *Social Marketing in the 21st Century*. Thousand Oaks, CA: Sage Publications; 2006.
10. Andreasen A. *Marketing Social Change: Changing Behavior to Promote Health, Social Development, and the Environment*. San Francisco: Jossey-Bass; 1995.
11. Siegel M, Doner L. *Marketing Public Health: Strategies to Promote Social Change*. Gaithersburg, MD: Aspen Publishers; 1998.
12. Dann S. Redefining social marketing with contemporary commercial marketing definitions. *J Bus Res*. 2010;63:147–53.
13. Nickelson J, Alfonso M, McDermott R, et al. Characteristics of 'tween' participants and nonparticipants in the VERB summer scorecard physical activity promotion program. *Health Educ Res*. 2010;26(2):225–38.

14. Hicks JJ. The strategy behind Florida's 'truth' campaign. *Tobacco Control.* 2001;10:3–5.

15. Cheng H, Kotler P, Lee NR. *Social Marketing for Public Health: Global Trends and Success Stories.* Burlington, MA: Jones & Bartlett Learning; 2011.

16. Siegel M, Lotenberg LD. *Marketing Public Health: Strategies to Promote Social Change.* Sudbury, MA: Jones and Bartlett Publishers; 2007.

17. Zaltman G. *How Customers Think: Essential Insights into the Mind of the Market.* Boston: Harvard Business School Press; 2003.

18. Rothschild M. Carrots, sticks and promises: a conceptual framework for the management of public health and social issue behaviors. *J Marketing.* 1999;63:24–37.

19. Thackery R, Brown KR. Creating successful price and placement strategies for social marketing. *Health Promot Pract.* 2010;11:166–8.

20. Grier S, Bryant C. Social marketing in public health. *Annu Rev Public Health.* 2005;26:319–39.

21. Kotler P, Andreasen A. *Strategic Marketing for Non-profit Organization.* Upper Saddle River, NJ: Prentice-Hall; 1996.

22. National Cancer Institute. 5 A Day for Better Health Program Evaluation Report: Executive Summary. Available at: http://dccps.nci.nih.gov/5ad_exec.html. Accessed March 20, 2013.

23. Hastings G. Competition in social marketing. *Social Marketing Quarterly.* 2003;9(3):6–10.

24. Kotler P, Lee NR. *Social Marketing, Influencing Behaviors for Good.* 3rd ed. Thousand Oaks, CA: Sage Publications; 2008.

25. Forthofer MS, Bryant CA. Using audience-segmentation techniques to tailor health behavior change strategies. *Am J Health Behavior.* 2000;24(1):36–43.

26. National Highway Traffic Administration. *Patterns of Misuse of Child Safety Seats: Final Report* (DOT HS 808-440). Washington, DC: U.S. Department of Transportation; 1996.

27. Administration NHTS. Federal Motor Vehicle Safety Standards; Child Restraint systems; Child restrain anchorage systems. In: Administration NHTS, ed. Vol Fed. Reg. 10785:1999.

28. Balch GI, Sutton SM. Keep me posted: a plea for practical evaluation. In: Goldberg ME, Fishbein M, Middlestadt SE, eds. *Social Marketing: Theoretical and Practical Perspectives.* Mahwah, NJ: Lawrence Erlbaum Associates; 1997:61–74.

29. Creswell J. *Research Design: Qualitative, Quantitative, and Mixed Methods Approaches.* Thousand Oaks, CA: Sage Publications; 2009.

30. Denscombe M. *Ground Rules for Social Science: Guidelines for Good Practice.* 2nd ed. New York: McGraw-Hill; 2010.

31. National Cancer Institute. Step 2: Developing and Pretesting Concepts, Messages, and Materials. *Making Health Communication Programs Work.* Available at: http://www.cancer.gov/cancertopics/cancer library/pinkbook/page6. Accessed March 20, 2013.

32. Strolla LO, Gans KM, Risica PM. Using qualitative and quantitative formative research to develop tailored nutrition intervention materials for a diverse low-income audience. *Health Educ Res.* 2006;21(4):465–76.

33. Green LW, Kreuter MW. *Health Promotion Planning: An Educational and Environmental Approach.* 2nd ed. Mountain View, CA: Mayfield; 1991.

34. National Cancer Institute. *Making Health Communication Programs Work: A Planner's Guide.* Bethesda, MD: National Cancer Institute; 2002. NIH Pub. No. 02-5145.

35. Steckler A, Linnan L, eds. *Process Evaluation for Public Health Interventions and Research.* San Francisco: Jossey-Bass; 2002.

36. Beresford SA, Curry SJ, Kristal AR, et al. A dietary intervention in primary care practice: The Eating Patterns Study. *Am J Public Health.* 1997;87:610–6.

37. Fishbein M. Editorial: great expectations, or do we ask too much from community-level interventions? *Am J Public Health.* 1996;86:1075–6.

38. Kristal AR. Choosing appropriate dietary data collection methods to assess behavior changes. In: Doner L, ed. *Charting the Course for Evaluation: How Do We Measure the Success of Nutrition Education and Promotion in Food Assistance Programs? Summary of Proceedings.* Alexandria, VA: U.S. Department of Agriculture Food and Nutrition Service; 1997:39–41.

39. Hornik R. Public health education and communication as policy instruments for bringing about changes in behavior. In: Goldberg ME, Fishbein M, Middlestadt SE, eds. *Social Marketing: Theoretical and Practical Perspectives*. Mahwah, NJ: Lawrence Erlbaum Associates; 1997:45–58.

40. Durlak JA. *School-Based Prevention Programs for Children and Adolescents*. Thousand Oaks, CA: Sage Publications; 1995.

41. Feinlieb M. Editorial: new directions for community intervention studies. *Am J Public Health*. 1996;86:1696–8.

42. Hornik RC, ed. *Public Health Communication: Evidence for Behavior Change*. Mahwah, NJ: Lawrence Erlbaum; 2002.

43. Basch CE, Sliepcevich EM, Gold RS, et al. Avoiding type III errors in health education program evaluations: a case study. *Health Educ Q*. 1985;12:315–31.

44. Bryant CA, Brown K, McDermott RJ, et al. Community-based prevention marketing: a new planning framework for designing and tailoring health promotion interventions. In: DiClemente RJ, Crosby RA, Kegler MC, eds. *Emerging Theories in Health Promotion Practice and Research: Strategies for Improving Public Health*, 2nd ed. San Francisco: Jossey-Bass; 2009:331–356.

45. Minkler M, Wallerstein N., eds. *Community-Based Participatory Research for Health From Pocess to Outcomes*. 2nd ed. San Francisco: Jossey-Bass; 2008.

46. Bond L, Hauf A. Community-based collaboration: an overarching best practice in prevention. *Counsel Psychol*. 2007;35:567–75.

47. Alfonso, ML, Nickelson J, Hogeboom D, et al. Assessing local capacity for intervention. *Eval Program Plann*. 2008;31:145–59.

48. Chinman M, Hannah G, Wandersman A, et al. Developing a community science research agenda for building community capacity for effective preventive interventions. *Am J Community Psychol*. 2005;35(3/4):143–57.

49. Donnermeyer JF, Plested BA, Edwards RW, et al. Community readiness and prevention programs. *J Community Dev Soc*. 1997;28(1):65–83.

50. Kelly K, Edwards R, Comello MLG, et al. The Community Readiness Model: a complementary approach to social marketing. *Marketing Theory*. 2003;3(4):411–425.

51. Bretthauer-Mueller R, Berkowitz JM, et al. Catalyzing community action within a national campaign: VERB™ community and national partnerships. *Am J Prev Med*. 2008;34(6S):S210–21.

52. Alfonso ML, McDermott RJ, Thompson Z, et al. Kentucky's *VERB™ Summer Scorecard*: change in tweens' vigorous physical activity 2004-2007. *Prev Chronic Dis*. 2001;8(5):A104.

53. Israel BA, Eng E, Schulz AJ, et al., eds. *Methods in Community-Based Participatory Research for Health*. San Francisco: Jossey-Bass; 2005.

54. Alfonso ML, Lopez I, Bryant CA, et al. Planned Approach to Community Health (PATCH): a review and discussion of PATCH in Sarasota County, FL. *Florida J Public Health*. 2001;12(1&2):19–26.

55. Eaton DK, Forthofer MS, Zapata LB, et al. Factors related to alcohol use among 6th through 10th graders: the Sarasota County Demonstration Project. *J School Health*. 2004;74(3):95–104.

56. Bryant CA, Brown KR, McDermott RJ, et al. Community-based prevention marketing: organizing a community for health behavior intervention. *Health Promot Pract*. 2007;8:154–63.

57. Wallerstein N, Duran B. The theoretical, historical, and practice roots of CBPR. In Minkler M, Wallerstein N, eds. *Community-Based Participatory Research for Health From Pocess to Outcomes*. 2nd ed. San Francisco: Jossey-Bass; 2008: 25–46.

58. Eng E, Moore KS, Rhodes SD, et al. Insiders and outsiders assess who is "the community": participant observation, key informant interview, focus group interview, and community forum. In: Israel BA, Eng E, Schulz AJ, et al., eds. *Methods in Community-Based Participatory Research for Health*. San Francisco: Jossey-Bass; 2005:77–100.

59. Stoecker R. Are academics irrelevant? approaches and roles for scholars in CBPR. In: Minkler M, Wallerstein, N, eds. *Community-Based Participatory Research for Health From Pocess to Outcomes*. 2nd ed. San Francisco, CA; 2008:107–20.

60. Sharpe PA, Burroughs EL, Granner ML, et al. Impact of a community-based prevention marketing intervention to promote physical activity among middle-aged women. *Health Educ Behav*. 2010;37:403–23.

61. World Health Organization. Global health promotion scaling up for 2015—A brief review of major impacts and developments over the past 20 years and challenges for 2015. Paper presented at the Sixth Global Conference in Health Promotion, Thailand, 2005. Available at: http://www.who.int/health promotion/conferences/6gchp/hpr_conference_background.pdf. Accessed March 20, 2013.

62. Centers for Disease Control and Prevention. Gateway to health communication and social marketing. 2012; Available at: http://www.cdc.gov/healthcommunication/. Accessed March 20, 2013.

63. Stableford S, Mettger W. Plain language: a strategic response to the health literacy challenge. *J Public Health Policy*. 2007;28:71–93.

64. Bernhardt JM. Communication at the core of effective public health. *Am J Public Health*. 2004;94(12):2051–2.

65. Wallack L. The role of mass media in creating social capital: a new direction for public health. In: Hofrichter R, ed. *Health and Social Justice: Politics, Ideology, and Inequity in the distribution of disease. A Public Health Reader*. San Francisco: Jossey-Bass; 2003:594–625.

66. Wymer W. Rethinking the boundaries of social marketing: activism or advertising? *J Bus Res*. 2010;63:99–103.

Prevention, Health Education, and Health Promotion

Lawrence W. Green, Judith M. Ottoson, and Maria L. Roditis

LEARNING OBJECTIVES

- To understand the central importance of health education and promotion in public health
- To become familiar with processes and techniques used in health promotion
- To fully appreciate the core mission of public health as prevention
- To gain perspective on the role of the community in public health promotion
- To better understand the functions of each: education, promotion, and prevention
- To be able to look at these functions holistically

Chapter Overview

Public health organizations use health education strategies to facilitate voluntary adaptations of behavior that are conducive to health.[1] **Health education** seeks to influence a range of behavior including participation in health-promoting activities, appropriate use of health services, health supervision of children, and adherence to appropriate medical and nutritional regimens.[2] **Health promotion** encompasses a broader set of educational, policy, organizational, environmental (especially social environmental), and economic interventions to support behavior and conditions of living conducive to health.[3] Designing and managing successful health education and health promotion interventions require strong institutional capacities in applied behavioral science, community assessment, and program administration.[3,4]

The health of populations varies with the interaction of behavior, environment, human biology, social conditions, and community organization. Various scientific and professional subspecialties and academic disciplines have emerged to address these complex interactions. These subspecialties include environmental epidemiology, behavioral ecology, behavioral medicine, health psychology, social medicine, medical geography, and social epidemiology. Application of the scientific knowledge and technologies developed within these subspecialties falls largely to health workers in the community, especially through the vehicle of health promotion and the work of health education specialists.

Public health education employs a combination of methods designed to predispose, enable, and reinforce voluntary adaptations of behavior that are conducive to health. It too has subspecialties such as patient education, school health education, population education, environmental education, sex education, family planning education, nutrition education, dental health education, mental health education, and occupational health education.[1] The broader efforts of community or population health promotion may go beyond voluntary changes in behavior. These broader efforts may include regulatory and environmental control strategies designed to channel, restrain, or support health-related behavior or quality of life for the person, the community, or a population.[2,3] Nonetheless, health education strategies are a core element of most health promotion efforts that target communities and population groups. Without the health literacy and an informed electorate that health education helps create, many health laws would never be passed, would be rescinded, or would not be enforced.

This chapter examines the health education and health promotion strategies used by public health organizations to improve community health. The chapter focuses first on the design and management of health education approaches directed at voluntary changes in behavior. It then examines linkages between health education strategies and the larger field of health promotion, with attention given to policy, regulatory, organizational, and environmental factors that enable health education strategies to achieve health promotion goals.

Public Health Education

Public, community, or population health education interventions are designed to inform, elicit, facilitate, and maintain positive health practices in large numbers of people. The practices in question may be those of individuals whose health is at risk, or those whose behavior influences the health risks faced by other individuals and populations, such as through exposures to environmental threats. "Inform, elicit, facilitate, and maintain" refer to the processes of change supported by increasing the understanding, predisposition, skills, and support that motivate individuals to undertake and sustain voluntary actions conducive to their health. These actions reflect the efforts of health education to affect three broad categories of factors that 1) predispose, 2) enable, or 3) reinforce behavior that is related to health.[3]

Whether in populations or with individuals, health education addresses current behavior such as the participation in health-promoting activities, appropriate use of health services, health supervision of children, and adherence to appropriate medical and nutritional regimens. Health education also addresses issues in child and youth development that create the cognitive and behavioral foundation for future health. Within their families and with peers at school, children form predispositions—knowledge, attitudes, and values—that can prevent or promote many of the health problems associated with later adult life. Good planning in health education ensures that programs combine these channels of influence appropriately to support voluntary patterns of health-related behavior.

Focus on Health Behavior

Human behavior relates to health in direct and indirect ways, as shown in **Figure 22.1**. The direct effect of behavior (personal and social) on health (arrow A) occurs when behavior exposes an individual, group, or population to more or less risk of injury, disease, or death. Sometimes, the exposure is subtle, as with small but repeated doses of a substance that may become addictive or cumulative in their effect. Drugs and fatty food are examples of this type of exposure. At other times, behavior may pose an immediate and excessive risk, such as eating a poisonous substance or infected food. Acute risks to health in food production, distribution, and consumption have been minimized by the environmental and regulatory controls that are administered by public health agencies.

Behavior influences health indirectly through health services (arrow B). This can happen in at least three ways. Individuals, groups, or organizations can do the following:

- Influence the distribution and delivery of services through action in the legislative and health planning process
- Use (or not use) available services in a timely and appropriate way
- Follow (or fail to follow) the medical or preventive regimens prescribed by their health service providers

Behavior also influences health indirectly through the environment (arrow C) to the degree that people will plan individual or community actions to bring about changes in the environment. Examples of behavioral influences on health through environment include the following:

- Participating in efforts to control toxic waste disposal
- Organizing a lead paint removal program in the neighborhood
- Voting on referenda or for elected officials in support of community water fluoridation
- Advocating drunk driving laws or other automobile safety provisions
- Writing letters to the editor of a local paper concerning food and drug labeling
- Signing a petition on air or water pollution controls
- Boycotting stores that sell cigarettes to minors

A. Behavior → Health
B. Behavior → Health Services → Health
C. Behavior → Environment → Health
D. Behavior → Health Services and Environment → Health

Figure 22.1   Linkages Between Behavior, Environment, Services, and Health
Source: Courtesy of Lawrence Green as adapted by James A. Johnson

Voluntary Behavior

Beneficial voluntary health behavior in children and adults can result from health education if it provides for a combination of planned, consistent, integrated learning opportunities and reinforcement. To achieve these ends, community or population health education systematically applies theories and methods from the social and behavioral sciences, epidemiology, ecology, administrative science, and communications. These approaches are informed by scientific evaluations of health education programs in schools, at work sites, in medical settings, and through community organization and the mass media. Further, indirect evidence is borrowed from experiences outside of the fields of health and education. Community development, agricultural extension, social work, marketing, and other enterprises in human services and behavior change all contribute to the understanding of planned change at the community level and in various populations.

Planned learning experiences that can influence voluntary changes in behavior, as distinct from incidental learning experiences, link the educational approach to community and population health. Health education is also distinguished from other change strategies that may be excessively manipulative or coercive. Behavioral changes resulting from education are by definition voluntary and freely adopted by people, with their knowledge of alternatives and probable consequences. Some behavioral change strategies may have unethical components. Behavior modification techniques, for example, qualify as health education only when people freely request them to achieve a specific behavioral result that they desire, such as controlling eating or smoking habits. Principles of planning for community health education call for the participation of consumers, patients, or citizens in the planning process, especially in diverse, multicultural communities.[5,6]

Mass media qualify as educational channels for community or population health up to the point that commercial or political interests control the messages strictly for profit or propaganda. The regulation of advertisers and the media may be necessary as a more coercive, economic, or legalistic strategy to protect consumers from, for example, deceptive advertising claims concerning the health value of food products. Such was the case when communities took action to restrict the advertising of certain foods and toys on Saturday morning television programs directed at young children. Several countries restrict the advertising of tobacco and alcohol in the mass media. Third world nations took action to restrict the marketing of powdered milk formula for bottle-feeding of babies because it was leading the public to use unsanitary water and bottles in place of breastfeeding, and to neglect the opportunity and need for exclusive breastfeeding.

Limits of Health Education

Some people may not have the resources or support necessary to make independent decisions and to take voluntary actions when some of the determinants of health are factors beyond their control. Not being born in a democratic country to loving parents with access to resources, for example, might set limits on their ability and will to act independently to control the determinants of their health. These limits must be recognized by public health organizations in designing and managing health education programs.

Social epidemiology identifies many barriers individuals face that affect their ability to make healthful choices at the individual level. For example, black males have higher rates of hypertension than found in the U.S. general population. While diet and exercise regimens may be useful, larger socioecological factors may be at play, such as socially inflicted trauma that may chronically trigger the stress response and thus promote hypertension, or inadequate health care.[1-3] Such considerations set limits on how much health education alone can achieve health objectives without placing undue responsibility for change on people who are relatively powerless to make such change. This excessive reliance on health education without changing social and environmental conditions has been referred to as "victim blaming." Combining health education with policy and regulatory actions that empower the relatively powerless and restrain the more powerful who might exploit them overcomes this risk of victim blaming.

Health education remains necessary even when the changes in health risks require regulatory or environmental controls on behavior. For example, health education in a democratic society must precede such controls as banning texting while driving or enforcement of wearing seatbelts to gain the public's understanding and support required to pass legislation. It also helps to gain the public's cooperation in abiding by the new regulations. Community health promotion, then, is the combination of health education with related organizational, environmental, and economic supports to foster behavior that is conducive to health.

Linking Health Education and Health Promotion

Population health and community health promotion require an understanding of health behavior that goes beyond the specific actions of individuals and includes more than educational interventions alone to change behavior. Lifestyle, a broader concept than behavior, describes value-laden, socially conditioned behavioral patterns. The lifestyle concept has a rich history of study in anthropology and sociology. Only in recent decades has it taken on special significance in epidemiology, population health, and community health promotion. It is a concept that public health administrators need to understand in managing the broad-ranging, complex, value-laden, and often politically charged interventions of health promotion. This section examines how health education strategies fit within the larger set of health promotion approaches that may be used by public health organizations to improve community health.

Lifestyle

The midcentury shift from acute infectious diseases to chronic, degenerative diseases as the leading causes of death in Western societies brought a new perspective to epidemiology. No longer could isolation and suppression of a single germ or agent control the predominant diseases. Now, the causes of most chronic diseases tend to be multiple and elusive. These causes defy simple environmental control measures because they involve people's pleasures and rewards, their social relationships and physical needs, and, for some, their habits and addictions.[2] They involve *lifestyle*, which encompasses discrete individual behaviors within the web of social relationships and culture in which they are conditioned over a lifetime and entwined. They require public health education within a broader strategy of health promotion.

Planning for Public Health Education and Health Promotion Programs

Public health administrators and practitioners require a comprehensive planning process to achieve sound health education and health promotion programming and effectiveness.[3] An understanding of the stages and components of health education planning is therefore requisite for public health administrators.

The published applications of the PRECEDE model include, for example, identifying factors that promote positive mental health behaviors among adults in Hong Kong;[7] developing an oral healthcare program for frail elders in Canada;[8] developing an intuitive eating (nondieting) program for weight management;[9] assessing factors that influence mammography use among community health workers;[10] nutrition and physical activity programs for seniors,[11] and for fourth graders;[12] the launch of a health-promoting hospital in rural South Africa;[13] improving hand hygiene compliance among hospital healthcare personnel;[14] deploying community health workers, counseling, and a self-care approach to reduce diabetes-related complication in urban African Americans;[15] assessing determinants of tobacco use among Cambodian Americans;[16] parent education for self-management of asthma;[17] increasing the use of booster seats for children 4–8 years of age;[18] predicting injury due to fatal motor crashes;[19] a screening program for scoliosis;[20] a community campaign on youth mental health in Australia;[21] the creation of a theory-guided model for HIV prevention outreach;[22] and developing a tobacco cessation program for U.S. veterans.[23]

Phases of Planning for Public Health Education and Health Promotion

An educational plan for community health or population health ideally begins with analyses of social issues or quality-of-life concerns (phase 1) and the determinants of these through phase 3 (**Figure 22.2**). These three phases "precede" the selection, development, and implementation of interventions for a program, whereupon the process "proceeds" through evaluation. It involves matching behavioral priorities with adequate methods. Here, the use of a combination of evidence, theory, and experience will be necessary, because the evidence is never complete in its applicability to every community or its generalizability to every population.[24,25]

Phase 1: Social Assessment. The ideal starting point in planning is an assessment or "social diagnosis" of the social concerns and assets of the community or population. Starting with social or quality-of-life issues rather than with epidemiologic or health problems ensures that the health planners appreciate the broader context of issues that are paramount in the community.[26] This step requires an understanding of the subjective concerns and values of the community, as well as objective data on social indicators such as unemployment, housing problems, teenage pregnancy, violence, and poverty.[27] Consideration of varying community perceptions should take place early in program development. Health programs are not likely to be successful without community support and participation in the planning process.[28,29]

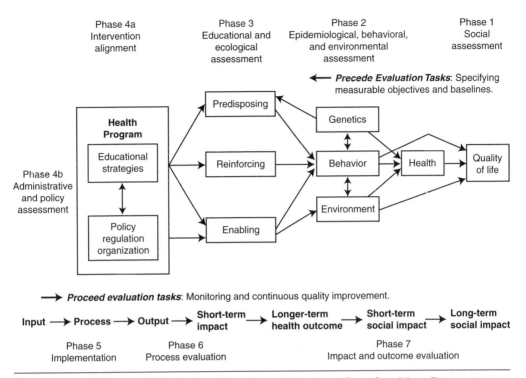

Figure 22.2 Evaluation Tasks Begin at Phase 1, and Continue Through as Many Diagnostic, Implementation, and Follow-up Evaluation Phases as Required

Phase 2: Epidemiological, Behavioral, and Environmental Assessment. The social concern or quality-of-life issues in the community or population can be analyzed for priority health problems embedded within them. Once the priority health problem is analyzed, addressing and solving that problem becomes the overall program goal, along with specific, quantified program objectives for a community's health risk factors and environmental risk conditions.[30] The agency sponsoring the program should use the most recent available demographic, vital, and sociocultural statistics to define the characteristics of the subpopulations experiencing the health problem. Planners can review the problem from the perspective of related agencies, a review of previously published reports, and the U.S. Department of Health and Human Services objectives for the nation.[30] They can gain perspective on the experience of the community with the health problem by reviewing similar data from other cities, states, or regions.

Citizens or lay participants in the planning process at this stage can help identify population subgroups within the community, such as adolescent mothers and preschool youth, who may have special problems and needs.[31] Information on these subpopulations can include geographic distribution; occupational, economic, and educational status; age and sex composition; ethnicity; health indicators, including age-specific morbidity; and service-utilization patterns.

Once the health problem has been defined and the program goal and high-risk subpopulations have been identified, a second part of the epidemiological assessment is the determination of behavioral problems or barriers to the community solution of the problem (Figure 22.2, phase 2). The following guidelines should be considered when performing the behavioral assessment:

- Specify the behaviors that are presumably contributing to the health problem as concretely as possible. Make an inventory of as many possible behavioral determinants as one can imagine.
- Identify the nonbehavioral factors (environmental, biologic, and technological factors) contributing to the problem as determinants for which strategies other than health education must be developed.
- Review research evidence on how the behaviors identified as possible causes are amenable to change through educational or environmental interventions and that such change will improve the health problem in question.
- For each health problem, identify one or more of the relevant dimensions of health behavior. For example, in prenatal care, one behavioral dimension is the timing or promptness of the care, which should begin with the first trimester of pregnancy.

The same questions can apply to the identified environmental factors influencing the health problem. An assessment should lead to the selection of specific behaviors and environmental determinants that will be the target of the educational and policy or organizational interventions. Rarely, if ever, does an agency have the resources necessary to influence all the behaviors and environmental factors contributing to a health problem. Therefore, an initial selection of some of the behaviors and environmental determinants should be made. The selection is often influenced by policies governing required services of the agency. Priorities might also consider legal and economic factors affecting the desired behaviors, agency resources and expertise available, political viability of the educational interventions, the possibility of continued funding, and the probability of quick program success. The reasons for selecting specific behaviors as the priority foci of the educational interventions should be justified.

The two most important objective criteria for the selection of priority behavioral and environmental targets for health education are: 1) evidence that the behavioral or environmental change will make a difference in the reduction of the health problem, and 2) evidence that the behavior or environmental factor is amenable to change.

Phase 3: Educational and Ecological Assessment.   Once the behaviors have been selected, they can be subjected to further analysis for assessment of their causes (Figure 22.2, phase 3). The following sets of factors should be considered as possible causes of each behavior:

- Predisposing factors—Knowledge or awareness, attitudes, beliefs, and values that motivate people to take appropriate health actions
- Enabling factors—Skills and the accessibility of resources that make it possible for a motivated person to take action
- Reinforcing factors—Support from providers of services, families, and community groups who reinforce the health behavior of an individual who is motivated and able to adopt the behavior but who will discontinue the behavior if it is not rewarded

Planners should consult representatives of the various segments within the agency and community who are potentially affected by the program. Failure to assess some of these factors and to develop a community health education program addressed to all three sets of these factors would seriously limit the impact of the program. Selecting the health education methods for a community health program follows almost automatically from a thorough identification and ranking of predisposing, enabling, and reinforcing factors influencing the health behaviors. Detailed procedures for assessing these from a combination of research evidence and theory are offered by the method of "intervention mapping."[4]

Phase 4: Intervention Alignment (4a) and Administrative and Policy Assessment (4b). The final phase of the process includes the alignment of interventions with the predisposing, enabling, and reinforcing factors, and an assessment of available resources to support the selected methods. The process of selecting or developing interventions to align or match with predisposing, enabling, and reinforcing factors calls first on evidence-based practices identified in systematic reviews of previous studies.[24,32] But there will never be sufficient evidence to cover all of the combinations of population characteristics, settings, and needs,[25,33] so theory must come into play as a second source for selecting and mapping interventions onto predisposing, enabling, and reinforcing factors.[4,26,34] Gaps will still remain in how well interventions match with the needs identified, so a third source of intervention candidates comes into play with the time-honored method of pooling ideas from other practitioners and health administrators who have planned similar programs for similar populations.[27,35] Woven through all of these considerations is a participatory patching process of filling gaps in the matching and mapping of interventions onto local population characteristics and circumstances with the advice and guidance of local residents and practitioners who have firsthand, indigenous experience in the locality.[28,36]

Resources required to deploy the chosen combination of interventions that will make up the program can be identified and obtained from organizations and agencies at national, state or provincial, and local levels, or developed locally for the specific program. Some examples of extant resources include citizens' groups, industry, labor organizations, religious groups, colleges, advertising agencies, drama groups, pharmacies, local facilities (e.g., libraries, health centers, hospitals, training centers, town halls, gathering places), personnel (e.g., volunteers, agency staff, social workers), communications resources (e.g., numbers of telephones and use of radios, billboards, local television and radio stations, newspapers, newsletters, organization bulletins, Internet/websites and social networking applications such as Facebook and Twitter), and funding sources available for the educational program through the health service agency itself and related organizations. This identification and assessment of available resources should lead to the further refinement of objectives, strategies, and methods. Advocacy for the reallocation of resources or the changes in policy required to support the program may be necessary at this phase of the planning process.[37]

The coordination and budgeting of resources into a timetable that corresponds to the community health program is the next step in the administrative assessment. Both require constructive participation by staff, other organizations, and area residents. By including other organizations and community members in the planning, one obtains their personal commitment to realizing program success, which can help eliminate duplication of services. Most importantly, their participation enables program planners to incorporate the interests, perspectives, and values of various stakeholders into the educational activities of the program. The principle of participation usually applies to representatives of related agencies, institutions, and organizations in the community; to the agency staff who will implement the program activities; and to community residents who live with the problem.

It should be noted that the assessment process used as part of health education planning is analogous to assessment processes that public health organizations may undertake for broader program purposes. Indeed, public health organizations increasingly undertake health education assessment efforts as part of larger public health assessment processes, and the public health program planning process has incorporated many of the behavioral and ecological concepts of health education and health promotion planning, just as health education planning has incorporated the concepts of social, epidemiological, and administrative diagnosis.[3,38]

Components of Public Health Education and Health Promotion

Cross-cutting concerns are an issue in all phases of planning, including the identification of the population in need, writing of clear objectives, and the use of methods and theories. These issues weave through the assessment phases discussed earlier and continue through organizational implementation and program evaluation in an iterative way, requiring the planner and practitioner to back up and fill out earlier steps with their new knowledge and understanding as their experience with the community or population grows. This process makes planning a technical and a socially negotiated process.

Priority Populations in Need. An early program planning task is the identification of the populations who are at risk, or those who are most affected by the health problem. These populations are the object and the intended beneficiaries of most of the educational and environmental interventions, and thus constitute the primary groups that planners should consult. It is the understanding and perspective of this group that focuses the social assessment and is deepened in subsequent rounds of epidemiologic, behavioral, educational-ecological, and administrative assessments. An iterative and deep understanding of the target population sidelines an ineffective "one size fits all" approach to packaged educational interventions.

The primary target population should receive direct communication designed to influence members' predisposition to accept the recommended health practices (the arrow from "Health Program" to "Predisposing" factors in Figure 22.2). Planners need to describe the primary target population by their geographic, occupational, economic, educational, age, sex, and ethnic distributions. Planners should consult or collaborate with representative persons from the described population and cooperating agencies in the assessment of needs and the further development of the educational plans. The characteristics of the target population that provide the basic analysis for the specification of community health programs are also the basis for the development of educational interventions.

Education must also be directed toward populations who are not affected by the health problem, but who are in a direct position to influence those who are. These "gatekeepers," role models, and social reinforcers—such as parents, spouses, teachers, peers, employers, and opinion leaders—are often an intermediate or additional target population for indirect communication to support their reinforcing role (see the arrow from "Health Program" to "Reinforcing" factors in Figure 22.2). To develop the enabling factors (see the arrow from "Health Program" to "Enabling" factor in Figure 22.2), planners can direct educational interventions toward these intermediate target groups. For example, one intermediate target group for community organization efforts would be directors of other agencies who control resources that would enable or facilitate the health behavior. Another intermediate target group might be employers, friends, or family members who would receive training, consultation, or supervision in reinforcing the recommended health behavior.

Objectives as Planning Tools.   At each of the assessment phases previously discussed, clear statements of objectives serve as a guiding tool not only for the planning, but also for the eventual evaluation of public health education programs. To illustrate the writing of objectives, we provide examples here of behavioral objectives (Figure 22.2, phase 2, Behavior).

The objectives for behavior change derive from the findings of the behavioral assessment. The proper statement of the objectives should lend purpose to the program plan and direction to its implementation.

Because education appears to be more abstract and difficult to define or measure than some of the other activities of community health programs, time spent on the formulation of objectives in educational planning is especially important. Objectives should be expressed as intended outcomes. They may apply to providers, to the organization or system, and to the consumers. Each objective should answer the following question: *Who* is expected to achieve or become *how much* of *what* by *when* and *where*?

The desired behaviors (what) should describe what the participants would do or not do as a result of the program that they could not or did not do (to the same extent) before the program. The conditions of the action should be stated in the following way:

- Who—Some logical or evidence-supported portion (percentage) of the target group who is expected to change
- How much or to what extent—An amount of behavioral change that will depend on available resources
- What—The action, change in behavior, or health practice to be obtained
- When, or how soon, or within what time period—Determined by the urgency of the health problem in the population and by the rate of change that can be expected from the amount and type of effort that is devoted to the program
- Where—Geographic, political, or institutional boundaries derived in part from the original description of the health problem

In most community health or population-based programs, "how much" refers to the number of people or percentage of the population expected to change their behavior as a result of the program. The numerator is the number expected to change and the denominator the number in need of change. For individuals, "how much" would refer to the level of accomplishment (e.g., number of monthly prenatal visits). Planners should word their objectives in such a way as to imply their assessment criteria. They should state the objectives in concrete terms with at least an implied, if not stated, scale of measurement that can be used to evaluate progress and achievement of the objective.

The test of good objectives is their ability to communicate realistic, expected results. Lucidity and precision in their formulation should accomplish several things. First, these objectives should provide limits to expenditure of time and effort on specific educational interventions. Second, they should identify criteria for measurement of program achievement. Third, they should lead to task analyses for selection, training, and supervision of staff. Finally, these objectives, like others, should provide orientation to cooperating agencies and to the general community. An excellent application of these procedures to injury prevention is provided in "Planning Models: PRECEDE-PROCEED and Haddon Matrix."[39]

Methods and Theories.   Having set priorities and selected strategies, the next step is to plan for the appropriate tools, tactics, and methods. Regardless of the setting in which the community health promotion program occurs, there are three basic types of strategies at its core:

1. Direct communications with the target population to *predispose* behaviors that are conducive to health—These include lectures and discussions, individual counseling or instruction, mass media campaigns, audiovisual aids, educational television, and programmed learning. Interpersonal or two-way communication and demonstration processes provide the most favorable environment for learning and generally have greater long-term behavioral effects. One-way communication, such as the use of pamphlets, may be appropriate in the early phases of a program or when other methods with more lasting outcomes are not feasible and when the audience is literate.
2. Training and community organization methods to *enable or reinforce* behaviors and environmental changes that are conducive to health—These include skills development, simulations and games, inquiry learning, small group discussion, modeling, and behavior modification, and communications with the role models and influential others who can reinforce the behavior.
3. Organizational methods to support behaviors and environmental changes that are conducive to health—These include community development, social action, social planning, and economic and organizational development. Such methods usually go beyond health education in supporting behavior.

A single educational intervention cannot be relied on to have a significant, lasting impact on an individual's health behavior. Only through repeated educational reinforcement by health staff, aides, community leaders, friends, and family, combined with environmental support or the removal of environmental barriers, can health education affect human behavior in the context of today's complex community health problems. Emerging theories applicable to these procedures and interventions are summarized variously in books and journals cited here and elsewhere in this chapter.[2–6,34,39,40]

Implementing Public Health Education and Health Promotion Programs

Once the planning operations have been developed and refined, the community health program can move toward implementation (Figure 22.2, phase 5).

Putting the Plan in Reverse

Planning for health education and health promotion programs works backward in the causal chain from the social assessment of ultimate outcomes (Figure 22.2, phase 1) to the administrative assessment of immediate targets of change (Figure 22.2, phase 4). The implementation of plans (phase 5) reverses the flow to work forward from the administrative assessment toward implementation and evaluation of educational and other interventions that influence changes that resolve health problems and ultimately meet the social concerns of the population (arrows from left to right at the bottom of Figure 22.2, phases 5–7). If the planning process has carefully paved the way from social concerns to educational programs—with adequate assessment, information, and social support—the road back should be a visible and viable one. The health educator or administrator approaches implementation with a well documented and supported plan in hand. If not, the usual bumps and twists in any implementation path may turn into impassable gaps and crevices.

Assessing Barriers and Facilitators to Implementation

To implement the educational plan, an assessment of factors that may impede or facilitate program activities and intended outcomes must be conducted. Both the barriers and facilitators to the program should be assessed.

Barriers. Barriers to the achievement of objectives can assume several forms. Some examples of social, psychological, and cultural barriers include citizen and staff bias, prejudice, misunderstanding, taboos, unfavorable past experiences, values, norms, social relationships, official disapproval, and rumors. Communication obstacles include illiteracy and local or professional vernacular. Examples of economic and physical barriers to enabling change include low income, inability to pay for prescribed drugs, lack of transportation to medical services, and long distances over difficult terrain to medical or health education facilities. Legal and administrative barriers include residency requirements to be eligible for services, legal requirements that the program operate within defined geographical boundaries, and policies or regulations that restrict program implementation.

Facilitators. Facilitators to the achievement of program objectives go beyond the mere absence of barriers. The predispositions of area residents who are favorable to the implementation of the program may include past and positive experiences with similar programs and high credibility of the program's sponsoring agency. Other capabilities facilitating the program might be high education levels of consumers, dynamic and supportive local leaders and organizations, skilled staff with experience, open channels of communication with consumers, and support from other agencies. In addition, some geographic and physical enabling factors may serve as program assets, such as population distribution, density, and access to facilities.

The introduction of new or unfamiliar schemes for promoting awareness and health behavior has its greatest opportunity for success when it is integrated into existing systems of knowledge transfer and influence within the community. Schools, local media, clubs, churches, neighborhoods, and ethnic associations are the most accepted channels of communication for their respective constituencies, but not necessarily for others who are not their constituents. In addition, planners should identify barriers in additional objectives that indicate how much and when the program will surmount each of the barriers.

Priorities for Implementation

Resources are often scarce in relation to the great needs in public health. When budgets are reduced, the first line item to get cut is often the health education component. To ensure the most economical use of the resources available, priorities among alternative educational activities must be considered. Related to this pressing need for efficiency is the need for effectiveness. For a program to be effective, the most effective combination of educational interventions and activities available must be selected and implemented strategically. The first step is to determine which effective procedures, based on evidence, are feasible, given limited staff, services, money, and time, and then to combine these resources to achieve the best implementation of the best combination of interventions in support of program objectives.[41]

The following guidelines can be used to set priorities:

- Obtain opinions and contributions from community members on priorities for educational services.
- Delineate the areas that will provide the greatest benefits to the most recipients.
- Phase program activities with a gradual beginning.
- Limit the number and range of activities, with initial emphasis on areas that are most amenable to quick and early success and activities requiring minimum staff training.
- Review the most recent scientific literature on the evaluation of health education methods relevant to the local program to guide these decisions on priorities.
- Develop a contingency plan to aid program survival in the event of future reduction of resources.

Beyond these general principles, the selection of educational efforts in strategic patterns or combinations depends on the particular circumstances of each site, the specific objectives, and the expectations for sustaining or institutionalizing the program.

Using Methods and Media

Methods, media, and materials can be pretested in the intended target audience to determine their acceptability, cultural relevance, and their convenience (e.g., time demands, personnel requirements, and situational concerns such as light and sound) to the particular group. They should also be selected based on their efficiency and effectiveness. Efficiency relates to fixed costs, continuing costs, space and maintenance requirements, and staff and time needed to convey a message. Presumed effectiveness is based on confidence in the ability to communicate messages, arouse attention and interest, promote interaction, use suitable repetition and message-retention techniques, and encourage desired attitudes and the adoption of practices.

Managing Human Resources for Health Education and Health Promotion

Some health workers and allied personnel may be uninformed about the methods of health education and health promotion; others may feel that educational efforts are too slow, complex, and of dubious efficacy. Training or continuing education for these workers can provide them with time to discuss their concerns and develop their competence and confidence. Training in health education and health promotion should be differentiated from technical training related to health and medical content. Health education and health promotion training underscores the attitudinal and behavioral factors essential to voluntary, long-term health maintenance, the cultural perceptions of the target population, and the necessity of well-planned and properly sustained action. Knowledge of these factors can help health workers achieve the health behavior changes required by the objectives of the community health program.

Although many health professionals are involved in various forms of health education, one group of professionals, certified health education specialist (CHES), has specialized training in the planning, implementation, and evaluation of public health education (for more information see http://www.nchec.org). CHES professionals are typically assigned the responsibility for planning, implementing, and evaluating community health education programs because they have specialized training in public health or community health education and experience in a community health agency or institution. Competencies tested for CHES include the following:

- Planning at the community level, including epidemiologic and sociological research methods, community organization, and health services administration
- Assessment and adaptation of communications to attitudinal, cultural, economic, and ethnic determinants of health behaviors
- Educational evaluation within the context of community health (as distinct from formal curriculum evaluation), including biostatistics, demography, and behavioral research methods

When these skills are not available within the staff of a community health agency, consultation for the planning and preparation stages of health education programs may be obtained from other organizations employing CHES professionals. Continuing education and in-service training are important to maintaining up-to-date knowledge and skills in all community health staff.

The CHES may work in a variety of different settings, such as public health departments, hospitals, voluntary agencies, educational institutions, or for-profit organizations. What links educators together in these various settings is their training and intent of facilitating voluntary actions by the public with regard to health. In some organizations, health educators work as part of a team with other health professionals to achieve intended outcomes. For example, a health educator may work as a team member with a physician, nurse, nutritionist, and social worker to develop and implement programs for maternal and child health. In other organizations, health educators may all work in the same department and be loaned to other departments, such as nursing or nutrition, to help plan and implement health education programs. Both models of organization have their advantages and disadvantages; the former promotes collaboration among health professionals, and the latter may allow health educators to support each other, but it isolates them from other health professionals. Careful consideration needs to be given to the placement of health education specialists.

Staff training may include orientation aimed at sensitizing staff members to their educational function and to the general objectives of the education program. It may also include preparation in recognizing educational opportunities, communication skills, and reinforcement techniques; training priorities for those staff members in contact with consumers; and continuing education.

Volunteers are not free of cost. Proper use of volunteers requires continuous, careful supervision and training. These items should be budgeted in the educational plan. A thorough plan for training volunteers might include content designed to foster their interest in health education and in the program's need for their insight into the attitudes, reactions, and daily lives of the target population. It can also include training in communications skills, teamwork roles, and limits of volunteers' responsibility and authority.

Data Collection and Records

Documenting the implementation process not only provides guidance for present action, but it also provides statistics and financial accounts that are useful for evaluation and future planning. Good records and documentation, supervisor reports on quality control, and other process evaluations can provide immediate feedback on whether things are working satisfactorily. Records provide for continuous monitoring of program impact; for supervision, training, and staff development; and for evaluation of program process and outcome. Peer review among health professionals helps to maintain quality control, but it must be based on standards and documentation of practice. Feedback on patients' or clients' utilization and satisfaction with health services should provide data for program adjustment and redirection. Population surveillance will aid in continuous health education planning and evaluation.

Information collection can be integrated into daily routines and may require coordination among various units and sites in order to provide meaningful data for future planning. Information collection that requires additional paperwork must always be weighed against other demands for time. Small additions and checklists may be integrated into existing records with little effort and with staff acceptance. For more intensive narrative reporting and recording, special efforts during limited time periods may be acceptable and may provide sufficient data without generating staff resistance and unmanageable amounts of paperwork. The educational plan should clearly identify the use and purpose of new forms and records.

Scheduling Implementation

Timing is crucial to the success of the educational plan of action. It requires an analysis of when, where, and who is responsible for implementation. This analysis will provide the starting and completion date required for each activity in relation to the total program. Consideration of the training required, production schedules for material, and staff loads guide the development of timetables. A task analysis and time sequence of activities should integrate the educational implementation with the total program plan. Planners should consider external events when scheduling to avoid conflict with community happenings, school openings, holidays, and related community schedules. The implementation stage is a logical progression from the previous stages of assessment, planning, and organizing.

Evaluating Public Health Education and Health Promotion Programs

Evaluation is the comparison of an object of interest against a standard of acceptability.[38] The evaluation of a health education program, then, is the systematic assessment of the operations or outcomes of a program against standards for the purposes of improving the program. These operations, outcomes, and standards are contained in the program objectives. The evaluation of a program needs to be guided by the standards of program evaluation promulgated by the American Evaluation Association: accuracy, feasibility, propriety, utility, and evaluation accountability. Evaluation needs to be not only technically well done and ethically conducted, but also feasible in cost and effort and directed toward program improvement.

The various levels of objectives developed in the assessment phases of planning—epidemiologic, behavioral, educational, and administrative—shape the dimensions and standards that are used during evaluation to determine the value (success or failure) of the program including its process, components, and outcomes. If the objectives were well developed during the planning stage, evaluation can proceed with ease, as compared with programs that have no explicit or transparent standards for judging their success or failure. The involvement of various stakeholders in determining the dimensions and standards used to judge program value is essential in the highly political context of program evaluation. If stakeholders do not accept the program components and standards as those they would use in judging value, they are not likely to accept or use the results of the evaluation.

Program evaluation, at the very least, is an assessment of the worth or merit of a program, a method, or some other object of interest. It may provide an estimate of the degree to which spent resources result in intended activity and the degree to which performed activities attain goals. The determination of whether the program has met its goals is based formally on program objectives; it may be informally based on subjective impressions and reporting. Evaluation can suggest which of several alternative educational strategies is the most efficient and which steps have an effect on the behavior specified. Evaluation provides accountability for time spent. Results can offer a sense of accomplishment to staff and consumers or sponsors of the program.

Formative and Process Evaluation

Formative evaluation is the earliest phase of process evaluation. Formative evaluation usually refers to preliminary assessments of the appropriateness of materials and procedures before beginning the program. Sources of data for formative evaluation include pretesting of materials, access to planning by relevant stakeholders, and adequate resources. Process evaluation refers to continuous observation and checking to see whether the program activities are taking place with the quality and at the time and rate necessary to achieve the stated objective. Process evaluation requires ongoing sources of data that often include budget reports on monthly expenditures in specific categories where rate of expenditures would indicate the amount of program activity relevant to the achievement of objectives.

Professional and/or participant consensus can provide the source of the standards of acceptability in formative and process evaluation. The data for process evaluation often come from routine records kept on encounters with consumers, patients, or clients. These might include, for example, clinic attendance records tabulated weekly or monthly for total numbers of patients. Staff can tabulate systematic samples of the records in more detail to estimate progress on such variables as broken appointment rates, sources of referral, and trimester of first visit for pregnant women. Another type of data available for process evaluation is administrative records. For example, administrators can tabulate personnel records to assess the number of home visits attempted, the number completed, the number of group sessions conducted, and the time allotted for various educational functions. These may become the numerators in evaluations with outcomes as the denominators, where the quotient shows an efficiency measure of, for example, home visits by staff per prenatal visit at the clinic.

Supervisors should conduct periodic reviews of personnel to assess staff performance. Time should be set aside on the agenda of staff and community meetings for consideration of strengths, weaknesses, and adaptation of ongoing programs. There should be a plan for charting records over time or comparing progress statistics with other programs or standards.

Outcome Evaluation

Outcome evaluation, sometimes referred to as *summative* or *impact evaluation*, assesses the achievement of program effects. Intended program effects are contained in objectives that were developed during the planning phase. The more precisely stated the objectives, the more meaningful and useful the evaluation. Outcome evaluation asks the following questions: What are the results of program efforts in the promotion of health behavior? Has there been any change in the attitudes of the clients toward recommended actions, change in their ability to carry out the recommended actions, or change in the resources and social support for such actions in the community? An outcome evaluation may also assess unintended program effects that may be either beneficial or harmful to intended recipients.

Data concerning program outcomes can be assessed with quantitative or qualitative approaches. Quantitative approaches attempt to measure the frequency or prevalence of intended outcomes; qualitative approaches are more concerned with explaining why and how outcomes occurred, whether or not they were intended. For quantitative measurement, planners or evaluators can obtain baseline information on a period prior to the program's inception for comparison with similarly gathered data during the program or following the program.

Evaluators should report on outcomes to the affiliated organizations, agencies, and institutions participating in the program and to the clients and general public. Reports can encourage their continued participation by noting their contribution to, or influence on, the program. Finally, practitioners should seek to publish case histories and reports in professional journals and newsletters for use by other departments, programs, or projects and to contribute to the advancement of professional knowledge, practice, and policies.

Beyond Internal Validity in Evaluations

Health education programs that have been evaluated and found effective in systematic reviews of rigorously controlled trials are deemed by officially designated bodies, such as the U.S. Preventive Services Task Force and the Task Force on Community Preventive Services, to be **evidence-based programs (EBPs)**. EBPs are typically evaluated in very controlled conditions that often bear too little resemblance to the everyday realities of public health agencies to be seen as applicable or generalizable. Additionally, EBPs often do not allow for flexibility in how the program is implemented. Health educators, however, regularly work in community settings where customization of a program is necessary to make it culturally appropriate, age appropriate, setting appropriate, and so on. Practitioners have to deal with the tension between ensuring a program is implemented as it was tested in the controlled experimental trials while also ensuring that it is implemented in a way that is effective for the community in which they are working.

One way to deal with this issue for future programs is to create programs that are inherently flexible and provide for further evaluation in their various applications and settings such that the results can be reported with particular attention to external validity considerations. We have suggested a method that: 1) outlines a limited set of key components of an EBP, 2) has a range of permissible adaptations that still retain the core components of the program, 3) states the theory and experience-based justifications for these deviations, and 4) provides through evaluation the practice-based evidence needed to supplement the usual "evidence-based practice" with more "practice-based evidence."[41–43]

Additionally, evaluating programs for external validity would ensure more feasible implementation across a number of settings. Such an evaluation should include ratings of:

- *Reach and representativeness of the program*, which includes assessments of participation, target audience, representativeness of settings, and representativeness of individuals
- *Implementation and consistency of effects*, which includes factors related to program or policy implementation and adaptation such as assessment of consistent implementation, staff expertise, program adaptation, and mechanisms related to data reported; factors related to outcomes for decision making such as reporting outcomes so they can be compared to other goals or guidelines, the reporting of adverse consequences, moderators that enhance or detract, sensitivity of the program, and cost
- *Maintenance and institutionalization*, which includes the assessment of long-term effects, the sustainability of the program, and information on rates of attrition[41]

We placed the late 20th-century social epidemiological concern with the "ecosocial" web of influences on behavior under the broader concept of "lifestyle."[44] Lalonde identified lifestyle as one of the four elements of his health field concept; the other elements include health services, human biology, and environment (which can be broken down further into physical environment and social circumstance).[45] Of these, lifestyle was seen by Lalonde as the most neglected component, and has since been estimated to be responsible for the largest proportion of the years of life that are prematurely lost in the more developed nations (**Figure 22.3**).[46] Tobacco use, diet (in combination with physical activity), and alcohol use are the three leading determinants of the

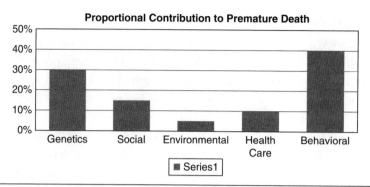

Figure 22.3   Proportional Contribution to Premature Death
Source: Adapted from McGinnis JM, Williams-Russo P, Knickman JR. The case for more active policy attention to health promotion. *Health Aff.* 2002;21(2):78–93.

leading causes of death in North America. Together, they account for some 38% of premature deaths.[47] To put these revealing statistics in more positive terms, the greatest gains in preventing premature death and disability can be achieved today through community supports or policies for more healthy lifestyles. Reducing risk means that chances of developing a disease are lowered. It does not guarantee that a disease will be prevented. Because several factors are involved in the development of disease, risk reduction usually involves several strategies or approaches.

Broad Supports for Lifestyle Change

Health education typically has been called on to alert the public to complex community health problems, but health education by itself can hardly be expected to solve such problems. The lifestyles in question are too embedded in organizational, socioeconomic, cultural, and environmental circumstances for people to be able to change their own behavior without concomitant changes or support in these circumstances. Health promotion combines health education with organizational, economic, and environmental supports for behavior and conditions of living that are conducive to health.

The entire burden for improved health or risk reduction must not be placed on the individual alone. The responsibility must be shared between individuals and their families; between families and their communities; and between communities and their state, provincial, and national governments. Each level of organizational influence on behavior must assume some responsibility for setting the economic and environmental conditions that will support healthful lifestyles. Families, for example, must set examples for children. Communities must provide facilities and pass local ordinances to encourage, enable, and reinforce healthful behavior. State and national governments and private organizations must assume responsibility for the production, sale, and advertising of foods and other substances that can be either helpful or harmful to health.

Health Promotion

Any program that has to deal with the complex problems related to lifestyle must address the social, environmental, economic, psychological, cultural, and physiological factors encompassed by the lifestyle in question. The first part of this chapter introduced the PRECEDE model of health education, but its presentation in Figure 22.2 included the additional elements of economic, organizational, and environmental supports for behavior that are conducive to health and applied as the PRECEDE-PROCEED model of health promotion.[2] This health promotion model, as shown in Figure 22.2, includes health education at its core along with other types of policy, organizational, and regulatory interventions. The combined model has been applied to health promotion programs at international, national, and local levels for planning and evaluating such complex interventions for such complex lifestyle problems.

Three levels and strategies used in public health serve to compare and contrast health education and health promotion approaches. This understanding paves the way for the various applications of the PRECEDE-PROCEED model.

Prevention Strategies

Three types of strategies can be used in each of the three prevention levels to accomplish health promotion goals:

- *Educational strategies* inform and educate the public about issues of concern, such as the dangers of drug misuse, the benefits of automobile restraints, or the relationship of maternal alcohol consumption to fetal alcohol syndrome.
- *Automatic protective strategies* are directed at controlling environmental variables, such as public health measures providing for milk pasteurization, fluoridation of water, and the burning or chemical killing of marijuana crops.
- *Coercive strategies* employ legal and other formal sanctions to control individual behavior, such as required immunizations for school entry, mandatory tuberculosis testing of hospital employees, compulsory use of automobile restraints, and arrests for drug possession or use.

Table 22.1 provides examples of community health programs and measures classified by level of prevention and category of prevention strategy. The examples illustrate traditional public health strategies and new strategies in community health promotion, with illustrations related to drug misuse prevention.

Health Promotion Includes Health Education

Our definition of health promotion as any combination of educational, organizational, environmental, and economic supports for behavior and conditions of living conducive to health,[1,2] views health education as an integral part of all health promotion interventions. Indeed, health education has a long history of advocating for the wider range of policy and socioenvironmental changes before Lalonde's Canadian initiative, and before the 1976 U.S. Health Information and Health Promotion Act that supported the *Healthy People* initiative in health promotion and disease prevention.[48] "Health promotion," as a related but more comprehensive term, has helped make that scope explicit. It follows that the interventions should be directed toward voluntary behavior at all levels—individuals, organizations, and communities. At the community, state or provincial, or national level, additional interventions may be legal, regulatory, political, or economic, and therefore potentially coercive. Nevertheless, to be successful, an informed electorate and a consenting public must support such interventions.

Such informed consent requires health education. Ideally, the coercive measures are focused on the behavior of those individuals whose actions may affect the health of others, such as the manufacturers, distributors, and advertisers of hazardous products; drunk or reckless drivers; smokers or irresponsible users of potentially lethal products such as hallucinatory drugs, environmental pollutants, firearms, and explosives. Even then, public health education is required to ensure the support of an informed public because taxes, prices, availability of services and products, cherished freedoms, and jobs may be affected by such regulations of health-related industries, sources, and users. For example, one part of a health promotion program for drug misuse prevention could target organizational change. Local public leaders could combine health education with various incentives (e.g., free program consultation services) and persuasion techniques (e.g., program promotion by local opinion leaders) in an attempt to increase the number of schools offering peer counseling programs for those persons who misuse drugs.

If the program also targeted political change, community organization techniques could be combined with health education activities to develop "concerned parent groups" in neighborhoods and to apply political pressure on local school, law enforcement, and government officials to support drug misuse prevention efforts. If the program directed other efforts toward economic change, health professionals and others could work with representatives of insurance carriers to initiate health insurance reimbursements for counseling and rehabilitation services.

The point is simple: When health education activities are combined with appropriate changes in organizations, political systems, and environmental and economic supports for behavior, the end result is more likely to be favorable than is the result achieved by a series of single, uncoordinated changes. Indeed, uncoordinated changes sometimes make things worse by throwing a community system out of balance and forcing an overreaction or overcompensation by elements in the community.

The relationships of health education and health promotion activities to the three prevention targets (lifestyle, environment, and health services) and the relationships of these targets to the health objectives set for the community, state, or nation are depicted in Figures 22.2 and 22.3. The various prevention targets are not isolated. The physical environment and the organization of services continually affect lifestyle. Furthermore, a successful program must effectively integrate and coordinate activities in relation to each of these targets. To facilitate the integration of activities within and between the prevention strategies, a planning framework is needed. The planning framework introduced in the first part of this chapter forces an encompassing and systematic analysis of public health problems in the context of social problems or quality-of-life concerns.

Organization of Health Promotion Within Public Health Institutions

Placing professional health educators and other health promotion specialists within the staffing and organization of public health organizations poses some quandaries. From what has been described here as the tasks of coordinating the necessary components of effective health education and health promotion, it would seem that personnel performing these functions should be distributed to specific program areas, such as maternal and child health, environmental health, or tobacco control. This would allow each health educator or other health promotion personnel to specialize in and learn the content, resources, and community capabilities of the area in which the work is to be done. However, in recent years, many public health organizations have not been able to afford a sufficient number of health education and other health promotion specialists to have one assigned to every problem area in which they are needed. The usual, preferred staffing arrangement, then, is to centralize or pool the health education and other health promotion staff in a unit that provides planning and organizing services or consultation to the other units within the organization.

The major trap to avoid in centralizing the health education and health promotion staff is turning them into a public relations unit serving the publicity needs of the organization. A separate and distinct public relations officer should serve the purpose of representing the agency to the community and should remain distinct from the health education and health promotion functions of representing the community's needs to the agency, as described in this chapter.

Future Outlook

There is no simple solution to such health-related lifestyle problems as tobacco use, alcohol misuse, drug misuse, and obesity. Such complex problems as these may defy even well planned preventive efforts. Nevertheless, the effects of well planned and systematically implemented preventive efforts are more likely to be successful than the single-focused, uncoordinated efforts that have typified many of the early attempts to address lifestyle, particularly those at the local level.

Specific, measurable objectives for the United States have been set in each of the past 4 decades in the *Healthy People* initiatives of the federal government. If these objectives were met each decade, the scope and intensity of health problems attributable to lifestyle, the environment, and inadequate health services would be appreciably reduced. These objectives can serve to concentrate the limited resources of communities where they can be most productive. To illustrate how community health programs can work toward the objectives, a planning framework encompassing lifestyle, environment, and services has been presented in this chapter.

Health education directed at individuals and decision makers has been demonstrated to influence population changes in simple behaviors such as one-time immunizations and more complex behaviors for those segments of the population that are highly motivated, more affluent, or more educated. Some of these successes have reduced risk factor prevalence for whole populations, such as the spectacular public health success with tobacco control,[49] but have had the regrettable effect sometimes of increasing disparities in those populations.[50] Health education can enhance its effect on more complex behaviors (lifestyles) and in poorer, less educated segments of a population by combining the best of tailored educational interventions with advocacy and organizational efforts to affect social environments, including political and economic systems. Applying the latest findings from the rapidly developing research in designing and evaluating prevention programs and ensuring the necessary quality and quantity of resources for programs will not guarantee success, but it will increase the probability of reaching the objectives set for a community.

Discussion Questions

1. Why is health education so important in public health? Why is health promotion important? How do they differ?
2. Identify and describe a health education or promotion initiative. What were the results?
3. Why is it important to measure outcomes in health promotion? Discuss.
4. Go to the website of your state health department and identify five programs that have been developed. What elements of this chapter do you see in these programs? Describe them and share with your class.
5. What is the skill set needed for someone working in health education?

References

1. Green LW, Ottoson JM. *Community and Population Health*. 8th ed. St. Louis, MO: McGraw-Hill; 1999.
2. Green LW, Hiatt RA, Hoeft KS. Behavioural determinants of health and disease. In: Detels R, Beaglehole R, Lansang MA, et al., eds. *Oxford Textbook of Public Health*, 6th ed. Oxford, UK: Oxford University Press; 2013.
3. Green LW, Kreuter MW. *Health Program Planning: An Educational and Ecological Approach*. 4th ed. New York: McGraw-Hill; 2005.
4. Bartholomew LK, Parcel GS, Kok G, et al. *Planning Health Promotion Programs: An Intervention Mapping Approach*. 3rd ed. San Francisco: Jossey-Bass; 2011.

5. Gorin SH, Arnold J., eds. *Heath Promotion in Practice.* San Francisco: Jossey-Bass; 2006.

6. Kline MV, Huff RF. *Health Promotion in Multicultural Populations: A Handbook for Practitioners and Students.* 3rd ed. Thousand Oaks, CA: Sage Publications; 2013.

7. Mo PK, Mak WW. Application of the PRECEDE model to understanding mental health promoting behaviors in Hong Kong. *Health Educ Behav.* 2008;35:574–87.

8. Dharamsi S, Jivani K, Dean C, et al. Oral care for frail elders: knowledge, attitudes, and practices of long-term care staff. *J Dent Educ.* 2009;73:581–8.

9. Cole R, Horacek T. Applying PRECEDE-PROCEED to develop an intuitive eating, nondieting approach to weight management program. *J Nutr Educ Behav.* 2009;41(2):120–6.

10. Kratzke C, Garzon L, Lombard J, et al. Training community health workers: factors that influence mammography use. *J Community Health.* 2010;35(6):683–6.

11. Burke L, Jancey J, Howat P, et al. Physical activity and nutrition program for seniors (PANS): protocol of a randomized controlled trial. *BMC Public Health.* 2010;10(1):751–7.

12. Slawta JN, DeNeui D. Be a fit kid: nutrition and physical activity for the fourth grade. *Health Promot Pract.* 2010;11:522–9.

13. Delobelle P, Onya H, Langa C, et al. Advances in health promotion in Africa: promoting health through hospitals. *Glob Health Promot.* 2010;(S2):33–6.

14. Aboumatar H, Ristaino P, Davis RO, et al. Infection prevention promotion program based on the PRECEDE model: improving hand hygiene behaviors among healthcare personnel. *Infect Control Hosp Epidemiol.* 2012;33(2):144–51.

15. Gary TL, Bone LR, Hill MN, et al. Randomized controlled trial of the effects of nurse case manager and community health worker interventions on risk factors for diabetes-related complications in urban African Americans. *Prev Med.* 2003;37:23–2.

16. Friis RH, Forouzesh M, Chhim HS, et al. Sociocultural determinants of tobacco use among Cambodian Americans. *Health Educ Res.* 2006;21:355–65.

17. Mancuso CA, Peterson MG, Gaeta TJ, et al. A randomized controlled trial of self-management education for asthma patients in the emergency department. *Ann Emerg Med.* 2011;57(6):603–12.

18. Rivara FP, Bennett E, Crispin B, et al. Booster seats for child passengers: lessons for increasing their use. *Inj Prev.* 2001;7:210–3.

19. Awadzi KD, Classen S, Hall A, et al. Predictors of injury among younger and older adults in fatal motor vehicle crashes. *Accident Anal Prev.* 2008;40(6):1804–10.

20. Mirtz TA, Thompson MA, Greene L, et al. Adolescent idiopathic scoliosis screening for school, community, and clinical health promotion practice utilizing the PRECEDE-PROCEED model. *Chiroprac Osteopathy.* 2005;13:25–35.

21. Wright A, McGorry PD, Harris MG, et al. Development and evaluation of a youth mental health community awareness campaign—The Compass Strategy. *BMC Public Health.* 2006;6(1):215.

22. Ford CL, Miller WC, Smurzynski M, et al. Key components of a theory-guided HIV prevention outreach model: pre-outreach preparation, community assessment, and a network of key informants. *AIDS Educ Prev.* 2007;19(2):173–86.

23. Duffy SA, Karvonen-Gutierrez CA, Ewing LA, et al. Veterans Integrated Service Network (VISN) 11 tobacco tactics team: implementation of the tobacco tactics program in the Department of Veterans Affairs. *J Gen Intern Med.* 2010;25:3–10.

24. Brownson RC, Baker EA, Leet TL, et al. *Evidence-Based Public Health.* 2nd ed. Oxford, UK: Oxford University Press; 2011.

25. Brownson RC, Colditz GA, Proctor EK. *Dissemination and Implementation Research in Health: Translating Science to Practice.* Oxford, UK: Oxford University Press; 2012.

26. Institute of Medicine. *An Integrated Framework for Assessing the Value of Community-Based Prevention.* Washington, DC: National Academies Press; 2012.

27. Gilmore GD, Campbell MD. *Needs Assessment Strategies for Health Education and Health Promotion.* 4th ed. Dubuque, IA: Brown & Benchmark; 2011.

28. Green LW. The theory of participation: a qualitative analysis of its expression in national and international health policies. In: Patton RD, Cissell WB, eds. *Community Organization: Traditional Principles and Modern Applications.* Johnson City, TN: Latchpins Press; 1990:48–62.

29. Minkler M, Wallerstein N, eds. *Community-Based Participatory Research for Health: From Process to Outcomes.* 2nd ed. San Francisco: Jossey-Bass; 2008.

30. U.S. Department of Health and Human Services. *Healthy People 2020.* Available at: http://www.healthypeople.gov. Accessed March 21, 2013.

31. Eakin EG, Bull SS, Glasgow RE, et al. Reaching those most in need: a review of diabetes self-management interventions in disadvantaged populations. *Diabetes Metab Res Rev.* 2002;18:26–35.

32. Briss PA, Brownson RC, Fielding JE, et al. Developing and using the Guide to Preventive Health Services: lessons learned about evidence-based public health. *Annu Rev Public Health.* 2004;25:281–302.

33. Green LW. From research to "best practices" in other settings and populations. *Am J Health Behavior.* 2001;25:165–78.

34. Glanz K, Rimer BK, Viswanath K, eds. *Health Behavior and Health Education: Theory, Research, and Practice.* 4th ed. San Francisco: Jossey-Bass; 2008.

35. D'Onofrio CN. Pooling information about prior interventions: a new program planning tool. In: Sussman S, ed. *Handbook of Program Development for Health Behavior.* Thousand Oaks, CA: Sage Publications; 2001.

36. Kreuter MW. PATCH: its origin, basic concepts, and links to contemporary public health policy. *J Health Educ.* 1992;23:135–9.

37. Maibach EW, Rothschild ML, Novelli WD. Social marketing. In: Glanz K, Rimer BK, Lewis FM, eds. *Health Behavior and Health Education: Theory, Research, and Practice.* 3rd ed. San Francisco: Jossey-Bass; 2002:437–61

38. Green LW, Lewis FM. *Measurement and Evaluation in Health Education and Health Promotion.* Palo Alto, CA: Mayfield; 1986.

39. Freire K, Runyan CW. Planning models: PRECEDE-PROCEED and Haddon Matrix. In: Gielen AC, Sleet DA, DiClemente RJ, eds. *Injury and Violence Prevention: Behavioral Science Theories, Methods, and Applications.* San Francisco: Jossey-Bass; 2006:127–58.

40. DiClemente RJ, Crosby RA, Kegler MC, eds. *Emerging Theories in Health Promotion Practice and Research: Strategies for Improving Public Health.* San Francisco: Jossey-Bass; 2002.

41. Green LW, Glasgow RE. Evaluating the relevance, generalization, and applicability of research: issues in external validity and translation methodology. *Eval Health Prof.* 2006;29:126–53.

42. Ottoson JM, Green LW. Reconciling concept and context: a theory of implementation. *Adv Health Educ Promot.* 1987;2:353–82.

43. Green LW, Ottoson JM. From efficacy to effectiveness to community and back: evidence-based practice vs practice-based evidence. In: Green L, Hiss R, Glasgow R, et al., eds. *From Clinical Trials to Community: The Science of Translating Diabetes and Obesity Research.* Bethesda, MD: National Institutes of Health; 2004:15–18.

44. Krieger N. Theories for social epidemiology in the 21st century: an ecosocial perspective. *Int J Epidemiol.* 2001;30:668–77.

45. Lalonde M. *A New Perspective on the Health of Canadians: A Working Document.* Ottawa, Canada: Government of Canada; 1974.

46. McGinnis JM, Williams-Russo P, Knickman JR. The case for more active policy attention to health promotion. *Health Aff.* 2002;21:78–93.
47. Mokdad AH, Marks JS, Stroup DF, et al. Actual causes of death in the United States, 2000. *JAMA.* 2004;291(10):1238–45.
48. Green LW, Allegrante JP. *Healthy People 1980–2020:* Raising the ante decennially, or just the name from health education to health promotion to social determinants? *Health Educ Behav.* 2011;38(6):558–62.
49. Eriksen MP, Green LW, Husten CG, et al. Thank you for not smoking: the public health response to tobacco-related mortality in the United States. In: Ward JW, Warren CS, eds. *Silent Victories: The History and Practice of Public Health in Twentieth-Century America.* New York: Oxford University Press; 2007:423–36.
50. Warner KE. Disparities in smoking are complicated and consequential. What to do about them? *Am J Public Health.* 2011;25:S5–7.

Evidence-Based Public Health Management and Practice

Ross C. Brownson

LEARNING OBJECTIVES

- To provide an overview of the principles of evidence-based public health (EBPH), including types of evidence, the role of transdisciplinary problem solving, and similarities and differences from clinical practice
- To describe six key characteristics of EBPH
- To identify analytic tools that assist in the EBPH process by describing the size of a problem, effective interventions, contextual conditions, and relative value of various approaches
- To describe a seven-stage framework for EBPH that, if implemented, has the potential to improve public health decision making and management
- To explore several barriers to implementing principles of EBPH in practice and some potential approaches for overcoming these challenges
- To describe several future issues that are likely to affect attempts to move forward in EBPH in the coming years

Chapter Overview

Despite the many accomplishments of public health, greater attention on evidence-based approaches is warranted. This chapter reviews the concepts of evidence-based public health (EBPH) and how they affect public health administration, on which formal discourse originated around the beginning of the 21st century. Key components of EBPH include making decisions based on the best available scientific evidence, using data and information systems systematically, applying program-planning frameworks, engaging the community in decision making, conducting sound evaluation, and disseminating what is learned. Three types of evidence have been described regarding the causes of diseases and the magnitude of risk factors, the relative impact of specific interventions, and how and under what contextual conditions interventions were implemented. Analytic tools (e.g., systematic reviews, economic evaluation) can be useful in accelerating the uptake of EBPH. A seven-stage, sequential framework (moving from community assessment to evaluation) may be useful in training practitioners and in promoting the greater use of evidence in day-to-day decision making. Challenges and opportunities (e.g., political issues, training needs) for disseminating EBPH are reviewed. Several future issues in EBPH include the need to expand the evidence base, overcome barriers to implementation, engage leadership, expand training opportunities, enhance accountability, and address disparities. To better bridge evidence and practice, the concepts of EBPH outlined in this chapter hold promise.

Introduction

Public health research and practice are credited with many notable achievements, including much of the 30-year gain in life expectancy in the United States over the 20th century.[1] A large part of this increase can be attributed to provision of safe water and food, sewage treatment and disposal, tobacco use prevention and cessation, injury prevention, control of infectious diseases through immunization and other means, and other population-based interventions.[2]

Despite these successes, many additional opportunities to improve the public's health remain. To achieve state and national objectives for improved population health, more widespread adoption of evidence-based strategies has been recommended.[3–8] Increased focus on evidence-based public health (EBPH) has numerous direct and indirect benefits, including access to more and higher quality information on what works, a higher likelihood of successful programs and policies being implemented, greater workforce productivity, and more efficient use of public and private resources.[5,9,10]

Ideally, public health practitioners should always incorporate scientific evidence in selecting and implementing programs, developing policies, and evaluating progress.[11,12] Society pays a high opportunity cost when interventions that yield the highest health return on an investment are not implemented.[13] In practice, intervention decisions are often based on perceived short-term opportunities, lacking systematic, planning and review of the best evidence regarding effective approaches. These concerns were noted in 1988 when the Institute of Medicine determined that decision making in public health is often driven by "crises, hot issues, and concerns of organized interest groups."[14, p. 4] Barriers to implementing EBPH include the political environment (including lack of political will), and deficits in relevant and timely research, information systems, resources, leadership, and the required competencies.[11,15–18]

Nearly every public health problem is complex,[19] requiring attention at multiple levels and among many disciplines. Partnerships that bring together diverse people and organizations have the potential for developing new and creative ways of addressing public health issues.[20]

Transdisciplinary research provides valuable opportunities to collaborate on interventions to improve the health and wellbeing of individuals and communities.[21,22] For example, tobacco research efforts have been successful in facilitating cooperation among disciplines such as advertising, policy, business, medical science, and behavioral science. Research activities within these multidisciplinary tobacco networks try to fill the gaps between scientific discovery and research translation by engaging a wide range of stakeholders.[23–25] A transdisciplinary approach has also shown some evidence of effectiveness in obesity prevention by engaging numerous sectors including food production, urban planning, transportation, schools, and health.[26,27]

As these disciplines converge, several concepts are fundamental to achieving a more evidence-based approach to public health practice. First, we need scientific information on the programs and policies that are most likely to be effective in promoting health (i.e., undertake evaluation research to generate sound evidence).[5,9,28,29] An array of effective interventions is now available from numerous sources including the Guide to Community Preventive Services,[30,31] the Guide to Clinical Preventive Services,[32] Cancer Control PLANET,[33] and the National Registry of Evidence-based Programs and Practices.[34] Second, to translate science to practice, we need to marry information on evidence-based interventions from the peer-reviewed literature with the realities of a specific real-world environment.[35,36] To do so, we need to better define processes that lead to evidence-based decision making, including a more transdisciplinary approach to problem solving. Finally, wide-scale dissemination of interventions of proven effectiveness must occur more consistently at state and local levels.[37]

This chapter includes six major sections that describe: 1) relevant background issues, including a brief history, definitions, an overview of evidence-based medicine, and other concepts underlying EBPH; 2) several key characteristics of an evidenced-based process that crosses numerous disciplines; 3) analytic tools to enhance the uptake of EBPH and the disciplines responsible; 4) a brief sketch of a framework for EBPH in public health practice; 5) a summary of barriers and opportunities for widespread implementation of evidence-based approaches; and 6) key future issues in EBPH. A primary goal of this chapter is to move the process of management and decision making toward a proactive approach that incorporates effective use of scientific evidence and data, while engaging numerous sectors and partners.

Historical Background and Core Concepts

Formal discourse on the nature and scope of EBPH originated in the late 1990s. Several authors have attempted to define EBPH. In 1997, Jenicek defined EBPH as the "conscientious, explicit, and judicious use of current best evidence in making decisions about the care of communities and populations in the domain of health protection, disease prevention, health maintenance and improvement (health promotion)."[38] In 1999, scholars and practitioners in Australia[6] and the United States[11] elaborated further on the concept of EBPH. Glasziou and colleagues posed a series of questions to enhance uptake of EBPH (e.g., "Does this intervention help alleviate this problem?") and identified 14 sources of high-quality evidence.[6] Brownson and colleagues described a six-stage process by which practitioners are able to take a more evidence-based approach to decision making.[5,11] Kohatsu and colleagues broadened earlier definitions of EBPH to include the perspectives of community members, fostering a more population-centered approach.[35] In 2004, Rychetnik and colleagues summarized many key concepts in a glossary for EBPH.[39] There appears to be a consensus that a combination of scientific evidence with values, resources, and context should enter into decision making.[3,5,39,40] A concise definition emerged from Kohatsu: "Evidence-based public health is the process of integrating science-based interventions with community preferences to improve the health of populations."[35, p. 419] More recently, Satterfield and colleagues examined evidence-based practice across five disciplines (public health, social work, medicine, nursing, psychology) and found many common challenges including: 1) how evidence should be defined, 2) how and when the patient's and/or other contextual factors should enter the decision-making process, 3) the definition and role of the experts or key stakeholders, and 4) what other variables should be considered when selecting an evidence-based practice (e.g., age, social class).[40]

Defining Evidence

At the most basic level, evidence involves "the available body of facts or information indicating whether a belief or proposition is true or valid."[41] The idea of evidence often derives from legal settings in Western societies. In law, evidence comes in the form of stories, witness accounts, police testimony, expert opinions, and forensic science.[42] Our notions of evidence are defined in large part by our professional training and experience. For a public health professional, evidence is some form of data—including epidemiologic (quantitative) data, results of program or policy evaluations, and qualitative data—for uses in making judgments or decisions (**Figure 23.1**).[43] Public health evidence is usually the result of a complex cycle of observation, theory, and experiment.[44,45] However, the value of evidence is in the eye of the beholder (e.g., usefulness of evidence may vary by stakeholder type).[46] Medical evidence includes not only research but characteristics of the patient, a patient's readiness to undergo a therapy, and society's values.[47] Policymakers seek out distributional consequences (i.e., who has to pay, how much, and who benefits)[48] and in practice settings, anecdotes sometimes trump empirical data.[49] Evidence is usually imperfect and, as noted by Muir Gray: "The absence of excellent evidence does not make evidence-based decision making impossible; what is required is the best evidence available not the best evidence possible."[3]

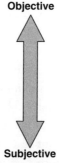

- Scientific literature in systematic reviews
- Scientific literature in one or more journal articles
- Public health surveillance data
- Program evaluations
- Qualitative data
  - Community members
  - Other stakeholders
- Media/marketing data
- Word of mouth
- Personal experience

Objective

Subjective

Figure 23.1 Different Forms of Evidence

Table 23.1   Comparison of the Types of Scientific Evidence

Characteristic	Type 1	Type 2	Type 3
Typical Data/Relationship	Size and strength of preventable risk–disease relationship (measures of burden, etiologic research)	Relative effectiveness of public health intervention	Information on the adaptation and translation of an effective intervention
Common Setting	Clinic or controlled community setting	Socially intact groups or community-wide	Socially intact groups or community-wide
Example	Smoking causes lung cancer	Price increases with a targeted media campaign reduce smoking rates	Understanding the political challenges of price increases or targeting media messages to particular audience segments
Quantity	More	Less	Less
Action	Something should be done	This particular intervention should be implemented	How an intervention should be implemented

Several authors have defined types of scientific evidence for public health practice (**Table 23.1**).[5,11,39] Type 1 evidence defines the causes of diseases and the magnitude, severity, and preventability of risk factors and diseases. It suggests that "*something* should be done" about a particular disease or risk factor. Type 2 evidence describes the relative impact of specific interventions that do or do not improve health, adding "*specifically*, this should be done."[5] It has been noted that adherence to a strict hierarchy of study designs may reinforce an "inverse evidence law" by which interventions most likely to influence whole populations (e.g., policy change) are least valued in an evidence matrix emphasizing randomized designs.[50,51] A study from Sanson-Fisher and colleagues showed the relative lack of intervention research (Type 2) compared with descriptive/epidemiologic research (Type 1). In a random sample of published studies on tobacco use, alcohol use, and inadequate physical activity, their team found that in 2005–2006, 14.9% of studies reported on interventions whereas 78.5% of articles were descriptive or epidemiologic research.[52] There is likely to be even less published research on Type 3 evidence—which shows how and under what contextual conditions interventions were implemented and how they were received, thus informing "*how* something should be done."[39] Studies to date have tended to overemphasize internal validity (e.g., well controlled efficacy trials) while giving sparse attention to external validity (e.g., the translation of science to the various circumstances of practice).[53,54]

Understanding the Context for Evidence

Type 3 evidence derives from the context of an intervention.[39] While numerous authors have written about the role of context in informing evidence-based practice,[9,39,46,55–59] there is little consensus on its definition. When moving from clinical interventions to population-level and policy interventions, context becomes more uncertain, variable, and complex.[60] One useful

Table 23.2 Contextual Variables for Intervention Design, Implementation, and Adaptation

Category	Examples
Individual	Education level
	Basic human needs*
	Personal health history
Interpersonal	Family health history
	Support from peers
	Social capital
Organizational	Staff composition
	Staff expertise
	Physical infrastructure
	Organizational culture
Sociocultural	Social norms
	Values
	Cultural traditions
	History
Political and economic	Political will
	Political ideology
	Lobbying and special interests
	Costs and benefits

*Basic human needs include food, shelter, warmth, and safety.

definition of context highlights information needed to adapt and implement an evidence-based intervention in a particular setting or population.[39] The context for Type 3 evidence specifies five overlapping domains (**Table 23.2**). First, there are characteristics of the target population for an intervention such as education level and health history.[61] Next, interpersonal variables provide important context. For example, a person with a family history of cancer might be more likely to undergo cancer screening. Third, organizational variables should be considered. For example, whether an agency is successful in carrying out an evidence-based program will be influenced by its capacity (e.g., a trained workforce, agency leadership).[9,62] Fourth, social norms and culture are known to shape many health behaviors. Finally, larger political and economic forces affect context. For example, a high rate for a certain disease may influence a state's political will to address the issue in a meaningful and systematic way. Particularly for high-risk and understudied populations, there is a pressing need for evidence on contextual variables and ways of adapting programs and policies across settings and population subgroups. Contextual issues are being addressed more fully in the new "realist review," which is a systematic review process that seeks to examine not only whether an intervention works but also *how* interventions work in real-world settings.[63]

Issues Associated with Public Health Evidence

There are a number of issues associated with public health evidence, such as *underpopulated, dispersed,* and *different.*[64,65] Underpopulated refers to relatively few well done evaluations of public health interventions. Dispersed means information for public health decision making may be found in different sources rather than well concentrated, as in clinical interventions. Different has to do with the nature of public health evidence, which is typically derived from nonrandomized designs or so-called "natural experiments."[66]

Triangulating Evidence

Triangulation involves the accumulation of evidence from a variety of sources to gain insight into a particular topic[67] and often combines quantitative and qualitative data.[5] It generally involves the use of multiple methods of data collection and/or analysis to determine points of commonality or disagreement.[68] Triangulation is often beneficial because of the complementary nature of information from different sources. Though quantitative data provide an excellent opportunity to determine how variables are related for large numbers of people, these data provide little in the way of understanding why these relationships exist. Qualitative data, on the other hand, can help provide information to explain quantitative findings, or what has been called "illuminating meaning."[68] There are many examples of the use of triangulation of qualitative and quantitative data to evaluate health programs and policies, including AIDS prevention programs,[69] occupational health programs and policies,[70] and chronic disease prevention programs in community settings.[71] These examples also illustrate the roles of numerous disciplines in addressing pressing public health problems.

Cultural and Geographic Differences

So far, most of the tenets of EBPH have been developed in a Western, European-American context[72] with logical positivism as its foundation.[73,74] Thus, the evidence certainly does not capture what's happening in other parts of the world. Even in Western countries (including the United States), information published in peer-reviewed journals may not adequately represent all populations of interest.

Audiences for EBPH

There are four overlapping user groups for EBPH as defined by Fielding.[75] The first includes public health practitioners with executive and managerial responsibilities who want to know the scope and quality of evidence for alternative strategies (e.g., programs, policies). In practice, however, public health practitioners frequently have a relatively narrow set of options. Funds from federal, state, or local sources are most often earmarked for a specific purpose (e.g., surveillance and treatment of sexually transmitted diseases, inspection of retail food establishments). Still, the public health practitioner has the opportunity, even the obligation, to carefully review the evidence for alternative ways to achieve the desired health goals. The next user group is policymakers at local, regional, state, national, and international levels. They are faced with macro-level decisions on how to allocate the public resources for which they are stewards. This group has the additional responsibility of making policies on controversial public issues. The third group is composed of stakeholders who will be affected by any intervention. This includes the public, especially those who vote, and interest groups formed to support or oppose specific policies, such as the legality of abortion, whether the community water supply should be fluoridated, or whether adults must be issued handgun licenses if they pass background checks. The final user group is composed of researchers on population health issues, such as those who evaluate the impact of a specific policy or programs. They develop and use evidence to answer research questions.

Similarities and Differences Between EBPH and Evidence-Based Medicine

The concept of evidence-based practice is well established in numerous disciplines including psychology,[76] social work,[77,78] and nursing.[79] It is probably best established in medicine. The doctrine of evidence-based medicine (EBM) was formally introduced in 1992.[80] Its origins can be traced back to the seminal work of Cochrane that noted many medical treatments lacked scientific effectiveness.[81] A basic tenet of EBM is to de-emphasize unsystematic clinical experience and place greater emphasis on evidence from clinical research. This approach requires new skills, such as efficient literature searching and an understanding of types of evidence in evaluating the clinical literature.[82] There has been a rapid growth in the literature on EBM, contributing to its formal recognition. Using the search term "evidence-based medicine" in PubMed, there were 255 citations in 1990, rising to 8,141 citations in 2011 (**Figure 23.2**). Even though the formal terminology of EBM is relatively recent, its concepts are embedded in earlier efforts such as the Canadian Task Force for the Periodic Health Examination[83] and the *Guide to Clinical Preventive Services*.[84]

There are important distinctions between evidence-based approaches in medicine and public health. First, the type and volume of evidence differ. Medical studies of pharmaceuticals

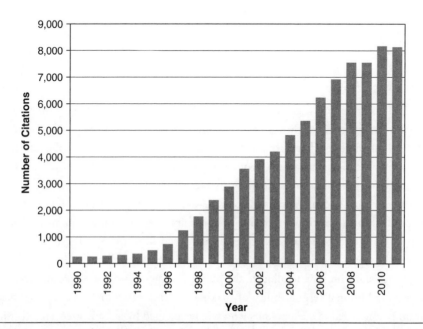

Figure 23.2   Citations for Evidence-Based Medicine

and procedures often rely on randomized controlled trials of individuals, the most scientifically rigorous of epidemiologic studies. In contrast, public health interventions usually rely on cross-sectional studies, quasi-experimental designs, and time-series analyses. These studies sometimes lack a comparison group and require more caveats in interpretation of results. Since the last half of the previous century, there have been more than 1 million randomized controlled trials of medical treatments.[85] There are many fewer studies of the effectiveness of public health interventions,[5,86] because they are difficult to design and often results derive from natural experiments (e.g., a state adopting a new policy compared to other states). EBPH has borrowed the term *intervention* from clinical disciplines, insinuating specificity and discreteness. However, in public health, we seldom have a single "intervention," but rather a program that involves a blending of several interventions within a community. Large community-based trials can be more expensive to conduct than randomized experiments in a clinic. Population-based studies generally require a longer time period between intervention and outcome. For example, a study on the effects of smoking cessation on lung cancer mortality would require decades of data collection and analysis. Contrast that with treatment of a medical condition (e.g., an antibiotic for symptoms of pneumonia), which is likely to produce effects in days or weeks, or even a surgical trial for cancer with endpoints of mortality within a few years.

The formal training of persons working in public health is much more variable than that in medicine or other clinical disciplines.[87] Unlike medicine, public health relies on a variety of disciplines and there is not a single academic credential that "certifies" a public health practitioner, although efforts to establish credentials (via an exam) are now underway. Fewer than half of public health workers have any formal training in a public health discipline such as epidemiology or health education.[88] This higher level of heterogeneity means that multiple perspectives are involved in a more complicated decision-making process. It also suggests that effective public health practice places a premium on routine, on-the-job training.

Key Characteristics of Evidence-Based Decision Making

There are a number of characteristics associated with evidence-based decision making, as summarized in **Box 23.1**. Achieving these characteristics would require a combination of scientific skills, enhanced communication, common sense, and political acumen.

Box 23.1   Characteristics of Evidence-Based Decision Making

- Using best available peer-reviewed evidence
- Using information systems
- Using program planning frameworks
- Using community
- Using sound evaluation
- Using input from key stakeholders

Using Best Available Peer-Reviewed Evidence

As one evaluates public health evidence, it is important to understand where to obtain the best possible scientific evidence. Examples are the scientific literature and guidelines developed by expert panels.

Once the issue to be considered has been clearly defined, the practitioner needs to become knowledgeable about previous or ongoing efforts to address the issue. This should include a systematic approach to identify, retrieve, and evaluate relevant reports on scientific studies, panels, and conferences related to the topic of interest. The most common method for initiating this investigation is a formal literature review. Many databases can facilitate such a review, the most common of which for public health purposes are MEDLARS, MEDLINE, PubMed, PsychInfo, Current Contents, HealthSTAR, and CancerLit. These databases can be subscribed to by an organization, can selectively be found on the Internet, or sometimes can be accessed by the public through institutions (such as the National Library of Medicine [http://www.nlm.nih.gov], universities, and public libraries). Many organizations also maintain websites that can be useful for identifying relevant information, including many state health departments, the Centers for Disease Control and Prevention (CDC), and the National Institutes of Health. It is important to remember that not all interventions (Type 2) studies will be found in the published literature.

Using Information Systems

Public health information systems have provided much evidence for decision making. For example, data are developed for local-level issues (e.g., SMART BRFSS) and efforts are underway to develop public health policy surveillance systems.[89–92]

Using Program Planning Frameworks

Program planning frameworks and theories can be used for public health decision making. An example is the ecological or systems models in which "appropriate changes in the social environment will produce changes in individuals, and the support of individuals in a population is seen as essential for implementing environmental changes."[93]

Engaging the Community

Community-based approaches involve community members in research and intervention projects and show progress in improving population health and addressing health disparities.[94,95] As a critical step in transdisciplinary problem solving, practitioners, academicians, and community members collaboratively define issues of concern, develop strategies for intervention, and evaluate the outcomes. This approach relies on stakeholder input,[96] builds on existing resources, facilitates collaboration among all parties, and integrates knowledge and action that seek to lead to a fair distribution of the benefits of an intervention for all partners.[95,97]

Using Sound Evaluation

Sound evaluation plans must be developed early in program development and should include formative and outcome evaluation. Qualitative and quantitative data may be used in framing an evaluation.[98]

Using Input from Stakeholders

Input from stakeholders is sought throughout the decision-making process. Stakeholders are those typically affected by the public health programs or policies. Examples are schools, worksites, healthcare settings, and broader community environments.

Analytic Tools and Approaches to Enhance the Uptake of EBPH

Several analytic tools and planning approaches can help practitioners in answering questions such as:[99]

- What is the size of the public health problem?
- Are there effective interventions for addressing the problem?
- What information about the local context and this particular intervention is helpful in deciding its potential use in the situation at hand?
- Is a particular program or policy worth doing (i.e., is it better than alternatives) and will it provide a satisfactory return on investment, measured in monetary terms or in health impacts?

Public Health Surveillance

Public health surveillance is a critical tool for those using EBPH. It involves the ongoing systematic collection, analysis, and interpretation of specific health data, closely integrated with the timely dissemination of these data to those responsible for preventing and controlling disease or injury.[100] Public health surveillance systems should have the capacity to collect and analyze data, disseminate data to public health programs, and regularly evaluate the effectiveness of the use of the disseminated data.[101] For example, documentation of the prevalence of elevated levels of lead (a known toxicant) in blood in the U.S. population was used as the justification for eliminating lead from paint and then gasoline and for documenting the effects of these actions.[102] In tobacco control, agreement on a common metric for tobacco use enabled comparisons across the states and an early recognition of the doubling and then tripling of the rates of decrease in smoking in California after passage of its Proposition 99,[103] and then a quadrupling of the rate of decline in Massachusetts compared with the other 48 states.[104]

Systematic Reviews and Evidence-Based Guidelines

Systematic reviews are syntheses of comprehensive collections of information on a particular topic. Reading a good review can be one of the most efficient ways to become familiar with state-of-the-art research and practice on many specific topics in public health.[105–107] The use of explicit, systematic methods (i.e., decision rules) in reviews limits bias and reduces chance effects, thus providing more reliable results upon which to make decisions.[108] One of the most useful sets of reviews for public health interventions is the *Guide to Community Preventive Services* (the *Community Guide*),[31,109] which provides an overview of current scientific literature through a well defined, rigorous method in which available studies themselves are the units of analysis. The *Community Guide* seeks to answer:

1. What interventions have been evaluated and what have been their effects?
2. What aspects of interventions can help guide users select from among the set of interventions of proven effectiveness?
3. What might this intervention cost and how does this compare with the likely health impacts?

A good systematic review should allow the practitioner to understand the local contextual conditions necessary for successful implementation.[110]

Economic Evaluation

Economic evaluation is an important component of evidence-based practice.[111] It can provide information to help assess the relative value of alternative expenditures on public health programs and policies. In cost–benefit analysis, all of the costs and consequences of the decision options are valued in monetary terms. More often, the economic investment associated with an intervention is compared with the health impacts, such as cases of disease prevented or years of life saved. This technique, cost-effectiveness analysis (CEA), can suggest the relative value of alternative interventions (i.e., health return on dollars invested).[111] CEA has become an increasingly important tool for researchers, practitioners, and policymakers. However, relevant data to support this type of analysis are not always available, especially for possible public policies designed to improve health.[49,112]

Health Impact Assessment

Health impact assessment (HIA) is a relatively new method that seeks to estimate the probable impact of a policy or intervention in nonhealth sectors, such as agriculture, transportation, and economic development, on the health of the population.[113] Some HIAs have focused on ensuring the involvement of relevant stakeholders in the development of a specific project. This latter approach, the basis of environmental impact assessment required by law for many large place-based projects, is similar to the nonregulatory approach that has been adopted for some HIAs. Overall, HIA, in both its forms, has been gaining acceptance as a tool because of mounting evidence that social and physical environments are important determinants of health and health disparities in populations. It is now being used to help assess the potential effects of many policies and programs on health status and outcomes.[114–116]

Participatory Approaches

Participatory approaches that actively involve community members in research and intervention projects[94,95,117] show promise in engaging communities in EBPH.[35] Practitioners, academicians, and community members collaboratively define issues of concern, develop strategies for intervention, and evaluate the outcomes. Stakeholders, or key players, are individuals or agencies that have a vested interest in the issue at hand.[118] In the development of health policies, for example, policymakers are especially important stakeholders.[119] Stakeholders should include those who would potentially receive, use, and benefit from the program or policy being considered. Three groups of stakeholders are relevant: people developing programs, those affected by interventions, and those who use results of program evaluations. Participatory approaches may also present challenges in adhering to EBPH principles, especially in reaching agreement on which approaches are most appropriate for addressing a particular health problem.[120]

An Approach to Increasing the Use of Evidence in Public Health Practice

Strengthening EBPH competencies needs to take into account the diverse education and training backgrounds of the workforce. The emphasis on principles of EBPH is not uniformly taught in all the disciplines represented in the public health workforce. For example, a public health nurse is likely to have had less training in how to locate the most current evidence and interpret alternatives than an epidemiologist. A recently graduated health educator with a master of public health (MPH) degree is more likely to have gained an understanding of the importance of EBPH than an environmental health specialist holding a bachelor's degree. Probably fewer than half of public health workers have any formal training in a public health discipline such as epidemiology or health education.[88] An even smaller percentage of these professionals have formal graduate training from a school of public health or other public health program. Currently, it appears that few public health departments have made continuing education about EBPH mandatory.

While the formal concept of EBPH is relatively new, the underlying skills are not. For example, reviewing the scientific literature for evidence or evaluating a program intervention are skills often taught in graduate programs in public health or other academic disciplines, and are building blocks of public health practice. The most commonly applied framework in EBPH is probably that of Brownson and colleagues (**Figure 23.3**), which uses a seven-stage process.[5,62,121] The process used in applying this framework is nonlinear and entails numerous iterations.[122] Competencies for more effective public health practice are becoming clearer.[123–125] For example, to carry out the EBPH process, the skills needed to make evidence-based decisions require a specific set of competencies (**Table 23.3**).[126] Many of the competencies on this list illustrate the value of developing partnerships and engaging diverse disciplines in the EBPH process.

To address these and similar competencies, EBPH training programs have been developed in the United States for public health professionals in state health agencies,[62,127] local health departments, and community-based organizations,[128,129] and similar programs have been developed in other countries.[121,130,131] Some programs show evidence of effectiveness.[62,129] The most common format uses didactic sessions, computer labs, and scenario-based exercises, taught by a faculty team with expertise in EBPH. The reach of these training programs can be increased by emphasizing a train-the-trainer approach.[121] Other formats have been used, including Internet-based self-study,[128,132] CD-ROMs[133] distance and distributed learning networks, and targeted technical assistance. Training programs may have greater impact when delivered by "change agents" who are perceived as experts yet share common characteristics and goals with trainees.[134] A commitment from leadership and staff to life-long learning is also an essential ingredient for success in training.[135]

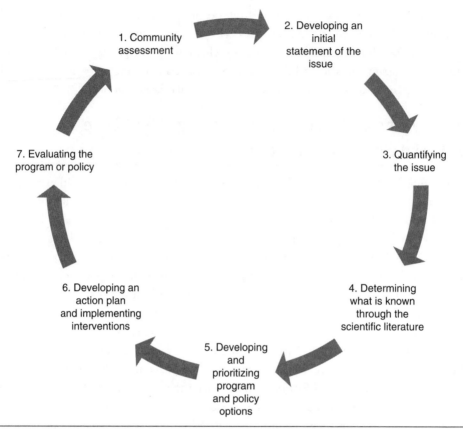

Figure 23.3   Training Approach for Evidence-Based Public Health
Source: Data from Brownson RC, Baker EA, Leet TL, Gillespie KN, True WR. *Evidence-Based Public Health.* 2nd ed. New York: Oxford University Press; 2011; and Brownson RC, Gurney JG, Land G. Evidence-based decision making in public health. *J Public Health Manag Pract.* 1999;5:86–97.

Implementation of training to address EBPH competencies should take into account principles of adult learning. These issues were recently articulated by Bryan and colleagues,[136] who highlighted the need to: 1) know why the audience is learning, 2) tap into an underlying motivation to learn by the need to solve problems, 3) respect and build upon previous experience, 4) design learning approaches that match the background and diversity of recipients, and 5) actively involve the audience in the learning process. A seven-stage, sequential framework to promote greater use of evidence in day-to-day decision making is briefly summarized in Figure 23.3.[11] It is important to note that this process is seldom a strictly prescriptive or linear one, but should include numerous feedback "loops" and processes that are common in many program planning models.

Future Outlook

The United States spends more than $30 billion annually on health-related research. A small portion of these expenditures is dedicated to research relevant to the practice of public health. Nonetheless, evidence for addressing a number of priority public health problems now exists.

Table 23.3   Potential Barriers and Solutions for Use of Evidence-Based Decision Making in Public Health[a]

Title	Domain[b]	Level[c]	Competency
1. Community input	C	B	Understand the importance of obtaining community input before planning and implementing evidence-based interventions.
2. Etiologic knowledge	E	B	Understand the relationship between risk factors and diseases.
3. Community assessment	C	B	Understand how to define the health issue according to the needs and assets of the population/community of interest.
4. Partnerships at multilevels	P/C	B	Understand the importance of identifying and developing partnerships in order to address the issue with evidence-based strategies at multiple levels.
5. Developing a concise statement of the issue	EBP	B	Understand the importance of developing a concise statement of the issue in order to build support for it.
6. Grant writing need	T/T	B	Recognize the importance of grant writing skills including the steps involved in the application process.
7. Literature searching	EBP	B	Understand the process for searching the scientific literature and summarizing search-derived information on the health issue.
8. Leadership and evidence	L	B	Recognize the importance of strong leadership from public health professionals regarding the need and importance of evidence-based public health interventions.
9. Role of behavioral science theory	T/T	B	Understand the role of behavioral science theory in designing, implementing, and evaluating interventions.
10. Leadership at all levels	L	B	Understand the importance of commitment from all levels of public health leadership to increase the use of evidence-based interventions.
11. Evaluation in 'plain English'	EV	I	Recognize the importance of translating the impacts of programs or policies in language that can be understood by communities, practice sectors, and policy makers.
12. Leadership and change	L	I	Recognize the importance of effective leadership from public health professionals when making decisions in the midst of ever changing environments.
13. Translating evidence-based interventions	EBP	I	Recognize the importance of translating evidence-based interventions to unique 'real-world' settings.
14. Quantifying the issue	T/T	I	Understand the importance of descriptive epidemiology (concepts of person, place, time) in quantifying the public health issue.

(continues)

Table 23.3 Potential Barriers and Solutions for Use of Evidence-Based Decision Making in Public Health[a] (continued)

Title	Domain[b]	Level[c]	Competency
15. Developing an action plan for program or policy	EBP	I	Understand the importance of developing a plan of action, which describes how the goals and objectives will be achieved, what resources are required, and how responsibility of achieving objectives will be assigned.
16. Prioritizing health issues	EBP	I	Understand how to choose and implement appropriate criteria and processes for prioritizing program and policy options.
17. Qualitative evaluation	EV	I	Recognize the value of qualitative evaluation approaches including the steps involved in conducting qualitative evaluations.
18. Collaborative partnerships	P/C	I	Understand the importance of collaborative partnerships between researchers and practitioners when designing, implementing, and evaluating evidence-based programs and policies.
19. Nontraditional partnerships	P/C	I	Understand the importance of traditional partnerships as well as those that have been considered nontraditional such as those with planners, department of transportation, and others.
20. Systematic reviews	T/T	I	Understand the rationale, uses, and usefulness of systematic reviews that document effective interventions.
21. Quantitative evaluation	EV	I	Recognize the importance of quantitative evaluation approaches including the concepts of measurement validity and reliability.
22. Grant writing skills	T/T	I	Demonstrate the ability to create a grant including an outline of the steps involved in the application process.
23. Role of economic evaluation	T/T	A	Recognize the importance of using economic data and strategies to evaluate costs and outcomes when making public health decisions.
24. Creating policy briefs	P	A	Understand the importance of writing concise policy briefs to address the issue using evidence-based interventions.
25. Evaluation designs	EV	A	Comprehend the various designs useful in program evaluation with a particular focus on quasi-experimental (nonrandomized) designs.
26. Transmitting evidence-based research to policy makers	P	A	Understand the importance of coming up with creative ways of transmitting what we know works (evidence-based interventions) to policy makers in order to gain interest, political support and funding.

[a]Adapted from Brownson et al.[121]

[b]C = community-level planning; E = etiology; P/C = partnerships and collaboration; EBP = evidence-based process; T/T = theory and analytic tools; L = leadership; EV = evaluation; P = policy;

[c]B = beginner; I = intermediate; A = advanced

Unfortunately, the translation from research to clinical or community applications often occurs only after a delay of many years.[37,137,138] To accelerate the production of new evidence and the adoption of evidence-based interventions to protect and improve health requires several actions.

Expanding the Evidence Base

The growing literature on the effectiveness of preventive interventions in clinical and community settings[31,32] does not provide equal coverage of health problems. For example, the evidence base on how to increase immunization levels is much stronger than how to prevent HIV infection or reduce alcohol abuse. A greater investment of resources to expand the evidence base is therefore essential. Even where we have interventions of proven effectiveness, the populations in which they have been tested often do not include subpopulations with the greatest disease and injury burden. Expanding the base of evidence requires reliance on well tested conceptual frameworks, especially those that pay close attention to dissemination and implementation. For example, RE-AIM helps program planners and evaluators to pay explicit attention to *r*each, *e*fficacy/effectiveness, *a*doption, *i*mplementation, and *m*aintenance.[139,140]

Overcoming Barriers to Dissemination and Implementation

More knowledge is needed on effective mechanisms to translate evidence-based practice to public health settings. Several important questions deserve answers:

- Why have some types of evidence languished while others have been quickly adopted?
- What dissemination and implementation strategies appear to be most cost-effective?
- How can funding agencies accelerate the replication and adaptation of evidence-based interventions in a variety of settings and populations?
- What specific processes best integrate community health assessment and improvement activities into health system planning efforts?
- How can we harness new tools, such as the Internet, to improve intervention effectiveness and dissemination?
- What changes in organizational culture that promote innovation and adoption of EBPH are feasible?
- How can we increase attention on external validity in the production and systematic reviews of evidence?

Engaging Leadership

As noted earlier, leadership is essential to promote adoption of EBPH as a core part of public health practice.[141] This includes an expectation that decisions will be made on the basis of the best science, needs of the target population, and what will work locally. In some cases additional funding may be required, but in many circumstances not having the will to change (rather than dollars) is the major impediment. Use of EBPH should be incorporated as part of performance reviews for key public health personnel and as part of explicit goals and objectives for all program directors.

Expanding Training Opportunities

More practitioner-focused training is needed on the rationale for EBPH, how to select interventions, how to adapt them to particular circumstances, and how to monitor their implementation. The Task Force on Workforce Development has recommended that the essential public health services[142] be used as a framework to build the basic, cross-cutting, and technical competencies required to address public health problems. As outlined in this chapter, a framework for EBPH is likely to be useful (Figure 23.3).[126,138] Because many of the health issues needing urgent attention in local communities will require the involvement of other organizations (e.g., nonprofit groups, hospitals, employers), their participation in training efforts is essential.

Enhancing Accountability for Public Expenditures

Public funds should be targeted to support evidence-based strategies. Grants made by public health agencies to outside organizations should contain language explicitly requiring use of such strategies, when they exist, to justify expenditure of funds. While the science base for many topics is still evolving, it is irresponsible not to use existing evidence in the design and implementation of proven public health interventions. Evaluations of such efforts can thus contribute to a better understanding of what works in different settings. Simultaneously, the adoption of EBPH by the public health system as a whole and its impact on the community's health should be tracked. A central criterion in the accreditation of public health departments, currently being implemented,[143] is the use of best evidence in every effort to improve health and health equity.

Understanding How to Better Use EBPH to Address Disparities

To what degrees do specific evidence-based approaches reduce disparities while improving overall current and/or future health? For many interventions there is not a clear answer to this question. Despite national health goals focusing on the elimination of health disparities, recent data show large and growing differences in disease burden and health outcomes between high- and low-income groups.[144] Most of the existing intervention research has been conducted among higher income populations, and programs focusing on elimination of health disparities have often been short-lived.[145] Yet, in both developed and developing countries, poverty is strongly correlated with poor health outcomes.[146] When enough evidence exists, systematic reviews should focus specifically on interventions that show promise in eliminating health disparities.[147,148] Policy interventions hold the potential to influence health determinants more broadly and could significantly reduce the growing disparities across a wide range of health problems.[149]

Summary

The successful implementation of EBPH in public health practice is both a science and an art. The science is built on epidemiologic, behavioral, and policy research showing the size and scope of a public health problem and which interventions are likely to be effective in addressing the problem. The art of decision making often involves knowing what information is important to a particular stakeholder at the right time. Unlike solving a math problem, significant decisions in public health must balance science and art, since rational, evidence-based decision making often involves choosing one alternative from among a set of rational choices. Success in public health problem solving relies on a transdisciplinary approach, leadership, and sound management practices. By applying the concepts of EBPH outlined in this chapter, decision making, and, ultimately, public health practice can be improved.

Discussion Questions

1. If one is seeking to find more Type 3 (contextual evidence), what are the methods for obtaining this information?
2. In understanding the seven-stage framework for EBPH, what are the core public health disciplines that might be most useful or informative within each of the seven stages?
3. Choose an important current public health problem. In addressing this problem, think about which disciplines outside of the health sector might be important for addressing the issue.
4. For the same problem, how might participatory approaches help you in engaging these various disciplines or sectors?
5. In addition to the barriers to EBPH covered in this chapter, consider barriers that might limit your ability to implement a transdisciplinary approach to evidence-based decision making. How might you begin to overcome these barriers?
6. Consider two future issues in EBPH. How might a public health practitioner best address these issues in a state or local public health agency? What immediate steps could be taken?

Acknowledgment

Parts of this chapter were adapted with permission, from the *Annual Review of Public Health*, Volume 30 ©2009 by Annual Reviews http://www.annualreviews.org. The author is also grateful for the input of Jonathan Fielding and Christopher Maylahn. The principles in this chapter were developed in part due to support from Cooperative Agreement Number U48/DP001903 from the Centers for Disease Control and Prevention (the Prevention Research Centers Program).

References

1. National Center for Health Statistics. *Health, United States, 2000 with Adolescent Health Chartbook.* Hyattsville, MD: Centers for Disease Control and Prevention, National Center for Health Statistics; 2000.
2. Centers for Disease Control and Prevention. *Public Health in the New American Health System. Discussion Paper.* Atlanta, GA: Centers for Disease Control and Prevention; 1993.
3. Muir Gray JA. *Evidence-Based Healthcare: How to Make Health Policy and Management Decisions.* New York and Edinburgh: Churchill Livingstone; 1997.
4. Brownson RC, Fielding JE, Maylahn CM. Evidence-based public health: a fundamental concept for public health practice. *Annu Rev Public Health.* 2009;30:175–201.
5. Brownson RC, Baker EA, Leet TL, et al. *Evidence-Based Public Health.* 2nd ed. New York: Oxford University Press; 2011.

6. Glasziou P, Longbottom H. Evidence-based public health practice. *Aust NZ J Public Health.* 1999;23(4):436–40.

7. McMichael C, Waters E, Volmink J. Evidence-based public health: what does it offer developing countries? *J Public Health (Oxf).* 2005;27(2):215–21.

8. Fielding JE, Briss PA. Promoting evidence-based public health policy: can we have better evidence and more action? *Health Aff (Millwood).* 2006;25(4):969–78.

9. Hausman AJ. Implications of evidence-based practice for community health. *Am J Community Psychol.* 2002;30(3):453–67.

10. Kohatsu ND, Melton RJ. A health department perspective on the Guide to Community Preventive Services. *Am J Prev Med.* 2000;18(1 Suppl):3–4.

11. Brownson RC, Gurney JG, Land G. Evidence-based decision making in public health. *J Public Health Manag Pract.* 1999;5:86–97.

12. McGinnis JM. Does proof matter? why strong evidence sometimes yields weak action. *Am J Health Promot.* 2001;15(5):391–6.

13. Fielding JE. Where is the evidence? *Annu Rev Public Health.* 2001;22:v–vi.

14. Institute of Medicine, Committee for the Study of the Future of Public Health. *The Future of Public Health.* Washington, DC: National Academies Press; 1988.

15. Anderson J. "Don't confuse me with facts...": evidence-based practice confronts reality. *Med J Aust.* 1999;170(10):465–6.

16. Baker EL, Potter MA, Jones DL, et al. The public health infrastructure and our nation's health. *Annu Rev Public Health.* 2005;26:303–18.

17. Haynes B, Haines A. Barriers and bridges to evidence based clinical practice. *BMJ.* 1998;317(7153): 273–6.

18. Catford J. Creating political will: moving from the science to the art of health promotion. *Health Promot Int.* 2006;21(1):1–4.

19. Murphy K, Wolfus B, Lofters A. From complex problems to complex problem-solving: transdisciplinary practice as knowledge translation. In: Kirst M, Schaefer-McDaniel N, Hwang S, et al., eds. *Converging Disciplines: A Transdisciplinary Research Approach to Urban Health Problems.* New York: Springer; 2011:111–29.

20. Roussos ST, Fawcett SB. A review of collaborative partnerships as a strategy for improving community health. *Annu Rev Public Health.* 2000;21:369–402.

21. Harper GW, Neubauer LC, Bangi AK, et al. Transdisciplinary research and evaluation for community health initiatives. *Health Promot Pract.* 2008;9(4):328–37.

22. Stokols D. Toward a science of transdisciplinary action research. *Am J Community Psychol.* 2006;38 (1-2):63–77.

23. Kobus K, Mermelstein R. Bridging basic and clinical science with policy studies: the Partners with Transdisciplinary Tobacco Use Research Centers experience. *Nicotine Tob Res.* 2009;11(5):467–74.

24. Kobus K, Mermelstein R, Ponkshe P. Communications strategies to broaden the reach of tobacco use research: examples from the Transdisciplinary Tobacco Use Research Centers. *Nicotine Tob Res.* 2007;9(Suppl 4):S571–82.

25. Morgan GD, Kobus K, Gerlach KK, et al. Facilitating transdisciplinary research: the experience of the transdisciplinary tobacco use research centers. *Nicotine Tob Res.* 2003;5(Suppl 1):S11–19.

26. Byrne S, Wake M, Blumberg D, et al. Identifying priority areas for longitudinal research in childhood obesity: Delphi technique survey. *Int J Pediatr Obes.* 2008;3(2):120–2.

27. Russell-Mayhew S, Scott C, et al. The Canadian Obesity Network and interprofessional practice: members' views. *J Interprof Care.* 2008;22(2):149–65.

28. Black BL, Cowens-Alvarado R, Gershman S, et al. Using data to motivate action: the need for high quality, an effective presentation, and an action context for decision-making. *Cancer Causes Control.* 2005;16(Suppl 1):15–25.

29. Curry S, Byers T, Hewitt M, eds. *Fulfilling the Potential of Cancer Prevention and Early Detection.* Washington, DC: National Academies Press; 2003.

30. Briss PA, Brownson RC, Fielding JE, et al. Developing and using the Guide to Community Preventive Services: lessons learned about evidence-based public health. *Annu Rev Public Health.* 2004;25:281–302.

31. Zaza S, Briss PA, Harris KW, eds. *The Guide to Community Preventive Services: What Works to Promote Health?* New York: Oxford University Press; 2005.

32. Agency for Healthcare Research and Quality. *Guide to Clinical Preventive Services.* 3rd ed. Available at: http://www.ahrq.gov/professionals/clinicians-providers/guidelines-recommendations/guide/guide-clinical-preventive-services.pdf. Accessed October 11, 2005, 2005.

33. Cancer Control PLANET. Links resources to comprehensive cancer control. Available at: http://www.cancercontrolplanet.org/. Accessed March 21, 2013.

34. Substance Abuse and Mental Health Services Administration. SAMHSA's National Registry of Evidence-based Programs and Practices. Available at: http://www.nrepp.samhsa.gov/. Accessed March 21, 2013.

35. Kohatsu ND, Robinson JG, Torner JC. Evidence-based public health: an evolving concept. *Am J Prev Med.* 2004;27(5):417–21.

36. Green LW. Public health asks of systems science: to advance our evidence-based practice, can you help us get more practice-based evidence? *Am J Public Health.* 2006;96(3):406–9.

37. Kerner J, Rimer B, Emmons K. Introduction to the special section on dissemination: dissemination research and research dissemination: how can we close the gap? *Health Psychol.* 2005;24(5):443–6.

38. Jenicek M. Epidemiology, evidence-based medicine, and evidence-based public health. *J Epidemiol Commun Health.* 1997;7:187–97.

39. Rychetnik L, Hawe P, Waters E, et al. A glossary for evidence based public health. *J Epidemiol Community Health.* 2004;58(7):538–45.

40. Satterfield JM, Spring B, Brownson RC, et al. Toward a transdisciplinary model of evidence-based practice. *Milbank Q.* 2009;87(2):368–90.

41. McKean E, ed. *The New Oxford American Dictionary.* 2nd ed. New York: Oxford University Press; 2005.

42. McQueen DV. Strengthening the evidence base for health promotion. *Health Promot Int.* 2001;16(3):261–8.

43. Chambers D, Kerner J. Closing the gap between discovery and delivery. *Dissemination and Implementation Research Workshop: Harnessing Science to Maximize Health.* Rockville, MD; 2007.

44. McQueen DV, Anderson LM. What counts as evidence? Issues and debates. In: Rootman I, ed. *Evaluation in Health Promotion: Principles and Perspectives.* Copenhagen, Denmark: World Health Organization; 2001:63–81.

45. Rimer BK, Glanz DK, Rasband G. Searching for evidence about health education and health behavior interventions. *Health Educ Behav.* 2001;28(2):231–48.

46. Kerner JF. Integrating research, practice, and policy: what we see depends on where we stand. *J Public Health Manag Pract.* 2008;14(2):193–8.

47. Mulrow CD, Lohr KN. Proof and policy from medical research evidence. *J Health Polit Policy Law.* 2001;26(2):249–66.

48. Sturm R. Evidence-based health policy versus evidence-based medicine. *Psychiatr Serv.* 2002;53(12):1499.

49. Brownson RC, Royer C, Ewing R, et al. Researchers and policymakers: travelers in parallel universes. *Am J Prev Med.* 2006;30(2):164–72.

50. Nutbeam D. How does evidence influence public health policy? Tackling health inequalities in England. *Health Promot J Aust.* 2003;14:154–8.

51. Ogilvie D, Egan M, Hamilton V, Petticrew M. Systematic reviews of health effects of social interventions: 2. Best available evidence: how low should you go? *J Epidemiol Community Health.* 2005;59(10):886–92.

52. Sanson-Fisher RW, Campbell EM, Htun AT, Bailey LJ, Millar CJ. We are what we do: research outputs of public health. *Am J Prev Med.* Oct 2008;35(4):380–85.

53. Glasgow RE, Green LW, Klesges LM, et al. External validity: we need to do more. *Ann Behav Med.* 2006;31(2):105–8.

54. Green LW, Glasgow RE. Evaluating the relevance, generalization, and applicability of research: issues in external validation and translation methodology. *Eval Health Prof.* 2006;29(1):126–53.

55. Castro FG, Barrera M, Jr., Martinez CR, Jr. The cultural adaptation of prevention interventions: resolving tensions between fidelity and fit. *Prev Sci.* 2004;5(1):41–5.

56. Kerner JF, Guirguis-Blake J, Hennessy KD, et al. Translating research into improved outcomes in comprehensive cancer control. *Cancer Causes Control.* 2005;16(Suppl 1):27–40.

57. Rychetnik L, Frommer M, Hawe P, Shiell A. Criteria for evaluating evidence on public health interventions. *J Epidemiol Community Health.* 2002;56(2):119–27.

58. Glasgow RE. What types of evidence are most needed to advance behavioral medicine? *Ann Behav Med.* 2008;35(1):19–25.

59. Kemm J. The limitations of 'evidence-based' public health. *J Eval Clin Pract.* 2006;12(3):319–24.

60. Dobrow MJ, Goel V, Upshur RE. Evidence-based health policy: context and utilisation. *Soc Sci Med.* 2004;58(1):207–17.

61. Maslov A. A theory of human motivation. *Psychol Rev.* 1943;50:370–96.

62. Dreisinger M, Leet TL, Baker EA, et al. Improving the public health workforce: evaluation of a training course to enhance evidence-based decision making. *J Public Health Manag Pract.* 2008;14(2):138–43.

63. Pawson R, Greenhalgh T, Harvey G, et al. Realist review—a new method of systematic review designed for complex policy interventions. *J Health Serv Res Policy.* 2005;10(Suppl 1):21–34.

64. Millward L, Kelly M, Nutbeam D. *Public Health Interventions Research: The Evidence.* London: Health Development Agency; 2003.

65. Petticrew M, Roberts H. Systematic reviews—do they 'work' in informing decision-making around health inequalities? *Health Econ Policy Law.* 2008;3(Pt 2):197–211.

66. Petticrew M, Cummins S, Ferrell C, et al. Natural experiments: an underused tool for public health? *Public Health.* 2005;119(9):751–7.

67. Tones K. Beyond the randomized controlled trial: a case for 'judicial review.' *Health Educ Res.* 1997; 12(2):i–iv.

68. Steckler A, McLeroy KR, Goodman RM, et al. Toward integrating qualitative and quantitative methods: an introduction. *Health Educ Q.* 1992;19(1):1–8.

69. Dorfman LE, Derish PA, Cohen JB. Hey girlfriend: an evaluation of AIDS prevention among women in the sex industry. *Health Educ Q.* 1992;19(1):25–40.

70. Hugentobler M, Israel BA, Schurman SJ. An action research approach to workplace health: integrating methods. *Health Educ Q.* 1992;19(1):55–76.

71. Goodman RM, Wheeler FC, Lee PR. Evaluation of the Heart to Heart Project: lessons from a community-based chronic disease prevention project. *Am J Health Promot.* 1995;9:443–55.

72. McQueen DV. The evidence debate. *J Epidemiol Community Health.* 2002;56(2):83–4.

73. Suppe F. *The Structure of Scientific Theories.* 2nd ed. Urbana, IL: University of Illinois Press; 1977.

74. Cavill N, Foster C, Oja P, et al. An evidence-based approach to physical activity promotion and policy development in Europe: contrasting case studies. *Promot Educ.* 2006;13(2):104–11.

75. Fielding JE. Foreword. In: Brownson RC, Baker EA, Leet TL, et al., eds. *Evidence-Based Public Health.* New York: Oxford University Press; 2003:v–vii.

76. Presidential Task Force on Evidence-Based Practice. Evidence-based practice in psychology. *Am Psychol.* 2006;61(4):271–85.

77. Gambrill E. Evidence-based practice: sea change or the emperor's new clothes? *J Social Work Educ.* 2003;39(1):3–23.

78. Mullen E, Bellamy J, Bledsoe S, et al. Teaching evidence-based practice. *Res Social Work Prac.* 2007;17(5):574–82.

79. Melnyk BM, Fineout-Overholt E, Stone P, et al. Evidence-based practice: the past, the present, and recommendations for the millennium. *Pediatr Nurs.* 2000;26(1):77–80.

80. Evidence-Based Medicine Working Group. Evidence-based medicine. A new approach to teaching the practice of medicine. *JAMA.* 1992;17:2420–5.

81. Cochrane A. *Effectiveness and Efficiency: Random Reflections on Health Services.* London: Nuffield Provincial Hospital Trust; 1972.

82. Guyatt G, Cook D, Haynes B. Evidence based medicine has come a long way. *BMJ.* 2004;329(7473): 990–1.

83. Canadian Task Force on the Periodic Health Examination. The periodic health examination. Canadian Task Force on the Periodic Health Examination. *Can Med Assoc J.* 1979;121(9):1193–254.

84. U.S. Preventive Services Task Force. *Guide to Clinical Preventive Services: An Assessment of the Effectiveness of 169 Interventions.* Baltimore: Williams & Wilkins; 1989.

85. Taubes G. Looking for the evidence in medicine. *Science.* 1996;272:22–24.

86. Oldenburg BF, Sallis JF, French ML, et al. Health promotion research and the diffusion and institutionalization of interventions. *Health Educ Res.* 1999;14(1):121–30.

87. Tilson H, Gebbie KM. The public health workforce. *Annu Rev Public Health.* 2004;25:341–56.

88. Turnock BJ. *Public Health: What It Is and How It Works.* 3rd ed. Gaithersburg, MD: Aspen Publishers; 2004.

89. Chriqui JF, Frosh MM, Brownson RC, et al. Measuring policy and legislative change. *Evaluating ASSIST: A Blueprint for Understanding State-Level Tobacco Control.* Bethesda, MD: National Cancer Institute; 2006.

90. Masse LC, Chriqui JF, Igoe JF, et al. Development of a physical education-related state policy classification system (PERSPCS). *Am J Prev Med.* 2007;33(4, Suppl 1):S264–76.

91. Masse LC, Frosh MM, Chriqui JF, et al. Development of a school nutrition-environment state policy classification system (SNESPCS). *Am J Prev Med.* 2007;33(4, Suppl 1):S277–91.

92. National Institute on Alcohol Abuse and Alcoholism. *Alcohol Policy Information System.* Available at: http://alcoholpolicy.niaaa.nih.gov/. Accessed March 21, 2013.

93. McLeroy KR, Bibeau D, Steckler A, et al. An ecological perspective on health promotion programs. *Health Educ Q.* 1988;15:351–77.

94. Cargo M, Mercer SL. The value and challenges of participatory research: strengthening its practice. *Annu Rev Public Health.* 2008;29:325–50.

95. Israel BA, Schulz AJ, Parker EA, et al. Review of community-based research: assessing partnership approaches to improve public health. *Ann Rev Public Health.* 1998;19:173–202.

96. Green LW, Mercer SL. Can public health researchers and agencies reconcile the push from funding bodies and the pull from communities? *Am J Public Health.* 2001;91(12):1926–9.

97. Leung MW, Yen IH, Minkler M. Community based participatory research: a promising approach for increasing epidemiology's relevance in the 21st century. *Int J Epidemiol.* 2004;33(3):499–506.

98. Land G, Romeis JC, Gillespie KN, Denny S. Missouri's Take a Seat, Please! and program evaluation. *J Public Health Manag Pract.* 1997;3(6):51–8.

99. Jacobs J, Jones E, Gabella B, et al. Tools for implementing an evidence-based approach in public health practice. *Prev Chronic Dis.* 2012;9:110324.

100. Thacker SB, Berkelman RL. Public health surveillance in the United States. *Epidemiol Rev.* 1988;10: 164–90.

101. Thacker SB, Stroup DF. Public health surveillance. In: Brownson RC, Petitti DB, eds. *Applied Epidemiology: Theory to Practice.* 2nd ed. New York: Oxford University Press; 2006: 30–67.

102. Annest JL, Pirkle JL, Makuc D, et al. Chronological trend in blood lead levels between 1976 and 1980. *N Engl J Med.* 1983;308:1373–7.

103. Tobacco Education and Research Oversight Committee for California. *Confronting a Relentless Adversary: A Plan for Success: Toward a Tobacco-Free California, 2006–2008.* Sacramento, CA: California Department of Public Health; 2006.

104. Biener L, Harris JE, Hamilton W. Impact of the Massachusetts tobacco control programme: population based trend analysis. *BMJ.* 2000;321(7257):351–4.

105. Hutchison BG. Critical appraisal of review articles. *Can Fam Physician.* 1993;39:1097–102.

106. Milne R, Chambers L. Assessing the scientific quality of review articles. *J Epidemiol Community Health.* 1993;47(3):169–70.

107. Mulrow CD. The medical review article: state of the science. *Ann Intern Med.* 1987;106(3):485–8.

108. Oxman AD, Guyatt GH. The science of reviewing research. *Ann N Y Acad Sci.* 1993;703:125–33.

109. Mullen PD, Ramirez G. The promise and pitfalls of systematic reviews. *Annu Rev Public Health.* 2006;27:81–102.

110. Waters E, Doyle J. Evidence-based public health practice: improving the quality and quantity of the evidence. *J Public Health Med.* 2002;24(3):227–9.

111. Gold MR, Siegel JE, Russell LB, et al. *Cost-Effectiveness in Health and Medicine.* New York: Oxford University Press; 1996.

112. Carande-Kulis VG, Maciosek MV, Briss PA, et al. Methods for systematic reviews of economic evaluations for the Guide to Community Preventive Services. Task Force on Community Preventive Services. *Am J Prev Med.* 2000;18(1 Suppl):75–91.

113. Harris P, Harris-Roxas B, Harris E, et al. *Health Impact Assessment: A Practical Guide.* Sydney: Australia: Centre for Health Equity Training, Research and Evaluation (CHETRE). Part of the UNSW Research Centre for Primary Health Care and Equity, UNSW; 2007.

114. Cole BL, Wilhelm M, Long PV, et al. Prospects for health impact assessment in the United States: new and improved environmental impact assessment or something different? *J Health Polit Policy Law.* 2004;29(6):1153–86.

115. Kemm J. Health impact assessment: a tool for healthy public policy. *Health Promot Int.* 2001;16(1): 79–85.

116. Mindell J, Sheridan L, Joffe M, et al. Health impact assessment as an agent of policy change: improving the health impacts of the mayor of London's draft transport strategy. *J Epidemiol Community Health.* 2004;58(3):169–74.

117. Green LW, George MA, Daniel M, et al. *Review and Recommendations for the Development of Participatory Research in Health Promotion in Canada.* Vancouver, British Columbia: The Royal Society of Canada; 1995.

118. Soriano FI. *Conducting Needs Assessments. A Multidisciplinary Approach.* Thousand Oaks, CA: Sage Publications; 1995.

119. Sederburg WA. Perspectives of the legislator: allocating resources. *MMWR.* 1992;41(Suppl):37–48.

120. Hallfors D, Cho H, Livert D, et al. Fighting back against substance abuse: are community coalitions winning? *Am J Prev Med.* 2002;23(4):237–45.

121. Brownson RC, Diem G, Grabauskas V, et al. Training practitioners in evidence-based chronic disease prevention for global health. *Promot Educ.* 2007;14(3):159–63.

122. Tugwell P, Bennett KJ, Sackett DL, et al. The measurement iterative loop: a framework for the critical appraisal of need, benefits and costs of health interventions. *J Chronic Dis.* 1985;38(4):339–51.

123. Birkhead GS, Davies J, Miner K, et al. Developing competencies for applied epidemiology: from process to product. *Public Health Rep.* 2008;123(Suppl 1):67–118.

124. Birkhead GS, Koo D. Professional competencies for applied epidemiologists: a roadmap to a more effective epidemiologic workforce. *J Public Health Manag Pract.* 2006;12(6):501–4.

125. Gebbie K, Merrill J, Hwang I, et al. Identifying individual competency in emerging areas of practice: an applied approach. *Qual Health Res.* 2002;12(7):990–9.

126. Brownson R, Ballew P, Kittur N, et al. Developing competencies for training practitioners in evidence-based cancer control. *J Cancer Educ.* 2009;24(3):186–93.

127. Baker EA, Brownson RC, Dreisinger M, et al. Examining the role of training in evidence-based public health: a qualitative study. *Health Promot Pract.* 2009;10(3):342–8.

128. Maxwell ML, Adily A, Ward JE. Promoting evidence-based practice in population health at the local level: a case study in workforce capacity development. *Aust Health Rev.* 2007;31(3):422–9.

129. Maylahn C, Bohn C, Hammer M, et al. Strengthening epidemiologic competencies among local health professionals in New York: teaching evidence-based public health. *Public Health Rep.* 2008;123 (Suppl 1):35–43.

130. Oliver KB, Dalrymple P, Lehmann HP, et al. Bringing evidence to practice: a team approach to teaching skills required for an informationist role in evidence-based clinical and public health practice. *J Med Libr Assoc.* 2008;96(1):50–7.

131. Pappaioanou M, Malison M, Wilkins K, et al. Strengthening capacity in developing countries for evidence-based public health: the data for decision-making project. *Soc Sci Med.* 2003;57(10):1925–37.

132. Linkov F, LaPorte R, Lovalekar M, et al. Web quality control for lectures: Supercourse and Amazon.com. *Croat Med J.* 2005;46(6):875–8.

133. Brownson RC, Ballew P, Brown KL, et al. The effect of disseminating evidence-based interventions that promote physical activity to health departments. *Am J Public Health.* 2007;97(10):1900–7.

134. Proctor EK. Leverage points for the implementation of evidence-based practice. *Brief Treatment Crisis Intervention.* 2004;4(3):227–42.

135. Chambers LW. The new public health: do local public health agencies need a booster (or organizational "fix") to combat the diseases of disarray? *Can J Public Health.* 1992;83(5):326–8.

136. Bryan RL, Kreuter MW, Brownson RC. Integrating adult learning principles into training for public health practice. *Health Promot Pract.* 2009;10(4):557–63.

137. Balas EA. From appropriate care to evidence-based medicine. *Pediatr Ann.* 1998;27(9):581–4.

138. Brownson RC, Baker EA, Leet TL, et al. *Evidence-Based Public Health.* New York: Oxford University Press; 2003.

139. Glasgow RE, Vogt TM, Boles SM. Evaluating the public health impact of health promotion interventions: the RE-AIM framework. *Am J Public Health.* 1999;89(9):1322–7.

140. Jilcott S, Ammerman A, Sommers J, et al. Applying the RE-AIM framework to assess the public health impact of policy change. *Ann Behav Med.* 2007;34(2):105–14.

141. Scutchfield FD, Knight EA, Kelly AV, et al. Local public health agency capacity and its relationship to public health system performance. *J Public Health Manag Pract.* 2004;10(3):204–15.

142. Centers for Disease Control and Prevention. *CDC Taskforce on Public Health Workforce Development.* Atlanta, GA: CDC; 1999.

143. Tilson HH. Public health accreditation: progress on national accountability. *Annu Rev Public Health.* 2008;29:xv–xxii.

144. Ezzati M, Friedman AB, Kulkarni SC, et al. The reversal of fortunes: trends in county mortality and cross-county mortality disparities in the United States. *PLoS Med.* 2008;5(4):e66.

145. Shaya FT, Gu A, Saunders E. Addressing cardiovascular disparities through community interventions. *Ethn Dis.* 2006;16(1):138–44.

146. Subramanian SV, Belli P, Kawachi I. The macroeconomic determinants of health. *Annu Rev Public Health.* 2002;23:287–302.

147. Masi CM, Blackman DJ, Peek ME. Interventions to enhance breast cancer screening, diagnosis, and treatment among racial and ethnic minority women. *Med Care Res Rev.* 2007;64(5 Suppl):195S–242S.

148. Peek ME, Cargill A, Huang ES. Diabetes health disparities: a systematic review of health care interventions. *Med Care Res Rev.* 2007;64(5 Suppl):101S–56S.

149. Brownson RC, Haire-Joshu D, Luke DA. Shaping the context of health: a review of environmental and policy approaches in the prevention of chronic diseases. *Annu Rev Public Health.* 2006;27:341–70.

Social Entrepreneurship and Public Health

Kristine Marin Kawamura, Nailya O. DeLellis,
and Ormanbek T. Zhuzzhanov

LEARNING OBJECTIVES

- To evaluate the variations among several definitions of social entrepreneurship, and distinguish critical differences and similarities among them
- To recognize the role of the principles of social entrepreneurship in public health and how those principles have been applied to enhance public health services
- To appreciate the role of leadership of individuals and of organizations in initiating and sustaining programs and interventions defined as social entrepreneurship in public health, and the extent of leadership training and educational opportunities available in this field
- To observe the variety of institutional settings and populations served by social entrepreneurship in public health
- To comprehend the wide range of organizational structures, financial supports, and interorganizational relationships of successful social entrepreneurship projects in public health

Chapter Overview

Problems facing the world's public health systems cannot be controlled or even managed by public health systems alone, nor are the problems they face the responsibility only of the public health systems. Rather, the public health challenges encountered and anticipated in all societies are the responsibility of all sectors in those societies. Social entrepreneurship is one important manifestation of how many individuals and organizations within societies may imagine solutions, collaborate to focus resources, and intervene to address public health problems.

Social entrepreneurship in public health is a growing benevolent force of ideas and actions. Pervading the entire spectrum of the public health system, social entrepreneurship enhances the efforts of private, nonprofit, and governmental public health entities. It augments centrally planned national and state public health systems with individually inspired movements to cross organizational boundaries, fill gaps, identify solutions, implement interventions, raise consciousness, and educate.

This chapter first explores the foundation of social entrepreneurship in the tradition of business entrepreneurship. Multiple definitions of social entrepreneurship are then provided, with the goal of providing a consensus definition that will prove useful in understanding the phenomenon. Qualities of social entrepreneurs are provided as a baseline for developing personal leadership competencies and assessing the effectiveness of individual visionaries. A framework for describing social entrepreneurship in public health is provided in order to position it within greater complexities of market, organizational, and governmental environments, and key principles are arrayed from the more salient proponents of the movement in public health. A significant portion of the chapter is dedicated to illustrations of sustained social entrepreneurship projects in public health, in an attempt to paint the broad array of missions, strategies, organizational structures, and funding sources utilized by social entrepreneurs to simultaneously achieve economic and social returns. Since one chapter cannot thoroughly portray the opportunities, excitement, and complexities of this growing field, it provides examples of leadership development programs and resources available to those interested in combining profits and purpose through leading or participating in social enterprises.

Social entrepreneurship is attracting growing amounts of investment, talent, and attention from many sectors. Combining the passion of a social mission with the determination, efficiency, and innovation of business, it offers an entrepreneurial approach to solving social problems at a time when governmental and philanthropic approaches have delivered less than expected. Social entrepreneurship may well lead the way forward in addressing global and local public health challenges, eradicating poverty, and building bridges across public and private, for-profit and nonprofit sectors, and achieving human flourishing around the world.

Defining Social Entrepreneurship

The term **social entrepreneurship** has become popularized in the media, referenced by public officials, loosely used in corporate cause branding initiatives, and utilized as the foundation for new university programs. It has motivated students and change agents to "change the world" and has informed the vision and strategies of leading companies such as Ashoka, the Skoll Foundation, and the Bill & Melinda Gates Foundation.

Most people can easily state that that social entrepreneurship is an activity conducted by a social entrepreneur, thus most organizations are known by their founder(s)—the social entrepreneur(s) willing to work long hours and years to fulfill their social mission. From the work of Nobel Peace Prize winner Muhammad Yunus of the Grameen Bank and Ashoka founder Bill Drayton, social entrepreneurs have gained household recognition. Social entrepreneurship signals the imperative to drive social change and transform our world with lasting benefits—yet its definition is still unclear. The name implies a blurring of sector boundaries, from innovative not-for-profit ventures and social purpose business ventures to for-profit community development banks and hybrid organizations in the quest to achieve a greater social mission.

This chapter first explores the questions: What does "social entrepreneurship" actually mean? What does a social entrepreneur actually do? Such definitions are necessary to: 1) contrast the strategies, practices, and investment requirements of social entrepreneurship to other entrepreneurial approaches; 2) identify additional support required to achieve social change through legislation and social policy; and 3) focus resources on building and strengthening a concrete and identifiable field.[1,2]

Starting with Entrepreneurship

Any definition of social entrepreneurship must begin with a definition of the entrepreneur, the noun of the term. The *Merriam-Webster Dictionary* defines entrepreneur as "a person who organizes and manages any enterprise, especially a business, usually with considerable initiative and risk."[3] At this level of definition, a social entrepreneur would therefore be one who organized and/or managed a business that features social goals.

Over time, richer definitions of the term *entrepreneur* have been developed. From the 18th-century economists Say and Schumpeter's definitions, the term suggested that entrepreneurs create value by shifting economic resources from lower to higher areas of productivity and greater yield.[4] In the 20th century, entrepreneurs began to be described as those who were innovators, agents of change within the larger economy who drove the creative destruction process of capitalism conceived by Joseph Schumpeter. In contemporary management theory, Peter Drucker focused the term *entrepreneur* on persons who would always search for change, respond to it, and then exploit the opportunity.[5] From agent of change to exploiters of change, entrepreneurs became known as resourceful risk takers who embody the spirit of innovation and who utilize others' resources to create value.[2,6–8] Furthermore, entrepreneurship is a market-based activity and profits are its indicators of success. The key goal is to create financial wealth for the entrepreneur and his or her investors. Entrepreneurship thereby acts as an engine of innovation and change that enables people, firms, and nations to succeed in an ever-changing, increasingly competitive, global marketplace.

Expanding Entrepreneurship with "Social"

How does a definition of entrepreneurship that incorporates the attributes of creating value, exploiting an opportunity, innovating, risk-taking, resourcefully utilizing resources, and delivering financial returns to the investor and entrepreneur apply to social entrepreneurship?

Is it simply a category within the genus "entrepreneurship"? Or, is it a new category of business that stands within, yet also outside of, traditional practices of business, government, and philanthropy?[i]

Social entrepreneurship requires that leaders adopt a business-like innovation approach to delivering social value. Leaders use business-like principles—notions such as value creation, innovation and change, and opportunity exploitation in their work—from for-profit business to maximize revenues from social programs. Furthermore, leaders also must strategically balance the conflicting demands of multiple stakeholders and moral considerations with seemingly impossible social problems, all the while exhibiting balanced judgment and a unity of purpose and action in the face of complexity.[2,9] Social entrepreneurship may therefore be defined as: 1) the recognition and "relentless" pursuit of new opportunities to further the mission of creating social value, 2) continuous engagement in innovation and modification, and 3) bold action undertaken without acceptance of existing resource limitations.[4]

Social entrepreneurship also, by definition, requires a replacement for the role and function of markets that guide and define business entrepreneurship. In the latter, markets are used to allocate resources among competing ventures. Supply and demand dictate prices, and competitors force leaders to strategically position their products and services to meet customers' needs in the pursuit of value measured in profits. Markets, however, do not do a good job in valuing social improvements, public benefits, or harms, or the benefits and costs involved in meeting the needs of people who cannot pay for the good or service.[4] Markets cannot be used to allocate resources or to measure if the entity is creating sufficient social value to justify the resources used to create the social value. This does not mean, however, that social entrepreneurism abdicate the creation of financial wealth, or profits.

A more complex model of social entrepreneurship suggests that social entrepreneurs create social value by utilizing the behaviors of innovativeness, proactiveness, and risk management.[10] However, they are constrained by three forces: their desire to achieve their social mission, constant environmental change, and the need to maintain sustainability of the organization (see **Figure 24.1**).

Noting Figure 24.1, sustainability resulting from a balance of the entrepreneurial drives of innovativeness, proactiveness, and risk management is not an end in itself. Social entrepreneurs seek market opportunities that enable them to create better social value for their clients. They become sustainable only when the organization continues—because of its social mission and the financial viability of the opportunity. Both guide the overall strategy and decision-making framework for the social entrepreneur. Of note is that social entrepreneurship also serves markets that are not otherwise served by for-profit organization, as it creates new models for the provision of products and services that cater directly to basic human needs that remain unsatisfied by current economic or social institutions.[8]

Social enterprises may therefore reflect a range of goals. Some purely focus on achieving a social mission, while others aim to produce financial results through social mission or have shared social and financial goals, where social gains are subordinate to financial ones.

---

[i] In this chapter, we assume that defining entrepreneurship is logically linked with defining "entrepreneur," because what entrepreneurs do is the activity of entrepreneurship. Defining either term assumes and implies the other.

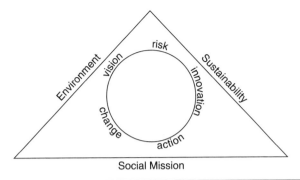

Figure 24.1 Wholistic Model of Social Entrepreneurship
Source: Courtesy of James A. Johnson.

Social entrepreneurship is also worthy of limits in definition. The following types of firms and related motives are not included as social enterprises: firms that would abandon their social goals if they create more profits, companies that use corporate social responsibility activities for marketing value, firms using cause branding to benefit the profitability of the business, or social activists who work to solve a social problem without business disciplines.[2]

Skills of the Social Entrepreneur Leader

Leaders of social enterprises couple the skills of business entrepreneurship with the passions of a social change agent. Like business entrepreneurs, social entrepreneurs are risk takers,[6] yet their main focus is creating social value rather than profits. Social entrepreneurs look for "trapped potential" in the communities and society around them—those situations where people are excluded, marginalized, or are suffering, and where they do not have the economic, psychological, or political power to transform their realities on their own. Social entrepreneurs tirelessly look for innovative solutions to major social issues that are not being solved by the government, philanthropy, or business sectors and then work to change the system, persuading entire societies to take new leaps. They want to create wide-scale, transformative benefit and ensure a better future for the targeted group and society at large.[1,11]

Like business entrepreneurs, social entrepreneurs are the key enabling figures for a business. They champion the cause and provide energy and enthusiasm to individuals, teams, and partners to move from the opportunity-recognition stage of an idea to implementation. They must work across boundaries and borders, sectors and disciplines, to succeed. They are also virtuous people who are passionately committed to a cause.[12] They are value driven and often serve as role models to others. They are society's change agents, described as "creators of innovations that disrupt the status quo and transform our world for the better."[13]

The social entrepreneur may be summarized as a passionate founder (or founders): 1) who aims to create social value, either exclusively or in a prominent way; 2) who recognizes a social/market opportunity, identifies a practical solution to a social problem, exploits the opportunity, and attempts to create value for an underserved population segment; 3) who employs innovation to create or deliver social value; 4) who balances risk-taking with resourcefulness, focus, and management while understanding constraints and opportunities of sustainability, social mission, and the greater complex environment; 5) who manages the competing challenges of social mission and financial returns to achieve sustainability of organization and mission; and 6) who serves as a role model to others, conscious of making direct, positive impacts in all their relationships, with clients, and in decision making.

Defining Social Entrepreneurship in Public Health

Building off this definition of social entrepreneurship, it can now be defined within public health. Social entrepreneurism in public health is sustained action taken to solve health-related problems, whether acute care, preventative, or research, that had previously been unaddressed, or unsuccessfully addressed, by government, the private sector, and the not-for-profit sector. Social enterprises, here, use collaboration among multiple organizations and the crossing of institutional or disciplinary boundaries to find or create solutions beyond the traditional. The scale of populations served may range from a small group of individuals, a neighborhood, or a village, to a nation or the entire world. Public health initiatives in the health sector focus on aging, disability, HIV/AIDS, reproductive rights, mental health, technology, post-trauma care, rehabilitation and prevention, disease treatment and prevention, and many other issues. Examples are numerous, ranging from neighborhood clinics that provide primary care to patients, reducing their use of hospital emergency rooms for routine matters,[14] to online games that teach children about good oral hygiene,[15] to libraries that employ entrepreneurial techniques to bring gender-based research into the clinical practice setting.[16]

This section provides a social entrepreneurship model for public health, where social enterprises fill the gaps between market (or commercial) solutions and government ones (see **Figure 24.2**). At the center of the model is the "iron triangle" of public health programs, policies, and initiatives, where initiatives are designed to improve access to care, quality of care, and/or cost efficiencies. The left-hand triangle represents the role of leaders in context of their community and societal environment. The leader typically has a passion for change and works within a community that serves as a host for the changes, where both are influenced or constrained by the present social norms and responsiveness to health needs and potential solutions. The right-hand triangle represents the interplay of social mission to serve public health ends, the resources required to fulfill this mission, and the need to balance social mission with financial returns for the initiative to achieve sustainable results and long-term impact at the levels of individual human beings, organization, and social community.

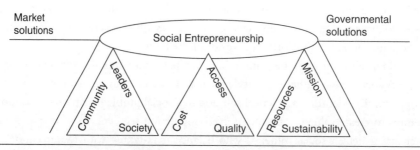

Figure 24.2   Model of Social Entrepreneurship in Public Health

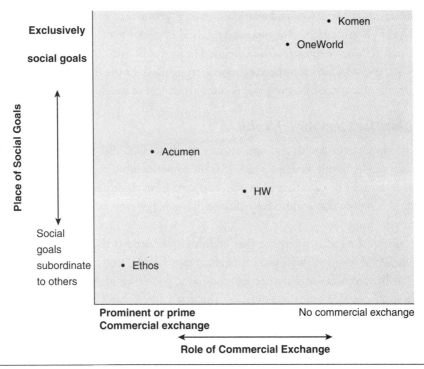

Figure 24.3 Range of Social Enterprises in Public Health
Source: Adapted from Peredo A, McLean M. Social Entrepreneurship: A Critical Review of the Concept. *The Journal of World Business.* 2006;41(1):56–65.

Social enterprises within public health are created to deliver a range of goals. Not only are they designed to strategically address one or more elements of the "iron triangle," they also may differ in emphasis on "social" (or social mission) and "entrepreneurship" (or profits). According to Peredo and McLean,[2] the enterprise's goals may range from being "exclusively social" at one end of the continuum to "exclusively profit, with social good as one of other subordinate goals" on the other end. Rearranging their classification into a two-dimensional model, **Figure 24.3** provides a map of social enterprises in public health and suggests their range of focus. Each firm is described in more detailed case studies in the following section.

Case Studies in Public Health

This section describes a small sample of a variety of types and scales of social entrepreneur projects in public health. Each of these social enterprises is headquartered in the Americas, and has been launched by a social entrepreneur—a social change leader—who has employed novel types of resources to meet the needs of a neglected or overlooked population sector and has successfully sustained operations for at least 5 years. Each differentiates themselves by their mission, strategy, and approach for delivering products and/or services within a gap left by the public and private sectors of the public health systems in which they function. They vary widely with regard to their organizational structure and relationships to governments, to for-profit companies, and to not-for-profit organizations. They have all received measurable success, though the measures employed may be outside those traditionally used in for-profit firms. Additionally, the founders and the firms have won awards or been otherwise recognized for the importance of their contributions, whether those contributions were on multinational or neighborhood levels.

The Institute for OneWorld Health

Today, vast disparities of wealth and opportunity divide nations and people across the globe in many areas of public health. Perhaps nowhere is the disparity more profound than in the area of health care. Infectious diseases that have been banished from wealthier nations still kill millions of the poorest people in the world. Many of these illnesses, however, can be easily prevented with vaccines or safe drugs.

One example of a social enterprise that addresses this need is the Institute for OneWorld Health. OneWorld meets all three aspects of the public health "iron triangle" in that they provide high-quality vaccines and drugs at a low cost to the poorest children in the developing world who suffer from treatable infectious diseases. The first United States–based nonprofit pharmaceutical company, OneWorld's mission is to "discover, develop, and deliver safe, effective, and affordable new treatments for diseases disproportionately affecting people in the developing world."[17] Target illnesses include visceral leishmaniasis, malaria, diarrhea, and Chagas disease.

OneWorld was founded in San Francisco, California, in 2000 by Drs. Victoria Hale and Ahvie Herskowitz and received 501(c)(3) tax-exempt status in 2001. Dr. Hale was formerly a reviewer of new drug applications for the U.S. Food and Drug Administration (FDA) and a research scientist at Genentech. She has also been an advisor to the World Health Organization for building ethical review capacity in the developing world, and has served as expert reviewer to the National Institutes of Health on the topic of biodiversity. Dr. Herskowitz was founder of Anatara Medicine, a modern integrative medicine practice that provides "Convergence Care."[ii] They passionately believed that the wonders and promise of modern medicine must meet the needs of everyone, not just a privileged few—and that it was the *responsibility* for those with the ability to conduct research and development and to provide lifesaving vaccines and medications to the poor. Thus, OneWorld takes the technology, medical science, and the insight of the "haves" to the poorest children in the world, while also addressing issues of access to medicine and global health advocacy.

OneWorld adopted a socioentrepreneurial business model that redesigned the whole value chain of drug delivery.[8] Large philanthropic foundations (e.g., the Bill & Melinda Gates Foundation, the Chiron Foundation, the Sapling Foundation, and the Lehman Brothers Foundation) and nongovernmental organizations (e.g., the Training in Tropical Disease program of the World Health Organization, or WHO/TDR) in the early years provided funding for the discovery and development stages of the pharmaceutical research and development (R&D) process.

[ii] A system designed to create a unified standard for personalized medicine by combining seven different lenses across the best of Western medical science with established Eastern and European medical traditions in order to address conditions arising from today's level of environmental, dietary, physical, and psychological toxicity.

Being a nonprofit also allowed OneWorld access to other forms of capital for which for-profit companies would not be eligible through partnerships where value was created for all the parties for the discovery stage of R&D: for example, in-licensing of promising new drug leads from for-profit pharmaceuticals, Orphan Drug Designation status from regulatory agencies, and donated patents for intellectual property that did not meet the established financial criteria for for-profit firms.[17] Innovative partnerships between universities, biotech companies, for-profit pharmaceutical companies, and/or contract manufacturing companies help OneWorld to bring compounds from discovery to the market.[iii] Furthermore, they attract research scientists and volunteers willing to donate time to compassion-based R&D efforts.

Measures of success include revenue growth, program expansion, and public awards. In 2010, revenues stood at $26 million in contributions and grants, up from $14 million in 2009. Approximately 80 cents on every program dollar is spent on their mission, including discovery, development, and delivery costs of drugs to poor children. The program has expanded from their first grant in 2002 to concentrate on four major disease areas, including diarrheal disease, malaria, kala-azar, and hookworm.

OneWorld has received many organizational awards, including:

- Inclusion in *The Global Journal*'s inaugural "Top 100 Best NGOs" list (2012)
- The "Social Responsibility Award" at the 2005 Pharmaceutical Achievement Awards[iv]
- The achievement award from the Social Enterprise Alliance and a spot on the panel at the Third Annual Conference on Borderless Giving sponsored by the Global Philanthropy Forum (2004)
- Being honored at the Skoll World Forum as one of the World's Top 50 Social Innovators by being named to the Phoenix 50 List (2004)[v]
- Being honored as one of the United States's Top 10 Social Enterprises by *Fast Company Magazine* (2008)[vi]

In social enterprises, the founder oftentimes receives public recognition that also brings greater "market" value to the institution. In 2003, Victoria Hale was named fellow by the Leadership Foundation of the International Women's Forum and one of five global laureates in health by the Tech Museum of Innovation; she was also selected as one of 10 outstanding global entrepreneurs by the Schwab Foundation for Social Entrepreneurship in Geneva, Switzerland.[vii] Dr. Hale spoke at the World Economic Forum in 2004 and 2006. In 2005, she was announced the winner of *The Economist's* Award for Social and Economic Innovation, which highlights

---

[iii] See the Institute for OneWorld Health website for examples: http://www.oneworldhealth.org/history.

[iv] Recognizes exemplary performance by a pharmaceutical industry company in the development and implementation of beneficial environmental, health, safety, and employment practices, and in the dedication of company resources to philanthropic causes.

[v] Recognizes innovators, entrepreneurs, and investors who are making significant contributions to building a more sustainable and equitable global economy and forging innovative business models focused on resolving social, environmental, and financial challenges.

[vi] Awarded to social enterprises for their bold and timely ideas and for innovative thinking.

[vii] Criteria include identifying practical solutions to social problems by combining innovation, research and scope, replicability, sustainability, direct positive impact, role modeling, mutual value added, resourcefulness, and opportunity.

the importance of individual thinking and innovation in the business world. In 2006, she was named a MacArthur Fellow and in 2007 was selected Woman of the Year by *Glamour Magazine*.

Like other "serial" social entrepreneurs, Dr. Hale has gone on to launch a new social enterprise called Medicines360, a nonprofit pharmaceutical company dedicated to developing medicines for women and children, including pregnant women.

Acumen Fund

Another form of social entrepreneurship firms are "impact investors," nonprofit venture capital firms whose main mission is profit making, yet who are committed to a social mission as a core decision-making criteria for investing. Impact investors aim to solve social or environmental challenges while generating financial profit. Typically founded by a passionate social investor, they use their investment strategy, board memberships, general partners, and innovative investment brands to attract capital that furthers the social missions of their funded firms, which provide public health and other basic services (balancing risk/return across the fund and meeting the wide range of basic community needs). Some examples include Ignia, Acumen Fund, Bamboo Finance, Grassroots Business Fund, New Ventures, Root Capital, and Small Enterprise Assistance Funds. A 2011 report by the Global Impact Investing Network, a Manhattan nonprofit focused on making impact investing more effective, collected data from 463 organizations (receiving or seeking impact investment funds) from 58 countries. The report claims their efforts resulted in 23,355 jobs at portfolio companies that generated $1.4 billion in revenue by serving nearly 8 million people, with 63% of reporting organizations profitable—and 92 million clients served through 1,931 micro-finance organizations, with 70% of reporting organizations profitable.[18]

Acumen Fund is a "social investor," or "social venture capital firm," that provides philanthropic funds (or "patient capital") to profit-oriented private ventures whose social mission is to serve the poor and deliver greater social benefits. Acumen may be considered a social enterprise that fulfills the access, cost, and quality aspects of the public health "iron triangle," because it extends access of needed solutions through low-cost, good-quality solutions that are provided by local business ventures to the poor. Its mission is to create a world beyond poverty by investing in social enterprises, emerging leaders, and breakthrough ideas. Acumen's vision is as follows:

> One day every human being will have access to the critical goods and services they need—including affordable health, water, housing, energy, agricultural inputs and services—so that they can make decisions and choices for themselves and unleash their full human potential and with this, dignity will start for every human being on earth.[19]

Acumen achieves both financial and social wealth by combining capitalism and philanthropy in an innovative way—adopting a market-oriented approach to development. Acumen takes donations from philanthropists as typical nonprofit organizations do, but invests them in a business-like way by lending or taking stakes in business models that deliver critical goods and services to the world's poor, improving the lives of millions. This approach leverages the power that globalization, technology, and markets plays in creating wealth for poor countries and helps to reduce the wealth gap between rich and poor countries—while creating sustainable value and societal change. Recipients of Acumen's loans or equity—private ventures aiming for profits—must serve the poor in a way that brings broader social benefits. Many ventures provide basic services such as clean water, health care, housing, and energy and are not seen as significant sources of market opportunity or tax revenues by traditional businesses or governments. Local people address the challenges of their local business climate (e.g., high costs, poor distribution systems, dispersed customers, limited financing options, and sometimes corruption) by creating imaginative business solutions and forming partnerships supported by investors willing to take on a risk–return profile that was unacceptable to traditional financiers.

Donor–investors do not get their money back, as all returns are reinvested in Acumen. The founder, Jacqueline Novogratz, provides hands-on management and review of all its investments. If the businesses do not deliver their solution in a manner that meets the needs of the local consumers and if they cannot repay their loans, the businesses are folded.

Acumen Fund was incorporated in 2001 with seed capital from the Rockefeller Foundation, Cisco Systems Foundation, and three individual philanthropists. With significant experience in traditional development companies and philanthropy,[viii] Jacqueline Novogratz exemplifies the passionate, committed, and experienced social entrepreneur who is driven to deliver both profits and social mission in the firms she funds. She spends half her time traveling, much of it reviewing and challenging business leaders, potential investments, and eventual end users throughout the developing world and constantly scrawling down conversations, analysis, and decisions in her infamous notebook. She raises donor money herself using the collected data and personal stories from her travels in fundraising.

By 2012, Acumen has invested $73 million in 65 enterprises in South Asia and Africa. Of these, 15 investments are in the health area, seeking to reduce costs and improve access to needed products and services. The businesses are wide in range, and include A to Z Textile Mills, a Tanzania-based company that has produced 29 million low-cost, long-lasting, antimalaria bed nets, and provided 7,000 jobs, mostly for women; Sustainable Healthcare Foundation (SHF), a nongovernmental organization providing comprehensive primary care to low-income communities in Kenya;[ix] Voxivia, an Internet and cell phone communication system that allows rural healthcare workers to call in patient's symptoms or conditions, providing officials with immediate information on disease outbreaks, and thus improve rural health care; and Sproxil, mobile technology that allows consumers to verify the authenticity of pharmaceutical products and combat the global counterfeit drug market.

Further Ssuccesses may be measured through Acumen's investments, which have created 55,000 jobs and impacted 88 million people. Forty-four Global Fellows and 22 East African Fellows have been trained in leadership development since 2006, of which two-thirds of alumni have launched or plan to launch a social enterprise in 5 years, which creates ripples of influence

---

[viii] Before launching Acumen Fund, Jacqueline Novogratz founded and directed The Philanthropy Workshop and The Next Generation Leadership program at the Rockefeller Foundation, and also founded Duterimbere, a micro-finance institution in Rwanda.

[ix] SHF's 80 franchise clinics treat nearly 300,000 patients each year for malaria, worms, respiratory infections, and diarrheal and other diseases, and provide living incomes to the nurses and community health workers who own them.

around the globe. Furthermore, Acumen developed an internal framework to measure financial, operational, social, and environment impact.

Susan G. Komen for the Cure

Breast cancer is the most common cancer among women in the United States, other than skin cancer. It is the second leading cause of cancer death in women, after lung cancer. In 2012, nearly 300,000 women are expected to be diagnosed with breast cancer and nearly 40,000 estimated to die. However, there are roughly 2.5 million survivors of breast cancer as well, a number increasing since the 1980s, probably due to enhanced screening and better treatment.[20]

Susan G. Komen for the Cure (formerly the Susan G. Komen Breast Cancer Foundation) is the world's largest grassroots network of breast cancer survivors and activists who are fighting to save lives, empower people, ensure quality care, and energize science to find cures for breast cancer.[21] Their vision is nothing short of a world without breast cancer. Komen was founded by Nancy G. Brinker who made a promise to her sister Susan G. Komen, who was dying of breast cancer, that she would work to do everything she could to rid the world of breast cancer. This personal experience had shown her that her sister's outcome may have been more favorable if she had been better educated and received greater depth and breadth of care for her illness. Nancy's vision, commitment, and passion along with her ability to assemble resources to address the needs of a huge target population and to differentiate the foundation's approach are all keys to Komen's success.

Komen is a consummate model of public health–oriented social enterprise dedicated to providing *access* to breast cancer solutions around the globe. Its approach is to focus on early detection through breast self-awareness (universal screening mammography and breast self-examination) as the primary method for fighting breast cancer, versus other strategies such as: medical consumerism (where patients make individual, evidence-based decisions in relationship with their doctors) or environmental research (which research environmental sources for breast cancer).[22,23] It also advocates for increasing expenditures on research, diagnosing, and treating breast cancer through corporate donors and federal governments. Komen is known by its logo, the pink ribbon, which symbolizes values of fear of breast cancer, hope, and the charitable goodness of people and business that publicly support the breast cancer movement.[23] Resembling a runner in motion, it also reflects the importance of Komen's well known Race for the Cure event, as well as the traditional color used for "femininity."

Since its inception in 1982, Komen has invested nearly $2 billion in breast cancer research, grants, advocacy, education, health services, and social support programs in the United States and through partnerships with institutions in more than 50 countries and a network of 124 affiliates worldwide—with key partners located in Italy, Germany, and Puerto Rico.[21] Critical activities are wide in range across the entire scope of public health, science, and human services involved with breast cancer. For example, they provide financial and emotional support to hundreds of thousands of patients and their families. They invest in research grants globally, funding a research portfolio of more than 500 active grants totaling almost $270 million, with such goals as basic, clinical, and translational research; postdoctoral fellowships; breast cancer disparities research; prevention strategies; screening technologies; and effective, personalized treatments for aggressive and metastatic diseases. Grants also are used to fund medical programs around the world, to distribute treatment and medical equipment, and to address other public health requirements. As they have grown, they have continued to launch innovative programs to address the issues of growth and changing needs. For example, they created a council, called Komen Scholars, of 68 world class researchers, clinicians, public health experts, and advocates to guide the programs and support the vision of Komen's Advisory Board. They have also launched the Susan G. Komen Global Health Alliance, which uses the influence of global leaders to make women's cancers a priority and to develop cancer screening and treatment programs in low-resource countries.

Komen has expanded its fundraising efforts to include major donors, foundations, and corporate contributions. In fact, total gross revenues in 2010 were $421 million with roughly 50% raised from contributions, 43% from the Komen Race for the Cure (the world's largest fundraiser for breast cancer), and the remainder from other public revenue.[24] Hundreds of corporations contribute to Komen, with nearly two dozen donating $1 million apiece, and others partnering in cause marketing activities. In 2010, Komen's 5-year average percentage of dollars spent on its mission was 84%, which earned it Charity Navigator's four-star rating. These mission dollars were allocated to education (34%), research (24%), screening (15%), administration (12%), fundraising (8%), and treatment (7%).[24]

Measurements of success used by Komen indicate "victory" over breast cancer, whereby: 1) the breast cancer death rate in the United States has fallen by more than 30% in 20 years; 2) the federal government now devotes more than $900 million each year to breast cancer research, treatment, and prevention (compared to $30 million in 1982); and 3) 5-year relative survival rates for women with early stage cancers (before they have left the breast) are at 99% (up from 74% in 1982). Komen also is known for the millions of people in its global community who are survivors, advocates, and researchers of breast cancer—those who share victories, fight for the cause, and work together to rid the world of breast cancer. Most importantly, the organization has helped to save millions of lives—with 2.5 million breast cancer survivors, the largest cancer-surviving group.[21,24]

Ethos Water

The lack of access to clean water is a major public health challenge. In fact, the World Health Organization estimates that 1.1 billion people worldwide lack access to clean water, roughly one in six people on Earth. Nearly 3.9 million people—equal to the entire population of Los Angeles—die each year from a water-related disease,[25] and of these, nearly 1.8 million people die from diarrheal diseases including cholera and infection with *Escherichia coli*. Of the 4,900 people dying every day, 90% of these are children under the age of 5 years, mostly in developing countries where water-related diseases are their leading cause of death because their immune systems are not fully developed.[25,26]

Furthermore, less than 1% of the world's fresh water is readily accessible for human use, with extreme disparities in use across countries and populations. Water use has grown 35-fold over the last 300 years, but mostly in rich countries; the average American uses 80 to 100 gallons of water at home each day, while the average African family uses about 5 gallons.[26]

There are numerous institutions and organizations representing different social enterprise forms working for clean water across the globe. One interesting (yet somewhat provocative) social enterprise model is Ethos Water, principally a commercial enterprise with a social mission that is subordinate to profitable goals. Peter Thum, working in South Africa as a McKinsey & Company strategy consultant, saw water issues and how they affected children, firsthand. This experience, coupled with his business background, courageous heart, and humanitarian concern, provoked an innovative business idea: to help children get clean water by selling expensive bottled water in the West.

Taking dream to plan, he and his partner Jonathan Greenblatt launched operations as a bottled water company in 2003 while simultaneously forming a nonprofit called Ethos International to invest funds. Monies would be used to raise awareness and fund safe water programs. Their strategy included creating a brand of water in a crowded marketplace that people really cared about; differentiating the product by sourcing it from natural sustainable springs; developing great packaging to compete effectively against brands like Evian and Fiji; distributing through cafes, health-food stores, and yoga studios in Southern California; targeting upscale consumers through retail selection and visible events such as the Academy Awards; and building a platform for raising awareness.[27] As a model they used Newman's Own, a for-profit social enterprise founded by actor Paul Newman and author A.E. Hotchner in 1982 that donates 100% of the proceeds, after taxes, to various educational and charitable organizations. Thum and Greenblatt also used brand as their platform for creating a community and spreading information about the need for clean water, where they connected consumer purchases with the greater social mission through the message of, "Buy water, help children get water."

Starbucks acquired Ethos Water in 2005 for $8 million, which gave it immediate access to more than 40 million consumers and grants for water-related programs. Post-acquisition, Starbucks established a partnership with Pepsi-Cola to market and produce Ethos through the North American Coffee Partnership and worked with IDEO, a design firm, to create a compelling bottle design for the emerging brand that could be manufactured to Pepsi's strict bottling guidelines (for which they received the 2007 American InHouse Design Award from *Graphic Design USA*).

Starbucks donates between 5 and 10 cents from every sale of Ethos bottled water to nongovernmental organizations working to increase access to clean drinking water, sanitation, and hygiene education programs in water-stressed countries. Additionally, they have created the Ethos Water Fund for large-scale grant provisions. They have been criticized, however, for using a less-than-holistic approach to social enterprise, because the bottles are not recyclable. Though more commercial than social in focus, this social enterprise differentiates itself in a crowded bottled-water marketplace with its social mission, and it brings attention and monies to a needed social cause.

Like many social entrepreneurs, Peter Thum has gone on to new social missions. After the Starbucks acquisition, he continued to work on the water crisis by founding Giving Water, which helps children in Kenya get water access. While in Kenya, he also saw the role that weapons played to endanger the development work and progress on issues such as economic growth, basic services, human rights, women's rights, children's rights, and the environment. In 2009, Thum founded Fonderie 47, whose mission is to reduce the impact and number of assault weapons and create a platform to engage leaders and raise awareness about the impact of guns on the body, mind, and spirit.[28] Fonderie 47 takes AK47s in Africa's war zones and transforms them into pieces of beauty—jewelry, watches, and accessories. By 2012, 4,004 guns had been destroyed and repurposed.

Hayes E. Willis Health Center of South Richmond

For decades many of the indigent and near indigent people in the part of Richmond, Virginia, known as Southside routinely sought health care at the emergency department of the Medical College of Virginia Hospitals (now part of the Virginia Commonwealth University Health System). While the emergency department provided primary care to many patients, some people elected to forego care. Accordingly, preventive care and preventive consultation for many in this vast system of neighborhoods was inadequate, intermittent, or nonexistent.

One solution to this problem was to create a primary care clinic in Southside Richmond that would be specifically designed with the needs of this population in mind.[14,29] A planning partnership was formed between the Medical College of Virginia (MCV) Hospitals and the City of Richmond's Department of Public Health. Together they formed the Richmond Urban Primary Care Initiative. After conducting an assessment to confirm the primary care needs of the community, a grant was sought and received from the Robert Wood Johnson Foundation, with matching funds from the Office of the Governor, to assist with the costs of planning. Participating in planning were numerous representatives from the hospital and other parts of the university, the state senate, state health agencies, city health agency, members of the community to be served, independent physicians from the area to be served, and others. Leading the process was an exceptionally dedicated physician, Dr. Hayes E. Willis, who was on the faculty of the Department of Family Medicine, School of Medicine, Virginia Commonwealth University.

Initially, when the clinic was established it was called the South Richmond Health Center. Subsequently, it was renamed the Hayes E. Willis Health Center of South Richmond in honor of Dr. Willis, its lead planner and first director, who died only a few years after the center was opened.[30] The center is located in a large strip mall in South Richmond, with free parking and on multiple bus routes. Initially, the center was a joint project of the MCV Hospitals and the Richmond City Health Department.[31] After several years of operation, however, with accord form the city, the hospital assumed sole ownership of the center.

Ongoing financial support for the center comes from reimbursements from Medicare and Medicaid, private insurance, Virginia Coordinated Care (a state-funded program for the indigent), and from copayments from those patients who have the means to make them. Although profit was not a motive in establishing the center, there are certain financial benefits that result when primary care patients are diverted from an emergency department to a primary care clinic.

Services provided by the center include financial screening for Medicaid/FAMIS and for Virginia Coordinated Care for the Uninsured, an on-site pharmacy, pediatrics, women's health, Spanish-speaking clinicians and support staff, screening for sexually transmitted diseases (STDs), and primary care for HIV patients.

In fiscal year (FY) 2011, the center had 3,742 patients, with a total of 10,053 patient visits to the center. In 2004, approximately 45% of the patients were not insured, and an additional 34% were Medicaid recipients. The Hayes E. Willis Health Center of South Richmond, as part of the Virginia Commonwealth University Medical Center, shares in the prestige of the Magnet status that the hospital was awarded in 2006 and again in 2011.[32]

Summary and Conclusions

Social entrepreneurship has emerged in many sectors of the economy. As it advances in public health, it has taken multiple forms, ranging from those in which social mission is the exclusive focus to those where profit making is nearly primary. In all sustainable cases of social entrepreneurship, however, financial and social wealth must be achieved. This chapter introduces several sustainable social enterprises that have achieved remarkable impact in addressing public health challenges and have been recognized for their excellence.

The principles of social entrepreneurship offered in this chapter have universal applicability in public health that will continue to be relevant as time progresses and as we learn from the successes and failures of founders and enterprises. New principles will emerge as the future of social entrepreneurship in public health unfolds.

As public and private leaders and global citizens recognize the remedies social entrepreneurship offers for many public health problems, leadership development, education, and training will be required. A list of higher education programs and a short set of information sources on social entrepreneurship are provided in the appendix at the end of this chapter (note that they constitute only a partial listing). Many more sources will be needed in the future as the full impact of social entrepreneurship activities are recognized and valued.

Future Outlook

The future of social entrepreneurship in public health looks bright. Awareness of social entrepreneurship principles is spreading. More and more businesses consider social entrepreneurship in public health as part of their mission. Colleges and universities are embracing social entrepreneurship in the form of public service by faculty, service learning by students, and as a growing aspect of their teaching and research missions. Government officials at all levels are becoming accustomed to hearing from and engaging with social entrepreneurs in public health. Philanthropies are focusing more resources on social enterprises in public health, and individuals too are becoming more aware of its current and potential value to society.

In the not-too-distant future, the success of social entrepreneurship efforts in public health may not be attributed exclusively to social entrepreneurs. As the principles and methods of social entrepreneurship are disseminated through the media, in-service training, and formal education, it will become more apparent that it takes social entrepreneurship spirit and attitude at all levels to be successful. Seeking solutions, crossing disciplinary and organizational boundaries, and innovating to establish new ways to address problems will become more second nature and commonplace than is now the case. As social entrepreneurship in public health is explored in greater depth around the world, however, new principles and practices must be defined in order to address the different cultural traditions and the political, social, and legal realities within different regions and nations.[33-35]

Although it is difficult to predict the future, it is likely that certain circumstances will result in predictable roles for social entrepreneurship in public health. If, for example, government shrinks its involvement with health care and prevention, the governmental sectors of the health-care system, the private sector, and the not-for-profit sector will be called upon to practice the principles of social entrepreneurship. On the other hand, if government were to increase its involvement with health care and prevention, it may result in less demand for social entrepreneurship in public health. In either case, however, social entrepreneurship in public health is expected to grow, in the former case more quickly and in the latter more slowly, but grow nevertheless, and far into the foreseeable future.

Discussion Questions

1. High-profile, charismatic leaders are often said to be essential to successful social entrepreneurship in public health. Others contend, however, that high-quality teamwork can accomplish far more in social entrepreneurship in public health than is possible even by talented individuals working alone. Please defend both points of view with one paragraph for each argument.
2. Some social enterprises in public health demand that recipients of service pay some amount of money or even volunteer their labor in exchange for service. If you believe there is merit in such practices, please explain why. On the other hand, if you believe such practices are not appropriate or not necessary, please explain why.
3. If a philanthropic foundation donates money to a not-for-profit hospital with the requirement that the hospital use the funds to treat chronic arthritis in indigent patients, is the foundation engaging in social entrepreneurship? Discuss your answer.
4. Some contend that social enterprises in public health must have impact on a large scale to truly be considered social entrepreneurship. Please discuss your opinion of this point of view.
5. Think of a population with health needs that are inadequately addressed by the government, the private sector, and the not-for-profit sector. Design an approach to addressing these health needs. Identify the business and social entrepreneurship roles and skills that will be needed to develop and implement this project.

Appendix: Resources for Social Entrepreneurship

Social Entrepreneurship Programs

There is a trend toward increasing the number and types of educational opportunities for studying social entrepreneurship at colleges and universities. The schools listed in this section are a sample of those offering either an undergraduate or graduate degree or focus on social entrepreneurship; some have a center for social entrepreneurship and others incorporate the topic into other areas, with a broader emphasis on entrepreneurship:

- Babson College F.W. Olin Graduate School of Business (MBA)
- Belmont University, Social Entrepreneurship Program (BA or BS)
- Brigham Young University Marriott School of Management Peery Social Entrepreneurship Program (MBA)
- Colorado State University College of Business Global Social & Sustainable Enterprise Graduate Program (MBA)
- Duke University Fuqua School of Business Center for the Advancement of Social Enterprise (CASE) (MBA)
- Indiana University–Bloomington Kelley Business School (MBA Certificate Program)
- Northwestern University Social Enterprise at Kellogg (SEEK) Program (MBA)
- New York University Reynolds Program in Social Entrepreneurship (undergraduate and graduate)
- Oxford University Saïd Centre School Skoll Centre for Social Entrepreneurship (graduate)
- Pace University Wilson Center for Social Entrepreneurship (undergraduate and graduate)
- Pepperdine University Graduate School of Education and Psychology, Master of Arts in Social Entrepreneurship and Change (graduate)
- Stanford University Graduate School of Business Social Innovation Program (MBA) and Executive Program in Social Entrepreneurship
- University of California at Berkeley Haas School of Business Center for Nonprofit and Public Leadership (MBA)
- University of Colorado at Boulder Deming Center for Entrepreneurship (MBA)
- Wake Forest University School of Business Social Entrepreneurship Initiative (MBA)
- Yale School of Management Program in Social Enterprise (MBA)

Social Entrepreneurship and Public Health

There are very few programs that integrate social entrepreneurship with public health as a field of study. Here are a few programs that offer services in this needed area of study:

- Harvard School of Public Health supports the Social Entrepreneurs in Health (SEIH) student organization that aims to provide students with the inspiration, skills, experiences, and networks needed to make a social impact through innovation and entrepreneurial pursuits in the fields of medicine and public health. They also collaborate with university initiatives to offer a range of programs in pursuit of the group's missions (e.g., social networking events, speaker series, career workshops, and fieldwork) and partner with other Boston-based schools and organizations to provide interdisciplinary social entrepreneurship opportunities. (See http://isites.harvard.edu/icb/icb.do?keyword=k3789)
- Unite for Sight offers a course called "Introduction to Global Health Careers" in a more general online global health course. One of its eight modules addresses the topic of social entrepreneurship in health care. (See www.uniteforsight.org/global-health-university/)

- University of North Carolina's (UNC) School of Public Health is collaborating with the Carolina Entrepreneurial Initiative at UNC's Kenan-Flagler Business School to offer a graduate certificate in entrepreneurship. The program currently has three tracks: artistic, life sciences, and public health entrepreneurship. Plans are underway for tracks in commercial and social entrepreneurship. The certificate requires completion of a 9-credit-hour course sequence taken in parallel with students' core degree programs.

Additional Resources

There are many resources regarding social entrepreneurship available on the Internet. Although none constitute a comprehensive clearinghouse of information, there are several that provide a solid foundation of valuable and impactful work occurring in this area, including:

- Ashoka—Innovators for the Public (http://www.ashoka.org)
- Aspen Institute and the Aspen Network of Development Entrepreneurs (http://www.aspeninstitute.org/policy-work/aspen-network-development-entrepreneurs)
- Echoing Green (http://www.echoinggreen.org)
- *Forbes Impact 30* Social Entrepreneurs (http://www.forbes.com/impact-30/lander.html)
- Schwab Foundation for Social Entrepreneurship (http://www.schwabfound.org)
- Skoll Foundation (http://www.skollfoundation.org)

As colleges and universities, philanthropic foundations, and other organizations enter the field of social entrepreneurship, the sources of information will multiply, so, too, will the training and educational opportunities. There is no space in this chapter for an exhaustive review of information clearinghouses and educational opportunities about this fast growing field, thus the offerings in this chapter are merely intended to be representative.

References

1. Martin RL, Osberg S. Social entrepreneurship: the case for definition. *Stanford Soc Innov Rev.* 2007; 5:28–39.
2. Peredo A, McLean M. Social entrepreneurship: a critical review of the concept. *J World Bus.* 2006; 41(1):56–65.
3. *Merriam-Webster Dictionary.* Care. Available at: http://www.merriam-webster.com/dictionary/care. Accessed March 22, 2013.
4. Dees JG. *The Meaning of "Social Entrepreneurship."* Palo Alto, CA: Stanford University; 1998.
5. Drucker PF. *Innovation and Entrepreneurship.* New York: Harper Collins; 1993.
6. Tan W, Tan T. *What Is the 'Social' in 'Social Entrepreneurship?'* Paper presented at: 48th World International Conference for Small Business, Belfast, Ireland; 2003.
7. Dess GG, Lumpkin GT, Eisner AB. *Strategic Management: Creating Competitive Advantages.* 5th ed. New York: McGraw-Hill Irwin; 2010.
8. Seelos C, Mair J. Social entrepreneurship: creating new business models to serve the poor. *Bus Horizons.* 2005;48:241–6.
9. Mort GS, Weerawardena J, Carnegit K. Social entrepreneurship: towards conceptualisation. *Int J Nonprofit Voluntary Sector Market.* 2003;8(1):76–89.
10. Weerawardena J, Mort GS. Investigating social entrepreneruship: a multidimensional model. *J World Bus.* 2006;41:21–35.

11. Ashoka. *About us.* Available at: https://www.ashoka.org/about. Accessed March 22, 2013.

12. Dees JG, Emerson J, Economy P. *Enterprising Nonprofits: A Toolkit for Social Entrepreneurs.* New York: John Wiley & Sons; 2001.

13. Skoll Foundation. *About.* Available at: http://www.skollfoundation.org/about/. Accessed March 22, 2013.

14. Garland SL. *Academic Medical Centers in a Safety Net Health Care Delivery System.* 2004. Available at: http://www.commed.vcu.edu/ppt05/garland04.ppt. Accessed March 28, 2012.

15. Aquafresh Amazing. *Nurdle World.* Available at: http://www.aquafresh.com/NurdleWorld/Play.aspx. Accessed March 22, 2013.

16. Alison MM. *Women's Health: Librarian as a social enterpreneur.* Available at: https://www.ideals.illinois .edu/handle/2142/4577. Accessed April 6, 2012.

17. Institute for OneWorld Health. *About us.* Available at: http://www.oneworldhealth.org/about-us. Accessed March 22, 2013.

18. Gelfand S, Bouri A, Fonzi CJ, et al. *Data Driven: A Performance Analysis for the Impact Investing Industry.* New York: GIIN and IRIS; 2011.

19. Acumen Fund. *About us.* Available at: http://www.acumenfund.org/about-us.html. Accessed March 22, 2013.

20. American Cancer Society. *Breast Cancer Overview.* Available at: http://www.cancer.org/Cancer/Breast Cancer/OverviewGuide/breast-cancer-overview-key-statistics. Accessed March 22, 2013.

21. Susan G. Komen for the Cure Orange County. *Home.* Available at: http://www.komenoc.org/site/c .mlI4IhNYJwE/b.1439181/k.BDB4/Home.htm. Accessed March 22, 2013.

22. Susan G. Komen. *Breast Self-Awareness Messages.* Available at: http://ww5.komen.org/BreastCancer/ BreastSelfAwareness.html. Accessed March 22, 2013.

23. Sulik GA. *Pink Ribbon Blues: How Breast Cancer Culture Undermines Women's Health.* USA: Oxford University; 2010.

24. Susan G. Komen for the Cure. *United Against Breast Cancer 2009–2010 Annual Report.* Available at: http://ww5.komen.org/uploadedFiles/SGKFTC_FY10AnnualReport.pdf. Accessed March 22, 2013.

25. Prüss-Üstün A, Bos R, Gore F, et al. *Safer Water, Better Health: Costs, benefits, and sustainability of interventions to protect and promote health.* Geneva: World Health Organization; 2008. Available at: http:// whqlibdoc.who.int/publications/2008/9789241596435_eng.pdf. Accessed March 22, 2013.

26. Clean Water for the World. Available at: http://cleanwaterfortheworld.org/. Accessed March 22, 2013.

27. *Bloomberg Businessweek.* Buy Water, Help Children. Available at: http://www.businessweek.com/ investor/content/mar2006/pi20060322_252796.htm. Accessed March 22, 2013.

28. The Gentlemen's Fund. Better Men Better World Search. Available at: http://www.thegentlemensfund .com/nominees/view/451. Accessed March 28, 2012.

29. Coles-Johnson A, Nurse manager. E-mail sent to N. DeLellis, Richmond: Hayes E. Willis Health Center of South Richmond; 2012.

30. Byrd B. South Richmond Health Center to be Renamed in Honor of the Late Hayes E. Willis M.D. Available at: http://www.govrel.vcu.edu/news/Advisories/1998/081398.htm. Accessed March 22, 2013.

31. Virginia Commonwealth University. *VCU Maps.* Available at: www.maps.vcu.edu/offcampus/willis center/index.html. Accessed March 21, 2012.

32. Virginia Commonwealth University. *Public Health Seminars.* Available at: http://www.publichealth.vcu .edu/. Accessed March 22, 2013.

33. Phillips SD. *Women's Social Activism n New Ukraine: Development and Politics of Differentiation.* Bloomington, IN: Indiana University Press; 2008.

34. Тихомиров А.В. Предпринимательство в здравоохранении. *Главный врач: хозяйство и право.* 2005;2:44–49.

35. Lebedev AA, Goncharova MV. Modernization of Public Health Organization: Social Entrepreneurship as an alternative to the commercialization of medical services. *Kazakstan Journal of Public Health.* 2011;4.

Disaster Preparedness and Public Health Response

Linda Young Landesman[i] and Cynthia B. Morrow

LEARNING OBJECTIVES

- To describe why disasters are a threat that the public health profession should be concerned about and prepared for
- To describe the public health role in disasters
- To understand the key public health implications of disasters
- To understand key responsibilities and tasks that public health performs during disasters

---

Chapter Overview

Public health has broad responsibilities to prepare for and respond to disasters. Carrying out these responsibilities effectively requires a multiorganizational response. Key public health responsibilities are disaster epidemiology and assessment, which are used as managerial tools as well as instruments of scientific investigation. In addition, public health organizations play essential roles in response, risk communication, implementation of necessary clinical and non-clinical interventions, recognition of and management of psychosocial effects of disasters, and mitigation of environmental threats. Although the challenges of managing public health threats are greater in developing countries than in the United States, essential elements of effective

---

[i]The author wishes to acknowledge the work of the coauthors on the original version of this chapter: Josephine Malilay, Richard A. Bissell, Steven M. Becker, Les Roberts, and Michael S. Ascher.

public health administration can be compromised substantially in the most devastating domestic disasters, creating imperatives for disaster preparedness.

Population-based management requires strong public health preparedness. Disasters have significant negative consequences for the community, resulting in increased morbidity and mortality, with physical and psychological impacts that may be reduced with adequate intervention. Public health professionals should augment their ability to respond to disasters for the following reasons:

- Natural disasters are having an increasing impact.
- There is a ubiquitous risk across the United States.
- Disasters have negative impacts on health but these impacts may be mitigated by a strong public health infrastructure.
- The effects of disasters can escalate, generating an increased need for public health intervention.
- The public's expectation of response has increased.
- Public health has the expertise to help communities handle the most common health-related problems in the aftermath of a disaster.

Across the globe, humankind is experiencing increased effects from natural disasters, as evidenced by events since the early 1990s.[1,2,3] On average, a disaster a day requiring external international assistance occurs somewhere in the world. In 2010 alone, more than 296,800 people died from natural disasters worldwide. As a consequence of these disasters, more than 2 million people were affected and economic damages associated with the disasters were reported to cost more than $100 billion.[4] One of the deadliest disasters in modern history occurred on January 12, 2010, when a catastrophic earthquake struck Haiti, killing more than 222,000 people. Less than 1 year after the earthquake, Haiti, crippled by a devastated infrastructure, experienced its first outbreak of cholera in more than a century. By late 2012, more than 605,000 cases of cholera were identified in Haiti and were associated with more than 325,000 hospitalizations and more than 7,600 deaths.[5]

This chapter reviews past and current threats that demonstrate the need for strong public health preparedness so that public health professionals can effectively intervene in response to natural and manmade disasters.

Definitions

Disasters have been defined as ecologic disruptions, or emergencies, of a severity and magnitude resulting in deaths, injuries, illness, and/or property damage that cannot be effectively managed by the application of routine procedures or resources and that result in a call for outside assistance. As the field of disaster study evolved, a common set of vocabulary emerged as well, notably distinguishing among hazards, emergencies, and disasters:[6]

- **Emergencies** are typically any occurrence that requires an immediate response. These events can be the result of nature (e.g., hurricanes, tornadoes, and earthquakes), they can be caused by technological or manmade error (e.g., nuclear accidents, bombing, and bioterrorism), or they can be the result of emerging diseases (e.g., West Nile virus in New York City).

- **Hazards** present the probability of the occurrence of a disaster caused by a natural phenomenon (e.g., earthquake, tropical cyclone), by failure of manmade sources of energy (e.g., nuclear reactor or industrial explosion), or by uncontrolled human activity (e.g., conflicts, overgrazing).
- **Incidents** are "an occurrence or event, natural or manmade, that requires a response to protect life or property. Incidents can, for example, include major disasters, emergencies, terrorist attacks, terrorist threats, civil unrest, wildland and urban fires, floods, hazardous materials spills, nuclear accidents, aircraft accidents, earthquakes, hurricanes, tornadoes, tropical storms, tsunamis, war-related disasters, public health and medical emergencies, and other occurrences requiring an emergency response."[7]
- **Natural disasters** are rapid, sudden-onset phenomena with profound effects, such as earthquakes, floods, tropical cyclones, and tornadoes. **Manmade disasters** are technological events not caused by natural hazards, such as fire, chemical spills and explosions, and airplane crashes. A type of manmade disaster, called a *complex emergency*, includes armed conflict and mass migration. No clear demarcation exists between the two categories. For instance, fire may be the result of arson, a manmade activity, but may also occur secondarily to earthquake events, particularly in urban areas where gas mains may be damaged. With increasing technological development worldwide, a category of disasters known as *natural-technological*, or *na-tech*, disasters, has been described in the literature. Na-tech disasters refer to natural disasters that create technological emergencies, such as urban fires resulting from seismic motion or chemical spills resulting from floods.[8]

The lifecycle of a disaster event is typically known as the disaster continuum, or emergency management cycle. In all phases of the disaster continuum (pre-impact, impact, and post-impact), actions to reduce or prevent injury, illness, or death can be taken by many partners, including public health, emergency management officials, and the population at risk. The basic phases of disaster management include prevention or mitigation, warning and preparedness, and response and recovery. In public health terms, **prevention** refers to actions that may prevent further loss of life, disease, disability, or injury. **Mitigation** includes the measures that are taken to reduce the harmful effects of a disaster by attempting to limit impacts on human health and economic infrastructure. **Warning**, or forecasting, refers to the monitoring of events to look for indicators that signify when and where a disaster might occur and what the magnitude might be. Recognition of these risks enhances the ability to mitigate and prepare. In **preparedness**, officials or the public itself plan a response to potential disasters and, in so doing, lay the framework for recovery.

In the United States, the **response** to disasters is organized through multiple jurisdictions, agencies, and authorities. The term *emergency management* is used to refer to these activities. The emergency management field organizes its activities by "sectors" such as fire, police, and emergency medical services (EMS). The response phase of a disaster encompasses emergency relief and is followed by recovery and rehabilitation or reconstruction. *Emergency relief* focuses attention on saving lives, providing first aid, restoring emergency communications and transportation systems, and providing immediate care and basic needs to survivors, such as food and clothing or medical and emotional care. *Recovery* includes actions for returning the community to normal, such as repairing infrastructure, damaged buildings, and critical facilities. *Rehabilitation* or *reconstruction* encompasses activities that are taken to counter the effects of the disaster on long-term development.[7]

All-Hazards Approach

In the United States, preparedness for disasters is based on an *all-hazards* approach. This approach integrates a common hazard management strategy when planning for all disasters. Given that the range of technological and natural hazards requires similar management strategies, an all-hazards approach fosters a consistent response to any type of event. By not having to develop, exercise, and remember different protocols for different scenarios, responding agencies can concentrate on strengthening broad-based response skills.

Public Health Problems

Disasters pose a number of unique public health and healthcare delivery problems. Examples include the need for warning and evacuation of residents; widespread "urban" search and rescue; triage and distribution of casualties; delivery of health services within a damaged or disabled healthcare infrastructure; and coordination among multiple jurisdictions, among all levels of government, and among private sector organizations. Because disasters pose unique healthcare problems, in order to be effective managers, public health professionals must be knowledgeable about information such as the lexicon of emergency management and the science of engineering and must be competent in a specialized set of skills. For example, although temporary deficiencies in resources may occur at certain times in any disaster, resource problems in U.S. disasters more often relate to how assets are used or distributed rather than to deficiencies.[9] In a foundational study of the impact of 29 major mass casualty disasters on hospitals, only 6% of the involved hospitals had supply shortages, and only 2% had personnel shortages.[10]

Disaster preparedness poses the quintessential public health dilemma—how to motivate people to prevent disaster-related health problems. It is human nature to say, "a major disaster will never happen here," and to fail to prepare. Healthcare organizations often do not give high priority to preparing for disastrous events, which are rare, when the general financial environment for healthcare is fragile. Furthermore, the benefits of preparedness often are not evident until after a disaster has occurred. In addition, economic constraints are often coupled with public apathy. Social scientists have noted that the public's perception of risk is often not correlated with actual risk, and that risks are usually downplayed. Many people continue to live in flood plains, even after repeated floods, and millions of people move to areas that are located on earthquake faults.

However, the benefits of effective prevention are demonstrated in a comparison of the morbidity and mortality statistics of Hurricane Andrew (Florida, 1992) and a hurricane that struck, without warning, off the Gulf Coast of Texas in 1900. Due to successful prediction, warning, and evacuation, the number of deaths following Andrew was less than two dozen. By contrast, 90 years earlier in Texas, 6,000 people were killed and 5,000 were injured.[11] As tragic as the outcomes of Hurricanes Katrina (2005) and Sandy (2012) were, many deaths were averted because of the warning and mass evacuation that took place in the days preceding the hurricanes, again demonstrating the benefits of prevention.

Natural Disasters

Across the United States, a massive number of people are at risk from three classes of natural disasters: floods, hurricanes, and earthquakes. The most frequently occurring and most rapidly increasing events around the globe and in the United States are floods, which hit every state in the United States.[12] Almost 30% of the U.S. population, 5 of its 10 most populous cities, and 7 of its 10 most populous counties live along the Atlantic, Pacific, and Gulf coastlines.[13] Further expected economic and population growth in these coastal counties will result in increasing population density along these vulnerable locations.[14] The significance of this shift is evident when the risk posed by hurricanes alone is examined. Because of climatic changes in western Africa, hurricane activity along the Atlantic Coast and the Gulf of Mexico is expected to become as frequent as that which occurred between 1940 and 1950.[2] During that decade, three category 4–5 hurricanes struck Miami, New Orleans, and the Gulf Coast. The National Oceanic and Atmospheric Administration noted an increasing trend in hurricane activity since 1995, consistent with a multidecade climate pattern that is predicted to last for many more years.

At least 70 million people face significant risk of death or injury from earthquakes because they live in the 39 states that are seismically active. Six major cities with populations greater than 100,000 located in California, the Pacific Northwest, Utah, and Idaho are within the seismic area of the San Andreas fault. Previous projections for a major earthquake in California, similar to nine others that occurred in the state over the past 150 years, suggest 20,000 deaths, 100,000 injuries, and economic losses totaling more than $100 billion.[15] Other parts of the country face serious risk because scientists are expecting a major earthquake along the New Madrid Zone in the heartlands of the United States. During 1811–1812 several temblors on that fault impacted an area encompassing about 5,500 square miles. Some believe a great New Madrid quake to be 30 years overdue.[16] Even in Utah, there is a 20% probability that a large earthquake of a magnitude of 7.5 will occur on some segment of the Wasatch front within the next 50 years.[17]

Manmade Disasters

Manmade or technological disasters can also have devastating impacts on the public's health. The most shocking U.S. manmade disaster occurred in 2001, with the collapse of the World Trade Center in New York City after a terrorist attack. More than 2,600 people died at the World Trade Center, 125 died at the Pentagon, and 256 died on the four planes involved in this coordinated attack. Further, many who witnessed the events or participated in the recovery suffered emotional and/or physical problems, even 10 years later.[18]

Japan escaped a catastrophic disaster at its Fukushima Daiichi nuclear reactors following a major earthquake on March 11, 2011. The plant's power supply and cooling mechanisms were disabled by a 49-foot tsunami and the three cores melted within the first 3 days. The response involved cooling the reactors and preventing the release of radioactive materials, by air or leaking contaminated water. More than 100,000 people were evacuated from their homes. Given the enormity of the cascading events, many more deaths were avoided by the extensive preparedness that is operational throughout Japan.[19] The actual and potential effects of manmade disasters will likely escalate, generating an increased need for public health intervention as the world's population grows, as population density increases, and as technology becomes more sophisticated. The need for public health information has spurred the development of readily available guidance.[20,21]

History of Public Health's Role

Although public health is late in contributing to disaster preparedness and response, epidemiology made an early contribution to the domain of disaster research. Noji first detailed the course of epidemiology's research contribution.[22] In 1957, Saylor and Gordon suggested using epidemiologic parameters to define disasters.[23] Almost a decade later, the Centers for Disease Control and Prevention (CDC) helped develop techniques for the rapid assessment of nutritional status in Nigeria. The 1970s brought the establishment of the Centre for Research on Epidemiology of Disasters in Belgium and specialized units within the World Health Organization (WHO) and the Pan American Health Organization (PAHO).

The earliest investigations of disaster response were conducted by sociologists who studied organizational behavior under stress. Other contributions have been made by psychologists, management scientists, architects, engineers, economists, and public administrators. Since the early 1980s, there has been increased attention and interest in organizing a public health response to disasters and conducting studies within the public health discipline. The eruption of Mt. St. Helens in 1980 accelerated the involvement of the U.S. federal government in organizing a response.[24,25] The United Nations (U.N.) declared the 1990s as the disaster decade—the International Decade for Natural Disaster Reduction—due to continued human losses across the globe.[26] The declaration for the decade spurred the development of educational and research programs in all phases of disaster management by a broad variety of academic disciplines. The decade came to an end on December 31, 1999, and was succeeded by the International Strategy for Disaster Reduction as adopted by resolution 54/219 of the General Assembly of the U.N. in 2000.[27]

Prior to the U.S. effort to enhance public health preparedness for bioterrorism in 1999,[28] the profession had reacted slower than other disciplines in organizing professional activities. In many locales across the country, the medical/health efforts of preparedness were not coordinated as part of the community's disaster response. Health departments were called in as an afterthought to handle problems that were part of their domain, rather than as part of the team planning the response. Federal recognition of the need for public health intervention resulted in directed federal funding for departments of health to improve their core abilities to respond to acts of bioterrorism, bringing public health intervention into the core of disaster preparedness and response. However, the significant public health impact of Hurricane Katrina resulted in the broadest recognition of the need for public health professionals to be an integral part of the emergency preparedness effort in every community.

The ability of public health professionals to respond in emergencies received heightened attention from the passage of the federal Pandemic and All Hazards Preparedness Act (PAHPA) in 2006.[29] PAHPA requires national implementation plans for public health emergency preparedness and response. The public health response is to be integrated with other first responder systems and periodically evaluated through drills and exercises.

The public health workforce must be capable of numerous technical tasks, detailed in PAHPA. In order to meet this challenge, the Association of Schools of Public Health and the CDC developed a set of public health competencies for emergency preparedness.[30] The competency model provides a standard for the public health workforce when carrying out their preparedness and response role. The model has application for public health organizations and non-public health entities where public health workers are employed. The capabilities of the model are built upon established competencies for the public health profession, core proficiencies established for health security or emergency managers, and skills that are position specific or professionally defined. The four domains of the model include activities involved in:

- Model leadership
- Communicating and managing information
- Planning for and improving practice
- Protecting worker health and safety

The science of public health has shown that morbidity and mortality as a result of earthquakes often vary from one country to another due to differences in building standards and population density rather than the magnitude of an earthquake. This is demonstrated by a comparison of the impact of earthquakes in North America and in other continents.

In California, where antiseismic building and land-use codes are well enforced, the Northridge earthquake of 1994 resulted in 57 deaths and almost 9,200 serious injuries.[31] As comparison, the enormous number of deaths and those left homeless from the 2010 quake in Haiti can be attributed to poor construction and insufficient and poorly enforced antiseismic regulations.[32] In contrast, the massive 8.8 magnitude quake that struck Chile in February 2010 only killed hundreds of people.[33] The standards used for construction were the determinate factor for a structure's survival. Further, in the tsunami following the 2004 Sumatra-Andaman earthquake, of the 225,000 deaths, it is not known how many could have been saved by warning systems that advise residents to seek higher ground.

Finally, the medical literature regarding disasters is full of anecdotal accounts of response. Reports substantiating the *effectiveness* of the reported preparedness are beginning to be published.[34,35,36,37]

Public Health's Current Role

Public health has a natural role in disaster preparedness and response. State departments of health, with responsibility as a major directing unit overseeing the public's health, already work in partnership with local health departments (LHDs) and other appropriate federal, state, and local agencies. Disaster response is more than an extension of daily tasks for public health professionals. In many states and localities, public health professionals coordinate the health response following natural and technological emergencies.[20]

Comprehensive preparedness planning should involve multiple partners within the local, state, federal, and even global community as mentioned earlier. Because it may take 24–48 hours or more for regional and federal resources to organize and deploy, the local community must be prepared to respond at the earliest warning and, as shown by Hurricanes Katrina and Sandy, continue interventions for months, especially in locations where housing is destroyed or impacted by flood water.

Many lessons can be learned about public health's role in natural disasters by looking at the impact of three major hurricanes. Due to its impact on realms where public health is core, including healthcare infrastructure, Hurricane Andrew (in 1992) demonstrated that public health professionals must be involved in preparedness and response operations. Hurricane Andrew was considered one of the most destructive disasters ever to affect the United States,[38, p. 243] leaving 175,000 Floridians homeless and water systems inoperable for at least a week.[11] The infrastructure of the healthcare system was also destroyed—59 hospitals were damaged, more than 12,000 patients needed to be examined, and pharmacies could not dispense medication.[39] To help in this situation, more than 850 public health nurses were deployed during the 2 months following the storm.[40] This lesson was magnified by Hurricane Katrina, where more than 400,000 Louisiana residents were displaced because of the mandatory evacuation orders and the flooding that followed the hurricane.[41] Public health activities in response to Hurricane Katrina included investigations of infectious disease, environmental assessments, morbidity and mortality surveillance, shelter-based surveillance, community health and needs assessments, location and follow up of displaced persons with tuberculosis, and broad utilization of immunization registries for displaced children.[42] In an assessment of the public health response, Greenough and Kirsch state, "The biggest health concern, however, was and will continue to be the inability of the displaced population to manage their chronic diseases."[43] When physicians' offices, mental health clinics, nursing homes, pharmacies, community clinics, and urgent care centers are closed, those individuals needing routine care or medication will seek care from emergency departments based in already stressed hospitals. Hurricane Sandy devastated the U.S. East Coast in fall 2012. The storm and storm surge destroyed entire communities located on the New York and New Jersey coasts. Tens of thousands of people were homeless or continued to live in buildings without power, water, or heat; 8 million homes lost power, with many losing water and heat for weeks before they were restored. One week after the storm struck, an increase in the number of exposures to carbon monoxide (CO) was reported to poison centers in eight states.[44] Volunteers found elderly and disabled residents unable to evacuate in their apartments weeks later. Yet only 100 or so died. Five weeks out, tens of thousands of homes remained inhabitable, many with mold growing and no end in sight.[45] For many years, there have been significant opportunities for disaster-related public health interventions. In two examples, strong planning was evident when the Los Angeles Department of Health provided important services following the 1994 Northridge earthquake and the New York City Department of Health and Mental

Health was crucial to the recovery of New York City following the collapse of the World Trade Center in 2001. In both cases, public health intervened when there were numerous environmental (e.g., water, air, sewage), clinical (e.g., personal and mental health, healthcare facilities, clinical operations), and educational (e.g., public information about safety, health, and environmental concerns) issues.[31,46]

With the increase in domestic natural disasters and international complex emergencies, there is greater recognition of the need for intergovernmental experts who understand disasters.

Being prepared is necessitated not only because of legal mandates, but also because of the devastating consequences if healthcare systems are unable to function. The Joint Commission prescribes standards and requirements that healthcare facilities must meet in order to remain accredited. These standards ensure that basic disaster plans are in place and that exercises of these plans are held on a regular basis.[47] The public health professional is involved in ensuring that essential health facilities are able to function after the impact of a disaster.[9,20] Essential facilities include hospitals, health departments, poison control centers, storage sites for disaster supplies, dispatch centers, paging services, and ambulance stations. Hurricane Katrina demonstrated the importance of developing advance creative solutions for the maintenance and continuation of home-based services (e.g., dialysis, intravenous antibiotics, visiting nurses services). Patients in all residential care facilities (e.g., long-term care, psychiatric, rehabilitation) may need to be evacuated and placed elsewhere. Public health also initiates arrangements to ensure that routine sources of medical care will be functioning after a disaster.

Public Health Personnel

Worldwide the growing number of humanitarian emergencies has resulted in an expanding need for skilled public health professionals. The application of public health principles in a domestic response differs from public health practice in an international response, but the competencies required of the profession are the same. The tasks involved in fostering the development of community self-sufficiency are also functionally different in developed countries where the medical response for emergency care is well organized through EMS. Conversely, in developing countries, that infrastructure often does not exist, resulting in public health personnel playing a more prominent role because virtually all of the problems resulting from disasters are related to the health of the populations. In complex humanitarian emergencies, public health personnel may be called on to:

- Conduct initial assessments of health needs
- Assist with risk communication
- Design and establish health activities
- Plan for the delivery of services
- Establish refugee camps
- Provide and monitor food supplies
- Supervise and monitor environmental health activities
- Monitor the protection of human rights

Functional Model of Public Health's Response in Disasters

In disaster preparedness and response, public health professionals are service providers, scientists, and administrators. The core functions of public health have specific application to the organizational model of disaster preparedness and response, providing a role for all public health professionals. Public health practitioners need to relate what public health can do to the framework of activities defined by the emergency management community. In order to function as part of the emergency management team and provide technical assistance to communities, public health professionals must incorporate specialized information that may not be directly related to health and seek out state-of-the-art resources from other scientific fields, such as earth science, engineering, and demography. This interface between the core components of professional training and the matrix of emergency management is called the *functional model* and defines public health's response in disasters.

The functional model provides a paradigm to identify disaster-related activities and is organized by each core area where public health has responsibility. The functional model is composed of six phases that correspond to the type of activities involved in preparing for and responding to a domestic disaster. The paradigm identifies the roles and responsibilities, operationalizes a typical disaster response, and categorizes the cycle of activities performed by the public health field. The functional model expands traditional public health partnerships because it requires public health professionals to collaborate and to work in an integrated fashion with other responding sectors. The components of the model follow:

- *Planning:* The goals of planning are to work cooperatively with other disciplines and understand the resources, skills, and tools that public health professionals bring to the impacted community.
- *Prevention:* Prevention involves primary, secondary, and tertiary efforts and includes the activities that are commonly thought of as "mitigation" in the emergency management model.
- *Assessment:* Assessments are short-term and long-term snapshots that help with decision making and enhance the profession's ability to monitor disaster situations. The goal of conducting assessments is to convey information quickly in order to recalibrate a system's response.
- *Response:* Response includes the delivery of services and the management of activities.
- *Surveillance:* Surveillance includes data collection and monitoring of morbidity and mortality.
- *Recovery:* Recovery includes activities of repairing and reconstructing those elements of a community damaged by the disaster and helping community members recover emotionally. Recovery has short- and long-term policy, political, and social implications.

Structure and Organizational Makeup of Disaster Response

When the healthcare sector responds to a disaster, it is most efficient to do so with the resources already at hand. However, because disasters overwhelm the local authority's ability to respond effectively in protecting human health, local assets often need to be supplemented by resources from organizations outside the area. Additionally, disasters typically generate needs that are beyond the breadth of any one type of healthcare organization. This tension between need and availability is overcome by planning for and mounting a *multi-organizational* response—one of the key characteristics of disaster operations in the health sector. This section provides a quick overview of the organizations that are typically involved in the health sector's response to disaster and describes how they interact with each other in disaster situations. **Table 25.1** lists the most important response organizations.

Structure and Operations of the EMS System

For most sudden-onset disasters, the first medical response is provided by the local or regional EMS system. The potential public health impact that can be contributed by EMS in times of disaster is substantial.[48] In most parts of the United States, EMS is provided by semiautonomous local agencies with regional or state oversight. This service is provided under the authority of the state health department in most, but not all, states, but is not provided directly by the health department. Essential elements of an EMS include the prehospital system composed of:

- Public access through the 911 emergency telephone system
- A dispatch communication system to ensure responders can locate the persons in need
- Trained responders (EMTs/medics)
- Ambulance and other transport services

The in-hospital system is composed of:

- Emergency departments
- Inpatient and other definitive care
- Facilities
- Personnel

In responding to a disaster, the function of coordinating and managing the multiple simultaneous activities, as well as managing the effective deployment of incoming resources, is of primary importance. Drabek et al. found that the coordination of multiple activities, resource inputs, and organizations was among the most difficult and crucial challenges in managing a disaster response.[49] A strong command and coordination system is imperative if emergency health services are to overcome the disruption to the normal operations of the system and to manage additional

Table 25.1   Key Disaster Response Entities

Organization	Functions and Definitions
Public Access System	Enables public to communicate response needs, typically through the 911 phone system
Fire Department	Finds and extricates victims; often provides on-scene incident management
Emergency Medical Services (EMS)	Assesses scene for medical needs, initiates triage of patients, assesses individual patients for status and treatment needs, initiates life-sustaining first aid and medical care, determines treatment destination, and transports patients to definitive care
National Response Framework	Defines principles, roles, and structures of U.S. national response to disasters
National Incident Management System (NIMS)	Comprehensive model for managing emergencies in the United States
Emergency Management Agency (EMA)	A state or jurisdictional agency tasked with preparedness and response for disasters and other emergencies; sometimes called the Office of Emergency Preparedness (OEP)
Department of Homeland Security	The coordinating agency for all federal agency responses to disasters
Department of Health and Human Services (HHS)	The federal action agency charged with lead responsibility for supporting health officials in disaster response
Assistant Secretary for Preparedness and Response (ASPR)	Offices have leadership roles in carrying out support functions for health and medical services as delegated by HHS
Centers for Disease Control and Prevention (CDC)	One of 13 major operational components of HHS; within the CDC, the Office of Public Health Preparedness and Response coordinates and supports CDC's response efforts
Federal Emergency Management Agency (FEMA)	Responsible for emergency management at the scene of a disaster through preparedness, mitigation response, and recovery activities
Emergency Support Function 8 (ESF#8)	The public health and medical function of the National Response Plan provides coordination between HHS operating divisions and ESF#8 interagency partners
National Disaster Medical System (NDMS)	A multiagency response system coordinated by the U.S. Public Health Service OEP with responsibility for responding to overwhelming medical needs in a disaster-struck state or territory
Disaster Medical Assistance Team (DMAT)	A trained unit of medical response personnel available to respond with the NDMS to a disaster scene
Office of the Surgeon General (OSG)	Deploys teams that carry out responsibility of ESF#8
American Red Cross (ARC)	Private voluntary national organization tasked by government to provide mass care and shelter to disaster victims
Private Volunteer Organization (PVO)	National and local volunteer groups that carry out response; groups have a broad range of functions and structures

incoming resources. First published as the FIRESCOPE Program in 1982, the Incident Command System (ICS) is the standard management structure used in disaster response across the United States. Through a system called "sectorization," the tasks and functions of those responding and the use of resources are divided into manageable components. As the size or type of the operation changes, these sectors allow for the ICS to be universally applied.

Organization of Public Health Emergency Response

The basis for all local public health emergency responses resides in the LHD (which is discussed in detail in the section on Bioterrorism). However, the public health sector is not nearly as uniformly organized for emergency responses as the EMS system is, with its broad variety of system designs. Furthermore, the health department is only one actor in the overall emergency response, which is usually coordinated by a public safety agency such as the emergency management authority, a sheriff's office, or a fire department. The best prepared health departments have well designed emergency or disaster response plans, complete with a thorough risk analysis, prognostication of probable health effects, and analysis of the resources needed (and available) to provide an appropriate response. The health departments that are well prepared are likely to have coordinated their plans with other response functions in the health sector (EMS and hospitals), and with other public safety efforts.

The public health response to local-level emergencies and disasters is inevitably a multidisciplinary effort. The American Red Cross (ARC) provides emergency shelter; basic health services for those residing in shelters; food services on site and in shelters; counseling, including mental health services or referrals; and family reunification. The public works department or a contracted commercial provider most often manages the potable water supply. Social services agencies work with the displaced, attend to psychosocial needs, and ensure that special needs populations such as the older adults, children, and individuals with disabilities receive the care required. Associations providing home care are often integrated into the emergency response plan to assist individuals with chronic diseases or special nursing needs. The health department is responsible, in most jurisdictions, for coordinating the efforts of the agencies listed in Table 25.1 on behalf of the public's health.

When the resources of the local jurisdiction are insufficient to meet the needs resulting from the disaster, local authorities have the option to call for additional help. The coordinating agency can seek help from surrounding jurisdictions (often referred to as mutual aid resources) or escalate a request to the state or federal level, or both. The call for outside aid is often called "escalate upward." All states have an emergency management authority (EMA), sometimes called an office of emergency preparedness (OEP). It is the responsibility of the EMA, under the authority of the governor's office, to coordinate the efforts of all state resources used during an emergency or disaster. These resources may be expansive and include the state's health department, housing and social services agencies, and public safety agencies (e.g., state police). In disasters of this magnitude, certain federal resources are made available to the states, such as the National Disaster Medical System, CDC (e.g., Epidemic Intelligence Service), and the U.S. Public Health Service (e.g., the Agency for Toxic Substances and Disease Registry). Local and state emergency management agencies typically convene at a command center away from the disaster site whose function is to coordinate the multiorganizational response of representatives of each pertinent response agency. Health departments should plan to participate in the command center activities as a full partner.

Like a local jurisdiction, states also have the ability to escalate upward if the disaster response requires more resources than the state can quickly provide. States in many regions of the country formed multistate regional mutual aid compacts through the Emergency Management Assistance Compact (EMAC). These nonfederal, interstate agreements facilitate a relatively rapid response due to geographic proximity.

Federal Response

Domestically, there are 40–70 presidential disaster declarations per year. The Robert T. Stafford Disaster Relief and Emergency Assistance Act (Stafford Act), passed by Congress in 1988, provides for orderly assistance by the federal government to state and local governments to help them carry out their responsibilities in managing major disasters and emergencies.[50] A disaster declaration must precede any federal aid whereby states make a request for federal assistance to activate a declaration. Most presidential declarations are made immediately following impact. However, if the consequences of a disaster are imminent and warrant limited predeployment actions to lessen or avert the threat of a catastrophe, a state's governor may submit a request even before the disaster has occurred. Although rarely used, the president may exercise his authority in certain emergencies and make a disaster declaration prior to state request in order to expedite the sending of federal resources. Under the Stafford Act, the president may provide federal resources, including medicine, food and other consumables, manpower and services, and financial assistance.

The U.S. Department of Homeland Security (DHS), established through the Homeland Security Act of 2002, coordinates federal programs and assists states through operational and/or resource coordination and on-scene incident command structures to respond to events that rise to the level of national significance. The Federal Emergency Management Agency has been designated by DHS to coordinate the federal government's response to emergencies.

To provide federal, state, and local guidance regarding a national emergency response, the DHS created the National Response Framework (NRF) in 2008. The NRF, with an all-hazards approach, provides national direction for managing and responding to domestic disasters and combines fundamental principles from previous federal response plans. Using established protocols, the NRF provides guidance for federal coordination with state, local, and tribal governments and with the private sector during incidents. The resources covered by the NRF are normally accessed by a request from a state's governor or the state's EMA to the DHS, referred to earlier as a presidential declaration. A core concept of the national response plan is that the responding federal resources work at the behest of, and in support of, the local or state jurisdiction that is in charge of managing the disaster response.[51]

Presidential Policy Directive 8

Historically, the president has issued executive orders, known as Presidential Policy Directives (or Presidential Decision Directives), to establish national policy about disasters. Recent major disasters, such as Hurricane Katrina, demonstrated that government needs the support of the entire community to mount an effective response. In 2011, President Obama signed Presidential Policy Directive 8 (PPD-8): National Preparedness to fulfill this vision. PPD-8 directs the federal departments and agencies to work with the whole community to prepare for and be resilient in disaster response.[52]

PPD-8 has six components. Key is the National Preparedness Goal (NPG).[53] The NPG defines the core capabilities that the United States needs to achieve the goal and emphasizes that entire communities must work together to best use resources and mount an effective response. The importance of this goal was illustrated following Hurricane Sandy in 2012. For weeks and months, local volunteer groups from around the region provided the full range of response activities (hygiene support, food, clothing, supplies, etc.) when resources of the official response couldn't meet the continuing need. The National Preparedness Goal is: "A secure and resilient nation with the capabilities required across the whole community to prevent, protect against, mitigate, respond to, and recover from the threats and hazards that pose the greatest risk."[53]

Another key component of PDD-8 is the National Preparedness System (NPS), which identifies the approach, resources, and tools needed for achieving the NPG. This system includes assessments of national risk and identification of threats and hazards. The Comprehensive Preparedness Guide (CPG) 101, Version 2.0.2 provides direction for conducting these assessments and for creating state emergency operations plans. In addition to the National Incident Management System (discussed in the next section), the NPS also provides for a program for managing remedial action. Those wanting more information about the status of achieving the NPG can examine the National Preparedness Report; public health and medical services are a content area examined in the report.[54]

National Incident Management System

To enhance the ability of the United States to manage domestic incidents, DHS established a single, comprehensive model for the national management of major incidents known as the National Incident Management System (NIMS). As the response to disasters begins and ends with local officials managing the events, responsibility for the response stays with state and local authorities. In a unified structure and standardized management plan, NIMS uses common terminology, concepts, principles, and processes so that execution during a real incident will be consistent and seamless. This framework was developed to enhance the ability of responders, the private sector, and nongovernmental organizations to work together effectively. Key components of NIMS include:

- Preparedness
- Communications and information management
- Resource management
- Command and management
- Incident command system
- Multiagency coordination systems
- Public information
- Ongoing maintenance and management

Public Health and Medical Capabilities

From the principle that an effective emergency response requires that responders have core capabilities, or skills, two sets of national standards provide that guidance for the public health and medical communities. The CDC developed 15 capabilities to serve as national public health preparedness standards. In 2011, the CDC issued this guidance to assist state and local public health departments in their strategic planning.[55] These standards will help public health agencies determine priorities for preparedness activities and include the following capabilities organized in six domains:

1. Biosurveillance incident management
   - Public health laboratory testing
   - Public health surveillance and epidemiological investigation
2. Community resilience
   - Community preparedness
   - Community recovery
3. Countermeasures and mitigation
   - Medical countermeasure dispensing
   - Medical materiel management and distribution
   - Nonpharmaceutical interventions
   - Responder safety and health
4. Incident management
   - Emergency operations coordination
5. Information management
   - Emergency public information and warning
   - Information sharing
6. Surge management
   - Fatality management
   - Mass care
   - Medical surge
   - Volunteer management

A complementary set of capabilities to guide emergency planning by the healthcare system was published in 2012 by the Office of the Assistant Secretary for Preparedness and Response.[56] The eight capabilities align with and complement the public health standards:

- Healthcare system preparedness
- Healthcare system recovery
- Emergency operations coordination
- Fatality management
- Information sharing
- Medical surge
- Responder safety and health
- Volunteer management

Vulnerable Populations

Federal guidance for caring for people vulnerable to the effects of disasters was strengthened following the tragic events that occurred in New Orleans after Hurricane Katrina. The plight of those at risk was amplified by the images of thousands stranded in the New Orleans Superdome without adequate supplies and the stories of nursing homes that were not evacuated and could not be reached because of the flooding.

Section 2814 of PAHPA (discussed earlier) requires that local, state, and federal communities include the needs of at-risk populations in their emergency planning. At-risk individuals include those who have additional needs in:

- Maintaining independence (need support to be independent in daily activities)
- Communication (have difficulty hearing or seeing communication)
- Transportation (cannot drive due to disability or do not have transportation)
- Supervision (need supervision to make decisions)
- Medical care (need trained medical care to manage condition)

In addition, key sections of the Post-Katrina Emergency Management Reform Act, passed by the U.S. Congress in 2006, require improved preparedness and response for people with disabilities. Specific requirements detail actions to enable disabled persons to stay in an emergency shelter with the general population. **Table 25.2** describes national guidance on preparedness for at-risk populations.

Voluntary Agencies

Of considerable importance to the successful provision of good public health response to a disaster is mass care. The ARC is the primary agency responsible for this function, which includes sheltering, feeding, emergency first aid, family reunification, and the distribution of emergency relief supplies to disaster victims. The ARC responds first through its local chapters, then state and regional chapters, which may call on national-level ARC resources if necessary.

A vast array of other voluntary agencies participates in disaster response with functions that contribute significantly to public health outcomes. Many of these are church affiliated, such as the Salvation Army, Mennonite Central Committee, and Catholic Relief Services. Some are dedicated solely to disaster-related functions, but most have more routine public service and emergency functions that are activated according to the needs of a specific disaster.

International Agencies

A vast array of agencies stands ready to respond to requests for international assistance to protect the public's health after disasters. Multinational U.N.-based organizations include WHO, United Nations Children's Fund (UNICEF), the U.N. High Commissioner for Refugees (UNHCR), and the World Food Programme. PAHO (WHO's regional affiliate for the Americas) has a highly organized Office for Emergency Preparedness and Disaster Relief Coordination, which helps coordinate international health sector response in the Americas. Many national governments have an agency that provides unilateral foreign disaster assistance, such as the U.S. State Department's Office of Foreign Disaster Assistance. Numerous voluntary agencies have gained

Table 25.2 National Standards in Preparedness and Response for At-Risk Populations

Organization	Guidance Name	What It Does	Source
FEMA	Comprehensive Preparedness Guide 301 (CPG-301): Emergency Management Planning Guide for Special Needs Populations	• Helps governments develop emergency plans for people with functional needs • Addresses planning considerations for range of hazards, security, and emergency functions • Provides general guidelines for developing a governmental household pets and service animals plan	http://www.fema.gov/
Americans with Disabilities Act (ADA) and ADA Amendments Act (2008)	ADA Amendments Act	• ADA requires equal access to all government programs • Broadened scope of the definition of "disability" • Allows people with functional needs to seek protection under the ADA, including all disaster plans developed for a community under Title II	http://www.ada.gov
ADA Guide for Local Governments	Making Community Emergency Preparedness and Response Programs Accessible to People with Disabilities	Provides guidance for making local emergency preparedness and response programs accessible to people with disabilities	http://www.usdoj.gov/crt/ada/emergencyprep.htm
1986 Superfund Amendment and Reauthorization Act (SARA), Title III	Local Emergency Planning Committees (LEPCs)	Directs the creation and membership of LEPCs	http://www.epa.gov/emergencies/content/epcra/epcra_plan.htm#LEPC
The Joint Commission	Emergency Management Standards of the Joint Commission	Oversees standard setting for healthcare facilities and accredits healthcare facilities	http://www.jointcommission.org
National Fire Protection Association (NFPA)	NFPA 99, 1600	Recommends safety codes and standards for the prevention of fires and other hazards	http://www.nfpa.org

(continues)

Table 25.2   National Standards in Preparedness and Response for At-Risk Populations (continued)

Organization	Guidance Name	What It Does	Source
Federal Communications Commission (FCC)	• Emergency Alert System (EAS) Rules (47 C.F.R. Part 11) Closed-Captioning Rules • (47 C.F.R. Section§ 79)	Regulations regarding the Emergency Alert System (EAS) and closed captioning	http://www.fcc.gov
FEMA	Guidance on Planning Integration of Functional Needs Support Services in General Population Shelters	Provides guidance for the implementation of practices so that individuals with disabilities can maintain their health, safety, and independence in a shelter whose residents are from the general population	http://www.fema .gov/pdf/about/ odic/fnss_guidance .pdf

Source: Adapted from National Organization on Disability. *Functional Needs of People with Disabilities: A Guide for Emergency Managers, Planners and Responders.* Washington, DC: National Organization on Disability Emergency Preparedness Initiative, 2009; and the Federal Emergency Management Agency. *Guidance on Planning for Integration of Functional Needs Support Services in General Population Shelters.* San Antonio, TX: BCFS Health and Human Services; 2010. Available at: http://www.fema.gov/pdf/about/odic/fnss_guidance.pdf. Accessed March 27, 2013.

considerable expertise in responding to post-disaster health needs across international borders. Examples include Médecins Sans Frontières (Doctors Without Borders), World Vision, Oxfam, and Save the Children.

Assessment in Disasters

Public health, at the local, state, and federal levels, has a major role in assessing and monitoring the nature of disasters and their impacts on communities. These assessments are important managerial tools in preventing morbidity and mortality and in organizing a response. The information provided in these assessments helps health officials or emergency managers make informed decisions about response and recovery activities.

During each phase of the disaster continuum, public health assessment for a disaster event is conducted by gathering information. These processes lead to an identification of: 1) the needs of the affected community after a disaster has occurred, 2) appropriate relief goods or services for that community, 3) epidemic levels of disease or injury if indicated, and 4) resources that may be needed by healthcare services in the disaster zone.

Emergency Information Systems

Information is critical to any response effort after a disaster has occurred. The need for objective and reliable information is underscored because disasters disrupt physical and social environments, may trigger threats to health, often cause ecologic changes and population displacement leading to overcrowding and situations in which sanitation and hygiene are compromised, and disrupt normal public health programs. Moreover, the potential for communicable diseases increases for vector-borne, waterborne, and person-to-person transmission. As such, accurate and reliable information is needed to aid decisions about immediate relief efforts, short-term responses, and long-term planning for recovery and reconstruction. These emergency information systems facilitate the monitoring of health events, diseases, injuries, hazards, exposures, and risk factors related to a designated event.

Several types of information are collected for decision making, and each type has multiple uses. Mortality data are tracked to assess the magnitude of the disaster event, to evaluate the effectiveness of disaster preparedness and the adequacy of warning systems, and to identify high-risk groups where more contingency planning is required. By reviewing information about casualties or the injured, emergency medical personnel and managers of critical care facilities can estimate needs for emergency care, evaluate predisaster planning and preparedness, and evaluate the adequacy of warning systems. Managers can assess information about morbidity to estimate the types and volume of immediate medical relief needed, to identify populations at risk for disease, to evaluate the appropriateness of relief activities, and to identify areas for further planning.

In addition to information that helps public health professionals understand the health effects of disasters, information concerning public health resources, particularly from LHDs, is important for emergency information systems. Using these data, officials can estimate the types and volume of supplies, equipment, and services required. Finally, information may be compiled about specific events related to and health outcomes associated with community hazards.

Surveillance

Public health surveillance is the ongoing and systematic collection, analysis, and interpretation of health data used for planning, implementing, and evaluating public health interventions and programs, closely integrated with the timely dissemination of these data to those who need to know. Surveillance data are used to determine the need for public health action and to assess the effectiveness of programs. A surveillance system includes a functional capacity for data collection, analysis, and dissemination linked to public health programs.[57, p. 164]

In the postdisaster setting, surveillance provides information that can serve as the basis for action during the immediate disaster and also for planning of future activities. For example, measles vaccination campaigns may be launched in shelters if potential outbreaks are identified. Surveillance is also conducted to investigate rumors, such as the occurrence of infectious disease, which commonly arise in the aftermath of a disaster event. Syndromic surveillance data can signal whether an outbreak is emerging or has occurred. If unusual increases of disease are observed, public health workers may be deployed to investigate and confirm diagnosis. Finally, surveillance is also conducted to monitor the effectiveness of response activities. For example, cases of acute diarrheal disease would be expected to decline with the use and implementation of water treatment interventions. A surveillance system that monitors diarrheal disease where water treatment has been implemented could indicate, as evidenced by rates of diarrheal disease, whether intervention was effective.

Surveillance systems measure hazards, exposures, and outcomes. A *hazard* surveillance is, by definition, an assessment of the occurrence of or distribution of levels of hazards and the trends in hazardous levels (e.g., toxic chemical agents, physical agents, or biologic agents) responsible for disease and injury. An example of the application of postdisaster hazard surveillance is the tracking of daily variations in respirable particulate matter (i.e., particles with a mass median aerodynamic diameter of ≤ 10 microns) after wildland fires. Federal thresholds are established for guiding those susceptible to pulmonary disease to take precautionary measures when the particles reach a certain size.

Surveillance may also assess *exposure.* In disaster settings, exposure may be based on physical or environmental properties of the disaster event, such as "ash fall" after volcanic activity or pesticide-contaminated soil unearthed by flood water.[58]

Surveillance most commonly looks for health *outcomes,* defined as a health event of interest, usually illness, injury, or death. Other types of surveillance systems may be based on the characteristics and objectives for establishing those particular systems.

Those establishing a surveillance system determine the variables of potential importance after a specific disaster event (i.e., diseases, injuries, and causes of death). Diseases that were endemic in the affected area prior to the disaster event should be included in the system because these would be expected to rise with increased population density, displacement, interrupted normal public health programs, and compromised sanitation and hygiene.

Facilitating the dissemination of information is critical to a successfully implemented surveillance system. Proper dissemination includes content reported in a format that would alert policy and decision makers, prevention program managers, the media, and the public about the required public health actions.

Data Collection

Accurate and reliable information is needed for planning relief, recovery, and evacuation activities for disaster response. Historical information may be used by emergency managers as a reference against which to compare phenomena exhibited by a given disaster event. Such information originates from a variety of sources, including existing community institutions (e.g., utility companies) and units created specifically to provide immediate response following a disaster. A decision maker will have a better idea about the severity of an event if historical information about the hazards, risks, and vulnerabilities of a particular area has been pre-gathered. Historical information is available from the local emergency management authority, geologic institutions, or international ministries responsible for natural resources and the environment.

During the relief phase, the following data help gauge appropriate relief efforts by emergency managers and public health officials:

- Demographic characteristics of the affected area and surrounding vicinities
- Casualty assessment, including deaths, injuries, and selected illnesses
- Assessment of the needs of the displaced population
- Coordination of volunteer assistance
- Management of facilities
- Storage and distribution of relief materials
- Communication systems

- Transportation systems
- Public information and rumor control
- Registration inquiry services
- Traffic and crowd control

Data for postimpact surveillance may be extracted from a variety of sources, including existing data sets (e.g., census and national health information systems), hospitals and clinics (e.g., hospital electronic medical records), community healthcare providers (e.g., patient records), temporary shelters (e.g., daily shelter census, medical logs at shelters), first-responder logs (e.g., DMAT patient logs), mobile health clinics (e.g., patient logs, records of prescription medications dispensed), and geographic information systems (e.g., locations of injured, where power is out, socially vulnerable communities).

The selection of an appropriate sampling method depends on the objectives of a collection system and the existence of a sampling frame. Population-based sampling techniques, when possible, should be employed. For instance, if all of the households in an affected area are identified and mapped prior to a disaster event, a simple random sample may be appropriate for a community-based needs assessment. If a sampling frame does not already exist, then a cluster design might be more appropriate. Other designs include a systematic or stratified sampling.

Measurements of Disasters

Objective measures are used to quantify environmental hazards and human impacts related to natural disasters. To indicate the severity of a disaster event, scales developed by other scientific disciplines such as seismology and meteorology are used to measure and describe the hazard from the public health standpoint. For example, the magnitude of an earthquake is indicated by the Richter scale, which provides a measure of the total energy released from the source of the earthquake. Similarly, the strength of tornadoes is measured by the Fujita scale.

Measuring the physical manifestations of a disaster event can indicate the size and severity of that event. For example, the height of a river can signal the scope of a flood event. Levels of pesticides in drinking water or sediment after severe flooding may lead to questions about acute and chronic exposure to toxic chemicals in na-tech events.

Measures of biologic effects indicate resulting impacts on human health and disease. In earthquake events, age-specific injury and death rates may be calculated in cases where a direct health outcome is associated with the event. Among displaced persons in shelters where an infectious disease outbreak may occur, laboratory typing of organisms in biologic samples such as blood and urine may indicate exposure to a disease-causing pathogen and confirmation of disease. In famine situations, anthropometric measurements, such as height-to-weight ratios among young children, may indicate the type and degree of malnutrition due to lack of food.

Applied Epidemiology

A systematic approach to assessing postdisaster conditions is based on the principles of epidemiology, the cornerstone of public health science. One application of epidemiology is the investigation of the public health consequences of natural disasters. Known as "disaster epidemiology," or "epidemiology in disaster settings," this discipline evolved as scientists realized that the effects of disasters on health were amenable to study by epidemiologic methods.[59] For example, cause-and-effect studies can be undertaken to identify the impact of disasters. Children and adolescents with environmental exposures following Hurricane Katrina experienced an increase of upper respiratory and lower respiratory symptoms.[60]

The ultimate aim of disaster epidemiology is to determine strategies to prevent or reduce deaths, injuries, or illnesses related to the disaster. Prevention strategies are often grouped into three categories:

1. *Primary prevention*, or prevention of the occurrence of deaths, injuries, or illnesses related to the disaster event (e.g., evacuation of a community in a flood-prone area, sensitizing warning systems for tornadoes and severe storms)
2. *Secondary prevention*, or the mitigation of health consequences of disasters (e.g., use of carbon monoxide detectors when operating gasoline-powered generators after loss of electric power, building a "safe room" in dwellings located in tornado-prone areas)
3. *Tertiary prevention*, minimizing the effects of disease and disability among the already ill, which is employed in persons with preexisting health conditions and in whom the health effects from a disaster event may exacerbate those health conditions (e.g., appropriate sheltering of persons with respiratory illnesses from haze and smoke originating from forest fires, sheltering elderly who are prone to heat illnesses during episodes of extreme ambient temperatures)

In the immediate aftermath of a disaster, a critical concern of relief authorities is the identification of the needs of an affected community, and epidemiologic studies can help provide that information. Public health authorities or emergency management officials can provide information for emergency planning, provide reliable and accurate information for relief decisions, and ultimately, match resources to requirements. Finally, managers can employ epidemiologic applications to evaluate the effectiveness of programs used to provide relief.

Behavioral Health Considerations in Disasters: Psychosocial Impacts and Public Health

When most people hear the word "disaster," they tend to picture the physical destruction images of injured people and collapsed buildings. As disasters can flatten trees, break bones, and tear houses apart, they can also profoundly affect individual wellbeing, family relations, and the fabric of community life. The psychosocial impacts of disasters range from mild stress reactions to serious problems such as substance abuse, depression, and posttraumatic stress disorder (PTSD).

The mental health sequelae of a disaster can be quite widespread. In terms of morbidity, the social and psychological impacts of a disaster can greatly exceed the direct toll of physical injuries. Furthermore, these less visible effects of disasters have historically affected the functioning of individuals and communities years after a disaster struck. Thus, any effort to help restore the health of a community that has suffered a calamity should incorporate mental health into response and recovery efforts.

Public health agencies and public health professionals are heavily involved in addressing the social and psychological impacts of disaster, and attention to these issues represents a core part of the public health profession's response to disaster.[61] In fact, at the federal level, the Department of Health and Human Services is a leader in the field of disaster mental health services. Staff of the Substance Abuse and Mental Health Services Administration's Emergency Services and Disaster Relief Branch in the Center for Mental Health Services helps to ensure that victims of presidentially declared disasters receive immediate, short-term crisis counseling and ongoing support for emotional recovery. Numerous other examples of public health involvement with mental health issues can be found at the federal, state, and local levels.

Behavioral Health Effects of Disaster

Disasters are life-changing experiences; these events are highly stressful, disruptive experiences for individuals, families, and entire communities. During a disaster, people may experience such traumatic stresses as loss of relatives, friends, and associates; personal injury; property loss; witnessing death or mass destruction; or having to handle bodies.[62] The period after a disaster can bring additional stresses, such as grieving for lost loved ones, changes to one's role in family and community, moving, cleaning and repairing property, and dealing with large bureaucracies to report loss.[63] Overall, experiencing a disaster "is often one of the single most traumatic events a person can endure."[61, p. 101]

People who have gone through a disaster may experience any of a range of emotional, physical, cognitive, and interpersonal effects, and the numbers of people experiencing stress reactions following a major disaster can be large. A list of common stress reactions to disaster is provided in **Exhibit 25.1**.

In general, the transient reactions that people experience after a disaster represent a normal response to a highly abnormal situation. People are exposed to situations that are well outside the bounds of everyday experience, and such situations place extraordinary demands—both physical and emotional—on people. Given the circumstances, mild to moderate stress reactions are common during the emergency and in the initial phases of recovery. These common stress reactions generally do not become chronic problems.[62] As a general rule, most individuals who are exposed to a disaster do not suffer prolonged psychological illnesses.

Importantly, common stress reactions should not be ignored in the planning and implementation of a comprehensive public health response to a disaster. Behavioral health programs and services should include informational and educational support about normal reactions, ways to handle reactions, and early treatment, where indicated, in addition to the many types of services required at family assistance centers and in long-term treatment.[20]

Persistent Effects

While most stress reactions after disaster tend to be transient, a portion of the population impacted by a disaster may suffer more serious, persistent effects. Research shows that behavioral health problems can result from exposure to both natural and technological disasters. These psychological problems include acute stress disorder (ASD), posttraumatic stress disorder (PTSD), depression, substance abuse, anxiety, and somatization. Other kinds of problems, including

---

Exhibit 25.1   Common Stress Reactions to Disaster

Emotional Effects	Cognitive Effects
Shock	Impaired concentration
Anger	Impaired decision-making ability
Despair	Memory impairment
Emotional numbing	Disbelief
Terror	Confusion
Guilt	Distortion
Grief or sadness	Decreased self-esteem
Irritability	Decreased self-efficacy
Helplessness	Self-blame
Loss of pleasure derived from regular activities	Worry
Dissociation (e.g., perceptual experience seems "dreamlike," "tunnel vision," "spacey," or on "automatic pilot")	Intrusive thoughts and memories
Physical Effects	**Interpersonal Effects**
Fatigue	Alienation
Insomnia	Social withdrawal
Sleep disturbance	Increased conflict within relationships
Hyperarousal	Vocational impairment
Somatic complaints	School impairment
Impaired immune response	
Headaches	
Gastrointestinal problems	
Decreased appetite	
Decreased libido	
Startle response	

Source: Reprinted from Young BH, Ford JD, Ruzek JI, et al. *Disaster Mental Health Services: A Guidebook for Clinicians and Administrators.* Menlo Park, CA: National Center for Posttraumatic Stress Disorder; 1998.

---

physical illness; domestic violence; and more general symptoms of distress, daily functioning, and physiological reactivity have also been documented.[61]

ASD is "characterized by posttraumatic stress symptoms lasting at least 2 days but not longer than 1 month post-trauma."[64, p. 7] In the aftermath of stressful events that are "both extreme and outside of the realm of everyday experiences," some individuals may experience a prolonged stress response known as PTSD.[65, p. 29] Unlike transient stress reactions seen among disaster survivors, PTSD is associated with much greater levels of impairment and dysfunction.[62]

While PTSD usually appears in the first few months after a trauma has been experienced, sometimes the disorder may not appear until years have passed. Likewise, PTSD's duration can vary, with symptoms diminishing and disappearing over time in some people and persisting for many years in others. It should also be noted that PTSD frequently occurs with—or leads to—other psychiatric illness, such as depression. This is known as comorbidity.[66,67]

Much is known about factors associated with the development of PTSD, and about factors that may reduce the likelihood of developing PTSD. A key factor, the nature of the trauma experienced (i.e., if the person's life was threatened or was exposed to terror, horror, and the grotesque), poses the greatest risk of PTSD.[68] According to Young et al., disaster-related variables associated with long-term adjustment problems include mass casualties, mass destruction, death of a loved one, residential relocation, and toxic contamination.[62] There is evidence that some pretrauma factors have an effect as well, such as a history of prior exposure to trauma.

As might be expected, what happens in a disaster survivor's life after the trauma also appears to affect the risk of developing PTSD.[69] For example, it appears that in many situations social support may play a role as a protective factor. While PTSD is usually associated with primary exposure to trauma, people who have not actually experienced a disaster themselves can still develop PTSD and related symptoms, such as spouses/significant others of disaster workers.[68]

In recent years, researchers have focused increasing attention on ethnocultural issues related to PTSD.[70] While a number of studies of disasters in the United States have found differing rates of PTSD or other disaster-related impairments among groups of different races or ethnicities, the PTSD construct has been found to have a universal dimension that makes it applicable across cultures. In fact, survivors of the Japanese earthquake-tsunami-radiation accident experienced similar distress to that seen in other devastating disasters.[71,72] As such, it is important to incorporate culturally sensitive assessment techniques in order to identify variants on expressions of distress.

Social Impacts of Disaster

In addition to having the potential to produce PTSD, ASD, depression, and other psychological effects, disasters can also profoundly affect the *social* health of communities. Postdisaster efforts must include interventions to restore support networks and the health of the community as a whole. The need for this was dramatically illustrated in Erikson's study of the 1972 Buffalo Creek disaster,[73] where a makeshift dam used by a coal mining company sent millions of gallons of waste- and debris-filled flood waters roaring into a mountain hollow known as Buffalo Creek, West Virginia. The Appalachian mountain community was devastated: 125 people were killed, many others were injured, hundreds of homes and other buildings were wrecked, and thousands of people were displaced. Survivors, many of whom had witnessed dead and dismembered bodies, suffered a wide array of impacts including nightmares, numbing, insomnia, guilt, despair, confusion, depression, and hopelessness. In addition to these individual effects, the disaster plus an ill-conceived relocation effort effectively destroyed the social support system that held together the formerly tight-knit community.

Resilience and Social Support

It is now recognized that the mental health outcomes of a community are partially dependent on the community's level of preparation. Becoming resilient, or capable of withstanding the stresses that accompany disasters, is a critical element in community preparedness. Experience has shown that the extent to which disasters cause serious, long-lasting mental health impacts can vary by disaster and by community. In some disasters, victims seem to fare well without long-lasting problems. In other disasters, they suffer major mental health problems both immediately and for several years after the disaster.

The impact of social support on recovery has been documented from the earliest research on the effects of disasters. Even 14 years after the Buffalo Creek, West Virginia disaster, the survivors still showed significantly higher rates of major depression, general anxiety, and lifetime PTSD as compared to the nonexposed group.[70] Yet, after the tornado in Xenia, Ohio, where 33 people were killed and between 1,000 and 2,000 people were injured, the population fared much better.[74]

What accounts for the dramatic difference between the results of Buffalo Creek and Xenia studies? One factor may be that whereas Buffalo Creek's tight-knit community network was obliterated by the flood, most of Xenia's extended support networks remained intact despite the damage caused by the tornado. Outcomes have been shown to be dependent not only on the highly complex nature of disaster situations but also on the often enormous variations among communities.

Natural Disasters and Technological Disasters

In recent years, there has been considerable discussion in the disaster research community regarding the similarities and differences between natural and manmade disasters. When comparing natural and human caused disasters, the two, suggest Green and Solomon, "are probably more alike than different."[75, p. 164] While both have in common an immediate threat and the potential for ongoing disruption, there is a huge difference in perceived and actual human control over the disasters. Natural disasters tend to be seen as part of nature over which we have no control. On the other hand, manmade disasters are, in principle, preventable. Because we expect to be able to control technology, technological disasters often produce higher levels of anger and distrust than natural disasters because blame and responsibility are often ascribed.

Services Provided After a Disaster

Public health professionals should work with local emergency planning committees to ensure that disaster and emergency plans adequately address potential social and behavioral health issues and that these concerns are appropriately incorporated into a community's disaster plans.

The numerous psychosocially oriented activities and services that are typically provided after a disaster are listed in **Table 25.3**. Public health professionals should also identify community resources/assets (citizen groups, associations, publications, specialists at nearby universities, etc.) and link them with mental health plans for assistance.[20] In addition, public health professionals should build community capacity to address social and psychological impacts.[20]

Activities and services provided in the aftermath of disaster need to be tailored to the community being served. This means involving stakeholders, community groups, and others in the development and delivery of services. In addition, special services and assistance should be geared toward vulnerable groups of the population and those with special needs, such as children, the elderly, and the disabled. Older adults may have more limited support networks, mobility impairment or

Table 25.3 Community Behavioral Services Needed Following a Disaster

Adult, adolescent, and child services

Assessments, crisis interventions, evaluations, and referrals

Bereavement counseling

Business counseling

Crisis counseling

Debriefing groups for healthcare and emergency workers

Drop-in crisis counseling

Emergency services in medical emergency departments

Family support center

Individual and group counseling

Mobile mental health crisis teams

Multidisciplinary services to designated community sites (police precincts, fire departments, temporary business locations)

Multilingual services

Outpatient mental health services and counseling

Ongoing support groups

Outreach to schools for students, parents, and teachers

Outpatient services

School presentations

Short-term treatment

Telephone triage

24-hour emergency psychiatric service

24-hour crisis hotline

Walk-in services

Weekly support groups

Source: Reprinted with permission. Landesman LY. *Public Health Management of Disasters: The Practice Guide.* 3rd ed. Washington, DC: American Public Health Association; 2012:218.

limitation, or illnesses. Finally, it is important to direct special attention to disaster workers who risk their own lives and their ability to provide for their families while being repeatedly exposed to mutilated bodies and life-threatening situations while doing physically demanding work.[76]

Public Health Aspects of Environmental Services During Disasters

General Principles

Assuming that following disasters, certain hazards move through the environment and cause harm to humans, post-impact environmental control measures must focus on preventing the hazardous situation, the transport of the hazard, or people being exposed to the hazard once they encounter it. For example, in malaria control, prevention activities would include stopping mosquito breeding by draining stagnant water, spraying for mosquitoes to avert the transport of pathogens, and getting people to use pesticide-impregnated bed nets or insect repellent to diminish their exposure. Whether the subject is diarrhea prevention or toxic waste control, these three types of preventive measures can apply.

As a general premise, no environmental measure functions perfectly 100% of the time. In developed countries, this is compensated by having multiple sanitary barriers between a hazard and a population. If, on a given day, any redundant measure is not functioning, the others will protect against the hazard. Most waterborne outbreaks in developed countries occur when a series of mishaps causes several public health barriers (e.g., filtration and chlorination) to fail.

A second sanitary principle is that distance aids safety. In general, the more dangerous a substance is and the more volume that exists, the more space is required between the substance and populations. Keeping hazardous material at a distance may cut down on human exposure because distance provides time for detection and for protective actions.

Within the context of an emergency situation, where people have been displaced from their homes and are sheltered in overcrowded conditions, these general premises of sanitary engineering become problematic. Resources are usually limited, and services must be established at very short notice. Moreover, where shelter is unavailable, displaced people are often shunted onto land where space to separate people and their nearest hazard is unavailable. Thus, the environmental practice becomes quite crude when applied to displaced populations and refugees. The principal hazard created within these settlements is usually feces. Because its creation is unavoidable, the public health task is to minimize fecal transport and to minimize the population's exposure, which in the case of fecally transmitted illnesses means minimizing oral ingestion.

During natural disasters, the usual task is either to protect or to restart the protective barriers that exist, or to promote changes in behavior that will compensate for the disrupted sanitary barriers. Examples of such messages include orders to boil water, warnings about foods that may have spoiled during electrical outages, or announcements regarding where potable water will be provided. For displaced populations, all basic services usually need to be restarted from scratch. During natural disasters, especially in developed countries, there may be few commonalties between the same types of crises in different locations. Typically, the infrastructure to provide safe water and food is in place, but it may be inoperative.

Sanitation

Since, during an emergency, the use of latrines or other excreta-containment facilities has been shown to prevent diarrheal illness more than any other environmental measure in undeveloped countries, one of the first disaster-response activities should be the establishment of a sanitation system. Mortality and morbidity rates among displaced populations in the first days and weeks of a crisis are often many times higher than rates among the same population once it is stabilized. Thus, providing some sanitation facilities during the first days of a crisis is critical. The goal is for everyone to use proper facilities all of the time. To do so, the appropriate type of facility needs to be identified that will be culturally sensitive to the affected population. For example, in some cultures, it may be important to include building separate latrines for men and women or separate latrines for children.

Personal Hygiene

The promotion of personal hygiene following a disaster is among the most difficult environmental interventions. Personal habits can influence a population's wellbeing, regardless of the infrastructure and resources provided, such as the poor hand-washing practices among relief workers which caused diarrhea during the Oklahoma City bombing. Regardless of the setting, several basic premises are universal—specifically, soap provides protection from diarrheal illness independent of any educational program that may accompany it.[77] As people need to be able to clean themselves after defecating, materials for cleansing (paper, sticks) should be made available along with water and soap.

Hand washing, particularly after defecating and before preparing food, has been shown to be protective against fecal–oral illnesses. No studies examining the impact of personal hygiene that were included in a recent review found health benefits associated with education alone, only with documented changes in behavior.[78] Therefore, any efforts to promote hand washing should have a simple monitoring component to ensure that increased hand washing is actually occurring.

To work, educational messages should be short and focused. All messages included in an educational campaign should promote measures known to prevent the specific health threat at hand, such as, "Boil your drinking water," and should focus on behaviors that are not presently practiced by a significant portion of the population.

Water Quality

Water quality is usually evaluated based on the presence of some bacterial measure, which indicates the possible presence of feces. Because human feces typically contain tens of millions of bacteria per gram, even minute amounts of feces in water are often detectable via bacterial monitoring. Fecal coliforms are a general category of bacteria that are empirically defined to match the characteristics of bacteria found in the stool of warm-blooded mammals. Finding no fecal coliforms in untreated water is a good indication that there are no fecal–oral bacterial pathogens present, although finding fecal coliforms in water does not prove that the water is dangerous. UNHCR considers water with less than 10 fecal coliforms per 100 mL to be reasonably safe, whereas water with more than 100 fecal coliforms per 100 mL is considered to be very polluted. Other indicator bacteria, such as *Escherichia coli*, fecal streptococci, or total coliforms, operate on the same premise that absence implies water safety. Although water sources may be of differing water quality, in many, if not most settings, the handling and storing of water by people will be the main determinant in water safety. Studies have shown that the dipping of water from household storage buckets causes considerable contamination, and that water quality deteriorates over time after the water is initially collected. The best assurance that clean water will stay clean is to add a chlorine residual to the water. This means that in unsanitary settings, or during times of outbreaks, it may be appropriate to chlorinate safe source water. **Exhibit 25.2** provides additional information about surface and ground water.

Exhibit 25.2   Getting and Treating Water in a Crisis Situation

Surface Water

Bucket collection: Where people collect water directly from water bodies in buckets, the only treatment of surface water that can easily be achieved is chlorination. Water can be chlorinated in the home or by health workers at the point of collection. Ideally, enough chlorine should be added to the bucket so that after 30 minutes, there is still at least 0.5 mg/L free chlorine in the water.

Pipe distribution: In systems that have many broken distribution pipes or during times of disease outbreaks, attempting to have 0.5 to 1.0 mg/L free chlorine is appropriate. During crises of conflicts, pressure intermittency in pipes allows water to be drawn in through cracks, resulting in cross-contamination responsible for most major waterborne outbreaks. Monitoring of chlorine is recommended to achieve a dose allowing free chlorine throughout the system.

Groundwater

Spring: A location where groundwater flows to the earth's surface of its own accord. To protect the water from contamination, build a spring box, which is a collection basin with an outflow pipe at or below the point where the water comes to the surface.

Wells: To prevent contamination with surface water, the well usually includes a skirt around the opening of the well, or a plate sealing off the surface at the top of the well. Where there is household water contamination or high risk of a waterborne outbreak, water disinfection of wells and springs with chlorine is advisable.

Wells can be of a variety of sizes and shapes, with a variety of pumps or devices to raise the water. Although many reasons relating to siting and construction errors can cause a well to never come into service, wells that operate for a time typically fail because of lack of maintenance and repair capacity. Thus, groups planning to build wells need to budget from the outset for parts and personnel to maintain the projects until local wealth and economic activity can sustain the water system, or until the wells are abandoned.

Water Quantity

In developing countries, by providing people with more water than they currently have, we can protect them against fecal–oral pathogens better than by providing people with cleaner water.[79,80] UNHCR purports that people need at least 15–20 liters of water per person per day (L/p/d) to maintain human health. Because of the importance of water to maintaining health, contaminated water sources should never be closed until equally convenient facilities become available.

During a crisis, water consumption should be estimated at least weekly. Often, the local utility or nongovernmental organization (NGO) providing water to a population collects these figures. Note that water consumption means what people receive, not what the water operators produce. Water can be lost or wasted during pumping and transport, and people may be prevented from getting adequate quantities because they do not have containers to hold water, leading to discrepancies between estimates of production and consumption. Therefore, sampling that documents people's use of water (such as household interviews) or the actual collection of water at watering points is a preferable method of assessing usage than to divide the water produced at a well or a plant by the number of people served. Cholera outbreak investigations have revealed that not owning a bucket puts families at increased risk of illness or death.[79] Thus, not only should the average water consumption be 15 L/p/d or more, but there should not be anyone with very low water consumption (< 5 L/p/d) in the population.

During natural disasters in areas with piped water, rapid surveys can quickly determine which areas are lacking in water service. Areas where service is expected to be cut for days or weeks are often vacated, or else water is transported to the area by vehicle.

Specific Outbreak Control Strategies for Epidemic Diarrheal Diseases

For several specific fecal–oral diseases, different combinations of environmental measures have been shown to be more effective than others. This becomes important when trying to choose the one or two messages to be included in a campaign and when available staff and resources limit the environmental programs that can be undertaken. **Exhibit 25.3** describes control strategies for four major diarrheal diseases.

Heating and Shelter

Although often not thought of as a health issue, heating and shelter have been essential components of disaster response. Although cold conditions are widely associated with the medical conditions of hypothermia and frostbite, symptoms of malaise and nutritional shortages probably result in more morbidity. Living in cold conditions, even with proper clothing, requires more caloric intake to maintain the same activity level. In general, approximately 1% more calories is needed for each degree below 20°C. Thus, someone whose house is 10°C requires 10% more food intake to sustain his or her activity level. Since food availability or intake rarely increases when energy is scarce, the metabolic response to cold is for people to slow down. Surveys in Bosnia and Armenia during the early 1990s found that many people were sleeping 18–20 hours per day.

In very cold climates, several things can be done to reduce the hardships associated with cold. High-energy foods such as oil can be made available. Plastic sheeting can be handed out to cover windows and unused doorways. Getting several people or households to share one common heated place can also be useful. In multistory buildings, the temperature in living areas can be dramatically increased by organizing structures so that each floor or apartment heats the same room, causing the heat loss from the floor below to pass into the heated room above. Blankets and sleeping bags can also help people conserve energy while sleeping. Educational messages should warn people about the signs of carbon monoxide poisoning and how to check for gas leaks where fuel is burned as a source of heat.

In warmer climates, sheeting to keep people dry during rainstorms and to provide shade in the daylight can be important for improving the quality of life. Sheeting can allow for the rapid construction of shelter and is often taken by displaced populations when they return home.

Vector Control

In the United States, mosquito spraying and mosquito monitoring can be a major component of a posthurricane public health program. In developing countries, rat control (particularly in food warehouses), mosquito spraying and eliminating breeding sites, distributing pesticide-impregnated bed nets, dipping cows, spraying for housefly and tsetse flies, setting fly traps, and delousing a population are often necessary.

Exhibit 25.3   Control Strategies for Epidemic Diarrheal Diseases

Cholera

Cholera is perhaps the most waterborne of all diarrheal diseases. Food has also been seen as the main route of transmission in many outbreaks, although food-borne outbreaks are typically less widespread and less rapidly occurring than waterborne outbreaks. Thus, the first task during a cholera outbreak is to make sure that the water people are consuming is chlorinated. In this setting, chlorinated water is considered to be water with a chlorine residual of at least 0.2 mg/L at the moment it is consumed. Where chlorination is not possible, a lemon per liter has been shown to be effective in killing the bacteria that causes cholera (*Vibrio cholerae*), as is boiling water. Because *Vibrios* grow well in unrefrigerated foods, efforts to ensure that people have the fuel needed to heat their food adequately are also called for. Adding acidic sauces such as tomato sauce to foods has been shown to be protective against food-borne cholera. Educational efforts should focus on getting people to consume only chlorinated or boiled fluids and eat only hot, cooked foods or peeled fruits and vegetables. Hand-washing practices among those who prepare food for others should also receive attention.

Typhoid fever

Typhoid is also a water- and food-borne disease caused by the bacteria *Salmonella typhi*. Ensuring that the water supply is chlorinated is the best assurance against a massive outbreak, as most large outbreaks are waterborne. Many smaller outbreaks are food-borne, with the hands of the food handlers being the primary hazard. Thus, food hygiene efforts should focus on hand washing among food handlers and ensuring that infected people do not prepare food for others. Although most people, once infected, stop passing the bacteria shortly after regaining their health, 10% of people will still be shedding 3 months after the onset of symptoms. Therefore, keeping food vendors with typhoid fever away from work until they are noncommunicable takes considerable effort.

Shigellosis

Outbreaks of *Shigella dysenteriae* type I have become quite frequent during periods of civil unrest in recent years. Case fatality rates for shigellosis can exceed 10%. Other forms of dysentery generally follow the same transmission patterns. Because the infective dose of *Shigella* species tends to be low, perhaps less than 100 organisms, hand-to-mouth or person-to-person transmission is more important to prevent than with many other waterborne diseases. Several epidemiologic studies have even linked *Shigella* transmission to flies. Strategies for control need to focus on a comprehensive personal hygiene program (soap and plentiful water made available, hand-washing promotion), along with water chlorination and food hygiene efforts. Secondary cases within the households of shigellosis patients are common, so outreach programs should focus education efforts on those households where cases occur.

Hepatitis E

Although hepatitis E is fairly uncommon, it disproportionately strikes refugee populations. During major outbreaks, water has been the main route of transmission, although the most common fecal–oral hepatitis, hepatitis A, is also transmitted by food and other routes. This illness is particularly lethal to pregnant women. Thus, control measures should focus on chlorinating water for the entire population and equipping and educating pregnant women about the need for personal and food hygiene.

Rat control is usually undertaken primarily to limit food and material losses. In addition, rats can transmit myriad diseases such as plague, leptospirosis, and salmonellosis, although the cost-effectiveness of health improvements through rat control is largely undocumented.

Mosquito control is often seen as an essential effort where malaria is a major cause of morbidity. Reducing breeding sites is an inexpensive and safe measure that is often undertaken either formally or informally. Spraying for mosquitoes has been done, but is often seen as expensive or environmentally unsound. Mosquito monitoring is widespread in the United States and can be a useful tool following storms and floods for assessing the risks of mosquito-borne illnesses.

Environmental Surveillance

Planning and organizing environmental surveillance is required before, during, and after any crisis occurs in order to reestablish the sanitary barriers that previously protected a stricken community. Displaced populations require food, water, and some type of sanitation services. Establishing and maintaining these services require a predictable set of material inputs (e.g., water, latrines, soap, food, fuel) and a set of culturally and socially appropriate messages to optimize the use of those materials. Evaluating the effectiveness of these efforts is critical to ensuring the success of an environmental response.

The monitoring process allows for an accurate estimate of how conditions are changing over time. More importantly, having a numeric estimate of service levels or service quality often improves the service either by making the monitored workers more conscientious or by adding political impetus. Often, the process of surveying keeps workers in touch with the people being serviced and enables them to notice ancillary issues to the parameters being measured.

Monitored information should be graphically displayed in a public location to increase everyone's awareness of the efforts underway. Programs for which the level of indicators is favorable will help inspire other programs. Programs that are not meeting their goals may generate suggestions, help, or even prodding from others. Certain parameters, such as fuel and soap availability, need to be monitored only when indicated. In some settings, such as when people are still in their houses and have electricity, people have all of the fuel they need so monitoring the average hours of electrical service is a more demonstrative indicator of their conditions.

Bioterrorism, Pandemic Influenza, and Emerging Infectious Diseases

In recent years, there has been a global recognition of the potential peril from bioterrorism and other emerging threats such as severe acute respiratory syndrome (SARS) and pandemic influenza. Terrorist activity within United States borders and around the world is increasing, and a number of experts suggest that the likelihood of a chemical or biological warfare attack (CBW) is also increasing.[81] In response to growing concerns for public safety, there has been a decade of federal funding to help the country prepare. Initial programs were created to bolster non-public health preparedness at federal, state, and local levels, while later funding specifically addressed the role of public health. Unfortunately, funding for public health preparedness has since dropped significantly; for example, Public Health Emergency Preparedness Cooperative Agreement funding was more than $1 billion in 2006 but fell to $619 million by 2012.[82]

Bioterrorism Agents

Some understanding of the specific agents that might be employed by terrorists will assist in adequate preparation for a bioterrorist incident. The CDC has developed a list of critical agents

Table 25.4   Critical Agents for Health Preparedness, Extracted from CDC

Category A	Category B	Category C
Anthrax	Brucellosis	Emerging infectious diseases
Botulism	Epsilon toxin of *Clostridium perfringens*	
Plague	Food safety threats	
Smallpox	Glanders	
Tularemia	Melioidosis	
Viral hemorrhagic fevers	Psittacosis	
	Q Fever	
	Ricin toxin	
	Staphylococcal enterotoxin B	
	Typhus	
	Viral encephalitis	
	Water safety threats	

Source: Centers for Disease Control and Prevention. Bioterrorism Agents/Diseases. Available at: http://www.bt.cdc.gov/agent/agentlist-category.asp. Accessed March 27, 2013.

for health preparedness (**Table 25.4**).[83] Category A has high impact and requires high preparedness. Category B has a lesser requirement for preparedness. Category C can be handled within current public health capacity.

One of the greatest threats concerning the agents listed in Table 25.4 is that dissemination of a biologic agent may go unnoticed at first, with the exposed individuals leaving the scene and not showing signs of illness for hours, days, or even weeks. While the first response to bioterrorism must be at the local level, subsequent public health management should be coordinated at local, state, and federal levels.

A Closer Look at the Threat List

The definition of the threat list depends heavily on who is being threatened and how the threat is perceived. The military definition focuses primarily on bacteriologic agents and toxins that have been weaponized in aerosol form by a nation interested in producing a large number of battlefield casualties. These are the prototypical weapons of mass destruction. The military's threat list is dynamic and depends on intelligence assessment. Thus, it is possible that an organism could be appropriate in theoretical terms as a threat but is not considered a threat because no one has developed a large-scale weapon for containment and dispersion.

The civilian threat list is much broader. Many normal public health threats overlap with the agents of bioterrorism, both in the nature of the outbreaks produced and in the nature of the response to control them. Pneumonic plague is a good example where a naturally occurring case generates a rapid and vigorous public health response to prevent further dissemination.

For the purposes of this discussion, it is clear that there are relative priorities among the diseases on the threat list. Of these diseases, only five agents (anthrax, smallpox, plague, botulism, and tularemia) are considered serious threats (Category A). The diseases can be categorized in three ways. The first are those diseases, such as anthrax, plague, and tularemia, that can be spread by an aerosolized release of bacteria, producing a respiratory or pulmonary disease. The second are those diseases where the dissemination is dependent on person-to-person transmission, such as smallpox. Finally, there are diseases that can be caused by contamination of food, water, or other ingested material, such as botulinum toxin.

Anthrax is considered, both in the scientific and popular literature, to be a highly efficacious biologic warfare agent for a number of reasons. First, it forms spores, which give it stability in aerosol. Second, it is relatively easy to disseminate using off-the-shelf technology. Third, if acquired by the respiratory route, the disease is frequently fatal. The U.S. response system was challenged in 2001 when anthrax was mailed to locations in Florida, New York City, and Washington, DC.

Smallpox, as mentioned previously, has the additional feature of being highly contagious in unimmunized populations, with a cycle of 10 to 14 days, an attack rate of up to 90%, and mortality rate as high as 35%. While an eradication program eliminated the natural illness from the planet and only two samples of the live virus were maintained in the United States and Russia, it is thought that smallpox virus is also held by North Korea, injecting uncertainty into any planning.

Plague, a respiratory-acquired illness, is also spread person to person. Because it occurs as an enzootic disease of rodents in the United States, it may be possible to obtain an isolate for use as a terrorist agent.

Botulism is likewise an environmental organism that can be easily cultured from soil. Its toxin has the disturbing clinical feature of necessitating intensive supportive care of its victims. Additionally, the treatment for it, in the form of an antitoxin, is limited in supply and availability.

Tularemia can be disseminated in water. In aerosol form, it produces a severely debilitating pneumonia, although it has a lower mortality rate than anthrax. Other agents are on longer threat lists. Q fever and *Brucella* generally produce mild illnesses that would not generate large-scale stress on medical systems or produce large-scale panic. The agents in the next rank of concern are routine public health threats such as viral encephalitis, cholera, *Salmonella*, and staphylococcal enterotoxin B.

Differences Between Overt and Covert Release

It is unlikely that terrorists would use an overt release, in the form of an announced event or something that is recognized at the time, as their mode for biologic terrorism. This type of release would allow treatment before the onset of disease. In the case of overt releases, an assessment of the threat is made before the response is initiated. In many cases, announced biologic threats are considered hoaxes, and a limited and tempered response is often activated based on an analysis of the situation, thus allowing for resolution of the incident without major difficulties.

A covert release of a biologic agent would present as illness in the community, and its detection would be dependent on traditional surveillance methods. Recent federal programs have enhanced such systems through syndromic surveillance and have increased the sensitivity of frontline medical practitioners to the importance of recognizing and reporting suspicious syndromes. For some diseases, early recognition and diagnosis is essential for preventing devastating outcomes. For example, with anthrax, treatment is usually only effective before the onset of severe symptoms. Covert release of a contagious agent has the potential for large-scale spread of disease before detection. A release in an airport or in a highly mobile population could disseminate a pathogen such as smallpox throughout most of the world before the epidemic would be recognized. To bring such an epidemic under control, a major multifocal international response would need to be activated.

The Role of Health Departments and Preparedness

LHDs are first-line responders for incidents involving suspected bioterrorism or emerging infectious diseases. In such situations, protocols should be developed to deal with the most likely agents. At the local or regional level, public health planning for a bioterrorism event can be modeled after planning models for pandemic influenza. A community that is well prepared for pandemic influenza will be well prepared for most of the Category A threats. Numerous steps must be taken to address these threats to a community, such as the steps listed on the checklists released by the Department of Health and Human Services to guide multisector preparedness for pandemic flu. The following list is a brief review of the essential elements in planning at a local level, regardless of the threat:

- Readiness and impact assessment: The state or local health department needs to consider the state of readiness of the community and the potential impact of the threat. In assessing readiness, all other components of planning listed here must be considered.
- Expansion of surveillance and epidemiology capacity: In order to maximize opportunities to mitigate the spread of disease, community plans should include an ongoing effort to enhance the capacity for surveillance. Strengthened surveillance will ensure: 1) the earliest possible recognition of disease, 2) ongoing assessments of the impact of the threat and subsequent disease, and 3) data to evaluate individual and community responses to population-based interventions.
- Communication: Preplanned strategies for communication with other community agencies and the public are critical. Effective communication, fundamental in any response, is unfortunately often wrought with problems during the crisis. Protocols for communication, internally within the LHD and externally with other response agencies and the public, must have built-in redundancy (e.g., Internet, land-based and cellular telephones, radios) and be regularly tested. Templates, such as sample press releases for communicating risk to the public, can be developed in advance. LHDs should test the capacity of their websites to provide up-to-date information to the public and conduct a drill of their hotline.
- Laboratory capacity for identification of the chemical or biologic agent: The LHD should establish linkages with a laboratory capable of identifying agents of concern, the state public health agency, and the CDC in advance of any reported incident.
- Infection control measures including isolation and quarantine: Isolation and quarantine are among the most complicated infection control measures that must be addressed in the LHD disaster plan. Discussions with local law enforcement and legal authorities to clarify

conditions for declaring a public health emergency, or issuing and executing court orders to protect the public's health, should be part of LHD planning. While LHDs may have powers under their normal authority, advance clarification is required about when it might be necessary to establish and use extraordinary legal powers.

- Mass provision of clinical interventions (vaccine or medications): Depending on the threat facing a community, clinical interventions such as vaccine for smallpox or antibiotics for a bacterial agent may be available to mitigate a biologic threat. Uniform protocols with respect to vaccine distribution or prophylactic antibiotic usage are advisable.
- Coordination and capacity assessment of the healthcare delivery system: Communication between the responders and coordination of the healthcare delivery system are essential to minimize the morbidity and mortality associated with a biologic threat. Preparedness plans should include a mechanism for surge capacity, including ongoing assessment of needs, identification of alternate triage and treatment sites, and local capacity for isolation.
- Workforce training and support: In addition to NIMS and ICS training, training plans should include the capacity for "just-in-time" refreshers for the public health workforce and the psychosocial support needed by responders and the public during the crisis.

In planning a response strategy, LHDs should identify key responders in the community, including emergency medical services, hazardous materials (hazmat), and police and fire agencies. Discussions about coordinating the response and surveillance should also take place with hospitals and poison control centers. In these incidents, individuals may appear at their local hospital with concerns about potential exposure. Finally, evaluation of the public health preparedness efforts is important.

The Public Health Laboratory Network[ii]

The Laboratory Response Network (LRN) was established in 1999 by the Association of Public Health Laboratories and the CDC to assist in the U.S. response to biological and chemical terrorism. The LRN is now an integrated national network of about 120 biological and chemical labs with the capacity to respond to bioterrorism, emerging infectious diseases, and other public health threats and emergencies.

The LRN supports surveillance and epidemiologic investigations by identifying disease, providing direct and reference services, and conducting environmental, rapid, and specialized testing. Five of the major threats (i.e., botulism, plague, anthrax, tularemia, poxvirus illnesses) occur naturally in the United States, and specimens for these diseases are routinely evaluated by public health laboratories. In addition, the standard techniques for detecting bacterial agents (i.e., Gram stain, culture on selective media, visual colony morphology, growth after heat shock, and confirmatory methods using phage and direct immunofluorescence) are well recognized for establishing definitive diagnosis. Methods such as isolation in cell culture, inoculation of animals, direct fluorescence methods, and electron microscopy are considered definitive methods in virology.

[ii] Section on the Public Health Laboratory Network reprinted with permission from Landesman LY. *Public Health Management of Disasters: The Practice Guide.* 2nd ed. Washington, DC: American Public Health Association; 2005.

The laboratory response network has three levels of performance designated as sentinel, reference, or national. Designation depends on the types of tests a laboratory can perform and how it handles infectious agents to protect workers and the public. Membership in the LRN is not automatic. State lab directors determine the criteria and whether public health labs in their states should be included in the network. Prospective reference labs must have the necessary equipment, trained personnel, and properly designed facilities, and be able to demonstrate testing accuracy.

Sentinel labs (formerly Level A) represent the thousands of hospital-based clinical labs that are on the front lines. In an unannounced or covert terrorist attack, sentinel labs could be the first to identify a suspicious specimen and screen out a presumptive case during routine patient care. A sentinel laboratory's responsibility is to recognize, rule out, and refer a suspicious sample to the right reference lab. They may assess risks for aerosol agents. They use Bio Safety Level (BSL) 2 techniques.

Reference labs (formerly Levels B and C) can perform tests to detect and confirm the presence of a threat agent. These labs, also called "confirmatory reference labs," ensure a timely local response in the event of a terrorist incident or other emergency. Rather than having to rely on confirmation from labs at the CDC, reference labs are capable of producing conclusive results. Reference labs can be county, state, or major state public health laboratories that perform direct fluorescence or phage testing, such as molecular diagnostics. Using BSL 3 techniques, reference labs have the safety and proficiency to confirm and characterize susceptibility and to probe, type, and perform toxigenicity testing.

National laboratories (formerly Level D) are the network of federal and private partners in the U.S. Public Health Service, Department of Defense, national laboratories, and industry that can perform research on and development of new techniques that are disseminated to the other levels of the network. National labs have unique resources to handle highly infectious agents and are responsible for definitive high-level characterization (seeking evidence of molecular chimeras) or identifying specific agent strains. The CDC and U.S. Army Medical Research Institute of Infectious Diseases (USAMRID) national labs, operating at BSL 4, handle the most dangerous agents.

If a covert event occurs that is not recognized immediately, the incidence of disease in the community would trigger public health to submit samples to the laboratory and report to the surveillance network. With an announced threat or an overt event, the situation would be reported to the Federal Bureau of Investigation, which would in turn determine which level of laboratory is required and transport samples to the nearest appropriate laboratory resource in the network.

Point-of-Dispensing Sites for Available Countermeasures to Bioterrorist Events

Preventive measures have the distinct advantage of decreasing the potential impact of a bioterrorist event before the threat occurs. In 2002, in the face of perceived increased threats of biologic terrorism, the U.S. government launched a national Smallpox Vaccination Program in an effort to immunize healthcare providers and thereby decrease the impact of a potential smallpox epidemic. The program resulted in the immunization of far fewer providers than planned, but it did set the stage for a response to a reintroduction of smallpox, natural or unnatural.

For the major bacterial threat agents, the administration of antibiotics is the key component of the response. In the event of a release of anthrax, there are several possible scenarios for the large-scale administration of antibiotics. In addition to antibiotics, a vaccine may be administered to at-risk individuals to cut down on the duration of antibiotic administration required.

Planning for point-of-dispensing sites includes preselection of ideal locations and needs assessments for staffing, security, and information technology. There are many considerations in choosing sites, including geographic distribution, population density, and the physical layout of the site. Factors to consider include the ability to ensure security at all entrance and exit points, access for parking, and accessibility for persons with disabilities. Performing exercises of point-of-dispensing plans is critical to identify potential problems, such as bottlenecks in client flow.

Part of the federal public health response has been the earmarking of a national stock (Strategic National Stockpile, or SNS) of antibiotics and vaccines for the major bioterrorist agents of threat, discussed in more detail later in this chapter. The long-term strategy for the SNS includes developing a "virtual supply" by contracting with manufacturers to provide large amounts of product on relatively short notice.

Pandemic Influenza

Influenza is a common but frequently serious disease known as "flu," annually affecting 5–20% of the U.S. population.[84] Severity and associated mortality rates vary from year to year. Influenza spreads rapidly and can be transmitted by individuals who are asymptomatic but infected, leading to the near simultaneous occurrence of multiple community outbreaks in an escalating fashion. Influenza infections are responsible for secondary complications such as pneumonia, dehydration, and worsening of chronic respiratory and cardiac problems. Despite the potential severity of epidemics, the effects of seasonal influenza are usually moderated because most individuals have some immunity to the recently circulating viruses either from previous infections or from vaccination.

Pandemic influenza occurs on average every 3 to 4 decades when a new strain of the flu, capable of causing significant morbidity and mortality, emerges. Three pandemics occurred in the 20th century, in 1918, 1957, and 1968. The first pandemic of the 21st century occurred with the 2009 H1N1 pandemic, involving a triple-reassortant swine-origin H1N1 virus that was a 4th-generation descendant of the 1918 influenza virus.[85] A key component in pandemic influenza is that the virus is capable of efficient human-to-human transmission. Many infectious disease outbreaks, including SARS, Ebola, and West Nile Virus, can have devastating effects. However, these disease outbreaks typically are limited in spreading to either localized areas or regions, or to certain at-risk populations because of demographic, climactic, or other factors. Influenza pandemics, by contrast, are explosive global events in which most, if not all, persons are at risk for infection worldwide. Pandemics are expected to begin in the fall to spring seasons and multiple waves are likely 3 to 12 months after the initial outbreak. Such events have the potential to quickly overwhelm countries and health systems that have not made adequate preparation.

Despite vast improvements in medical technology since the 1918 "Spanish Flu" epidemic, where 675,000 died in the United States and 20–40 million people died worldwide, modern trends increase the potential for illnesses and deaths due to influenza. Modern travel patterns will result in quicker spread, with increased impact because of the susceptibility to infection in all age groups. This was evident with 2009 H1N1 when infections were first noted in Mexico but rapidly spread to the United States, with transmission likely facilitated by U.S. school children and their families traveling on spring break to Mexico.

Distinguishing Pandemic from Seasonal Influenza

Virologists and epidemiologists predict that new flu pandemics will continue to occur three to four times a century at irregular intervals.[86, p. 23] Several epidemiological features distinguish pandemic influenza from seasonal influenza. The infrequency and unpredictable timing of these events are explained by the fact that influenza pandemics occur only when a new influenza A virus emerges for which people have no immunity, which then spreads globally infecting the unexposed who are susceptible to infection. By contrast, seasonal influenza virus strain variants are modified versions of influenza A viruses that already are in widespread circulation. Therefore, there usually is some level of preexisting immunity to strain variants. Because of the frequent appearance of new variants, virus strains contained in influenza vaccines must be updated annually.

Why Influenza Pandemics Occur

Influenza viruses are fragile viruses that are primarily divided into two types: "A" and "B" viruses. Only type A viruses are known to cause pandemics. Influenza viruses have the ability to modify (drift) or replace (shift) two key viral proteins on the viral surface. Drift and shift have a profound impact the ability of the virus to stimulate an immune response, because these proteins are the main targets for the immune system. Drift, a continuously evolving process of mutation to the virus genome, results in the emergence of variant strains of virus. The amount of change can be subtle or dramatic, but eventually one of the new variant strains becomes dominant, usually for a few years, until a new variant emerges and replaces it. In essence, drift affects the influenza viruses already in worldwide circulation. This process allows influenza viruses to change and reinfect people repeatedly through their lifetime and is the reason the influenza virus strains in vaccines must be updated each year. Shift occurs when existing viral proteins are replaced by significantly different proteins.

Pandemic viruses can also arise when some of the genes from animal influenza viruses mix or reassort with some of the genes from human influenza viruses, creating a new hybrid virus. This can occur when a single animal is simultaneously coinfected by a human influenza virus and an avian influenza virus. In this situation, genes from the human and avian viruses can mix and create a virus with the surface proteins derived from the avian virus (hence, creating a new subtype) and the internal proteins derived from the human virus, enhancing the transmissibility of the hybrid virus. Reassorted viruses have been frequently identified and are thought to have been responsible for the 1957 and 1968 pandemic viruses.

Novel influenza viruses occasionally emerge among humans as part of the natural ecology and biology of influenza viruses. Large reservoirs of influenza viruses circulate among other animal species, notably wild birds. Wild birds are considered the ultimate reservoir for influenza viruses because they usually harbor the virus without becoming sick and readily transmit the virus to domestic chickens or ducks, probably via the fecal–oral route. Normally, animal influenza viruses do not infect humans. However, avian influenza viruses can sometimes "jump" the species barrier and directly infect humans.

A new threat vis-à-vis emergence of novel influenza viruses is the ability to genetically modify avian influenza viruses. This issue was hotly debated in 2012 when two teams of researchers modified H5N1 avian influenza to study the capability of efficient respiratory transmission, a trait that still does not exist with naturally occurring H5N1 avian influenza.[87]

Why Control by Vaccination Is Problematic

Widespread use of influenza vaccine can reduce the burden of mortality and morbidity. However, the timely availability of sufficient vaccine for influenza in the U.S. population has been problematic, because the industry manufacturing vaccine is shrinking for economic reasons and because of the decentralized distribution system in the United States. The challenges facing production and distribution of a vaccine for a novel strain are even greater. Once approved, its manufacture could strain an already troubled vaccine-manufacturing program. Current methods necessitate that manufacturers make advance predictions about the demand and the type of vaccine to produce. Further, when a new influenza strain spreads worldwide, sufficient vaccine will not be available for months due to current manufacturing capabilities. This scenario played out in 2009. Despite early recognition of the novel virus, with molecular diagnostics available in early spring 2009 and mobilization of federal agencies to expedite the vaccine-manufacturing and licensing process, vaccine was not widely available until late fall 2009, after the second wave had already peaked in most parts of the world.[85] To further complicate the issue, widespread unfounded fears of vaccine safety (in part associated with mistrust in the expedited process) contributed to supply-and-demand mismatches across the country.

In addition to manufacturing problems, the traditional delivery system for influenza vaccines in the United States is highly decentralized, with public health agencies having limited information about ordering by providers in the private sector and manufacturers' distribution of available vaccine. This lack of centralized oversight inhibits advance planning for or providing advance direction about redistribution during influenza vaccine shortage. In response to the 2009 pandemic, the federal government launched the national influenza 2009 H1N1 vaccination campaign. The entire vaccine purchasing (with four manufacturers) and distribution process was centralized, with the federal government procuring all of the vaccine for distribution to state health departments. Despite this centralized process, vaccine distribution challenges were still problematic across the country. In anticipation of demand greatly exceeding initial supply, the Advisory Committee on Immunization Practices issued prioritization strategies to target the most at-risk populations and healthcare and emergency medical services personnel.

With respect to antivirals, in February 2005, WHO recommended that countries stockpile antiviral medications to protect against the avian flu circulating in Asia, with the assumption that once an epidemic started, there would be high global demand for the limited supply of antivirals. As part of the United States' prepandemic planning efforts, the federal government had purchased 50 million treatment courses of antiviral drugs—oseltamivir and zanamivir—for the SNS, and states had purchased 23 million antiviral regimens. By late April 2009, the SNS released 25% of supplies to counter a pandemic, including antivirals and N-95 masks.[88] An additional 13 million doses of antivirals were ordered by HHS later that month. In addition to concerns about supply, there were concerns that novel influenza viruses might develop resistance to these antiviral medications, making a control strategy that depends on their use less than ideal. The 2009 H1N1 virus was resistant to both amantadine and rimantadine.

Public Health Planning and Preparedness for Pandemic Flu

The goal of *all* preparedness activities is to reduce morbidity and mortality, and to minimize social disruption and economic losses. In an influenza pandemic, all categories of responders (first responders, public health, and healthcare professionals) will become ill and the outbreak will be prolonged, occurring over months. For these reasons, planning should address the continuity of operations of essential services in the face of a marked decrease in available workforce. Furthermore, regional and federal assets, usually counted on in a natural disaster, are likely to be limited because of demand and the difficulty of moving things around the country given widespread outbreaks.

While much can be done to improve the readiness of communities, pandemic planning must be flexible, as assumed widely variable attack rates will drive a specific community's need for federal supplies. Ensuring that each community has robust surveillance and laboratory testing in place is an important step. Laboratories need to be prepared to handle a surge of specimens and to verify that their testing algorithms are adequate. Plans for traditional "shoe leather" public health should include contact tracing and legally vetted procedures for isolation and quarantine.

Population-based vaccine and antiviral distribution are a significant undertaking in any circumstance. Because of limited supply, procedures have to be established to: 1) acquire and take delivery of the drugs; 2) prioritize who will receive available drugs; 3) track supplies, their distribution, and use; 4) conduct mass vaccination clinics; and 5) track adverse events due to vaccination. Further, vaccination for a novel virus may require two doses of vaccine, 30 days apart, to achieve maximum immunity. Thus, any prophylaxis plan should address tracking and recall of individuals receiving novel flu vaccine.

During a pandemic, hospitals should prepare for an increase in inpatient medical care. Even a mild pandemic could produce a significant increase in demand for inpatient beds, intensive care unit (ICU) beds, and ventilators. With an anticipated high attack rate, staff absenteeism is expected to be high and there will be limited availability of critical resources. As an example of increased demand of critical resources, even though the 2009 pandemic was mild, local capacity for extracorporeal membrane oxygenation was threatened as physicians desperately struggled to save lives by developing new approaches to manage life-threatening cases of influenza.[89] Hospital preparations should address: 1) surge capacity issues; 2) the role of triage centers, volunteers, and home care; 3) guidance for hospital employees; 4) infection control guidelines; 5) mass mortality issues; 6) support for staff and their families; and 7) tracking hospital resources.

Communications is critical throughout a pandemic. In advance of any case in the United States, strategies for communicating risk-reduction behaviors must be shared across all media. These include social distancing, hand washing, and "respiratory etiquette." Further, planning should include communications about seeking care and vaccine and/or antiviral distribution. It is critical that key messages be communicated uniformly with "one voice."

Federal Preparedness Activities

The HHS provides up-to-date information about national and global activities relating to seasonal and pandemic flu at http://www.flu.gov. The CDC, as part of the global preparedness effort, has established cooperative agreements for surveillance in other countries and is supporting WHO activities. To ensure vaccine security and supply, HHS has provided funding to research cell-based influenza vaccine and to promote the expansion and diversification of U.S. influenza vaccine production. Finally, antiviral drugs are being added to the Strategic National Stockpile.

The Federal Pandemic Influenza Preparedness and Response Plan can serve as a foundation for the federal response to seasonal flu vaccine shortages. The federal plan provides guidance on assuring and expanding production capacity for influenza vaccine, increasing the use of influenza vaccination, stockpiling influenza antiviral drugs in the SNS, enhancing U.S. and global disease detection and surveillance infrastructures, supporting public health planning and laboratories, and improving healthcare system readiness at the community level.[90]

Future Outlook

Public health organizations carry out a broad and complex set of responsibilities in preparing for and responding to disasters and acts of bioterrorism. Carrying out these responsibilities requires a multiorganizational effort. Disaster epidemiology and assessment are important components of the public health response, as these activities support scientific investigation and disaster-management decision making. Public health organizations also play critical roles in preventing and controlling the psychosocial effects of disasters. The emerging threats of bioterrorism and global disease through pandemic influenza call attention to the importance of public health organizations in disaster preparedness and response initiatives, creating new risks and responsibilities for organizations along the continuum of public health practice settings. The contemporary public health environment demands informed decision making and effective management in response to the health threats posed by manmade and natural disasters.

Discussion Questions

1. Why should public health professionals be involved in disaster preparedness and response?
2. During weak economic periods, with budget cuts to public health services, does public health's role in preparedness and response change? Does it matter if you live in an area prone to devastating hazards?
3. Is an all-hazards approach to disasters better than preparing for each type of disaster? Why or why not?
4. Discuss the differences and similarities of natural and human-caused disasters. Give examples.
5. Why is it important to involve all sectors, public, private, and nonprofit in a coordinated effort? If this is not done, what might be the limitations of the response?
6. Discuss how monitoring disease and events are an essential element of preparedness. Give an example from recent events or outbreaks around the world.

References

1. Nishenko SP, Bollinger GA. Forecasting damaging earthquakes in the Central and Eastern United States. *Science.* 1990;249:1412–6.

2. Gray WM. Strong association between West African rainfall and U.S. landfall of intense hurricanes. *Science.* 1990;249:1251–6.

3. GRID Arendal Collaborating Centre with United Nations Environment Programme. *Trends in Natural Disasters.* Available at: http://www.grida.no/graphicslib/detail/trends-in-natural-disasters_a899. Accessed March 28, 2013.

4. Universite Catholique de Louvain, Brussels, Belguim, EM-DAT: The Office of Foreign Disaster Assistance/CRED International Disaster Database. Available at: http://www.emdat.be/. Accessed March 31, 2013.

5. World Health Organization. Epidemiologic Alert: Cholera Situation Update, 2 November 2012. Available at: http://ncw.paho.org/hq/index.php?option=com_docman&task=doc_view&gid=19243&Itemid=. Accessed March 31, 2013.

6. Gunn SWA. *Multilingual Dictionary of Disaster Medicine and International Relief.* Dordrecht, The Netherlands: Kluwer Academic Publishers; 1990.

7. Federal Emergency Management Agency. *National Response Framework Glossary.* Available at: http://www.fema.gov/glossary#D. Accessed March 31, 2013.

8. Showalter P, Myers MF. Natural disasters in the United States as release agents of oil, chemicals, or radiological materials between 1980–1989. *Risk Analysis.* 1994;14:169–82.

9. Auf der Heide E. *Community Medical Disaster Planning and Evaluation Guide.* Dallas, TX: American College of Emergency Physicians; 1996.

10. Quarantelli EL. *Delivery of Emergency Medical Care in Disasters: Assumptions and Realities.* New York: Irvington Publishers, Inc.; 1983.

11. Lyskowski R, Rice S. *The Big One: Hurricane Andrew.* Kansas City, MO: The Miami Herald Publishing Co.; 1992.

12. Federal Emergency Management Agency. *Flood Facts.* Available at: http://www.floodsmart.gov/floodsmart/pages/flood_facts.jsp. Accessed April 2, 2013.

13. U.S. Department of Commerce, Economics and Statistics Administration, U.S. Census Bureau. *Coastline Population Trends in the United States: 1960 to 2008.* Available at: http://www.census.gov/prod/2010pubs/p25-1139.pdf. Accessed April 2, 2013.

14. Federal Emergency Management Agency. *Strategic Foresight Initiative: Getting Urgent About the Future.* Available at: http://www.fema.gov/pdf/about/programs/oppa/demography_%20paper_051011.pdf. Accessed March 31, 2013.

15. Federal Emergency Management Agency. *Earthquake Fast Facts.* Available at: http://www.fema.gov/hazard/earthquake/facts.shtm. Accessed March 31, 2013.

16. Missouri Department of Natural Resources. *Facts about the New Madrid Seismic Zone.* Available at: http://www.dnr.mo.gov/geology/geosrv/geores/techbulletin1.htm. Accessed March 31, 2013.

17. Utah Earthquake Preparedness Information Center. *Earthquakes: What You Should Know When Living in Utah.* Salt Lake City, UT: Federal Emergency Management Agency; 2011.

18. National Commission on Terrorist Attacks Upon the United States. *The 9/11 Commission Report: Final Report of the Nation's Commission on Terrorist Attacks Upon the United States: Executive Summary.* Available at: http://www.9-11commission.gov/report/911Report_Exec.htm. Accessed March 31, 2013.

19. World Nuclear Association. Fukushima Accident 2011. Available at: http://www.world-nuclear.org/info/fukushima_accident_inf129.html. Accessed March 31, 2013.

20. Landesman LY. *Public Health Management of Disasters: The Practice Guide.* 3rd ed. Washington, DC: American Public Health Association; 2012.

21. Landesman LY. *Public Health Management of Disasters: The Pocket Guide.* Washington, DC: American Public Health Association; 2005.

22. Noji E, ed. *The Public Health Consequences of Disaster.* New York: Oxford University Press; 1997.

23. Saylor LE, Gordon JE. The medical component of natural disasters. *Am J Med Sci.* 1957;234:342–62.

24. Buist AS, Bernstein RS, eds. Health effects of volcanoes: an approach to evaluating the health effects of an environmental hazard. *Am J Public Health*. 1986;76(3):1–90.

25. Bernstein RS, Baxter PJ, Falk H, et al. Immediate public health concerns and actions in volcanic eruptions: lessons from Mount St. Helens eruptions, May 18–October 18, 1980. *Am J Public Health*. 1986;76(3):25–37.

26. Resolution 44/236 of the General Assembly of the United Nations, 1989. Available at: http://www .un.org/ga/search/view_doc.asp?symbol=A/RES/44/236&Lang=E&Area=RESOLUTION. Accessed April 2, 2013.

27. Resolution 54/219 of the General Assembly of the United Nations, 1999. Available at: http://www .un.org/ga/search/view_doc.asp?symbol=A/RES/54/219&Lang=E. Accessed April 2, 2013.

28. Rotz LD, Koo D, O'Carroll PW, et al. Bioterrorism preparedness: planning for the future. *J Public Health Manage Pract*. 2000;6(4):45–9.

29. Pandemic and All-Hazards Preparedness Act (PAHPA, Public Law109-417). Available at: http://www .gpo.gov/fdsys/pkg/PLAW-109publ417/pdf/PLAW-109publ417.pdf. Accessed March 31, 2013.

30. Gebbie KM, Weist EM, McElligott JE, et al. Implications of preparedness and response core competencies for public health. *J Public Health Manage Pract*. 2013;19(3):224–30.

31. Carr SJ, Leahy SM, London S, et al. The public health response to Los Angeles' 1994 earthquake. *Am J Public Health*. 1996;96(4):589–90.

32. AlertNet. *Haiti earthquake 2010*. Available at: http://www.trust.org/alertnet/crisis-centre/crisis/haiti-earthquake-2010. Accessed March 31, 2013.

33. Subsecretaría del Interior de Chile. *Informe final de fallecidos y desaparecidos por comunas*. Available at: http://www.interior.gob.cl/filesapp/listado_fallecidos_desaparecidos_27Feb.pdf. Accessed March 31, 2013.

34. Bissell RA, Pinet L, Nelson M, et al. Evidence of the effectiveness of health sector preparedness in disaster response: the example of four earthquakes. *Fam Community Health*. 2004;27(3):193–203.

35. Quereshi KA, Gershon RRM, Merrill JA, et al. Effectiveness of an emergency preparedness training program for public health nurses in New York City. *Fam Community Health*. 2004;27(3):242–9.

36. Imai T, Takahashi K, Hoshuyama T, et al. Substantial differences in preparedness for emergency infection control measures among major hospitals in Japan: lessons from SARS. *J Infect Chemo*. 2006;12(3):124–31.

37. Wolmer L, Hamiel D, Laor N. Preventing children's posttraumatic stress after disaster with teacher-based intervention: a controlled study. *J Am Acad Child Adolesc Psychiatry*. 2011;50(4):340–8.e2.

38. Ginzburg HM, Jevec RJ, Reutershan T. The public health services response to Hurricane Andrew. *Public Health Rep*. 1993;108(2):241–4.

39. Lewis P. *Final Report: Governor's Disaster Planning and Response Review Committee*. Tallahassee, FL: Governor's Disaster Planning and Response Review Committee; 1993.

40. Landesman LY. The availability of disaster preparation courses at US schools of public health. *Am J Public Health*. 1993;83(10):1494–5.

41. Daley WR. Public health response to Hurricane Katrina. *MMWR*. 2006;55(2);29–30. Available at: http://www.cdc.gov/mmwr/preview/mmwrhtml/mm5502a1.htm. Accessed March 31, 2013.

42. Toprani A, Ratard R, Straif-Bourgeois S, et al. Surveillance in hurricane evacuation centers—Louisiana, September–October 2005. *MMWR*. 2006;55(2);32–5. Available at: http://www.cdc.gov/mmwr/preview/mmwrhtml/mm5502a3.htm. Accessed March 31, 2013.

43. Greenough PG, Kirsch TD. Public health response—assessing the needs. *N Engl J Med*. 2005;353:1544–6.

44. Centers for Disease Control and Prevention. Notes from the field: carbon monoxide exposures reported to poison centers and related to Hurricane Sandy—Northeastern United States, 2012. *MMWR*. 2012;61(44):905.

45. Hurricane Sandy: covering the storm. *The New York Times*, November 6, 2012. Available at: http://www.nytimes.com/interactive/2012/10/28/nyregion/hurricane-sandy.html. Accessed March 31, 2013.

46. Holtz TH, Leighton J, Balter S, et al. The public health response to the World Trade Center disaster. In: Levy BS, Sidel VW, eds. *Terrorism and Public Health: A Balanced Approach to Strengthening Systems and Protecting People*. New York: Oxford University Press; 2003:19–48.

47. The Joint Commission. *Comprehensive Accreditation Manual for Hospitals: The Official Handbook.* Oakbrook Terrace, IL: Joint Commission Resources, Inc; 2009.

48. Bissell R, Becker BM, Burkle FM, Jr. Health care personnel in disaster response: reversible roles or territorial imperatives? *Emerg Med Clinics North Am.* 1996;14(2):267–88.

49. Drabek TE, Tamminga HL, Kilijanek TS, et al. *Managing Multiorganizational Emergency Response: Emergency Research and Rescue Networks in Natural Disaster and Remote Area Setting.* Boulder, CO: Natural Hazards Information Center, University of Colorado; 1981.

50. Robert T. Stafford Disaster Relief and Emergency Assistance Act, Public Law 93–288.

51. U.S. Department of Homeland Security. *National Response Framework, January 2008.* Available at: http://www.fema.gov/pdf/emergency/nrf/nrf-core.pdf. Accessed March 31, 2013.

52. Presidential Policy Directive/PPD 8. Available at: http://www.fas.org/irp/offdocs/ppd/ppd-8.pdf. Accessed March 31, 2013.

53. U.S. Department of Homeland Security. *National Preparedness Goal. September, 2011.* Available at: http://www.fema.gov/sitcs/default/files/orig/fema_pdfs/pdf/prepared/npg.pdf. Accessed March 31, 2013.

54. U.S. Department of Homeland Security. *National Preparedness Report, March 30, 2012.* Available at: http://www.nasemso.org/documents/NationalPreparednessReport_20120330_v21.pdf. Accessed March 31, 2013.

55. Centers for Disease Control and Prevention, Office of Public Health Preparedness and Response. *Public Health Preparedness Capabilities: National Standards for State and Local Planning, March 2011.* Available at: http://www.cdc.gov/phpr/capabilities/DSLR_capabilities_July.pdf. Accessed March 31, 2013.

56. Office of the Assistant Secretary for Preparedness and Response, Hospital Preparedness Program. *Healthcare Preparedness Capabilities: National Guidance for Healthcare System Preparedness, January 2012.* Available at: http://www.phe.gov/preparedness/planning/hpp/reports/documents/capabilities.pdf. Accessed March 31, 2013.

57. Thacker SB, Berkelman RL. Public health surveillance in the United States. *Epidemiol Rev.* 1988;10: 164–90.

58. Baxter PJ, Ing R, Falk H, et al. Mount St. Helens eruptions, May 18 to June 12, 1980: an overview of the acute health impact. *JAMA.* 1988;246:2585–9.

59. Cuny F. Introduction to Disaster management, lesson 1: the scope of disaster management. *Prehospital Disaster Med.* 1992;7(4):400–9.

60. Rath B, Young EA, Harris A, Perrin K, et al. Adverse respiratory symptoms and environmental exposures among children and adolescents following Hurricane Katrina. Public Health Rep. 2011;126:853–60.

61. Gerrity ET, Flynn BW. Mental health consequences of disasters. In: Noji EK, ed. *Public Health Consequences of Disasters.* New York: Oxford University Press; 1997:101–21.

62. Young BH, Ford JD, Ruzek JI, et al. *Disaster Mental Health Services: A Guidebook for Clinicians and Administrators.* Menlo Park, CA: National Center for Posttraumatic Stress Disorder; 1998.

63. Murphy SA. Health and recovery status of victims one and three years following a natural disaster. In: Figley CR, ed. *Trauma and Its Wake: Traumatic Stress Theory, Research, and Intervention.* New York: Brunner/Mazel Publishers; 1986:133–55.

64. Fullerton CS, Ursano RJ, eds. *Posttraumatic Stress Disorder: Acute and Long-Term Responses to Trauma and Disaster.* Washington, DC: American Psychiatric Press; 1997:3–18.

65. Hobfoll SE, et al. Conservation of resources and traumatic stress. In: Freedy JR, Hobfoll SE, eds.*Traumatic Stress: From Theory to Practice.* New York: Plenum Press; 1995:29–47.

66. Karam EG. Comorbidity of posttraumatic stress disorder and depression. In: Fullerton CS, Ursano RJ, eds. *Posttraumatic Stress Disorder: Acute and Long-Term Responses to Trauma and Disaster.* Washington, DC: American Psychiatric Press; 1997:77–90.

67. Hoffman KJ, Sasaki JE. Comorbidity of substance abuse and PTSD. In: Fullerton CS, Ursano RJ, eds. *Posttraumatic Stress Disorder: Acute and Long-Term Responses to Trauma and Disaster.* Washington, DC: American Psychiatric Press; 1997:159–74.

68. Fullerton CS, Ursano RJ. Posttraumatic responses in spouse/significant others of disaster workers. In: Fullerton CS, Ursano RJ, eds. *Posttraumatic Stress Disorder: Acute and Long-Term Responses to Trauma and Disaster.* Washington, DC: American Psychiatric Press; 1997:59–75.

69. O'Brien LS. *Traumatic Events and Mental Health*. Cambridge, England: Cambridge University Press; 1998.

70. Green BL. Cross-national and ethnocultural issues in disaster research. In: Marsella AJ, Friedman MJ, Gerrity ET, eds. *Ethnocultural Aspects of Posttraumatic Stress Disorder: Issues, Research, and Clinical Applications*. Washington, DC: American Psychological Association; 1996:341–61.

71. France-Presse A. Suicides in Japan spiked after earthquake: survey. *The Straits Times*, March 9, 2012, Available at: http://www.straitstimes.com/BreakingNews/Asia/Story/STIStory_775753.html. Accessed March 29, 2012.

72. Kim Y. Great East Japan earthquake and early mental-health-care response. *Psychiatry Clin Neurosci.* 2011;65(6):539–48, Available at: http://onlinelibrary.wiley.com/doi/10.1111/j.1440-1819.2011.02270.x/full. Accessed April 3, 2013.

73. Erickson K. *Everything in Its Path: Destruction of Community in the Buffalo Creek Flood*. New York: Simon and Schuster; 1976.

74. Taylor VA. *Delivery of Mental Health Services in Disasters: The Xenia Tornado and Some Implications* (The Disaster Research Center Book and Monograph Series #11). Columbus, OH: Disaster Research Center, The Ohio State University; 1976.

75. Green BL, Solomon SD. The mental health impact of natural and technological disasters. In: Freedy JK, Hobfoll SE, eds. *Traumatic Stress: From Theory to Practice*. New York: Plenum Press; 1995:163–80.

76. Ursano RJ, McCaughey BG, Fullerton CS. Trauma and disaster. In: Ursano RJ, McCaughey BG, Fullerton CS, et al. *Individual and Community Responses to Trauma and Disaster: The Structure of Human Chaos*. Cambridge, England: Cambridge University Press; 1994:3–27.

77. Peterson AE, Roberts L, Toole MJ, et al. The effect of soap distribution on diarrhoea: Nyamithuthu refugee camp. *Int J Epidemiol.* 1998;27(3):520–4.

78. Esrey S, Potash JB, Roberts L, et al. Effects of improved water supply and sanitation on ascariasis, diarrhoea, dracunculiasis, hookworm infection, schistosomiasis, and trachoma. *Bull World Health Org.* 1991;69(5):609–21.

79. Centers for Disease Control and Prevention. Mortality among newly arrived Mozambican Refugees—Zimbabwe and Malawi," *MMWR.* 1992;42(24):468–77.

80. Hatch DL, Waldman RJ, Lungu GW, et al. Epidemic cholera during refugee resettlement in Malawi. *Int J Epidemiol.* 1994;22(6):1292–9.

81. Hood E. Chemical and biological weapons: new questions, new answers. *Environ Health Perspect.* 1999;107(12):931–2.

82. Centers for Disease Control and Prevention. *Report on Public Health Preparedness*. Available at: http://www.cdc.gov/phpr/pubs-links/2012/documents/2012%20State-By-State_Preparedness_Report.pdf. Accessed April 2, 2013.

83. Centers for Disease Control and Prevention. *Bioterrorism Agents/Diseases*. Available at: http://www.bt.cdc.gov/agent/agentlist-category.asp. Accessed April 2, 2013.

84. Department of Health and Human Services. "About Seasonal Flu." Available at: http://www.pandemicflu.gov/. Accessed December 16, 2012.

85. Farley M. 2009 H1N1 influenza: a twenty first century pandemic with roots in the early twentieth century. *Am J Med Sci.* 2010;340(3):202–8.

86. World Health Organization. *Avian Influenza: Assessing the Pandemic Threat*. Available at: http://whqlibdoc.who.int/hq/2005/WHO_CDS_2005.29.pdf. Accessed April 2, 2013.

87. Kraemer JD, Gostin LO. The limits of government regulation of science. *Science.* 2012;335(6072):1047–9.

88. Centers for Disease Control and Prevention. *The 2009 H1N1 Pandemic: Summary Highlights, April 2009–April 2010*. Available at: http://www.cdc.gov/h1n1flu/cdcresponse.htm. Accessed April 2, 2013.

89. Morrow C. Personal communication with local hospitals. 2009.

90. American Public Health Association. *Developing a Comprehensive Public Health Approach to Influenza Vaccination*. Washington, DC: Author; 2004.

Public Health and Healthcare Quality

Cheryll D. Lesneski, Peggy A. Honoré, and Carolyn Clancy

LEARNING OBJECTIVES

- To articulate the gaps in quality in public health
- To define public health quality
- To name the nine aims for improvement of quality in public health
- To describe the concept of characteristics of quality
- To identify priority areas for improving public health quality
- To list major events in the history of quality in public health and health care
- To explain any differences in the evolution of quality in health care and public health
- To describe some quality improvement efforts in public health and health care

---

Chapter Overview

Quality as a path to population health improvements has taken center stage as the nation sets a course of action for better care, better health, and lower cost. The role of public health is critically important since multiple factors, beyond and greater than the delivery of medical services, affect population health improvements. Realizing these goals require an alignment of quality initiatives between public health and health care and specifically require improved patient outcomes, emphasis on prevention, focus on the upstream determinants of health, and reduction in healthcare costs.

In a 2010 Commonwealth Fund study, quality in the United States healthcare system ranked sixth when compared to seven other countries.[1] Reports also document the system as lagging in making care safe, promoting healthy lifestyles, and making data available to fully identify and assess health disparities that persist across racial, ethnic, and socioeconomic boundaries.[2] Health care is the fastest growing sector in the U.S. economy and, in 2010, represented 17.9% of the gross domestic product (GDP). Translating this to a personal level, the country is spending roughly $8,400 per capita on health care annually.

While these statistics reflect the burden on the nation of actual medical care costs, the public health system shares the responsibility for improving the health and wellbeing of the nation. The public health mission, after all, is to assure conditions in which people can be healthy.[3] The ethical practice of public health directs the public health system to primarily address the fundamental causes of disease and the prerequisites for health, and to seek and apply information in the development and implementation of effective policies and programs that protect and promote health.[4] Historically, the public health system achieved health improvement goals in the areas of communicable diseases, vehicle safety, tobacco control, cardiovascular diseases, cancer, and maternal and child health. Many of these improvements were accomplished through population-level interventions that influence environmental factors for disease prevention such as policies for bans on smoking, laws for traffic safety, and regulations for reportable diseases and vaccination. Policy development is in fact one of the essential public health services,[2] and recent research provides evidence that an environmental approach to prevention through the use of policies is more cost-effective when compared to clinical or nonclinical strategies.[5]

Chronic underfunding of the public health system in the United States explains some of the underperformance of public health agencies since the 1990s.[6] Public health researchers have also discovered wide variation in the availability and quality of public health services across many communities.[7] Addressing the quality of public health services is vital, and expectations for improvements in population health create a sense of urgency for public health to focus on eliminating system quality deficiencies. Moreover, keeping people healthier will reduce the need and the overall costs of health care.

Future gains will result from the ability of system leaders to continually improve and transform public health practices to meet changing population health needs. This chapter presents and compares past and present efforts to improve the quality of the U.S. public health and healthcare systems. It also studies current initiatives and future directions of the Department of Health and Human Services to accelerate quality, spearhead a national public health quality movement, and promote national quality and prevention strategies across all levels of the public health and healthcare systems.

History of Quality in Health

Responding to the arbitrary and chaotic medical education system and practice of medicine in colonial America, the American Medical Association was established in 1847 to promote tougher, standardized medical education requirements.[8] In the absence of any requirements for practicing medicine, many simply advertised their abilities to treat illnesses or injuries with woefully inadequate training and skills. A Council on Medical Education was formed in 1904 and Abraham Flexner was given the task of reporting on medical education in the United States and Canada, requiring an expansive transformation of medical schools. In 1911, Ernest Codman, a Harvard medical surgeon, took up the mantle of improving hospital care with the use of metrics to evaluate the source of any medical problem by collecting demographic, diagnostic, treatment, and outcome data on hospitalized patients, even observing patients for up to 1 year post-discharge. Using these data, Codman was able to identify clinical problems and establish systems to improve care. The American College of Surgeons adopted his "End Result System" and set minimum standards for medical care in a hospital setting. Hospital safety and care have absorbed much of the attention to quality in the field of health care since these early days.[9]

Assuring appropriate skills by medical care providers was one of the first steps in the quest for healthcare quality. State examining boards, medical diplomas, and licensures by medical associations were well established by the middle of the 19th century. These efforts were continued well into the 20th century, with laws such as the Health Professions Educational Assistance Act of 1963 and the 1976 charter for the Graduate Medical Education National Advisory Committee.[10]

The classic Welch-Rose Report of 1915 established the blueprint for education and training of the public health workforce. The report recommended collaboration for education with medical schools, but simultaneously proposed the creation of separate schools of public health. Nearly 100 years later in 2011, in an effort to improve the quality of public health education, the Association of Schools of Public Health (ASPH) formed an initiative called *Framing the Future: The Second Hundred Years of Public Health Education*. The mission for this effort is to reconsider the role of public health education, and its task force is charged with developing a new vision for public health education.[11]

Healthcare quality standards and performance requirements have advanced through laws, regulations, and presidential commissions (**Table 26.1**). As presented in Table 26.1, the history of quality in health care includes an impressive array of governmental, institutional, and professional policies and initiatives aimed at promoting quality and safety in the delivery of healthcare services. The list includes a notable collection of laws enacted specifically to address healthcare quality. Most noteworthy is the 1986 Healthcare Quality Improvement Act and its mandate for the establishment of the Agency for Healthcare Research and Quality (AHRQ), which has roots dating back to the 1968 creation of the National Center for Healthcare Services Research and Development.[9] A review of Table 26.1 reveals the absence of comparable policies and organizational structures specifically created to address **public health quality**. Policies are an effective means for building political and public support that can advance important health issues, yet interest for quality in public health has not garnered the attention needed to stimulate such national action as observed for healthcare quality.

The dramatic economic burden and negative patient outcomes attributable to the healthcare delivery system are issues that drive attention to improving quality in medical settings; however, greater attention should be given to the potential impact of public health quality on reducing those burdens through population-level interventions and programs. Additionally, the focus of the public health mission on preemptive measures such as prevention versus the reactive interventions of medicine illustrate how improving quality in public health could decelerate cost and prevent, or at a minimum curtail, the explosion of medical treatments.

Table 26.1   Milestones in the History of Quality in Health

Year	Healthcare Quality	Public Health Quality
	1800s	
1847–1872	**1847:** American Medical Association (AMA) was founded. **1864:** Hawaii was the first state to pass a law that mandated registration. Registration laws provided that practitioners were to register with either the county medical society or county official to practice in that state.	**1850:** Report of the Sanitary Commission of Massachusetts by Lemuel Shattuck, a blueprint for the development of a public health system **1872:** American Public Health Association (APHA) was founded.
1876–1889	**1876:** First state examining board was created in Texas. **1876:** First law mandating examination of candidates seeking to practice in the state, whether they were medical graduates or not. This law was first passed in Texas. **1889:** First law making a diploma in medicine a prerequisite for certification was passed in Florida.	
	1900s	
1915		Release of the Welsh-Rose Report on public health research and education. The report has been viewed as the basis for the critical movement in the history of the institutional schism between public health and medicine, because it led to the establishment of schools of public health.
1906–1926	**1906:** The Food and Drug Administration (FDA) undertook national regulation of medication. **1910:** The Flexner report was a wake-up call to reform quality of medical education. It was a commentary on the condition of medical education in the early 1900s and gave rise to modern medical education. It triggered much-needed reforms in the standards, organization, and curriculum of North American medical schools. **1918:** The Hospital Standardization Program of American College of Surgeons was developed in the public interest and was financed by the college through its practicing surgeons and offered without cost to the populace. Faced by rising costs and the interests of other groups who sought a role in the standardization of hospitals, the college relinquished this task to the Joint Commission on Accreditation of Hospitals in 1955.	**1920s–1930s:** APHA's appraisal form of public health agencies to assess immediate results of services

1926	**1926:** The Medical Group Management Association (MGMA) was formed. The mission of the association was to continually improve the performance of medical group practice professionals and the organizations they represent.	**1943:** APHA Evaluation Schedule measured needs, resources, degree of success in applying resources to needs by public health agencies
1946	Healthcare Financial Management Association (HFMA) was formed. Its major focus was on the intersection of cost and quality.	**1945:** APHA Emerson Report on landmark recommendations to improve public health practice after World War II
1951–1953	**1951:** The Joint Commission on Accreditation of Hospitals was founded. It started with providing accreditation of hospitals, but over the years has expanded to providing accreditation to ambulatory health care, behavioral healthcare organizations, homecare organizations, critical access hospitals, and laboratories. With the provision of more services, the name changed to The Joint Commission on Accreditation of Healthcare Organizations in 1987, but is now simply known as The Joint Commission.	**1950–1970:** APHA Policy Statements on mission redefinition for public health practice **1953:** Association of Schools of Public Health (ASPH) was established
1963–1979	**1963:** Health Professions Education Assistance Act **1965:** Medicare was institutionalized, mandating principles central to hospital operations, staff credentialing, round-the-clock nursing care, and utilization review. **1966:** Avedis Donabedian's Structure, Process, Outcome model was introduced and widely used as a framework for quality. **1966:** Current Procedural Terminology (CPT) was developed by the AMA. **1967:** National Commission on Health Manpower **1968:** National Center for Health Services Research (NCHSR) and Development was established by the Department of Health and Human Services (HHS) in response to growing concerns over cost and quality.	**1975:** Council on Education for Public Health (CEPH) was established by APHA and ASPH. In the late 1970s, CEPH responded to requests from practitioners and educators to undertake accreditation of community health/preventive medicine programs and to a request from APHA to assume the additional responsibility for community health education programs. In 2005, these separate programmatic categories were combined into a single category of public health programs. **1979:** Model Standards for Community Preventive Health Services were published by the Centers for Disease Control and Prevention (CDC) and instituted in public health agencies around the nation.

(continues)

Table 26.1 Milestones in the History of Quality in Health (continued)

Year	Healthcare Quality	Public Health Quality
	1970: World Health Organization implemented ICD-9 Codes for hospitals. The International Classification of Diseases (ICD) is the classification system used to code and classify mortality data from death certificates.	
	1971: Commission on Medical Malpractice	
	1972–2003: Amendments to Social Security Act focused on healthcare quality (i.e., establishment of professional standards review organizations, quality of medical care provided, and quality control peer review program)	
	1973: American College of Medical Quality was founded.	
	1976: Charter for Graduate Medical Education National Advisory Committee	
1980–1983	Introduction of Diagnosis-Related Groups Implementation of quality improvement organizations by the Social Security Administration (SSA): The Centers for Medicare and Medicaid Services (CMS) has made it mandatory for every state to have Quality Improvement Organizations (QIO). The mission of the QIO Program is to improve the effectiveness, efficiency, economy, and quality of services delivered to Medicare.	
1986	The Healthcare Quality Improvement Act was passed to address professional review activities and requirements for information reporting into the National Practitioner Data Bank.	
1987–1989	Institute for Healthcare Improvement (IHI) was founded. Dartmouth Institute for Health Policy and Clinical Practice was founded.	**1988**: The Institute of Medicine (IOM) released its "Future of Public Health" report, declaring the U.S. public health system was in disarray.
	1989: Agency for Healthcare Policy and Research (AHCPR) was created to replace the NCHSR with a specific mission to enhance quality.	
1990	The National Committee for Quality Assurance (NCQA) was founded.	Assessment Protocol for Excellence in Public Health (APEXPH) was established by the National Association of County and City Health Officials (NACCHO) and applied to local public health agencies for organizational assessment and improvement and community needs assessment.

1990–1992	IOM National Roundtable on Health Care Quality defines quality of health care. Healthcare quality improvement initiative was established. Healthcare Effectiveness Data and Information Set (HEDIS) measures were introduced. Use of healthcare quality report cards begins.
1996	President's Advisory Commission on Consumer Protection and Quality in the Health Care Industry was established, and 2 years later released its final report *Quality First: Better Health Care for All Americans*. Committee on Quality of Health Care in America was established by IOM.
1999–2001	**1999:** Healthcare Research and Quality Act changed name of AHCPR to Agency for Healthcare Research and Quality (AHRQ) and mandated AHRQ to produce a National Healthcare Quality report and National Healthcare Disparities report. **1999:** IOM's *To Err Is Human: Building a Safer Health System* was released. **1999:** Malcolm Baldrige National Quality Award was extended to healthcare organizations. **1999:** The National Quality Forum (NQF) was founded.

2000–2013

| 2001 | The report, *Crossing the Quality Chasm*, was released by IOM. |
| 2003 | IOM released *Priority Areas for National Action Plan: Transforming Healthcare Quality*. In this report, the committee recommends a set of 20 priority areas to focus on to improve the quality of health care delivered to all Americans. The CMS Quality Measurement and Health Assessment Group launched a project in October 2003 to implement a more standardized and efficient management system for the development and maintenance of quality measures. This is known as Measures Management System. It is composed of a set of business processes and decision criteria that CMS-funded measure developers follow in the development, implementation, and maintenance of quality measures. |

1990s: Baldrige award was offered to the public sector.

2000: National Public Health Performance Standards, a voluntary public health system assessment program, was instituted by the CDC.

IOM's *Future of Public Health in the 21st Century* report was released. This report was a follow up to the report that was first published in 1988.

(*continues*)

Table 26.1   Milestones in the History of Quality in Health (continued)

Year	Healthcare Quality	Public Health Quality
2005–2006	Tax Relief and Health Care Act of 2006 established the Physician Quality Reporting System (PQRS) to include an incentive payment for eligible professionals who satisfactorily report data on quality measures for covered professional services furnished to Medicare beneficiaries.	2005: National Board of Public Health Examiners was established as a program to certify public health students and professionals in mastery of public health knowledge.
2007		Public Health Accreditation Board (PHAB) was formed. It is a nonprofit organization dedicated to advancing the continuous quality improvement of tribal, state, local, and territorial public health departments.
2008–2010	2010: Passage of the Patient Protection and Affordable Care Act (ACA) 2010: Mandate to AHRQ for a National Quality Strategy included in ACA	HHS Office of the Assistant Secretary of Health (OASH) released the following reports: 2008: Consensus Statement on Quality in the Public Health System 2008: OASH created the Public Health System, Finance, and Quality Program, charged to develop concepts for quality in the public health system. 2008: First Certified in Public Health (CPH) exam was administered by the National Board of Publics Health Examiners (NBPHE). It announced the award of the inaugural certification to more than 500 qualifying professionals. 2010: Priority Areas for Improvement of Quality in Public Health
2011	AHRQ released the National Quality Strategy as mandated by the ACA.	2011: Public Health Accreditation Board initiated voluntary accreditation of public health agencies.
2012–2013	U.S. transition from ICD-9 to ICD-10 codes in hospitals. The transition is occurring because ICD-9 produces limited data about patients' medical conditions and hospital inpatient procedures. ICD-9 has outdated terms and is inconsistent with current medical practice.	ASPH Education Continuum Framing task force was created to reconsider the role of public health education.

Quality Chasms

Gaps in quality impede expected performance of the U.S. public health and healthcare systems and do not advance improvements in population health. In 1999, the Institute of Medicine Committee on Quality of Health Care in America published a ground-breaking report, *To Err Is Human: Building a Safer Health System*, on the avoidable medical errors resulting in 44,000–98,000 deaths yearly.[12] Twelve years later, researchers employing more sophisticated and rigorous quality reviews, detected at least 10 times more confirmed adverse events. This finding indicated that one in three hospital admissions would experience an adverse event, an indication of escalating medical errors over the years since the *To Err Is Human* report.[13] A variety of approaches have been used to improve the quality of health care during the past 50 years, and although some successes have been demonstrated, the complex problems of systematic and sustainable improvements in healthcare services remain major challenges. The estimated annual costs of medical errors that harm patients amounted to $17.1 billion in 2008.[14] However, as noted by AHRQ, hospitals that are transparent by revealing errors can help to build safer systems.[15]

Problems associated with attaining consistent, quality healthcare services have been widely reported. Less known perhaps, but equally as important to the health of Americans, are the gaps in performance by the U.S. public health system in the delivery of quality preventative and health-promoting services, so vital to improving the nation's health. To demonstrate this importance, research published in 2010 showed that over the 50-year period from 1950 to 2000, the reductions by at least 50% in 7 of the 10 leading causes of death could be attributed to the combined diffusion of innovations in both public health and medical care.[16] In spite of the heavy reliance that the nation has on public health for improving the quality of the U.S. health system, the IOM reported in 1988 in *The Future of Public Health* on the disarray of the U.S. public health system.[3] A lack of focus, underfunding, and inability to prepare and respond to urgent health issues were identified as major problems.

During the 20th century, the nation's public health system made remarkable achievements, increasing life expectancy at birth by 62% from 47.2 years in 1900 to 76.8 years in 2000. Ten public health achievements are credited with this increase:[17]

- Vaccination
- Tobacco control
- Prevention and control of infectious diseases
- Maternal and child health programs
- Motor vehicle safety
- Cardiovascular disease prevention
- Occupational safety
- Cancer prevention
- Childhood lead poisoning prevention
- Public health preparedness

Many of these accomplishments targeted one or more of the leading causes of death in the past century, resulting in a decline of age-adjusted death rate from 881.9 per 100,000 to 741.0 per

100,000. However, the Centers for Disease Control and Prevention (CDC) declared in 2001 that the public health system was "structurally weak in every area,"[18, p. iii] citing the 20% increase in drug-resistant tuberculosis cases worldwide, the escalating rates of chronic diseases that are largely preventable, and the unhealthy future for many of today's youth as a result of tobacco use and obesity. The CDC report made recommendations to rectify the weaknesses found in the system by moving to ensure a skilled public health workforce, a robust information and data system, and effective health departments and laboratories.[18]

Following the 2001 terrorist attacks in New York City, Congress allocated $3 billion over a 3-year period to strengthen public health agencies' infrastructure, primarily through programs administered by the CDC.[19] In addition to improving public health agencies' ability for preparedness and response to manmade or natural disasters, the funding was also intended to improve detection of broader threats to the public's health while also modernizing the entire public health system.[20] In efforts to measure preparedness, readiness, and improvements following the influx of new revenues, researchers at RAND discovered in 2004 wide variation in seven of California's local public health jurisdictions, even though California was considered to be in the top tier for preparedness services.[16] These findings are similar to those found across the nation, as documented in the 2004 Trust for America's Health report, *Ready or Not? Protecting the Public's Health in the Age of Bioterrorism*.[21] Wide variation in medical care has been indicative of waste, inefficiency, and quality of care issues. This is important since the RAND researchers contend that in their study the varied preparedness response capabilities point to similar problems of public health inefficiencies and lack of quality.

Following significant investments in rebuilding the public health infrastructure, gaps in performance persist. The Trust for America's Health follow-up report, *Ready or Not? 2011: Protecting the Public's Health from Diseases, Disasters, and Bioterrorism*,[22] attributed the gaps once again to insufficient funding, noting that an upward trajectory in preparedness by the public health system since 2001 was cut short by the U.S. economic crisis starting in 2007. This crisis led to cuts in local, state, and federal funding for public health systems and reduced or eliminated public health programs and staffing.[22]

Other signs of the **quality chasm** in the performance of public health systems are apparent. United States ranks number one in terms of healthcare spending per capita compared to other developed nations in 2006. However, the nation ranked 39th for infant mortality, 43rd for adult female mortality, 42nd for adult male mortality, and 36th for life expectancy, causing many to question why there is marginal improvement in outcomes when the country's expenditure in health care is so high.[22]

Evidence-based public health practice paired with a focus on quality and quality-improvement methods is needed to address existing and emerging health challenges of the 21st century, such as obesity, climate change, and the chronic disease epidemic. Statistics showing that the U.S. obesity rate is ranked as the sixth highest out of 70 other nations[23] and that 1 in 4 adults and 1 in 15 children in the United Sates have multiple concurrent chronic conditions[24] convey the urgency for public health–coordinated efforts with medical care to reverse these troubling trends.

A quality priority for public health is the application of evidence in the formation of policies, management decisions, and public health program implementation. An alternate scenario continues in parts of public health practice where decisions to improve the population's health are based on short-term demands and anecdotal evidence.[25] The IOM reported similar decision-making behavior in public health agencies in its 1988 report, noting that crises and hot topics were primary drivers for decisions about public health priorities. The 1988 IOM committee also found that, under the configuration at the time, the public health system was incapable of meeting its key responsibilities to protect and promote the public's health and was incapable of fully applying scientific knowledge and organizational skills, nor could it generate new knowledge, methods, and programs—a very critical indictment of the state of the U.S. public health system.[3]

Patient Protection and Affordable Care Act

Eliminating quality chasms by improving quality across all sectors of health received a boost with the passage and signing into law by President Barack Obama of the Patient Protection and Affordable Care Act (ACA) of 2010. Quality, access to care, and expectations for improvements in population health are the cornerstones of the ACA. A glimpse at the Congressional intent of the ACA is found in the opening title, "Quality, Affordable Healthcare for all Americans." While comprehensive health insurance reform is a central theme of the ACA, this historic law does include a mandate for the AHRQ to develop a National Strategy for Quality Improvement in Health Care (National Quality Strategy).[23]

The ACA stipulates that the National Quality Strategy include priorities that address improvements in health outcomes, patient care, payment policy, healthcare data, and the reductions in medical errors and preventable admissions. Title IV of ACA, Prevention of Chronic Disease and Improving Public Health, calls for "modernizing disease prevention and public health systems, increasing access to clinical preventive services, creating healthier communities, and support for prevention and public health innovation."[26, pp. 9–10] To fulfill this call to action, the ACA mandated the development of a National Prevention and Health Promotion Strategy (National Prevention Strategy) by the U.S. Surgeon General.[23, p. 464]

The ACA also authorizes the Health Resources and Services Administration (HRSA) and the CDC to coordinate programs and funding streams to build incentives that promote interactions between public health agencies and community health centers and encourage tax-exempt hospitals to treat primary care and community health as priorities and promote programs that address community needs.[23] With the release in 2011 of the National Quality Strategy and the National Prevention Strategy, unprecedented opportunities now exist for the public health and healthcare systems to work in a coordinated approach to strengthening quality across all sectors of the healthcare industry and other areas that influence the determinants of health.

The three broad national aims of the National Quality Strategy—better care, healthy people/healthy communities, and affordable care—provide a structure for integrating quality in healthcare and public health interventions. The seven priorities of the National Prevention Strategy—tobacco-free living, preventing drug abuse and excessive alcohol use, healthy eating, active living, injury- and violence-free living, reproductive and sexual health, and mental and emotional well-being—provide a focus where national attention can be directed for aligning public health and healthcare initiatives. The *Healthy People 2020* Leading Health Indicators (**Table 26.2**) also

Table 26.2 *Healthy People 2020* Leading Public Health Indicators

Access to Health Services
Clinical Preventive Services
Environmental Quality
Injury and Violence
Maternal, Infant, and Child Health
Mental Health
Nutrition, Physical Activity, and Obesity
Oral Health
Reproductive and Sexual Health
Social Determinants of Health
Substance Abuse
Tobacco

Source: Reproduced from U.S. Department of Health and Human Services. *Healthy People 2020* Leading Health Indicators. Available at: http://www.healthypeople.gov/2020/LHI/socialDeterminants.aspx. Accessed March 28, 2013.

present priority areas for health where the alignment of public health and healthcare forces can produce synergy and accelerate rates of improvement.[27] These three national strategic plans (National Quality Strategy, National Prevention Strategy, *Healthy People 2020*) facilitate the rigorous, systematic approach to quality needed to address the broad array of public health deficiencies that many have documented.[28]

Fundamental Definitions, Frameworks, and Characteristics of Quality

In the mid 1920s, three men laid the groundwork for today's quality improvement movement: Walter Shewhart, W. Edwards Deming, and Joseph Juran.[29] Shewhart's work focused on studying and controlling processes, making quality relevant to production as well as the finished product. Shewhart contributed the concepts of process control to the emerging quality field, maintaining that the discovery and elimination of the causes of variation created greater efficiency and effectiveness. He mentored Juran, founder of the American Society for Quality, and Deming, perhaps the best known of the three quality giants. Juran coined the term "Big Q," adding management and service to the traditional quality focus on products and their production. He created the "Pareto principle," or the 80/20 rule, to help quality managers focus on the vital few issues that significantly affect quality (the 20%) instead of the "useful many" (the 80%), which do not lead to new levels of quality. His book, *Managerial Breakthrough*, evolved into Six Sigma and Lean.[30] Deming is best known for his white paper, "If Japan Can, Why Can't We?", based on his revolutionary work to reconstruct Japan' successes in the auto and electronics markets by applying Deming's principles of **continuous quality improvement (CQI)**.[28] Key features of the CQI movement are presented in **Table 26.3**.

Table 26.3   Elements of CQI

Philosophical Elements	Structural Elements
Strategic focus—have mission vision, and values as well as measurable objectives	Process improvement teams
Customer focus—emphasis on customer, external and internal, satisfaction, and health outcomes	CQI tools—flowcharts, cause and effect diagrams, histograms, Pareto charts, run charts, control charts, and regression analysis
Systems view—analysis of the whole system	Quality councils
Data-driven or evidence-based analysis—gather objective data about system operation and performance	Organizational leadership
Implementer involvement—involve the owners of each and every system component to reach mutual understanding of the system and its processes	Statistical analysis
Multiple causation—identify the multiple root causes of system phenomena	Customer satisfaction measures
Process optimization—optimize processes to meet customer needs	Benchmarking
Continual improvement—ongoing system analysis, even when satisfactory performance occurs	Redesign of processes
Organizational learning—expand the capacity of the organization to generate process improvements and foster personal growth	

Source: Reproduced from Sollecito W, Johnson J. (Eds.). *Continuous Quality Improvement in Health Care.* 4th ed. Burlington, MA: Jones & Bartlett Learning; 2012.

These quality geniuses and many others helped to revolutionize the field of quality improvement, and their achievements in industry are now being duplicated in many areas of health care. Well known to many in health care is the framework for studying quality in the healthcare system developed in 1966 by Avedis Donabedian. **Figure 26.1** presents the major components of his model that links structure, process, and outcomes to the study and pursuit of quality in health care.

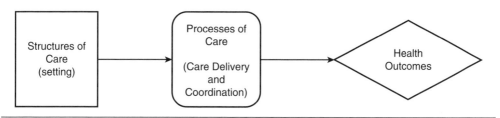

Figure 26.1   Donabedian's Quality Framework
Source: Reproduced from Conceptual Frameworks and Their Application to Evaluating Care Coordination Interventions Closing the Quality Gap: A Critical Analysis of Quality Improvement Strategies (Vol. 7: Care Coordination). Technical Reviews, No. 9.7. McDonald KM, Sundaram V, Bravata DM, et al. Rockville (MD): Agency for Healthcare Research and Quality (US); 2007 Jun.

In this model the structures of health care are the physical and organizational aspects of care settings (e.g., facilities, equipment, personnel, finance). The processes of patient care are dependent on the structures for resources and mechanisms needed to produce patient care activities. Processes are performed in order to improve patient health in terms of recovery, restoring function, survival, and patient satisfaction. The final components in the model are the outcomes of medical care that are produced by the structures and processes.[31] The framework is useful for assessing the multiple components of the healthcare system that contribute to good outcomes and point to areas for improvement when outcomes are less than satisfactory.

During the 1990s, not-for-profit organizations focused on helping healthcare providers and institutions improve the quality of their services began to flourish by teaching the tools of improvement developed by Juran, Shewhart, Deming, and Donabedian. Notable among these organizations are the Institute for Healthcare Improvement (IHI) and the National Initiative for Children's Healthcare Quality (NICHQ).

National attention to quality issues in the U.S. healthcare system intensified in 1996 with the establishment of the President's Advisory Commission on Consumer Protection and Quality in Health Care. In its 1998 report, *Quality First: Building Better Health Care for All Americans*, the commission recommended strategies to build quality into the system through the development of national quality goals, aims, and priorities to guide decision making across all sectors of the health industry.[32] In response, two IOM reports on healthcare quality followed as the world transitioned into the 21st century. In 1999, *To Err Is Human: Building a Safer Health System,* declared that health care in America was not as safe as it should be, or could be, noting that deaths from preventable medical errors were killing as many as 98,000 people yearly in hospitals.[12] The report declared that medical errors are not the result of a "bad apple" but faulty systems, processes, or conditions.[12] Such errors are preventable and are best addressed through a comprehensive improvement strategy where there should be a role for public health. For example, some states have recently established policies for hospitals to report healthcare-acquired infections to state public health agency databases. The following four areas were recommended in the IOM's 1998 report as actions to reduce medical errors by government, health care providers, industry and consumers:[3]

- Establishing a national focus to create leadership, research, tools, and protocols to enhance the knowledge base about safety
- Identifying and learning from errors by developing a nationwide public mandatory reporting system and by encouraging healthcare organizations and practitioners to develop and participate in voluntary reporting systems
- Raising performance standards and expectations for improvements in safety through the actions of oversight organizations, professional groups, and group purchasers of health care
- Implementing safety systems in healthcare organizations to ensure safe practices at the delivery level

In 1990, the IOM defined quality health care as "the degree to which health services for individuals and populations increase the likelihood of desired health outcomes and are consistent with current professional knowledge."[33] The IOM Committee on Quality of Health Care in America expanded on that work in 2001 with a sweeping redesign of the health caresystem. In the report, *Crossing the Quality Chasm: A New Health System for the 21st Century*,[34] six quality aims for patient care were introduced as a fundamental tool for achieving and measuring quality in health care. The IOM described the aims as characteristics that should be present when delivering patient care, as follow:

- *Safe*—avoiding injuries to patients from the care that is intended to help them
- *Effective*—providing services based on scientific knowledge to all who could benefit and refraining from providing services to those not likely to benefit
- *Patient-centered*—providing care that is respectful of and responsive to individual patient preferences, needs, and values and ensuring that patient values guide all clinical decisions
- *Timely*—reducing waits and sometimes harmful delays for those who receive and those who give care
- *Efficient*—avoiding waste, in particular waste of equipment, supplies, ideas, and energy
- *Equitable*—providing care that does not vary in quality because of personal characteristics such as gender, ethnicity, geographic location, and socioeconomic status

The six aims are used by AHRQ to describe characteristics of quality in health care.[2] Commonwealth Fund also incorporated the six aims into their methodology for ranking the performance of health systems internationally.[1] Both examples illustrate the translation of this concept for quality characteristics to the practice of measuring and improving quality.

Describing Public Health Quality

In a renewed effort to address the weaknesses in public health quality, quality in public health was defined 7 years after the release of *Crossing the Quality Chasm*.[34] With the leadership of the Assistant Secretary for Health, the HHS Public Health Quality Forum (Quality Forum) was launched, and in 2008 the *Consensus Statement on Quality in the Public Health System* was published. The Quality Forum defined quality in public health as "the degree to which policies, programs, services, and research for the population increase desired health outcomes and conditions in which the population can be healthy."[35] The *Consensus Statement* also established nine quality aims (**Table 26.4**) to aid entities across all sectors of public health (e.g., state and local health departments, tax-exempt hospitals, nonprofit organizations) with identifying and applying standard quality characteristics to public health work, and to ensure uniformity of improvement efforts.[33] The aims clarify fundamental strategies important to fulfilling the public health mission.

The concept of quality characteristics used in health care and public health is modeled on the definition of quality established by the Internal Organization for Standardization (ISO) as "a set of features and characteristics of a product or service that bear on its ability to satisfy stated or implied needs.[36] Essentially, given the broad scope of public health activities and difficulty often experienced when attempting to articulate the role of public health, the aims aid in focusing attention on a key set of critical and reasonable characteristics that should be present when fulfilling a public health mission. In essence, the aims are what should be used to measure for quality in the public health system similar to how *color, taste,* and *smell* represent characteristics

Table 26.4   Aims for Improvement of Quality in the U.S. Public Health System

Public Health Aim	Definition
Population-Centered	Protecting and promoting healthy conditions and health for entire populations
Equitable	Working to achieve health equity
Proactive	Formulating policies and sustainable practices in a timely manner, while mobilizing rapidly to address new and emerging threats and vulnerabilities
Health-Promoting	Ensuring policies and strategies that advance safe practices by providers and the population and that increase the probability of positive health behavior and outcomes
Risk-Reducing	Diminishing adverse environmental and social events by implementing policies and strategies to reduce the probability of preventable injuries and illnesses or negative outcomes
Vigilant	Intensifying practices and enacting policies to support enhancements to surveillance activities (technology, standardization, systems thinking/modeling)
Transparent	Ensuring openness in the delivery of services and practices, with particular emphasis on valid, reliable, accessible, timely, and meaningful data that are readily available to stakeholders, including the public
Effective	Justifying investments by using evidence, science, and best practices to achieve optimal results in areas of greatest need
Efficient	Understanding costs and benefits of public health interventions to facilitate the optimal use of resources to achieve desired outcomes

Source: Data from McDonald KM, Sundaram V, Bravata DM, et al. *Closing the Quality Gap: A Critical Analysis of Quality Improvement Strategies* (Vol. 7: Care Coordination). Rockville, MD: Agency for Healthcare Research and Quality; 2007. (Technical Reviews, No. 9.7.) 5, Conceptual Frameworks and Their Application to Evaluating Care Coordination Interventions. Available at: http://www.ncbi.nlm.nih.gov/books/NBK44008/. Accessed March 29, 2013.

of quality drinking water or how the six IOM aims for patient care represent quality in their corresponding aspects of health. Fundamentally, a system lacking the nine public health characteristics lacks quality and is unable to mount efforts to fuel desperately needed improvements in the system. Accordingly, areas identified as having public health quality deficiencies should be targeted for quality-improvement efforts. Similar to how AHRQ and the Commonwealth Foundation use the IOM aims for patient care to measure for quality, the **public health quality aims** should be used as well.

The nine aims also represent preemptive approaches to improving health versus the more reactive nature of medical care. Application of the public health quality aims can occur in a variety of ways:

- Advancing quality concepts in existing and future public health programs
- Providing policymakers with a useful standardized guide for examining public health programs and services
- Helping public health leaders articulate in clear terms the public health mission
- Creating a focal point to frame and promote consistency when implementing and measuring quality improvement (QI) initiatives across the public health system

Table 26.5   Application of the Public Health Quality Aims

Aims for Improvement of Quality	Program activities that align with the nine aims
Population-Centered	Conduct routine epidemiological studies
Equitable	Assessment of subpopulations by sex, race, medical condition
Proactive	Develop substantial infrastructure to monitor vaccine safety post-licensure and at all stages of vaccine development
Health-Promoting	Identifying persons at risk for vaccine adverse reactions and developing and implementing contraindications
Risk-Reducing	Identify people at increased risk and develop "next generation" vaccines with improved safety profile
Vigilant	Engage in activities through multiple departments (U.S. Department of Veterans Affairs, Department of Defense) and HHS agencies to detect and prevent adverse reactions
Transparent	Convene National Vaccine Advisory Committee Safety Working Group for public meetings
Effective	Development of the next generation Pertussis vaccine (whole cell→acellular)
Efficient	Provide infrastructure such as CDC's Vaccine Safety Datalink and FDA's Post-Licensure Rapid Immunization Safety Monitoring Network

Source: Data from Brownson RC, Baker EA, Leet TL, et al. *Evidence-Based Public Health Practice.* New York: Oxford University Press; 2003.

- Identifying QI projects by helping public health practitioners detect performance gaps in their public health programs, services, policies, and research
- Identifying gaps in terms of quality of public health services offered[37]

An example of the application of the quality aims to test for conformity in an existing public health program, the National Vaccine Safety program of the HHS, is provided in **Table 26.5**.[25]

Identification of quality measures that are aligned with the aims and appropriate measurement criteria are logical next steps in continuing to develop concepts for quality in public health. The National Quality Forum recently advanced this by including the nine public health quality aims as a criterion for the endorsement of population health measures.[38]

Continuous Quality Improvement (CQI) in Health Care and Public Health

Continuous quality improvement is "a structured organizational process for involving personnel in planning and executing a continuous flow of improvements to provide quality health care [and public health] that meets or exceeds expectations."[28, p. 4] Elements of CQI were presented earlier in this chapter in a discussion of W. Edwards Deming, considered by many to be the founder of CQI and the quality management philosophy. Continuous improvement of quality of health services, both in the healthcare and public health arenas, has become a necessary and integral aspect of the business and operational strategy of the 21st century health organization.

A successful model for CQI in health care was developed by the IHI, under the leadership of Don Berwick. The IHI is an independent, not-for-profit organization that focuses on sustaining good health and improving the quality of healthcare delivery systems.[39] This group has committed to achieving astonishing goals, such as their campaign to save 5 million lives. The aim of the 5 Million Lives Campaign supported the improvement of medical care in the United States and the reduction of rates of morbidity and mortality resulting from illness, medical harm, or surgical complications. IHI asked hospitals participating in the campaign to prevent 5 million occurrences of medical harm during a 2-year period, 2006–2008, and provided a set of steps and recommendations to help hospitals achieve their goals. The IHI triple aim framework is another approach for optimizing the performance of the health system.[40] This framework helps organizations focus simultaneously on three important dimensions of quality in health systems:

- Improving the patient's experience of care in terms of safety, quality, and satisfaction
- Improving the health of populations
- Reducing the per capita cost of health care

IHI's methods for improving quality combine *The Model for Improvement* with collaborative learning strategies, packaged into an educational program on quality known as the Breakthrough Series. The Model for Improvement (MFI) incorporates four major modules:

- What are we trying to accomplish? In this step the team develops a measurable aim and sets a timeframe for accomplishing this aim.
- How will we know that a change is an improvement? Here, measures are established to quantify that changes were undertaken and the effect on the outcome of those changes.
- What changes can we make that will result in an improvement? Applying the best available knowledge from evidence-based strategies to consensus statements or expertise from those working in the system helps to assure that selected changes will lead to expected improvements.
- Applying Plan–Do–Study–Act cycles. Repeated cycles of these steps test change(s) in real time.

Measuring Quality

Healthcare quality measurement systems have evolved over the years and serve several primary purposes. They are used to provide information to consumers of health care about the quality and type of healthcare available, helpful to them as they make choices about healthcare services and providers. Quality measurement systems also serve to hold healthcare systems accountable for the quality of their healthcare services to their many consumers. Such systems inform public health initiatives and public policy to protect and promote health. Lastly, these measurement systems are helpful in identifying gaps in performance and potential areas for quality improvement projects within healthcare and public health organizations. Although useful in reporting on accountability and gaps in performance, the major health measurements systems historically emphasized assessment and reporting and did not address the important need for leaders of healthcare systems to manage performance improvement. To manage improvement, healthcare professionals require systems that help them understand the gaps in their performance and measure changes that close that gap and achieve the mission of the organization. **Table 26.6** offers an overview of some of the major measurement systems within the healthcare system; improvement functions are now showing up in a number of major systems.

The Joint Commission, established in 1951, used minimum standards from the American College of Surgeons to initially evaluate hospitals.[9] The standards became more rigorous over

Table 26.6   Major Health Quality Measurement Systems in the United States

Name and Description	Primary Function	Uses	Developed For	Developed By
Health Employer Data Information System (HEDIS)	Accountability and Selection	Measures to evaluate healthcare insurance plans	Health Plans and Employers	National Committee for Quality Assurance (NCQA)
Foundation for Accountability (FACCT), 1995–2004	Accountability and Selection	Quality measures to help consumers evaluate the quality of the health care they receive, choose a provider, and manage their own health care	Consumers of health care (the public, Ford, GM, Chrysler, Leap Frog, NCQA)	FACCT—National organization whose mission is to improve health care in the United States
Consumer Assessment of Healthcare Providers and Systems (CAHPS)	Selection	Measures of consumers' satisfaction with the healthcare services they receive	Consumers of health care	Agency for Health Care Policy and Research (AHCPR)
The Joint Commission 2011 Accountability Measures	Accountability and Improvement	Measures to assess the performance of hospitals	Hospitals	The Joint Commission
The Joint Commission Oryx System, National Hospital Quality Measures, 1997	Accountability and Improvement	Measures to evaluate and report on performance of hospitals	Hospitals	The Joint Commission
National Quality Measures Clearinghouse	Widespread access to quality measures to healthcare community and other interested parties	Public resource for evidence-based quality measures and measure sets	Healthcare stakeholders, including practitioners, providers, health plans, purchasers, and consumers	Agency for Healthcare Research and Quality (AHRQ)

time and incorporated the Donabedian structure-process-outcome framework to comprehensively assess the quality of hospital care. The ORYX system was launched in 1997 by The Joint Commission and was the first national collection and reporting of standardized measures on hospital performance. At the start of the 21st century, The Joint Commission incorporated elements of CQI into their accreditation requirements. In 2002, accredited hospitals collected and reported on two of four core measures sets for heart attacks, heart failures, pneumonia, and pregnancy. Public reporting of these metrics occurred in 2004. By 2011, more than 40 improved accountability measures, expected to be moved into ORYX, have been adopted and cover areas of care for heart attack, heart failure, pneumonia, surgery, children's asthma, inpatient psychiatric services, venous thromboembolism, and stroke. The practice of measuring the quality of care and using these measures to inform improvement efforts, to influence payment, or to increase transparency is now moving from hospital settings into other healthcare settings, not only in the United States, but around the world.[41] By 2009, hospitals were achieving high marks on many of the standardized measures, and variation among hospitals was reduced decidedly. Not all measures, however, led to improvement in patient outcomes; hence, new criteria for measures established higher standards for quality in accreditation and accountability programs. The goal for these new metrics is to increase the likelihood that patient outcomes will improve when action is taken to improve the measures.[38]

The National Committee for Quality Assurance (NCQA) worked with corporate leaders and health plan quality leaders to develop standards for health maintenance organizations (HMOs) in the early 1990s. Healthcare Effectiveness Data and Information Set (HEDIS) was established to allow the comparison of health plans on effectiveness of care received by their members.[42] HEDIS became an official part of the NCQA accreditation process in 1999.

A similar system of standardized and robust quality measures for public health is not in existence today. A voluntary public health accreditation process, promoted rigorously and supported financially by the Robert Wood Johnson Foundation and CDC, has been established. A nonprofit organization, the Public Health Accreditation Board (PHAB), is the lead agency in overseeing the accreditation process for governmental public health departments. Domains, standards, and measures have been established. For example, domain one requires public health departments to conduct and disseminate assessments focused on population health status and public health issues facing the community, a requirement that embodies a number of public health quality aims—population-centered, proactive, and transparent. A number of standards have been developed to assure accurate implementation of this domain, including the participation of the agency in a collaborative process resulting in a comprehensive community health assessment. One of the multiple measures identified for assuring that this standard is in place: Participate in or conduct a tribal/local partnership for the development of a comprehensive community health assessment of the population served by the health department.[43] The measures listed throughout the accreditation document are for the purpose of quality assurance and are subjective in nature; that is, they are determined by the reviewers' personal judgment of how the service was performed. They differ from the accreditation measures in the ORYX system, for example, where quantitative measures are required. It is generally accepted in the health community that, "[q]uality assurance is the systematic monitoring and evaluation of the

Table 26.7   Examples of Public Health Quality Indicators from Los Angeles Department of Health

Indicator	Quality Dimension	Public Health Quality Aim
Ratio of California Children's Services patients to nurse providers	Structure	Population-Centered
Proportion of confirmatory test results for reportable diseases that hospital and other private labs reported to the Department of Health Services	Process	Risk-Reducing Vigilant Transparent
Proportion of patients with newly diagnosed active tuberculosis (TB) for whom ≤ 12 months of therapy are indicated or who complete recommended therapy within 12 months	Intermediate Outcome	Proactive Risk-Reducing
Percent reduction in TB case rates in the community	Outcome	Population-Centered Proactive

Source: Derose S, Asch S, Fielding J, et al. Developing quality indicators for local health departments: experience in Los Angeles County. *Am J Prev Med.* 2003;25(40):347–57.

performance of an organization or its programs to ensure that standards (usually set by public health experts) of quality are being met."[23, p. 455] Quality assurance methods help to pinpoint areas for improvement; however, prioritization of the areas for improvement are necessary to assure that resources address the vital few instead of the useful many, as Juran instructed with the 80/20 Pareto principle discussed earlier in this chapter.

The Los Angeles Department of Health Services undertook the task of developing quality measures in 2003 to assess quality in both public and personal health care.[44] Applying Donabedian's framework, structural, process, and intermediate and ultimate outcome indicators were identified following an extensive literature review on a variety of public health quality and performance topics. A final set of 111 indicators were identified, 61 of which were recommended based on their capacity to assess and improve quality at the health agency. Examples of indicators from each dimension of the measurement framework appear in **Table 26.7** and are mapped to the appropriate quality domain and public health quality aims.

A similar effort to identify outcome and process indicators occurred in the Florida Department of Health from 2007–2010. Measures for process and outcomes were identified, but linkages between the selected process and outcome metrics were missing, creating concern that changes in processes driven by measurement requirements would not necessarily result in improved outcomes.[45]

Priority Areas for Improvement

A vision for "building better systems to give all people what they need to reach their full potential for health"[46] was the major message from the Assistant Secretary for Health in the 2010 HHS report, *Priority Areas for Improvement of Quality in Public Health.*[44] The *Consensus Statement* produced by the HHS Public Health Quality Forum addressed the 1998 call for action.[35] A logical next step was the identification of priority areas for improvement of public health quality. The following six priority areas for improvement of quality in public health are presented in the priority areas document:

- *Population health metrics and information technology*—Improve methods and analytical capacity to collect, evaluate, and disseminate data that can be translated into actionable information and outcomes in population health at the local, state, and national levels.
- *Evidence-based practices, research, and evaluation*—Bridge research and practice and institutionalize evidence-based approaches to achieve results-based accountability.
- *Systems thinking*—Advance systems thinking in public health. Foster systems integration strategies by analyzing problems using systems science methodologies (e.g., network analysis) while taking into account the complex adaptive nature of the public health system.
- *Sustainability and stewardship*—Strengthen system sustainability and stewardship through valid measures and reporting of performance and quality.
- *Policy*—Strengthen policy development and analysis processes and advocacy to ensure that evidence is integrated into policymaking to improve population health.
- *Workforce and Education*—Develop and sustain a competent workforce by ensuring that educational and skills content are appropriately aligned with core and discipline-specific cometencies.[44]

These six priority areas for improvement are seen as primary drivers of public health quality. They are linked to key interventions called secondary drivers and, given that connection, facilitate the highest likelihood of enhancing the achievement of desired levels of public health services and outcomes. A causal driver diagram, modeled on the Institute of Healthcare Improvement system for Breakthrough Goals and Drivers, is presented in **Figure 26.2** to demonstrate this pathway to improvement success. The diagram illustrates the process of selecting and implementing improvement interventions in areas that can drive change. Figure 26.2 illustrates how reductions in tobacco use (the desired outcome) are accelerated when quality improvements are targeted at three of the public health priority areas—evidence-based practices, policy, and systems thinking—that serve as the primary drivers. Completing the model are the secondary drivers that cascade to support the primary drivers with specific interventions that influence improvements in the primary drivers and achievement of desired outcomes. For example, Figure 26.2 illustrates that social marketing and public service announcement (PSA) campaigns conform to characteristics of population centeredness and health promoting. PSAs are also documented evidence-based (a primary driver) interventions that aid in reducing tobacco use. The intervention (also in Figure 26.2) to create programs to increase excise taxes on tobacco is characteristic of the system being proactive and is also an evidence-based strategy for reducing tobacco use.

As this illustrates, supporting the primary drivers with secondary drivers framed by the public health quality aims ensures that improvements meet the characteristics of quality in public health. Measuring improvement is accomplished when quality measures are identified for the secondary driver interventions (Figure 26.2). Agencies desiring to improve by conforming to the quality aims of being population-centered, proactive, health-promoting, risk-reducing, and vigilant are guided by this process.

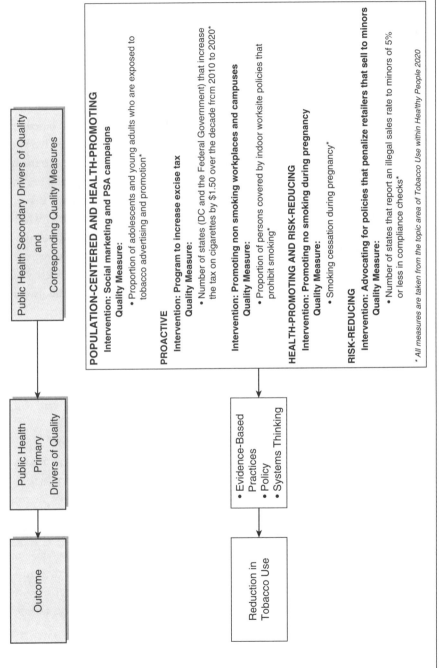

Figure 26.2   Public Health Quality Driver Diagram

Future Outlook

The IOM referred to public health agencies as the backbone of the U.S. public health system. That backbone is sagging under the impact of complex health issues requiring complex solutions. Reducing the threats to health and promoting the protective factors that improve health require a redesign of the public health system.

References throughout this chapter indicate that improving the public's health entails an intersectoral approach, because it involves addressing complex health issues that require transdisciplinary skills to effectively solve these challenging health problems. For this to be accomplished, integration of clinical care with community preventive services and health promotion is needed. It will also require experts in the emerging science of system design, a field based on knowledge from operations research, human factors engineering, and complex adaptive systems. The field of system design looks at the best ways of providing services that are extremely interdependent and centered on human needs.[46] By applying it to the practice of public health, headway in the best methods, techniques, and knowledge base can be made toward desired system redesign. For example, addressing the obesity epidemic involves academicians whose research skills can be used to build evidence that policymakers should use when developing national food, nutrition, agriculture, and physical activity policies. This evidence from research also should influence employers who establish work wellness programs, health providers who help patients develop individually adapted health behavior change programs, and schools that implement physical education programs.[47]

Strategic directions found in the National Quality Strategy and National Prevention Strategy aid in facilitating needed new directions and for achieving national goals such as those in *Healthy People 2020*. The recent release of the Centers for Medicare and Medicaid Services State Innovation Models Funding Opportunity Announcement serves as an ideal opportunity for leadership in states across the nation to demonstrate their ability to take giant steps forward with improving the health of the population.

Applying the quality aims in this part of the public health system is only possible with a highly skilled public health workforce that is educated in the disciplines of public health and in innovative formats that may emerge through efforts of the ASPH Framing the Future Task Force.

Many times public health programs operate in silos. The IOM recently made multiple recommendations for the integration of public health and primary care as both areas contribute to the common elements of preventing disease and promoting health. The IOM reported that this important work is often carried out in relative isolation, despite the fact that the integration of public health and primary care could enhance the capacity of both sectors to fulfill their mission.[48] Leadership and continuous quality improvement are two major components for successfully transforming the current health system from silos to a health system that embraces broader participation.

The *Consensus Statement*[35] and the *Priority Areas for Improvement of Quality in Public Health*[44] establish a common focus and a solid framework that assists with a number of vital tasks facing organizations committed to assuring conditions that promote health and direct resources toward prevention to reduce the burden of illness and disease. The vital tasks include identifying gaps in performance that inhibit quality, promoting a common set of goals for public health systems across all levels of government, and identifying areas for improvement where the application of CQI practices and system redesign are employed to ensure successful ventures.[18] Public health systems, as they are currently configured (typically a local governmental entity with jurisdiction over one geographic region), are stymied in their efforts to gain traction on the complex problems of modernity. The quality aims and priority areas, coupled with a competent workforce and broader partner engagement, are approaches that offer great opportunities for advancement of population health.

Discussion Questions

1. Why are we concerned about quality in the field of public health?
2. Define quality in public health and discuss the quality aims. Can you identify public health programs that achieve some of the quality aims?
3. How can we apply the quality aims to improve public health systems?
4. Explain why an intersectoral approach to health is essential in today's world. Who would you include in an intersectoral initiative to address obesity in your community?
5. Describe components of the National Quality Strategy and National Prevention Strategy.
6. What role do the *Healthy People 2020* Leading Health Indicators play in advancing quality?
7. Discuss examples of quality chasms presented in this chapter. Are you aware of other quality gaps to improve individual or population health?
8. What is the value of leading health indicators? Have we seen improvement in some of these indicators over time?
9. Discuss the major milestones of quality in health systems. What do you consider as being the missing elements in milestones for public health quality?
10. What is meant by the phrase, "continuous quality improvement"?
11. Explain the value of using the Expanded Chronic Care Model. Can you apply this to any work you are currently or have previously been involved with?
12. What are three major healthcare quality measurement systems and what purpose do they serve?
13. What is system design? Do you see a need to redesign the current health system? Why?

References

1. Davis K, Schoen C, Stremikis K. *Mirror, Mirror on the Wall: How the Performance of the U.S. Health Care System Compares Internationally, 2010 Update.* Available at: http://www.commonwealthfund.org/~/media/Files/Publications/Fund%20Report/2010/Jun/1400_Davis_Mirror_Mirror_on_the_wall_2010.pdf. Accessed March 29, 2013.
2. Agency for Healthcare Research and Quality. *National Healthcare Quality Report.* Available at: http://www.ahrq.gov/research/findings/nhqrdr/nhqr11/nhqr11.pdf. Accessed March 29, 2013.
3. Institute of Medicine. *The Future of Public Health.* Washington, DC: National Academies Press; 1988.
4. Public Health Leadership Society. *Principles of the Ethical Practice of Public Health.* Available at: http://www.apha.org/NR/rdonlyres/1CED3CEA-287E-4185-9CBD-BD405FC60856/0/ethicsbrochure.pdf. Accessed March 29, 2013.

5. Choski DA, Farley TA. The cost effectiveness of environmental approaches to disease prevention. *N Engl J Med.* 2012;367(4):295–7.

6. Trust for America's Health. *Investing in America's Health.* Available at: http://www.healthyamericans .org./report/94/. Accessed March 31, 2013.

7. Mays GP, McHugh MC, Shim K, et al. Institutional and economic determinants of public health system performance. *Am J Public Health.* 2006;96(3):1019–26.

8. Luce JM, Bindman AB, Lee PR. A brief history of health care quality assessment and improvement in the US. *West J Med.* 1994;160:263–8.

9. Chassin MR, O'Kane M. *History of the Quality Improvement Movement.* Available at: http://www2.aap .org/sections/perinatal/pdf/1quality.pdf. Accessed March 31, 2013.

10. Robinson WA. Historic and personal reflections on HCQIA, perspectives of a former federal executive. *J Leg Med.* 2012;33;43–61.

11. Association of Schools of Public Health. *Framing the Future: The Second Hundred Years of Public Health Education Task Force.* Available at: http://www.asph.org/document.cfm?page=1184. Accessed March 31, 2013.

12. Institute of Medicine. *To Err Is Human: Building a Safer Health System.* Available at: http://www .iom.edu/~/media/Files/Report%20Files/1999/To-Err-is-Human/To%20Err%20is%20Human%20 1999%20%20report%20brief.pdf. Accessed March 31, 2013.

13. Chassin MR, Loeb JM. The ongoing quality improvement journey: next stop, high reliability. *Qual J.* 2011;30(4):559–68.

14. Van Den Bos J, Rustagi K, Gray T, et al. The $17.1 billion problem: the annual cost of measurable medical errors. *Health Affairs.* 2011;30(4):596–603.

15. Clancy C. *Revealing Medical Errors Helps Chicago Hospitals Build a Safer Health System.* Available at: http://www.ahrq.gov/consumer/cc/cc071012.htm. Accessed March 31, 2013.

16. Rust G, Satcher D, Fryer GE, et al. Triangulating on success: innovation, public health, medical care, and cause-specific US mortality rates over a half century (1950–2000). *Am J Public Health.* 2010;100(S1):S95–S104.

17. Centers for Disease Control and Prevention. The Ten Great Public Health Achievements. *MMWR.* 2011;60(19):619–23. Available at: http://www.cdc.gov/mmwr/preview/mmwrhtml/mm6019a5.htm. Accessed March 31, 2013.

18. Centers for Disease Control and Prevention. *Public Health's Infrastructure.* Available at: http://www.uic .edu/sph/prepare/courses/ph410/resources/phinfrastructure.pdf. Accessed March 31, 2013.

19. Lurie N, Wasserman J, Stoto J, et al. Local variation in public health preparedness: lessons from California. *Health Affairs.* 2004;doi 10.1377/hlthaff.W4.341.

20. Hearne S, Segal L. Leveraging the nation's anti-bioterrorism investments: foundation efforts to ensure a revitalized public health system. *Health Affairs.* 2003;22(4):230–4.

21. Trust for America's Health. *Ready or Not? Protecting the Public's Health in the Age of Bioterrorism.* Available at: http://healthyamericans.org/reports/bioterror04/BioTerror04Report.pdf. Accessed March 31, 2013.

22. Trust for America's Health. *Ready or Not? 2011 Protecting the Public from Diseases, Disasters, and Bioterrorism.* Available at: http://healthyamericans.org/report/92/. Accessed March 31, 2013.

23. Central Intelligence Agency. *The World Fact Book.* Available at: https://www.cia.gov/library/ publications/the-world-factbook/rankorder/2228rank.html. Accessed March 31, 2013.

24. Robert Wood Johnson Foundation. *Chronic Care: Making the Case for Ongoing Care.* Available at: http://www.rwjf.org/en/research-publications/find-rwjf-research/2010/02/chronic-care.html. Accessed March 31, 2013.

25. Brownson RC, Baker EA, Leet TL, et al. *Evidence-Based Public Health Practice.* New York: Oxford University Press; 2003.

26. *Patient Protection and Affordable Care Act.* Available at: http://docs.house.gov/energycommerce/ ppacacon.pdf. Accessed March 31, 2013.

27. U.S. Department of Health and Human Services. *Healthy People 2020 Leading Health Indicators.* Available at: http://www.healthypeople.gov/2020/LHI/socialDeterminants.aspx. Accessed March 31, 2013.

28. Honoré PA, Wright D, Berwick DM, et al. Creating a framework for getting quality into the public health system. *Health Affairs.* 2011;30(4):737–45.

29. Smith JL. *The History of Modern Quality.* Available at: http://www.peoriamagazines.com/print/6196. Accessed March 31, 2013.

30. *Juran, The Source for Quality.* Available at: http://www.juran.com/our-legacy/#JMJ. Accessed March 31, 2013.

31. McDonald KM, Sundaram V, Bravata DM, et al. *Closing the Quality Gap: A Critical Analysis of Quality Improvement Strategies* (Vol. 7: Care Coordination). Rockville (MD): Agency for Healthcare Research and Quality (US); 2007 Jun. (Technical Reviews, No. 9.7.) 5, Conceptual Frameworks and Their Application to Evaluating Care Coordination Interventions. Available at: http://www.ncbi.nlm.nih.gov/books/NBK44008/. Accessed March 31, 2013.

32. President's Advisory Commission on Consumer Protection and Quality in Health Care. *Quality First: Building Better Health Care for All Americans.* Available at: http://archive.ahrq.gov/hcqual/final/append_a.html. Accessed March 28, 2013.

33. Lohr KN, ed., Institute of Medicine. *Medicare: A Strategy for Quality Assurance.* Washington, DC: National Academies Press; 1990.

34. Institute of Medicine. *Crossing the Quality Chasm: A New Health System for the 21st Century.* Washington, DC: National Academies Press; 2001.

35. U.S. Department of Health and Human Services. *Consensus Statement on Quality in the Public Health System.* Available at: http://www.apha.org/NR/rdonlyres/EAA91110-FA31-41F6-935B-A0BB8CFFF294/0/PHQFConsensusStatement92208.pdf. Accessed March 31, 2013.

36. International Organization of Standards. *Terminology.* Available at: http://www.issco.unige.ch/en/research/projects/ewg96/node69.html. Accessed March 31, 2013.

37. Honoré PA. Quality in the Public Health System. Presentation, National Association of Local Boards of Health, Omaha, NE. August, 5, 2010.

38. National Quality Forum. Measure Evaluation Criteria and Additional Guidance for Population Health Metrics. Available at: http://www.qualityforum.org/Home.aspx Accessed January 2, 2012.

39. Institute for Healthcare Improvement. *About IHI.* Available at: http://www.ihi.org/about/pages/default.aspx. Accessed March 31, 2013.

40. Institute for Healthcare Improvement. *IHI Triple Aim Initiative.* Available at: http://www.ihi.org/offerings/Initiatives/TripleAim/Pages/default.aspx. Accessed March 31, 2013.

41. Chassin M, Loeb J, Schmaltz S, et al. Accountability measures—using measurement to promote quality improvement. *New Engl J Med.* 2010;363(7):683–8.

42. Public Health Accreditation Board. *PHAB Standards and Measures Version 1.0.* Available at: http://www.exploringaccreditation.org/index.php/accreditation/standards/. Accessed March 31, 2013.

43. Derose S, Asch S, Fielding J, et al. Developing quality indicators for local health departments: experience in Los Angeles County. *Am J Prev Med.* 2003;25(40),347–57.

44. U.S. Department of Health and Human Services. *Priority Areas for Improvement of Quality in Public Health.* Available at: http://www.hhs.gov/ash/initiatives/quality/quality/improvequality2010.pdf. Accessed March 31, 2013.

45. Florida Department of Health. *2012 County Performance Snapshot Standards and Measures Fact Sheet: DOH 5-Step Performance Improvement Process.* Available at: http://www.doh.state.fl.us/hpi/pdf/2012_CHD_PIP_Fact_Sheet05_2012.pdf. Accessed March 29, 2013.

46. Colgrove J, Fried L, Northridge M, et al. Schools of public health: essential infrastructure of a responsible society and a 21st century health system. *Public Health Rep.* 2010;125:8–14.

47. Centers for Disease Control and Prevention. *The Guide to Community Preventive Services.* Available at: http://www.thecommunityguide.org/pa/behavioral-social/schoolbased-pe.html. Accessed March 31, 2013.

48. Institute of Medicine. *Primary Care and Public Health: Exploring Integration to Improve Population Health.* Available at: http://www.iom.edu/Reports/2012/Primary-Care-and-Public-Health.aspx. Accessed March 31, 2013.

Global Health Challenges and Opportunities

Leiyu Shi and James A. Johnson

LEARNING OBJECTIVES

- To better understand global health and its importance to public health administration
- To gain an awareness of the influence of globalization on global health
- To identify major global health challenges
- To gain an appreciation for the roles and activities of key world health stakeholders
- To better foresee future challenges and opportunities in global health

---

Chapter Overview

Global health care and global public health are changing rapidly as our patterns of society evolve. For instance, today, the aging population is increasing, countries around the world are experiencing a rise in chronic illnesses and infectious diseases amongst their populations, governments must recognize the higher possibility of bioterrorism, physicians are enhancing their focus on patient care, and the advancement of medical technology and evidence-based research in health care has dramatically changed the way health care is delivered. Many of these changes are products of globalization, a movement defined as being "driven by global exchange of information, production of goods and services more economically in developing countries and increased interdependence of mature and emerging world economies."[1] Globalization has radically altered the lives, and health, of people worldwide, often in a positive manner. Despite global health advocacy and despite the rising affluence attained by many in the global economy, the highest attainable standard of health has not been realized by the majority of people on the planet. Life expectancy in the 38 poorest countries is less than 50 years, almost the same as it was in the United States in 1900.[2] Along with the changes occurring with globalization come challenges, some of which are described in detail in this chapter.

Defining Global Health

Global health has been defined as "the area of study, research and practice that places a priority on improving health and achieving **equity** in health for all people worldwide."[3] Global health strives for a worldwide improvement in health status, a reduction of health disparities, and defense against threats that transcend national borders.[4] For example, an increase in travel and communications has spurred an important and positive exchange of goods and services between countries, but at the same time, created an increasing threat of transmission of infectious diseases across borders.

Economic, political, legal, social, cultural, religious, and physical differences and barriers among groups and nations contribute to these challenges of health and equity. Global health affects individual nations but also has a global political and economic impact.[5] It is a field of study, research and practice that includes not only the medical field, but also social science disciplines, including demography, economics, epidemiology, political economy and sociology. Global health endeavors to promote health for all people, regardless of individual differences.[1] The application of these principles to the domain of mental health is called global mental health, and is also an important and changing field.[6,7] Johnson and Stoskopf describe mental illness as accounting for 14% of the global burden of disease and within noncommunicable diseases, they account for 28% of the disability-adjusted life years and thereby more than cardiovascular disease.[8]

Why Is Global Health Important?

As Barry Bloom, former Dean of the Harvard School of Public Health, stated, "the huge disparities in health that exists between countries remain one of the great moral and intellectual problems of our time."[8] Global health aims to aid individuals living in a wide variety of places and facing different socioeconomic factors of health. Attempts to solve global health problems must anticipate and address the long-term effects of diseases, not just react to crises. When focusing on a specific disease, the global health community must consider all pertinent issues and work cooperatively to reduce its impact on societies and nations. For example, infectious diseases can cause severe pregnancy complications and death.[9] Therefore, any global health initiatives to control these infectious diseases must take into account the vulnerability of pregnant women, and any initiatives aimed at improving maternal and child health must acknowledge and act against the contributing burden of infectious diseases (see **Exhibit 27.1** for more examples of the importance of global health).

Exhibit 27.1   Why Global Health Is Important

Humanitarian Issues	• Neglected tropical diseases cause significant morbidity, affecting more than 1 billion people per year, almost exclusively in low-income countries. Inexpensive preventative treatments exist for several of these diseases, but without global health commitment, populations at risk do not receive potentially life-saving drugs.[*] • In 2011, an estimated 34.2 million people were living with HIV/AIDS, a prevalence of 0.8% among the world's adult population. Global health efforts aimed at controlling new HIV infection have been somewhat successful, but greater cooperation and resources will be necessary to stop HIV/AIDS.[†]
Equity Issues	• In 2010, 49.1 million Americans under the age of 65 lacked health insurance, even though three-quarters of those individuals come from working families.[‡] • Racial and ethnic minorities, even though the vast majority (more than 80%) are American citizens, are more likely to be uninsured.[‡] • In 1990, the Commission on Health Research for Development estimated that only 5% of the funds spent worldwide on health research was intended to address the health problems in low- and middle-income countries, where 93% of preventable deaths were occurring. Today, the imbalance has narrowed slightly, although it is still often referred to as the "10/90" gap.[§]

[*]USAID, Neglected Tropical Diseases Program. *About the Neglected Tropical Diseases Program.* Available at: http://www.neglecteddiseases.gov/about/index.html. Accessed March 30, 2013.
[†]Kaiser Family Foundation. *U.S. Global Health Policy.* Available at: http://www.globalhealthfacts.org/. Accessed March 30, 2013.
[‡]Kaiser Family Foundation. *Key Facts About Americans Without Health Insurance.* Available at: http://www.kff.org/uninsured/upload/7451-07.pdf. Accessed March 30, 2013.
[§]Global Forum for Health Research. *10/90 Gap.* Available at: http://www.globalforumhealth.org/about/1090-gap/. Accessed March 30, 2013.

As described in Johnson and Stoskopf[8] and supported by World Health Organization (WHO) research, the top 10 causes of death are as follows:

1. Heart disease
2. Cerebrovascular disease
3. Respiratory infection
4. HIV/AIDS
5. Chronic pulmonary disease
6. Perinatal conditions
7. Diarrheal disease
8. Tuberculosis
9. Malaria
10. Respiratory tract cancers

Each of these warrants a central role for public health and many can only be fully addressed with a global effort, while others require local interventions that are culturally appropriate.[2] A summary of global health statistics, as derived by the Kaiser Family Foundation, is provided in **Table 27.1**.

Table 27.1   Global Health Statistics

12 million	People living with tuberculosis worldwide (in 2010)
8.8 Million	New cases of tuberculosis
1.4 Million	Tuberculosis deaths
34.2 million	People living with HIV/AIDS worldwide (2011)
1.7 million	AIDS deaths
16.6 million	AIDS orphans (2009)
54%	Percentage of people in low- and middle-income countries receiving necessary antiretroviral (ARV) therapy (2011)
94.3 million	Cases of malaria worldwide (2010)
345,960	Malaria deaths worldwide (2010)
15%	Worldwide percentage of babies born with low birth weight (2005–2010)
16.2%	Worldwide percentage of malnourishment in children under 5 years of age (2005–2011)
$990	Global average per capita annual expenditure for health (2009)
57/1000	Child (0–5) mortality rate worldwide (2010)

Source: Data from Kaiser Family Foundation's *U.S. Global Health Policy.* Available at: http://www.globalhealthfacts.org/data/topic/default.aspx?all=1. Accessed March 30, 2013.

It is important to address global health issues for a variety of reasons—humanitarian, equity, direct impact on individuals and countries, **indirect impacts,** attainability, and universality.

Humanitarian

An estimated 1.8 million people died from AIDS in 2010, the vast majority of them in developing countries, and more than 16 million children have been orphaned as a result of AIDS.[10,11] Another 3 million people die annually from tuberculosis (TB) or malaria, both of which can be treated with proper medical care.[5] Global health also seeks to cure often overlooked, but still very important, neglected tropical diseases (NTDs):

> According to WHO estimates, the global burden of the NTDs for all ages, 21 million DALYs [disability-adjusted life years], is just over half as large as the global burden of malaria. Just over a third of this burden falls in those aged 10–24 years, and, in Africa, the NTDs cause 6% of the total burden for young people, compared with 3% for malaria and 9% for HIV/AIDS.[12]

Overall, working to solve global health problems will help avert the needless suffering and preventable deaths of millions of adults and children.

Equity

Equity in health care is an important and difficult objective for global health. Achieving equity is a challenge for even the richest countries in the world. In the United States, the Patient

Protection and Affordable Care Act (ACA) of 2010 was meant to make the U.S. healthcare system more accessible and fair for all citizens. President Barack Obama signed the bill into federal law, despite the resistance of the general public to healthcare reform (for fears of systematic change and rising costs, amongst other reasons). This legislation continues to be challenged in the federal Appellate and Supreme Courts by dissatisfied states and parties.[3]

Globally, more money is spent on diseases that affect a smaller number of primarily wealthier people than a large number of impoverished people;[13] for instance, it can be argued that the high burden of neglected tropical diseases continues because the people affected do not represent a profitable market for treatment development, leading to inequitable health outcomes. Many therefore argue that more resources need to be provided to these causes, as profitability should not infringe on the ability of all people to receive adequate health care. However, there is also growing similarity in the list of diseases that commonly affect people in high- and low-income countries. Working to solve widespread, universal health problems may help distribute healthcare money and resources more fairly across the globe.

There is also tension between global hopes for health equity and countries' and companies' needs to promote market competition and development. However, there are some strategies to balance these sometimes oppositional goals. For instance, tiered pricing is one strategy to ensure equitable access to medicines for populations in need; in tiered pricing, drugs and vaccines are sold in developing countries at prices deemed fair, meaning they are systematically lower than the prices paid for the same product in industrialized countries. This strategy "has received widespread support from industry, policymakers, civil society, and academics as a way to improve access to medicines for the poor."[14,15] While the acceptance of strategies like this represents great progress, the question of how to achieve equity in other areas and amongst all people is still a critical issue in global health.

Direct Impact on Individuals and Countries

In an increasingly connected world, diseases can move across borders as freely as people and products. Infectious diseases emerging in far corners of the world can pose almost immediate threats in the United States, which has already seen the arrival of diseases such as severe acute respiratory syndrome (SARS), avian flu, and drug-resistant TB. Many countries have become more aware of this threat and are working together to address it. The United Nations and its constituent organizations have global focus initiatives for global health issues, and WHO conducts disease surveillance and coordinates health activities between governments. In the United States, the Office of Global Affairs addresses global health and international matters from within the Department of Health and Human Services (HHS).[16]

Indirect Impacts

Global health should also matter to Americans for reasons other than its impact on their own health. For example, rising incidence of diseases like HIV/AIDS, malaria, and TB contribute to poverty and political instability in many countries. In turn, poverty and instability can have political and economic consequences worldwide. As articulated by Ottersen et al.:

> Globalization has tightened the links of interdependence binding together states, societies, and economies; this has both increased the degree to which we face shared health threats, and opened up new opportunities for collaborative action by a diverse range of sectors. New players also bring new resources, interests, and agendas to the table: today, non-state actors, such as private firms and civil society organizations, wield significant influence, alongside sovereign nation states and intergovernmental organizations.

While there is little doubt that globalization will continue, countries' responses to its effects will greatly impact global health.

Attainability

Is global health attainable? In the hope of providing some answers, the Institute of Medicine (IOM) has made recommendations and issued a report regarding the U.S. commitment to global health. In the report, the committee states that global health

> can be attained by combining a population-based promotion and disease-prevention measures with individual-level clinical care. The ambitious endeavor calls for an understanding of health determinants, practices, and solutions, as well as basic and applied research on disease and disability including risk factors.[17]

Universality

To meet these and other challenges, the United Nations formulated a set of goals to help guide the international community in the new millennium that started in 2000. The intermediate goals are to be achieved or substantially addressed by the year 2015. Longer term goals that seek to galvanize the world in a collective effort to eradicate poverty and health disparities are under consideration. The Millennium Development Goals (MDGs) are presented in **Table 27.2**.[18]

All eight of the goals relate to health in some way. Some delineate a specific health challenge such as child mortality, maternal health, HIV/AIDS, and malaria, while others address the social and environmental determinants of health.

Global health efforts also must be local efforts. The notion of "think globally, act locally" is most appropriate and necessitates training and education, capacity building, economic empowerment, and coordination at all levels of society.[2]

Working to address global health problems will be difficult, but much can be accomplished through commitment and cooperation amongst many different actors. Coordinated, creative approaches will be necessary to tackle major global health challenges.

Global Health Organizations

As described by Johnson, much of the work of public health occurs globally through international organizations.[19] Many of these exist under the auspices of larger governing bodies such as individual governments and partnerships among larger groups of nations. As Johnson stated,

Table 27.2   The Millenium Development Goals and Their Related Targets

Goal	Targets
Goal 1: Eradicate Extreme Hunger and Poverty	**Target 1.** Halve, between 1990 and 2015, the proportion of people whose income is less than $1 a day **Target 2.** Halve, between 1990 and 2015, the proportion of people who suffer from hunger
Goal 2: Achieve Universal Primary Education	**Target 3.** Ensure that, by 2015, children everywhere, boys and girls alike, will be able to complete a full course of primary schooling
Goal 3: Promote Gender Equality and Empower Women	**Target 4.** Eliminate gender disparity in primary and secondary education, preferably by 2005, and in all levels of education no later than 2015
Goal 4: Reduce Child Mortality	**Target 5.** Reduce by two thirds, between 1990 and 2015, the under-5 mortality rate
Goal 5: Improve Maternal Health	**Target 6.** Reduce by three-quarters, between 1990 and 2015, the maternal mortality ratio
Goal 6: Combat HIV/AIDS, Malaria, and Other Diseases	**Target 7.** Have halted by 2015 and begun to reverse the spread of HIV/AIDS **Target 8.** Have halted by 2015 and begun to reverse the incidence of malaria and other major diseases
Goal 7: Ensure Environmental Sustainability	**Target 9.** Integrate the principles of sustainable development into country policies and programs and reverse the loss of environmental resources **Target 10.** Halve, by 2015, the proportion of people without sustainable access to safe drinking water and basic sanitation **Target 11.** Have achieved by 2020 a significant improvement in the lives of at least 100 million slum dwellers
Goal 8: Develop a Global Partnership for Development	**Target 12.** Develop further an open, rule-based, predictable, nondiscriminatory trading and financial system **Target 13.** Address the special needs of the least developed countries **Target 14.** Address the special needs of landlocked developing countries and small island developing states **Target 15.** Deal comprehensively with the debt problems of developing countries through national and international measures in order to make debt sustainable in the long term

Source: Data from Millenium Project: Goals, Targets, and Indicators. Available at http://www.unmilleniumproject.org/goals/gti.htm.

"These entities are formed to benefit the global community in matters pertaining to public health, security, and other human needs and interests."[19, p. 170] Riegelman declares, since the founding of the World Health Organization in 1948, global public health efforts have grown, and this growth has been more dramatic in the 21st century.[20] A proliferation of governmental and nongovernmental organizations have become engaged in global health activities. The World Bank and other multilateral financial institutions are the largest funding source for global health, yet major donors such as the Bill and Melinda Gates Foundation and the Clinton Global Initiative assert a significant leadership role as well. International organizations vary in type, governance, role, and limitations as shown in **Table 27.3**.

Table 27.3 Global Public Health Organizations

Type of Agency	Structure–Governance	Role(s)	Limitations
World Health Organization	United Nations Organization Seven "Regional" semi-independent components e.g., Pan American Health Organization covers North and South America	Policy Development- e.g., tobacco treaty, epidemic control policies Coordination of services e.g., SARS control, vaccine development Data collection and standardization e.g., Measures of healthcare quality, measures of health status	Limited ability to enforce global recommendations, limited funding and complex international administration
International Organizations with focused agenda	UNICEF UNAIDS	Focus on vaccinations Focus on AIDS	Limited agendas and limited financing
International Financing Organizations	The World Bank Other multilateral regional banks e.g., InterAmerican and Asian Development Banks	World Bank is largest international funder increasingly supports "human capital" projects and reform of health care delivery systems and population and nutrition efforts Provides funding and technical assistance primarily as loans	Criticized for standardized approach with little local modifications
Bilateral Governmental Aid Organizations	USAID Most other developed countries have own organizations and contribute a higher percentage of their gross domestic product	Often focused on specific countries and specific types of programs such as the United States' focus on HIV/AIDS, and maternal and child health	May be tied to domestic politics and global economic, political or military agendas

Major Global Health Challenges

A few diseases are widely considered to be important global health issues; the most commonly cited and focused-on global diseases today include HIV/AIDS, tuberculosis, and malaria. HIV/AIDS receives huge amounts of global health funding, because of its perceived status as "the most thoroughly global of diseases."[21] Tuberculosis is also a continuing global health threat, causing significant morbidity and mortality; out of an estimated 8.8 million cases of tuberculosis in 2010, 1.4 million people died.[22] More than 1 million people die annually from malaria.[23] Other diseases, such as dengue fever, cholera, and shigellosis, may receive less attention, but that are no less deadly, especially in developing countries. These so-called "neglected diseases" sicken and kill millions each year.[5]

Both the well known and unknown global health threats can cause significant morbidity and mortality, but global health attempts to address the humanitarian, equity, direct, and indirect effects of these diseases are often hindered. Serious attempts to improve global health will have to overcome many of the following challenges.

Wellness, Prevention, and Health Promotion

While infectious disease remains an important global health issue, chronic diseases have recently become more prominent and widespread; healthcare systems must now adjust, as the previous focus on acute care is ill suited for the treatment of chronic disease. Health care has begun to recognize the importance of community wellness and health promotion for chronic condition prevention.[3,24] Growth in wellness care is not only evident in the United States and other countries with a high burden of chronic disease, but is quickly becoming a worldwide trend. The growing demand for wellness treatments, products, and programs can be attributed to several factors: the increasing age and diversity of the population, people seeking more cost-effective alternatives to acute episode health care, and increased globalization and awareness of wellness and health promotion.[25] Furthermore, at the domestic level, the U.S. government is supporting health promotion with the establishment of the National Center for Chronic Disease Prevention and Health Promotion and the Division of Adult and Community Health that will participate in the National Expert Panel on Community Health Promotion.[24] The shift in healthcare emphasis from acute care to prevention and wellness will require adaptation, openmindedness, and innovative, new practices designed to provide better global health care in this new disease landscape.

Rise in Chronic Diseases and Aging Populations

As previously noted, chronic diseases have become more prominent worldwide. Research from the American Academy of Family Physicians states, "chronic diseases are the single greatest threat to our nation's health and to our health care system."[26] With the increase in chronic illness and the urgent need to shift from an acute care model to chronic care model, a major challenge involves finding how best to respond to this changing nature of health problems.[27] Much of the rise in chronic condition prevalence is due to the higher life expectancy in today's society, and in conjunction, an increase in affluence-related diseases stemming from a higher standard of living. Prevalence worldwide does not seem to be subsiding and in fact is expected to grow throughout the 21st century.[8] **Exhibit 27.2** provides a snapshot of world health data on this phenomenon, along with predictions.

The aging of the population results in an increased prevalence of chronic and long-term conditions such as heart disease, diabetes, cancer, and degenerative diseases. These conditions often require multiple types of care and services. For example, the elderly or chronically ill may have needs in the areas of social welfare funding, adapted housing, special transportation, and home care or family support in addition to their physical health requirements. They face the problem of high medical costs despite insurance coverage, and, especially for long-term care, the costs are estimated to continue to increase well beyond the rate of inflation in the future. Many of these patient needs remain unmet. Furthermore, each individual's needs and desires differ; health care cannot be a one-size-fits-all solution, adding to the already difficult task of providing long-term

---

Exhibit 27.2   Chronic Disease Worldwide

Prevalence of diabetes

	2000	**2030**
World	171,000,000	366,000,000

7.4 million: the number of people who died from cancer worldwide in 2004. Today, cancer causes 1 death in every 8. If current trends continue, this could rise to 1 death in every 6.6 by 2015.

13 years: the deficit in average life expectancy for men in eastern Europe compared with those living elsewhere in Europe in 2005. Almost half of this excess mortality is due to cardiovascular diseases, and 20% is due to injuries.

150 million: the number of people globally experiencing financial catastrophe because of the cost of health care.

Source: Reproduced from Johnson JA, Stoskopf CH. *Comparative Health Systems: Global Perspectives.* Sudbury, MA: Jones and Bartlett Publishers; 2010.

---

care for a complex and heterogeneous population.[3,28] As a result, these new healthcare needs affect the demand for services and change the nature of the healthcare delivery system to a point that the current acute care model cannot adequately meet the chronic disease burden.

Infectious Diseases and Challenges of Globalization

Additionally, the rise of chronic illness and long-term care does not indicate a reciprocal decline in infectious diseases. After World War II, the availability of vaccines and antibiotics, along with improved public health policies, led the United States into an era of significant decline in the morality rate and increase in life expectancy. However, infectious diseases have begun to reassert themselves, currently representing approximately 25% of the annual deaths worldwide.[29,30]

Bacterial and viral infectious diseases such as tuberculosis, Hepatitis C, and HIV/AIDS are on the rise globally. The AIDS epidemic began in Africa, but continues to spread widely through India, Russia, China, and Latin America. Many strains of bacteria are becoming more drug resistant due to the overuse and misuse of antibiotics.[3] The rapid spread of new pathogens from other parts of the world, such as SARS, West Nile virus, and H1N1, magnifies the limitations of global public health.[30] Resistance to medical advice and distrust of government have been an issue in the administration and budget allocations for H1N1 vaccines, reviving an old debate about individual risk versus the good of the population.[31] Global surveillance networks are being developed and implemented to enhance monitoring of disease threats and enable better risk communication to populations through the media or other technologies.[3] The global distribution of disease shows that infectious disease and health care are directly linked to globalization, and need to be considered through a global perspective.

While globalization can be socially and economically beneficial, it also has great potential to contribute to the prevalence of major health problems.[3] Infectious diseases cannot be viewed as problems of developing countries, for although that is where the current burden is highest, the world is too interconnected to regard these issues as distant threats. With global trade, tourism, international relations, and migration, there are more opportunities than ever for rapid bacterial or viral spread, causing diseases that can affect millions of people worldwide. Responding to these pressing international health issues caused by globalization is a major challenge.[27,30]

Bioterrorism and the Transformation of Public Health

Increased threats of bioterrorism have spurred countries to develop new emergency infrastructure and to better coordinate functions and information that would be necessary in case of an attack. The public health field has undergone changes and modification as a result of the rise of bioterrorism concerns; for example, the new threat of nuclear weapons that involve biological and chemical materials has garnered major concern among states. Public health is also essential to protecting the American public against other types of disasters that threaten their health and wellbeing, such as the terrorist attacks in 2001 or the aftermath of Hurricanes Katrina and Sandy. The CDC is the domestic office that often takes the lead on protecting the public against any potential threat or outbreak.[3]

One major challenge of bioterrorism preparedness is the need for public health agencies to build partnerships and relationships with communities and state and local governments to ensure that future emergency responses will be effective on all levels. Moreover, public health agencies must organize around and effectively implement core public health functions in order to protect the health and safety of individuals and communities. These tenets will be essential in the case of a bioterrorism attack or other public health emergency. Furthermore, Johnson, Kennedy, and Delener,[32] in discussing bioterrorism, and Johnson and Johnson,[33] discussing natural disasters, describe critical success factors for all communities to consider when anticipating and addressing either human-caused or natural disasters. These include training and education; mitigation of confusion, fear, and panic; time management; building a response capacity; economic empowerment; and coordination at all levels.

Additionally, while the threat of bioterrorism is worrisome, it can and has helped spur important changes in public health practice. This renewed attention has supported advocates seeking to reestablish necessary but suffering public health infrastructure, such as workforce development, improved communication systems, and the advancement of surveillance and research; these investments will, in turn, strengthen our ability to respond to threats of bioterrorism and help address other public health issues as well.[3]

Health Professions Workforce

The future of the healthcare workforce is another challenge to public health. The situation in many places is dire; "The World Health Organization (WHO) estimates that the world faces a shortage of 4.5 million health professionals required for delivering essential health care services to populations in need."[34] Several factors have contributed to this workforce inadequacy. First, there is a highly inequitable distribution of healthcare professionals between and even within countries. It is often a challenge for some countries, especially lower income states, to retain their own native health professionals. This phenomenon, known as **brain drain**, is defined as "the migration of health personnel in search of the better standard of living and quality of life, higher salaries, access to advanced technology and more stable political conditions in different places worldwide."[35] While this inclination is certainly understandable, it has left many low-income areas without adequate health services. Additionally, the current workforce is also insufficient to keep up with the increasing population and demand for services worldwide. Some progress has been made with the WHO's "Global Code of Practice on the International Recruitment of Health Personnel,"[36] which was adopted by 193 member states of the World Health Assembly in May 2010 to address the global shortage of health professionals, with tenets including developing measures to educate and retain health workforce and developing sustainable health systems.[34] In order to cope with these deficits, task shifting has occurred, leading to an increasing number of healthcare practitioners (but not physicians), like nurse practitioners, physician assistants, and community health workers, providing important services and helping to address the professional shortage.[3]

The structural makeup of the healthcare workforce in the United States is also experiencing changes due to a decline in inpatient hospital care and an increase in the elderly population, leading to different market demands for certain types of healthcare workers (e.g., an increase in a need for geriatric specialists and home health aides).[3,37] Another shift is occurring as an increasing number of women and people of minority racial/ethnic backgrounds enter the healthcare field. The female participation rate in the health workforce increased from 42.3% to 58.4% from 1979 to 2008, and women are major contributors in all areas of the healthcare field.[37] The increase in minority participation has led to the creation of a more culturally diverse and sensitive healthcare workforce.

Health care is also affected by the distribution of professionals geographically and amongst medical specialty areas, and a shortage of certain types of practitioners, including nurses, general physicians, pharmacists, technicians, and therapists, also threatens the country's ability to provide high-quality health care to all its citizens. There is also a need for continuing education and training for healthcare professionals, especially in fast growing areas like geriatric care where the current number of specialists falls far short of demand. Additionally, the shortage of personnel in key areas creates difficulty in providing important training and practicing of the team-based approach to health care often necessary to address complicated healthcare issues.[3,37]

Focus on Quality

Since the early 2000s, health care has been trying to increase focus on patient quality of care and satisfaction, which has made the healthcare market more competitive and medical practice more dependent on the patient's choice. For example, according to Gauthier and Rogal, "states have passed legislation or established regulations to ensure that adequate provider networks are maintained and patients have adequate access to specialists through referrals."[38] However, there are still many challenges to achieving patient satisfaction. Dissatisfaction can often be due to extrinsic factors including care regulations and restrictions, lack of incentives for better performance, the predominance of the acute care medical model, and issues of paternalism amongst physicians.[3,38] While these situations can certainly be frustrating for both provider and patient, it is important that the provider continues to do everything possible to ensure top care and make the patient as comfortable as possible.

New Frontiers in Biomedical Technology

Medical technology is advancing rapidly and will greatly impact the broader realm of health care and the care given to individual patients. New technologies such as rational drug design, safer surgical and imaging procedures, genetic testing, gene therapy, and therapeutic vaccines can bring great changes to treatment for many diseases like cancer, AIDS, and neurological conditions. However, in order to best use quickly progressing technology to achieve better medical management and efficiency, it will be necessary to facilitate information sharing between providers and consumers; it will also require that providers adopt important new technology in a timely and useful manner.[3] On the other hand, while many of these novel therapies can save lives and improve health, it will be essential to conduct proper monitoring activities and to consider ethics and cultural acceptance during their introduction to ensure they are being used in a safe and socially acceptable manner. Political debate has already arisen between stakeholders and ethicists who argue about the use of some novel approaches to therapy. Several major fields of novel therapies are currently under development:

- *Genomics and gene therapy/stem cell therapy.* The possibility for greater usage of these methods in clinical diagnostics and treatment has raised great hopes and great emotion.[3] Gene therapy, which seeks to deliberately alter a small part of the body's genetic code to activate, inactivate, or replace a gene related to a medical condition, holds great promise, but is still in its infancy. Eventually, scientists hope that gene therapy can replace mutated genes that function improperly and stop disease symptoms or add genes that can help fight off other diseases.[39] Researchers and doctors also see great promise in the pluripotent nature of stem cell therapies for people who suffer from a variety of debilitating diseases, such as type 2 diabetes, chronic obstructive pulmonary disease (COPD), spinal cord injury, macular degeneration, blood diseases, and amyotrophic lateral sclerosis (ALS), but this research is also still fairly new. In opposition to the ongoing research efforts, many groups and individuals have expressed worry about the consequences of misusing such technology and the morality of this type of exploration. There is particular resistance among some people to using human embryonic stem cells, which have the most medically useful development potential, but are taken from a human fetus, which defies many peoples' religious or ethical beliefs.[40]
- *Organ transplantation.* Recently, there has been an increase in demand of organ transplant donors.[3] In certain cases, this demand has led to the commercialization of human organs as a trade good, and therefore the World Health Assembly in 1991 set forth the important guiding principles emphasizing voluntary donation, noncommercialization, and preference of cadaveric over living donors.[41] Still, the demand for organ transplants exceeds the supply, and people needing a transplant often face extremely long wait times, sometimes dying during the process.[42] Xenotransplantation (animal to human transplantation) is another possibility in medicine that needs to be monitored. WHO has set some regulatory control in this field.[41]
- *Tissue engineering/regenerative medicine.* This is another frontier of medicine that needs further research and regulation. Today, autologous cells or other stem cells are used for end-stage organ failure or other clinical uses.[3] The process still raises ethical issues and is still in its infancy.

Overall, the medical field is undergoing a rapid and impressive period of technological progress. While research raises ethical and social concerns that should be appropriately considered and addressed, such conflict should not be seen negatively. According to an article written for *Community Genetics*:

> Skepticism or ambivalence on the part of publics are not necessarily problems to overcome in the interest of scientific progress, but rather should be mobilized to enhance open and public debates about the nature of genomics research, medicine, and related social and ethical issues.[43]

Another challenge in new technology and research is that the cost of clinical technology is high and funding for purchase and implementation is often difficult to secure. There has been research reporting that healthcare organization redesign to speed the adoption of medical technology helps broaden access to innovative treatments; however, there is a lack of funding and many are still in trials.[44] Medicare often has denied coverage of new technology, especially when still undergoing clinical trials, which has driven other funding agencies to do the same.[44] Furthermore, Americans, more so than Europeans and Canadians, tend to believe that new clinical technology will be able to solve serious medical problems.[45] But technology, no matter how innovative, does not guarantee better access to health care and may be using up a greater share of resources and funding than is optimal for the healthcare practice.[45]

While people often think of new drugs or treatments when considering important medical advances, the field of computer technology and informatics is also rapidly changing the medical profession. Information technology, health informatics, e-health, m-health, electronic medical records, telemedicine, and virtual physician visits are all new terms for areas of research that arose with the computer age.[3]

Many of these innovations have spurred the exchange of ideas and education of health consumers or patients. Today, patients have access to significant medical information through services like WebMD and Medscape. Smart phones and the Internet can now be used to help monitor and evaluate treatment, even from afar. There are several programs described in the scientific literature addressing the possibility of using telemedicine for continuing medical education and consultations in remote areas of the world.[46]

Public health challenges of this new information technology include regulation, policies, and protocols and license regulation.[47] The new availability of detailed and complicated medical information to consumers can raise questions, fears, and doubts that must be addressed by the physician. Doctors facing this kind of increased patient demand for information and services may have their decisions questioned, which could lead either to improved communication between parties or to the overuse of testing and referrals, meant to please the patient even if not necessary (and possibly to avoid a lawsuit). Misuse of medical resources should be avoided, but direct-to-patient marketing of new drugs and the ability to self-diagnose can lead to significant pressure on the doctor to satisfy the patient, regardless of medical likelihood.

Additionally, computers have increased transparency about hospital quality indicators and physicians' backgrounds, giving patients perhaps better information for making their medical provider choices. Another great challenge to the proper use and progress of telemedicine is the protection of individual or patient privacy/confidentiality; medical computer technology has led to increasing access to medical records, which can be medically helpful or dangerous. While there are several laws designed to protect personal medical data in the United States, such as provisions in the Health Insurance Portability and Accountability Act (HIPAA) of 1996,[3,48] the law must continue to evolve with emerging technology to stay relevant and useful.

Another challenge of new technology is trying to distribute its beneficial effects equally. Most often, major new technological advances are first available at high prices to consumers and practitioners in high-income countries. Sinha and Barry describe this major issue for global technology and innovation:

> Creating appropriate products for low-resource settings requires not only a rethinking of what is considered a health technology, but also cross-disciplinary innovation and in-depth understanding of the particular needs of each country. Location-specific needs assessment will help ensure that more appropriate devices reach people in need and will support parallel efforts to deploy novel devices, processes, or information technologies to cost-effectively reduce disease incidence.

Health Systems

As described by Johnson and Stoskopf, "health systems in the 21st century are facing many new challenges as they seek to provide health care for growing populations with increasingly complex medical conditions."[8] Many countries are seeking to make improvements in this area, yet progress continues to be hamstrung by many issues such as politics, economics, and emerging social and natural events that put stress on health systems.

The four functional components of a healthcare delivery system, as described by Shi and Singh, are financing, insurance, delivery, and payment; these components can be provided by the government, private health insurance, or managed care systems.[3] However, without these four basic components, there is inequality of health care, particularly among the poor and the unemployed, unless the government or other actors intervene. Healthcare inequalities can increase disparities in health conditions and outcomes, such as increasing malnutrition, heart disease, and type 2 diabetes. As summarized by Zere et al., "Equity in health is defined as minimizing avoidable inequalities in health and its determinants—including but not limited to healthcare—between groups who have different levels of underlying social advantage or privilege."[49]

When these delivery systems fail to provide care to citizens, gaps have often been filled by altruism through volunteerism, hospital charity care, and other relief supplied through nongovernmental organizations (NGOs), churches, and other groups. Globally, this informal charity care has often become a huge part of the health system of low-income countries, with many NGOs and religious groups seeking to help improve health outcomes. However, critics believe that charity is not enough to sustain a functional health system. According to Ooms and Hammonds, "There is a global responsibility for global health and there are obligations of justice (beyond charity) to help fulfill (not merely respect or even protect) the right to health in other countries; these are obligations of global health justice."[42]

Particular social groups acutely feel inequality caused by malfunctioning health systems. For instance, WHO acknowledges the health inequality often faced by women and has sought to address this imbalance through the third Millennium Development Goal, promoting gender equality and empowering women. Important health system reform to restore functional care delivery will be needed in many parts of the world to achieving more equal health outcomes. Johnson and Stoskopf, in a recent comparative study of health systems in 20 countries worldwide, concluded that there is a critical need to focus resources and efforts on strengthening health systems development.[8] Furthermore, WHO advocates for and provides assistance to countries seeking to improve their health systems. In *Comparative Health Systems: Global Perspectives*, Johnson and Stoskopf[8] summarize the "health systems building blocks" promoted by WHO as critical success factors for health system development and sustainability, as shown in **Table 27.4**.

Global Economic Activity and Trade

In the increasingly globalized economy, the manufacture, transport, and sale of medical implements has become increasingly important for the health system and the economy of a country. While this trade has many positive effects, it increases the need for regulation to ensure proper usage and progress to ensure proper implementation. The Global Health Initiative of the U.S. Department of Health and Human Services describes a need for regulatory systems to monitor global manufacturing and supply chains to ensure the safety of medical products, food, and

---

Table 27.4 Health Systems Building Blocks (Critical Success Factors)

Service Delivery	**Medical Technology**
Good health services are those that deliver effective, safe, quality personal and non-personal health interventions to those who need them, when and where needed, with minimum waste of resources.	A well-functioning health system ensures equitable access to essential medical products, drugs, vaccines, and technologies of assured quality, safety, efficacy, and cost-effectiveness, and their scientifically sound and cost-effective use.
Health Workforce	**Health Financing**
A well-performing health workforce is one that works in ways that are responsive, fair, and efficient to achieve the best health outcomes possible, given available resources and circumstances (i.e., there are sufficient staff, fairly distributed; they are competent, responsive, and productive).	A good health financing system raises adequate funds for health, in ways that ensure people can use needed services and are protected from financial catastrophe or impoverishment associated with having to pay for them. It provides incentives for providers and users to be efficient.
Health Information	**Leadership and Governance**
A well-functioning health information system is one that ensures the production, analysis, dissemination, and use of reliable and timely information on health determinants, health system performance, and health status.	Leadership and governance involves ensuring that strategic policy frameworks exist and are combined with effective oversight, coalition building, regulation, attention to system design, and accountability.

Source: Data from WHO Framework.

other products that enter the United States.[50] Internationally, there is a need to improve manufacturing standards for these products, which will help ensure health and safety while providing positive economic effects as demand increases. As stated by WHO Director General, Margaret Chan, while discussing health in a post-2015 global agenda, "This is a world in which the international systems that govern trade, financial markets, and business relations can have a greater impact on the opportunities of citizens, also for better health, than the policies of their sovereign governments."[51]

During the recent global recession, many countries' public health infrastructure suffered. However, it has also been seen that public health investment is often the wisest choice to be made even by economically challenged countries. As described by Johnson, some low-income countries, such as Costa Rica, Vietnam, Cuba, and Chile, have exceeded the health indicators of higher income countries "by making policy choices that embrace fundamental health promotion and education."[2, p. 326]

Evidence-Based Health Care

Today, the United States and other countries are seeing a strong push for evidence-based practice in health care; evidence-based medicine is meant to ensure better and more equitable medical outcomes through the adherence to specific treatment and practice guidelines. In order to even monitor care and to measure progress and collect data, the government will need to establish uniform, standardized research methods for data collection and classification across different settings. If research methods and strict data regulations are not determined, the results may be unreliable; unreliable data can lead to confusion about best practices, and patients may then be subject to unnecessary risks. Much of this research has been promoted by specialized government agencies; in the United States, the Agency of Healthcare Research and Quality (AHRQ), in collaboration with other medical societies, has published medical guidelines that have been used to measure "quality of care" in healthcare facilities, and it has helped to promote the dissemination of information on quality of care to the public.[52]

Standard of care is another challenging issue. Standard is a constantly evolving concept; what is considered "standard" care today will almost certainly not be standard in a few years in light of new research, science, or expert opinion. Global health may also require the adoption of a single standard of care by different medical communities across the world, further complicating the issue. In this area, some progress has been made. WHO has established the Global Patient Safety Campaign, including a Hand Hygiene Campaign followed by the Safe Surgery Save Lives Campaign.[53] The desire to provide equitable and quality health care to all people of the world would be greatly aided by the adoption of certain standards of care, but the reality of costs and availability of support staff and other services that impact the care in poorer nations will hinder its implementation.

Finally, even in settings where evidence-based medical research has been conducted and substantiated, practitioner disregard of evidence-based practice regulations and procedures may result in the delay of new knowledge dissemination or decrease the availability of funding for worthy treatments and procedures. Healthcare professionals should become more familiar with evidence-based health care to better address patients' health issues and improve quality of life.[3,45]

Future Outlook and Opportunities

Global health is constantly evolving. Globalization continues to march forward, leaving the world more interconnected than ever, and health is in no way immune to this influence. Even today, health care is still often seen as a domestic issue, but countries must acknowledge the important influence global events can have domestically and locally. Shi and Singh stress that a "nation is not isolated from global events and the underdeveloped state of healthcare delivery in poorer countries."[3] Global health affects the spread of infectious disease, the success of preventive health efforts, and the diaspora of healthcare workers around the world. Fortunately, many organizations are working to mitigate this. One example is the work of WHO and UNAIDS in the area of HIV/AIDS. See **Box 27.1** for a description of their joint efforts and goals.

Global health takes into account the cultural beliefs that prohibit certain practices that are commonplace in other parts of the world, and acknowledges the importance of cultural communication for health and wellness. Global health realizes that health systems in different countries, while differing greatly in funding, implementation, and prioritization, all share certain commonalities and can all work for common goals of patient safety and healthcare quality.

As indicated by Johnson and Stoskopf, governments and the private sector in all countries will have to work in partnership to ensure the sustainability of vital health services and important health-promotion initiatives.[8] Furthermore, countries will need to realize their interconnectedness with the rest of the world as they face global pandemics and macro problems such as climate change. Global health acknowledges that progress does not come without controversy and seeks to implement new practices and technology in a way that is ethical and fair. Overall, global health has begun to reshape the health system as any individual knows it; these changes bring great challenges for countries seeking to protect the health and wellness of their citizens, but can also lead to great opportunities for health advancement and international cooperation. Global health can mean many things to many different people, but it cannot be ignored.

Discussion Questions

1. What is global health, and why should we study it in a public health administration course?
2. Identify and discuss major challenges in global health. Are there any you would like to add that have not been addressed in this text? Please give examples.
3. Why is globalization such a significant force shaping global health? How might this be even more significant in the future?
4. What are health systems building blocks, and why would they be considered "critical success factors" for global health development?
5. Read **Box 27.2** then discuss how working in public health in a border region might be a challenge. What would you do as a public health administrator to assure a more effective workforce? Give examples of other border areas around the world that might pose their own unique challenges, such as conflict zones, religious animosity, and refugee situations.

Box 27.1   The Evolving Global Health Strategy on HIV/AIDS

James Allen Johnson, IV
Karl E. Peace Endowed Research Assistant
Jiann-Ping Hsu College of Public Health
Georgia Southern University

In 2011, the 64th World Health Assembly unanimously adopted a new, comprehensive strategy to combat HIV. The Global Health Sector Strategy on HIV/AIDS, 2011–2015 provides a framework that guides actions by WHO and governments around the world during this critical time for the future of the HIV response. According to UNAIDS estimates, if the WHO's existing HIV treatment recommendations were fully implemented through 2015, at least 4.2 million new HIV infections would be averted and 2 million lives could be saved. Under the new strategy, WHO aims to promote even greater innovation in HIV prevention, treatment, testing, and care services so that countries can achieve the goal of universal access to HIV/AIDS services.

Better Integration, Broader Outcomes

Every day, more than 7,000 people are newly infected with HIV and about 5,000 die from AIDS. More accessible and affordable treatment and prevention are urgently needed. Delivery of HIV prevention, testing, treatment, and care services must be better linked and integrated with other health services such as those for maternal and child health, tuberculosis, and hepatitis, among others.

Global Goals Can Be a Reality

The Global Health Sector Strategy on HIV/AIDS outlines four strategic directions for 2015:

- To optimize HIV prevention, diagnosis, treatment, and care outcomes
- To leverage broader health outcomes through HIV responses
- To build strong and sustainable health systems
- To address inequalities and advance human rights

The Global Health Sector Strategy for HIV/AIDS, 2011–2015, is closely aligned with the UNAIDS Strategy 2011–2015, which has been developed in parallel. The strategy augments the UNAIDS Strategy by facilitating the health sector contribution to achieving the UNAIDS vision of zero new infections, zero AIDS-related deaths, and zero discrimination. Rolling out the strategy has required a robust global effort, but when fully implemented, will enable countries to attain the Millennium Development Goal related to HIV by 2015.

The strategy builds on the achievements and experiences of the "3 by 5" initiative and the five strategic directions of the WHO HIV/AIDS Universal Access Plan, 2006–2010. Furthermore, it takes into consideration the broad global HIV health and development architecture, including the UNAIDS Strategy and Outcome Framework and existing commitments to achieving universal access and the Millennium Development Goals. By identifying existing and agreed-upon global targets to motivate countries to plan for bold HIV/AIDS responses through 2015, the strategy provides guidance to countries on how to prioritize their HIV and broader health investments. In an effort to facilitate multilevel collaboration, the strategy provides a framework for concerted WHO action at the global, regional, and country levels and across all relevant WHO departments.

Source: Adapted from World Health Organization. New global strategy on HIV set to prevent millions of infections, deaths. Available at: http://www.who.int/hiv/mediacentre/feature_story/hiv_strategy/en/index.html. Accessed March 31, 2013.

Box 27.2   Multicultural Public Health Challenge in U.S.–Mexican Border Region

Barry Thatcher
Professor
New Mexico State University
and
Editor-in-Chief
Journal of Rhetoric, Professional Communication, and Globalization

The U.S.–Mexico border region is a dynamic cultural space with multiple languages (Spanish, Spanglish, and English) and a variety of complexly related cultural, economic, and linguistic groups (Mexican, Anglo, cross-border, and Latino/Hispanic). Since U.S. federal laws now mandate delivering health care and managing healthcare institutions using culturally appropriate methods,* public health workers would be well served to develop multicultural competencies for border contexts.

Since all U.S.–Mexico border states (California, Arizona, New Mexico, and Texas) were part of Mexico in the 19th century, many Mexican American (or Latino/Hispanic) residents who live there can easily trace their ancestry back five or six generations to the border region. They are often prominent farmers and ranchers, physicians, entrepreneurs, and important business, government, and industrialists. This group adapted itself (often reluctantly) to the change in nationality in the mid-1800s from Mexican to American. Many in this group have complex identities and often identify themselves as New Mexicans or Texans, integrating cultural and social patterns from the United States and the U.S.–Mexico border area but not often from Mexico. They rarely travel to Mexico or find themselves with Mexican nationals. Many in this group have lost their Spanish through the generations and are increasingly aligning themselves with predominant U.S. cultural values. Many distance themselves from the other Mexican groups discussed next. Others may self-identify as Hispanic or Latino, depending on the state. In New Mexico and west Texas, Hispanic is the preferred term, but in California and most of Texas, the preferred term is usually Latino; Arizona is mixed in this preference. In terms of culture, especially as related to health care, this group is often indistinguishable from predominant U.S. values.

The next multicultural group of the U.S.–Mexico border region is the recent immigrant, most of whom come from Mexico, but others from Guatemala and Central America. Those from Mexico speak Spanish as a first language, approach medicine and health care based on the traditions in Mexico, identify themselves as Mexican (as opposed to Hispanic/Latino), and associate themselves mostly with other recent Mexican immigrants. If possible, they frequently travel to Mexico where many family members still live. This group is represented by multiple classes and income levels, although a high percentage are working class and laborers. This group is the one most plagued by problems with immigration; many are undocumented and lack health coverage. This subgroup is usually accustomed to more folklore-like medical care such as *curanderos* (healers) and to self-medical treatment because of limited economic capacity.

A third group, the most complicated and disparate, is called Generation 1.5; this group is caught between the two groups discussed previously. They are often American-born, U.S. citizens, but their parents or grandparents are from Mexico. This group speaks Spanish as a first language, but learned English fluently at school and at work. When they travel to Mexico to visit family, they are capable linguistically but uncomfortable culturally or socially. They often rapidly acculturate to a specific set of predominant American values such as individualism and equality, which they often hold in an uneasy tension with the more Mexican values of family and social hierarchy. However, this group inherits many of the assumptions about medicine and health care from their Mexican parents, but they are grounded locally in U.S. bureaucratic and healthcare culture. It is common to observe this group—especially children—accompanying their parents or grandparents to the healthcare institution to translate linguistically and culturally. This group also varies more in their self-identification: Some may hide their Spanish or Latino characteristics because of their desire to integrate better into the United States, while others may openly identify themselves as Mexican American and insist on speaking Spanish. There are many variations and gradations of this group, depending on their historical, social, and cultural connections to either Mexico or the United States.

(continues)

Box 27.2   Multicultural Public Health Challenge in U.S.–Mexican Border Region (continued)

A fourth group is the Mexican national who emigrates to the United States legally because of better business opportunities, or more recently, to escape the drug-related violence. This group is usually middle or upper class, has been educated in private Mexican schools, and often speaks formal English learned in Mexico. This group is often accused of viewing the Latinos, Generation 1.5, or Mexican American groups with some disdain, accusing them of selling out their Mexican heritage, but Mexican nationals rarely can distinguish among the three groups. Mexican nationals present complicated relations with the U.S. healthcare context. They do not identify well with the recent immigrant or Generation 1.5 because of economic class differences and they share more economic, social, and educational values with the predominant U.S. middle class, but because of their deep connections to Mexico, they do not connect well with Anglo-Americans either. They are usually educated in international perspectives on health care, not only from the United States, but also Europe and even Asia. This group most likely eschews the *curandero* and folk medical traditions from Mexico and is probably adept at understanding the science of medicine and health care.

A fifth group is the cross-border, bilingual and bicultural group. This subgroup is composed mostly of Mexican nationals or Mexican Americans, and they function equally well on either side of the border. For example, a growing percentage of students at New Mexico State University and University of Texas–El Paso are Mexican nationals from Ciudad Juarez, right across the border of El Paso, Texas. In fact, many midlevel managers and engineers live in El Paso and work in the manufacturing plants or *maquilas* in Ciudad Juárez. Both groups travel across the border daily. They are mostly bilingual, though many have Spanish as their first language, and they work effectively on either side. An important component of this group is the cross-border health care. Many in this group will seek basic medical services in Mexico because they are much cheaper and often of better quality but seek U.S. services for complicated or risky care.

The final major group on the U.S.–Mexico border is the Anglo-Americans, *güeros* (whites), or Caucasians who are relatively latecomers to the border region. After the cession of one-third of the Mexican territory to the United States in the mid-1800s, Anglo-Americans began to arrive. According to official census, they account for about one-third of the population in Southern New Mexico and 18% in west Texas. This is a catchall term for anyone whose skin is somewhat white and who is not Hispanic, African American, or Asian. This group has some interesting divisions and history. A vast majority of Caucasians cannot distinguish among the five groups discussed here, simply confusing a 6th generation Mexican American with a recent immigrant or Mexican national. Very few whites speak Spanish except for those originating from the Mormon colonies in Northern Mexico or who are from bicultural families. As a de facto minority in race/ethnicity but part of the majority in terms of social class, the whites often mix seamlessly with the same economic class of Mexican Americans but rarely mix with the immigrant class and are awkward with some of those in G1.5. Most white New Mexicans, for example, speak some Spanish, just enough to get by in common places, but bilingualism is an exception.

A major lesson learned from these six groups is that skin color and racial characteristics are extremely unreliable at identifying where a specific person might map onto this template. Six patients at a health clinic could fit all six groups but in complex ways. Some suggestions for public health workers and other healthcare professionals follow. First, rarely do Anglos speak only Spanish, although many Mexican nationals can pass as Anglos with their fair skin and blue or green eyes, so be careful here. Second, unless there are other indications, one can generally assume people speak English, but be sensitive if they do nt. If they do speak English, they are usually part of the Mexican American, G1.5, or Mexican national groups—who will generally speak more formally. If they only speak Spanish, they are usually recent immigrants, new G1.5 residents, or Mexican nationals. Next, get some history: such as where they were born and where their parents and the family members were born, where they were educated, and what kinds of health care they prefer.

*See http://minorityhealth.hhs.gov.

References

1. Koplan JP, Bond TC, Merson MH, et al. Consortium of universities for global health executive board: towards a common definition of global health. *Lancet*. 2009;373:1993–5.

2. Johnson JA. International health education and promotion. In: Minelli MJ, Breckon DJ, eds. *Community Health Education*. Sudbury, MA: Jones and Bartlett Publishers; 2009.

3. Shi L, Singh DA. *Delivering Health Care in America: A Systems Approach*. 5th ed. Burlington, MA: Jones & Bartlett Learning; 2012.

4. Macfarlane SB, Jacobs M, Kaaya EE. In the name of global health: trends in academic institutions. *J Public Health Policy*. 2008;29:383–401.

5. Families USA. Why Global Health Matters. Available at: http://www.familiesusa.org/issues/global-health/matters/. Accessed March 31, 2013.

6. Patel V, Prince M. Global mental health—a new global health field comes of age. *JAMA*. 2010;303: 1976–7.

7. Raviola G, Becker AE, Farmer P. A global scope for global health—including mental health. *Lancet*. 2011;373:1993–5. Available at: http://www.lancet.com/journals/lancet/article/PIIS0140-6736(11)60941-0/fulltext. Accessed March 31, 2013.

8. Johnson JA, Stoskopf CH. *Comparative Health Systems: Global Perspectives*. Sudbury, MA: Jones & Bartlett Learning; 2010.

9. Bergström S. Daily deaths due to pregnancy complications: more than all deaths from AIDS, malaria and tuberculosis combined: the scandal of our time. 2nd International Conference on Global Public Health. Kristiansand, Norway. October 8–10, 2008.

10. World Health Organization. *Global Health Observatory: HIV/AIDS*. Available at: http://www.who.int/gho/hiv/en/. Accessed March 30, 2013.

11. Avert. *Children Orphaned by HIV and AIDS*. Available at: http://www.avert.org/aids-orphans.htm. Accessed March 31, 2013.

12. Gore FM, Bloem PJN, Patton GC, et al. Global burden of disease in young people aged 10–24 years. *Lancet*. 2011;377(9783):2093–102.

13. Global Forum for Health Research. 10/90 Gap. Available at: http://www.globalforumhealth.org/about/1090-gap/. Accessed March 31, 2013.

14. Moon S, Jambert E, Childs M, et al. A win-win solution?: A critical analysis of tiered pricing to improve access to medicines in developing countries. *Global Health*. 2011;12(7):39.

15. Wall S. Fuelling a hands-on approach to global health challenges. *Global Health Action*. Available at: http://www.globalhealthaction.net/index.php/gha/article/view/1822/1761. Accessed March 31, 2013.

16. U.S. Department of Health and Human Services. Global Health. Available at: http://globalhealth.gov. Accessed March 31, 2013.

17. Institute of Medicine, Committee on the U.S. Commitment to Global Health. *The US Commitment to Global Health: Recommendations for the Public and Private Sectors*. Washington, DC: National Academies Press; 2009. Available at: http://www.ncbi.nlm.nih.gov/books/NBK23794. Accessed March 31, 2013.

18. World Health Organization. *Millennium Development Goals (MDGs)*. Available at: http://www.who.int/topics/millennium_development_goals/about/en/index.html. Accessed March 31, 2013.

19. Johnson JA. Nongovernmental and global health organizations. In: Johnson JA, ed. *Introduction to Public Health Management, Organizations, and Policy*. Clifton Park, NY: Delmar-Cengage; 2013.

20. Riegelman R. *Public Health 101: Healthy People—Healthy Populations*. Sudbury, MA: Jones and Bartlett Publishers; 2010.

21. Colvin CJ. HIV/AIDS, chronic diseases and globalisation. *Global Health*. 2011;7:31.

22. World Health Organization. *Tuberculosis*. Available at: http://www.who.int/mediacentre/factsheets/fs104/en/. Accessed March 31, 2013.

23. Birn AE, Pillay Y, Holtz T. *Textbook of International Health: Global Health in a Dynamic World*. 3rd ed. Oxford, UK: Oxford University Press; 2009.

24. Navarro AM, Voetsch KP, Liburd LC, et al. (2007). Charting the future of community health promotion: recommendations from the National Expert Panel on Community Health Promotion. *Prev Chron Dis.* 2007;4(3):A68. Available at: http://www.ncbi.nlm.nih.gov/pmc/articles/PMC1955396/?tool=pmcentrez. Accessed March 31, 2013.

25. Global Spa Summit. *Wellness is no passing fad: Global market estimated at nearly $2 Trillion.* Available at: http://blog.globalspasummit.org/2010/06/wellness-is-no-passing-fad-global-market-estimated-at-nearly-2-trillion/. Accessed March 31, 2013.

26. American Academy of Family Physicians. Public health issues. Available at: http://www.aafp.org/online/en/home/clinical/publichealth.html. Accessed March 31, 2013.

27. Boufford JI, Lee PR. *Health policies for the 21st century: Challenges and recommendations for the U.S. Department of Health and Human Services.* Available at: http://www.milbank.org/uploads/documents/010910healthpolicies.html. Accessed March 31, 2013.

28. Blok C, Luijkx K, Meijboom B, et al. Improving long-term care provision: towards demand-based care by means of modularity. *BMC Health Serv Res.* 2010;10:278–91.

29. Morens DM, Folkers GK, Fauci AS. The challenge of emerging and re-emerging infectious diseases. *Nature.* 2004;430:242–9.

30. Pompe S, Simon J, Wiedemann PM, et al. Future trends and challenges in pathogenomics. *Eur Molecular Biol Org.* 2005;6(7):600–6.

31. Centers for Disease Control and Prevention. *2009 H1N1 and Seasonal Flu and African American Communities: Questions and Answers.* Available at: http://www.cdc.gov/h1n1flu/african_americans_qa.htm#ref. Accessed March 31, 2013.

32. Johnson JA, Kennedy MH, Delener N. *Community Preparedness and Resonse to Terrorism: The Role of Community Organizations and Business.* Westport, CT: Praeger; 2005.

33. Johnson JA, Johnson JA. Applied social sciences and public health in disaster response: comparative analysis of New Orleans, Haiti, and Japan. *Nat Soc Sci J.* 2012;39(2):52–9.

34. Taylor A, Hwenda L, Larsen B, et al. Stemming the brain drain: a WHO global code of practice on international recruitment of health personnel. *New Engl J Med.* 2011;365(25):2348–51.

35. Dodani S. Brain drain from developing countries: how can brain drain be converted into wisdom gain? *J Soc Med.* 2005;98(11):487–91.

36. World Health Organization. *Global Code of Practice on the International Recruitment of Health Personnel.* Available at: http://www.who.int/hrh/migration/code/code_en.pdf. Accessed March 31, 2013.

37. Segal L, Bolton T. Issues facing the future health care: The importance of demand modeling. *Aust New Zealand Health Policy* 2009;6:12. Available at: http://www.anzhealthpolicy.com/content/6/1/12. Accessed March 31, 2013.

38. Gauthier AK, Rogal DL. *The challenge of managed care regulation: Making markets work?* Available at: http://www.hcfo.org/pdf/managedcare.pdf. Accessed March 31, 2013.

39. National Institutes of Health. *Genetics Home Reference: What Is Gene Therapy?* Available at: http://ghr.nlm.nih.gov/handbook/therapy/genetherapy. Accessed March 31, 2013.

40. National Institutes of Health. *Stem Cell Information: Frequently Asked Questions.* Available at: http://stemcells.nih.gov/info/. Accessed March 31, 2013.

41. World Health Organization. *Human Organ Transplantation.* Available at: http://www.who.int/transplantation/organ/en/. Accessed March 31, 2013.

42. Ooms G, Hammonds R. Taking up Daniels' challenge: the case for global; health justice. *Health Human Rights.* 2010;12(1):29–46.

43. Cunningham-Burley S. Public knowledge and public trust. *Community Genetics.* 2006;9(3):204–10.

44. Fennel ML. The new medical technologies and the organizations of medical science and treatment. *Health Serv Res.* 2008;43(1):1–9. Available at: http://www.ncbi.nlm.nih.gov/pmc/articles/PMC2323138/pdf/hesr0043-0001.pdf. Accessed March 31, 2013.

45. Deyo RA. Marketing, media, wishful thinking, and conflicts of interest: inflating the value of new medical technology. *Permanente J.* 2009;13(2):71–6.

46. Geissbuhler A, Bagayoko CO, Ly O. The RAFT network: 5 years of distance continuing medical education and tele-consultations over the Internet in French-speaking Africa. *Int J Med Inform.* 2007;76:351–6.

47. Sarhan F. Telemedicine in healthcare 1: exploring its uses, benefits and disadvantages. *Nurs Times.* 2009;105(42):10–3.

48. U.S. Department of Health and Human Services. *Health Information Privacy.* Available at: http://www .hhs.gov/ocr/privacy/. Accessed March 31, 2013.

49. Zere E, Moeti M, Kirigia J, et al. Equity in health and healthcare in Malawi: analysis of trends. *BMC Public Health.* 2007;7:78.

50. USAID. *Fact Sheet: The U.S. Government's Global Health Initiative (GHI).* Available at: http://transition. usaid.gov/ghi/factsheet.html. Accessed March 31, 2013.

51. World Health Organization. *The Place of Health on the Post-2015 Development Agenda.* Available at: http://www.who.int/dg/speeches/2012/mdgs_post2015/en/index.html. Accessed March 31, 2013.

52. Agency for Healthcare Research and Quality. *Quality and Patient Safety.* Available at: http://www.ahrq .gov/qual/. Accessed March 31, 2013.

53. World Health Organization. *Patient Safety.* Available at: http://www.who.int/patientsafety/en/. Accessed March 31, 2013.

Glossary

adaptive leadership a relational, social process through which the leader first addresses stakeholders, communities, and those responsible for issues to carefully define their thoughts and feelings about an issue

administration includes all costs related to public health department management such as human resources, information technology, supplies, finance, and facilities; also includes expenses related to health reform and policy development not otherwise embedded in program areas

all-hazards preparedness and response includes disaster preparedness programs (including bioterrorism), and the costs associated with disaster response such as shelters and emergency healthcare facilities

assessment involves obtaining data to define the health of populations and the nature of health problems

assurance includes the oversight responsibility for ensuring that essential components of an effective health system are in place

biostatisticians focus primarily on statistical theory, techniques, and methods to identify and analyze health problems, to evaluate the effectiveness of health services, and to analyze data for planning and policy development; often are employed in the research divisions of pharmaceutical companies and academic medical centers and in specialized federal public health agencies

block grant allocation of financial resources to broad domains of activity that are largely determined by the grant recipients; allocated exclusively to state governments, which are charged with disbursing funds appropriately to specific programs and providers

brain drain global migration of health personnel in search of a better standard of living and quality of life, higher salaries, access to advanced technology, and more stable political conditions

capacities resources and relationships necessary to carry out the important processes of public health; made possible by the maintenance of the basic infrastructure of the public health system, and by specific program resources

case definition developed to clarify the health-related event being monitored and improve the comparability of reports from different data sources; may have several components, including clinical, epidemiologic, and behavioral information; may also distinguish between confirmed, probable, and suspect occurrences according to their degree of conformity with the event of interest

categorical grants-in-aid targeted at specific public health services and population groups; allow federal agencies to exercise more control over how public health funds are spent than do block grants, which allow greater levels of state discretion in resource use

Certified in Public Health (CPH) a voluntary, individual-level credential created to brand and elevate the field of public health, because the United States does not currently require any license to practice public health; the CPH examination is required by some schools (for graduation) and programs, many of which provide full or partial financial support for eligible students, alumni, faculty, and staff to become credentialed

choropleth map a type of map in which a given area, or polygon, is shaded with different colors to depict variations of features

chronic disease diseases of long duration and generally slow progression, such as heart disease, stroke, cancer, chronic respiratory diseases, and diabetes; the leading cause of mortality worldwide

civic vitality the strength of social networks within a community, region, province, or country; reflected in the institutions, organizations, and informal social practices that people create to share resources and build attachments with others

cloud computing a model for enabling ubiquitous, convenient, on-demand network access to a shared pool of configurable computing resources that can be rapidly provisioned and released with minimal management effort

coaching occurs regularly between individuals—supervisors, peers, and direct reports—working together in organizations to improve performance

community-based organizations (CBOs) organizations that have regular full-time staff, rely on volunteers, or combine professional and volunteer staffs and are often affiliated with local charity, religious, or political institutions; some CBOs address a specific health or other social problem; others are more concerned with the general health and wellbeing of the community

community-based prevention marketing (CBPM) a program planning framework that blends social marketing techniques and community organization principles into a synergistic design to tailor, implement, evaluate, translate, and disseminate public health intervention among selected audience segments; an amalgamation of the strengths of community organizing and social marketing

community engagement continuum provides convening organizations with insight on engaging constituent groups based on their history with each constituent group; within this continuum the five levels of input and community participation are outreach, consultation, involvement, collaboration, and shared leadership

community health workers (CHWs) frontline public health workers who are trusted members of and/or have an unusually close understanding of the community served; CHWs serve as liaisons between the medical and public health worlds and the communities in which they work, conducting outreach, imparting health information in more accessible formats, supporting community members in navigating the health system, and facilitating access to important health-enabling resources

competencies acceptable levels of performance, the skills needed to perform the work, and the actual conditions under which the work is executed; can be used to develop educational curricula, establish standards for professional certification, write job descriptions, and evaluate performance

competition any environmental or perceptual force that impedes an organization's ability to achieve its goals; anything that limits resources, diverts attention from the subject of the initiative, or calls for contrary behaviors

computer networking general nature of the connection and the underlying technologies used to handle the communications; its technology classes are wide area networking (WAN), local area networking (LAN), and storage area networking (SAN)

consequentialism *see* **utilitarianism**

constituency in addition to the meaning of a body of voters, a group of supporters or patrons and a group served by an organization or institution; a clientele

constituency engagement is art and science of establishing an organization's relationships to the public it serves, the governing body it represents, and other health-related organizations in the community

continuous quality improvement (CQI) to improve quality through ongoing strategic focus, customer focus, systems view, data-driven or evidence-based analysis, implementer involvement, identification of the multiple root causes of system phenomena (multiple causation), process optimization, organizational learning, and continuous system analysis even when satisfactory performance occurs

core functions denoted as assessment, policy development, and assurance

cultural competence an integrated pattern of learned beliefs and behaviors that can be shared among groups to improve the health of people from a variety of racial backgrounds, ethnicities, and religions and to eliminate health disparities; includes thoughts, styles of communicating, ways of interacting, views on roles and relationships, values, practices, and customs and is further influenced by factors such as physical and mental ability, occupation, and socioeconomic status

data granularity refers to the level of aggregation, or distance from individual events of the fact tables

disasters ecologic disruptions, or emergencies, of a severity and magnitude resulting in deaths, injuries, illness, and/or property damage that cannot be effectively managed by the application of routine procedures or resources and that result in a call for outside assistance

disaster response organized through multiple jurisdictions, agencies, and authorities

discretionary programs operate through a fixed appropriation of federal revenue that is subject to periodic updates, adjustments, and revisions; generally much more sensitive to political bargaining and governmental financing obligations than are entitlement programs

disease registries an often rigorous and resource-intensive surveillance approach by which all cases of a disease, or type of disease, are ascertained for a defined population (typically a geographic area)

doctor of public health (DrPH) training that provides an opportunity for deeper specialization and development of research skills; a practice degree, supporting a higher level of leadership or innovation in service organizations

emergencies any occurrence that requires an immediate response; these events can be the result of nature (e.g., hurricanes, tornados, and earthquakes), technological or manmade error (e.g., nuclear accidents, bombing, and bioterrorism), or emerging diseases (e.g., West Nile virus in New York City)

emotional intelligence (EI) comprised of the personal-emotional-social components of general intelligence; tends to be used with a variety of psychological assessment instruments

enable skills and the accessibility of resources that make it possible for a motivated person to take action

endemic always present

entitlement programs benefits to broad classes of individuals; funds are allocated to states in amounts based on a proportion of the expenditures incurred by states in serving eligible recipients

environmental health specialists ensure a safe and healthy environment through the control and management of air and water quality, food safety, toxic substances, solid wastes, and workplace hazards; job titles for individuals working in environmental health are extremely varied, but include scientist, engineer, geologist, hydrologist, toxicologist, risk assessor, industrial hygienist, and sanitarian

environmental protection includes lead poisoning and air quality programs, solid and hazardous waste management, and water quality and pollution control; also includes food service and lodging inspections

epidemic occurring occasionally

epidemiologists those who study of the distribution and determinants of health-related states or events in specified populations and the application of this study to the control of health problems

equity minimizing avoidable inequalities in health and its determinants—including but not limited to health care—between groups who have different levels of underlying social advantage or privilege

essential public health functions (or services) public health activities that should be undertaken in all communities

essential services provide a working definition of public health and a guiding framework for the responsibilities of local public health systems

ethics the study of right and wrong actions; ethical theories offer norms or principles of good conduct that aim to guide us about how to live our lives, how to treat one another, and how, all things considered, we should act

evidence some form of data—including epidemiologic (quantitative) data, results of program or policy evaluations, and qualitative data—for use in making judgments or decisions; public health evidence is usually the result of a complex cycle of observation, theory, and experiment

evidence-based programs (EBPs) typically evaluated in very controlled conditions that often bear too little resemblance to the everyday realities of public health agencies to be seen as applicable or generalizable; additionally EBPs often do not allow for flexibility in how the program is implemented

evidence-based public health (EBPH) making decisions based on the best available scientific evidence, using data and information systems systematically, applying program-planning frameworks, engaging the community in decision making, conducting sound evaluation, and disseminating what is learned

federalism the separation of federal and state powers to preserves the balance of power among national and state authorities

fiscal federalism assigns responsibility for specific functions to national, state, and local levels of government and puts in place proper financing mechanisms to fulfill those functions

formative research understanding the wants, needs, and desires of a priority population; studies that are conducted to understand the problem and the audience, and to develop and assess reactions to proposed strategies, including products, service-delivery approaches, messages, and materials

geocoding the process by which GIS software matches each record in an attribute database with the geographic files; the GIS software converts each address in the attribute file to a point on a map

geographic information system (GIS) automated computer packages that integrate several functions, including the incorporation, storage, and retrieval of data with a spatial or geographic component

global health the area of study, research, and practice that places a priority on improving health and achieving equity in health for all people worldwide—striving for a worldwide improvement in health status, a reduction of health disparities, and defense against threats that transcend national borders

hazard the probability of the occurrence of a disaster caused by a natural phenomenon (e.g., earthquake, tropical cyclone), by failure of manmade sources of energy (e.g., nuclear reactor, industrial explosion), or by uncontrolled human activity (e.g., conflicts, overgrazing)

health behavior an action taken by a person to maintain, attain, or regain good health and to prevent illness; reflects a person's health beliefs; common health behaviors include exercising regularly, eating a balanced diet, and obtaining necessary inoculations

health centers provide access to primary care services for vulnerable and underserved populations; serve as important sources for health education, counseling, and social support services

health data include the costs of data collection, data analysis (including vital statistics analysis), report production, monitoring of disease and registries, monitoring of child health accidents and injuries, and death reporting

health education seeks to influence a range of behavior including participation in health-promoting activities, appropriate use of health services, health supervision of children, and adherence to appropriate medical and nutritional regimens

health impact assessment (HIA) a relatively new method that seeks to estimate the probable impact of a policy or intervention in nonhealth sectors, such as agriculture, transportation, and economic development, on the health of the population

health information systems (HISs) support a wide variety of public health system objectives, including epidemiologic disease and risk factor surveillance; medical and public health outcomes assessment; facility and clinic administration (billing, inventory, clinical records, utilization review); cost-effectiveness and productivity analysis; utilization analysis and demand forecasting; program planning and evaluation; quality assurance and performance measurement; policy development, analysis, and revision; clinical and managerial research; and health education and health information dissemination

health laboratory operate as a first line of defense to protect the public against diseases and other health hazards; provide clinical diagnostic testing, disease surveillance, environmental and radiological testing, emergency response support, applied research, laboratory training, and other essential services to the communities they serve

health promotion encompasses a broader set of educational, policy, organizational, environmental (especially social environmental), and economic interventions to support behavior and conditions of living conducive to health; strategies focused on lifestyle and personal behaviors including physical activity, nutrition, and tobacco and alcohol consumption

health protection strategies to protect the health and wellbeing of the population, including environmental and regulatory activities

health surveys periodic or continuous collection of information to serve as a surveillance mechanism, providing data on health conditions, risk factors, or health-related knowledge, attitudes, and behaviors for the time period in which the surveys are conducted

Healthy People **initiative** 10-year plans, beginning in 1980, outlining certain key national health objectives to be accomplished during each period of time; initiatives have focused on the integration of medical care with preventive services, health promotion, and education; integration of personal and community health care; and increased access to these integrated services

Hippocratic tradition concentrating on the patient rather than the disease and emphasizing prevention; represents medicine as a professional vocation that uses and adapts healing methods and regimes based on empirical observation

human resources management to select and develop an engaged workforce capable of meeting organizational and community goals; consists of an array of functions including job analysis, recruitment and selection, orientation and onboarding, compensation and benefits, employee and labor relations, coaching, training, performance appraisal, workforce planning, management and leadership development, diversity, mentoring, and culture enrichment

humours blood, black bile, yellow bile, and phlegm reflected the essential elements of the physical universe: fire, earth, air, and water; health was achieved when all four were in perfect balance or equilibrium

improving consumer health includes all clinical programs such as those for Alzheimer's disease, adult day care, medically handicapped children, AIDS treatment, renal disease, breast and cervical cancer treatment, TB treatment, emergency health services, and assistance to local health departments

incidents occurrences or events, natural or manmade, that require a response to protect life or property, including major disasters, emergencies, terrorist attacks, terrorist threats, civil unrest, wildland and urban fires, floods, hazardous materials spills, nuclear accidents, aircraft accidents, earthquakes, hurricanes, tornadoes, tropical storms, tsunamis, war-related disasters, public health and medical emergencies and other occurrences requiring an emergency response

infectious disease caused by pathogenic microorganisms, such as bacteria, viruses, parasites, or fungi and can be spread, directly or indirectly, from one person to another

infrastructure the basic support for the delivery of public health activities; its components are skilled workforce, integrated electronic information systems, public health organizations, resources, and research

injury prevention includes programs such as consumer product safety, fire injury prevention, defensive driving, child abuse prevention, occupational health, and boating and recreational safety

Institute of Medicine (IOM) an independent nonprofit organization within the National Academy of Sciences that empanels committees of the nation's top scholars and practitioners to study health policy issues and to report findings

job analysis collection of data from a variety of sources, determined by job content (tasks and duties), job requirements (knowledge, skills, and attributes a candidate should possess), and job context (purpose of the position, responsibilities of the employee, working conditions, and supervision arrangements)

job description begins by listing the job title, department, grade or classification, and supervisor title; the next section includes a job summary, which is a brief paragraph outlining the specific duties performed in the job; the final portion is a job task section that identifies all of the tasks required for the job

leadership assures that an organization has an appropriate vision of the future informed by boundary-spanning and external connections

leadership assessment instruments designed to inform the leader about his or her style, behaviors, perspective, biases, and beliefs in relation to the larger, outside world

lifestyle describes value-laden, socially conditioned behavioral patterns, which encompass discrete individual behaviors within the web of social relationships and culture in which they are conditioned over a lifetime and entwined

local health department (LHD) an administrative or service unit of local or state government, concerned with health, and carrying some responsibility for the health of a jurisdiction smaller than a state; the public health government entity at a local level, including a locally governed health department, state-created district, department serving a multicounty area, or any other arrangement with governmental authority and responsibility for public health functions at the local level

macro societal and institutional level

managed care health insurance plans that contract with healthcare providers and medical facilities to provide care for members at reduced costs; providers include health maintenance organizations (HMOs) and preferred provider organizations (PPOs)

management the process of working with and through others to achieve organizational or program objectives in an efficient and ethical manner; focus is on the present, assuring that operations that support the vision and mission are run efficiently and effectively

manmade disasters technological events not caused by natural hazards, such as fire, chemical spills and explosions, and airplane crashes; a type of manmade disaster, called a complex emergency, includes armed conflict and mass migration

marketplace model assumes that individuals and groups are constantly interacting to satisfy their needs; all policy actors are both suppliers and demanders, since they must *exchange* some commodity

in the marketplace to "purchase" the other goods that they want; policy marketplace features disparities in power; the currency used in exchanges can be money and other financial resources, but it can also include superior leadership, more effective organization, more and higher quality information, or other types of exchange

master of public health (MPH) a degree that includes a basic introduction to epidemiology, biostatistics, environmental health, behavioral science, and management; graduates can also specialize in one of these fields, or in a program area such as maternal and child health, international health, or public health laboratory science

matching requirements federal matching component that requires the state grantees to contribute a specified amount of state funds in order to secure federal funds through the program

Medicaid a federal program that finances the delivery of clinical preventive services, prenatal care, case management services, communicable disease screening and treatment services, family planning services, and childhood developmental screening services

Medicare a federal program that provides healthcare coverage for the elderly and disabled populations

metadata data about data

micro individual actor level

mission defines where and organization currently exists in terms of what its purpose is and how it intends to accomplish that purpose; why the organization exists, what business it is in, who it serves, and where it provides its products or services

mission statement identifies the organization's reason for being; provides guidance in decision making, ensuring that the organization stays on the track that its leaders have predetermined

mitigation measures that are taken to reduce the harmful effects of a disaster by attempting to limit impacts on human health and economic infrastructure

Model State Emergency Health Powers Act (MSEHPA) five basic public health functions to be facilitated by law: preparedness, surveillance, management of property, protection of persons, and public information and communication

motivation include employee development, mentoring, job training, quality management, and recruitment

national health objectives *see Healthy People* initiative

National Notifiable Diseases Surveillance System (NNDSS) a major source of population-wide data, this system captures information on disease incidence for more than 65 diseases for which accurate and timely information is essential to effective prevention and control

natural disasters rapid, sudden-onset phenomena with profound effects, such as earthquakes, floods, tropical cyclones, and tornadoes

needs assessment an evaluation of the current state of health and care systems; provides data on the breadth, severity, and seriousness of health problems

network development establishing and maintaining relationships, communication channels, and exchange systems that promote linkages, alliances, and opportunities to leverage resources among constituent groups

new federalism federal courts have begun to hold that federal police powers should be circumscribed, with more authority returned to the states

nondecision a phenomenon defined as a decision to do nothing, which itself has political and policy impacts

nondelegation conventionally, representative assemblies may not delegate legislative or judicial functions to the executive branch; this doctrine holds that the legislative branch of government should undertake policy-making functions (because assemblies are politically accountable), whereas the judicial branch should undertake adjudicative functions (because courts are independent)

notifiable diseases communicable diseases; other occurrences, including animal bites, birth defects, cancer diagnoses, elevated blood lead levels, poisonings, and illness clusters, are often reportable; diseases, conditions, and events of importance designated by public health as notifiable, are required to be reported by persons with knowledge of their occurrence

nutritionists those who plan and supervise the preparation and service of institutional meals, assist in the prevention and treatment of illnesses by advising on healthy eating habits, and evaluate dietary trends in the population

operational planning finding the best methods, processes, and systems to accomplish the mission/vision, strategies, goals, and objectives of the organization in the most effective, efficient way possible;

focuses on internal resources, systems, processes, methods, and considerations

organizational commitment employees' belief in the goals and values of the organization, willingness to exert considerable effort on behalf of the organization, and desire to continue to work with the organization

organizational culture a pattern of shared basic assumptions that the group learned as it solved its problems that has worked well enough to be considered valid and is passed on to new members as the correct way to perceive, think, and feel in relation to those problems

organizational ethics focuses on the mission, values, and systems within an agency that create a climate for ethical behavior, practices, and policies

outcomes the immediate and long-term changes (or lack of change) experienced by individuals and populations as a result of public health processes and their effects on health status, risk reduction, social functioning, or consumer satisfaction

outcome evaluation assessment of the presence of anticipated and hoped for effects that can be immediately and closely linked to programmatic effects

pass-through entity the initial recipient who provides funds to another recipient; still considered the recipient of the grant, but the assistance provided in the grant may be "passed on" to another recipient, who is called a subrecipient; this process is used when the federal granting agency does not have the organizational capability to provide assistance directly to the final recipient and hence requires administrative support from an intermediate entity

Patient Protection and Affordable Care Act (ACA) an act passed in 2010, with many provisions and goals, including investments in public health and prevention; the public health workforce; expansion of coverage, awareness, and access to clinical preventive services; wellness programs; public health research and data; and the development of a national quality improvement plan

performance appraisals inform organizational decisions that determine salary, promotions, transfers, layoffs, demotions, and terminations; also provide the mechanism and opportunity for employees to receive useful coaching and suggested changes in behavior, attitudes, knowledge, and skills

performance management the active use of performance data in making management decisions, using performance standards and measures, reporting of progress, and quality improvement

performance measurement the selection and use of quantitative measures to reflect critical aspects of activities, including their effect on the public and other public health customers; the regular collection and reporting of data to track work that is performed and results that are achieved; the selection and use of quantitative measures of public health system capacities, processes, and outcomes to inform public health leaders and managers and the public about critical aspects of the public health system; the specific quantitative representation of a capacity, process, or outcome that is deemed relevant to the assessment of performance

physicians those who practice in public health come from almost every specialty of medicine, but mainly the primary care specialties, including pediatrics, obstetrics, internal medicine/infectious disease, emergency medicine, and pathology

planning a process that uses macro and micro environmental factors and internal information to engage stakeholders to create a framework, template, and outline for section, branch, or organizational success; planning can be strategic or operational or a combination of both

police powers the inherent authority of the state (and, through delegation, local government) to enact laws and promulgate regulations to protect, preserve, and promote the health, safety, morals, and general welfare of the people; to achieve these communal benefits, the state retains the power to restrict, within federal and state constitutional limits, private interests—personal interests in liberty, autonomy, privacy, and association, as well as economic interests in freedom of contract and uses of property

policy development includes developing evidence-based recommendations and analysis to guide public policy as it pertains to health

politics "who gets what, when, how"; the use of political power to get and use resources for the benefit of individual and group interests

population health a comprehensive way of thinking about the current and future scope of public health; utilizes an evidence-based approach to analyze the determinants of health and disease, along with options for intervention and prevention to preserve and improve health; the physical, mental, and social wellbeing of defined groups of individuals and the differences (disparities) in health between population groups

predispose knowledge or awareness, attitudes, beliefs, and values that motivate people to take appropriate health actions

preparedness officials or the public itself plan a response to potential disasters and, in so doing, lay the framework for recovery

prevention actions that may prevent further loss of life, disease, disability, or injury

preventive services include counseling, screening, and immunization

principled leadership model based on ethics and principles that embrace higher and less self-centered values

Privacy Rule prohibits the disclosure of individually identifiable health information, otherwise known as protected health information (PHI), without the consent of the patient (or guardian), except for three purposes: payment, medical treatment, or healthcare operations (e.g., care coordination, case management, quality assessment).

processes what is done to, for, with, or by defined individuals or groups to identify and address community or population-wide health problems

professional accountability being bound by the professional norms and codes and any moral and ethical codes related to serving the public; performing according to professional standards and ethics

professional development training and education, mentoring programs, and employee involvement in organizational improvement and decisions

professional ethics focuses on this important relationship between the individual officials and the community

protected health information (PHI) consists of individually identifiable health data that are transmitted or maintained in electronic media and related to the physical or mental health of an individual, the healthcare services provided to an individual, or the payment for those services provided to the individual

public health consists of organized efforts to improve the health of populations, with the goal to reduce disease and improve health in a population; society's desire and specific efforts to improve the health and wellbeing of the total population, relying on the government, the private sector, and the public, and by focusing on the determinants of population health

public health finance a field of study that examines the acquisition, utilization, and management of resources for the delivery of public health functions and the impact of these resources on population health and the public health system; its primary focus is on the resources needed for the delivery of essential public health services and how those resources are acquired and managed

public health law the study of the legal powers and duties of the state, in collaboration with its partners (e.g., health care, business, the community, the media, and academe), to assure the conditions for people to be healthy (e.g., to identify, prevent, and ameliorate risks to health in the population) and the limitations on the power of the state to constrain the autonomy, privacy, liberty, proprietary, or other legally protected interests of individuals for the common good; the prime objective of public health law is to pursue the highest possible level of physical and mental health in the population, consistent with the values of social justice

public health nurses distinct from other nursing specialties by their focus on populations rather than individuals and on disease prevention rather than acute or chronic care

public health partnerships coordinated efforts among public health organizations to address health problems and risks faced by broad segments of a community's population

public health quality the degree to which policies, programs, services, and research for the population increase desired health outcomes and conditions in which the population can be healthy

public health quality aims the nine aims of public health quality are to be population-centered, equitable, proactive, health-promoting, risk-reducing, vigilant, transparent, effective, and efficient

public health systems research (PHSR) a field of study that examines the organization, financing, and delivery of public health services in communities, and the impact of these services on public health

public health workforce those working in governmental public health agencies and official voluntary or not-for-profit public health agencies, community-based private organizations, healthcare organizations, and businesses; individuals whose primary work focus is delivery of one or more of the essential services of public health, whether or not those individuals are on the payroll of an official, voluntary, or not-for-profit public health agency

public policy encompasses the intentional actions or inactions by government to address a problem affecting the public

public policy ethics examines the ethical dimensions of particular government actions or decisions, and provides a framework for deliberation and public justification

quality assurance a minimum acceptable requirement for a process or output as the criteria for taking corrective action if that minimum is not met

quality chasm gaps in quality and performance in health care and public health

quality improvement a set of techniques used to make sustainable changes to a set of processes or a system that enhance the delivery of services

quality of health services includes quality-regulation programs such as health facility licensure and certification, regulation of emergency medical systems, health-related boards or commissions, and licensing boards; also includes the development of health access planning and financing activities

quarantine in the past, the systematic isolation of travelers and ships for a period of 40 days, hence the name quarantine; the contemporary public health practice of isolation

recruitment the process of attracting, screening, selecting, and onboarding a qualified person for a job

reinforcing factor support from providers of services, families, and community groups who bolster the health behavior of an individual who is motivated and able to adopt the behavior but who will discontinue the behavior if it is not rewarded

resource allocation the federal government's power to tax and to spend to fund public health initiatives

sanitation ensuring healthful environmental conditions

scope a measure of breadth of coverage across any of the dimensions

sentinel surveillance convenience sampling of data that are designed to characterize the magnitude of a public health problem in a larger population

separation of powers doctrine each branch of government—legislative, judicial, executive—possesses a unique constitutional authority to create, enforce, or interpret health policy

service-oriented computing (SOC) through computing standards, such as Extensible Markup Language (XML), Simple Object Access Protocol (SOAP), and Web Service Description Language (WDSL) that govern the structure, transmission, and description of services, makes implementing complex service-based systems practical

social determinants of health nonmedical factors that affect the average and distribution of health within populations, including distal determinants (political, legal, institutional, and cultural factors) and proximal determinants (socioeconomic status, physical environment, living and working conditions, family and social network, lifestyle or behavior, and demographics)

social entrepreneurship the recognition and "relentless" pursuit of new opportunities to further the mission of creating social value, continuous engagement in innovation and modification, and bold action undertaken without acceptance of existing resource limitations

social marketing undertaking commercial marketing activities, institutions, and processes as a means to induce volitional behavioral change in a targeted audience on a temporary or permanent basis to achieve a social goal

strategic planning finding the best future for an organization and determining how the organization will evolve to realize that future

surveillance a primary mechanism through which health agencies generate and process information for use in management, policy, and practice; continuous and systematic collection, analysis, interpretation, and dissemination of descriptive information for monitoring health problems

syndromic surveillance early outbreak detection, which can create the opportunity for rapid intervention to interrupt infectious disease transmission and prevent morbidity and mortality; syndromic systems tally sets of signs and symptoms into defined syndromes (e.g., gastrointestinal, respiratory, and neurologic illnesses), and clusters in data captured by the system trigger a public health investigation

systems model complex, interrelated, cyclical process of feedback and subsequent modification

systems perspective a multi-level, multi-participant view of public health as a complex adaptive system that is highly interconnected and interdependent in its relationship to individuals, communities, and the larger society, including the global community, yet capable of changing and learning from experience and its environment

transformational leadership embraces the core principles of the total quality management, continuous quality improvement, and systems thinking

Turning Point Model State Public Health Act (MSPHA) a tool for state, local, and tribal governments to revise or update public health statutes and administrative regulations; seeks to transform and strengthen the legal framework to better protect and promote the public's health

utilitarianism a theory that claims that whether an action is right or wrong depends on its consequences—for example, whether it produces a net amount of benefit or utility, whether it benefits more people than it harms, or whether it produces the greatest good for the greatest number

virtue ethics approach to business management that values honesty, loyalty, sincerity, courage, reliability, trustworthiness, and benevolence

vision an aspiration of what the organization intends to become; the shared image of the future organization that places the organization in a better position to fulfill its mission

vital statistics data provided through contracts between the National Center for Health Statistics and vital registration systems operated in the various jurisdictions legally responsible for the registration of vital events—births, deaths, marriages, divorces, and fetal deaths

warning forecasting; refers to the monitoring of events to look for indicators that signify when and where a disaster might occur and what the magnitude might be in order to mitigate and prepare

WIC Women, Infants, and Children program provides federal grants to states for supplemental foods, healthcare referrals, and nutrition education for low-income pregnant, breastfeeding, and nonbreastfeeding postpartum women, and to infants and children up to age 5 years who are found to be at nutritional risk

workforce enumeration system for assessment, advocacy, and accountability of the public health workforce through the collection of data that depict the number and characteristics of those providing the essential public health services

workforce plan identifies the number and types of qualified personnel necessary to develop an organization's strategic plan, strategies and tactics

Index

Note: *Page numbers followed by b, e, f, or t indicate material in boxes, exhibits, figures, or tables, respectively.*

E

P

S

X

Y

Z